T0075319

# Applications of Biomedical Engineering in Dentistry

Lobat Tayebi
Editor

# Applications of Biomedical Engineering in Dentistry

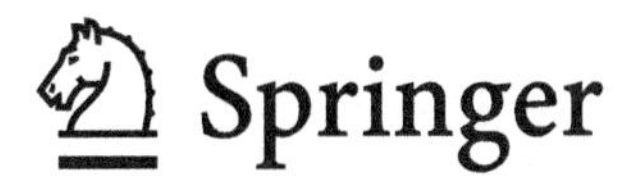

*Editor*
Lobat Tayebi
Marquette University School of Dentistry
Milwaukee, WI, USA

ISBN 978-3-030-21582-8 ISBN 978-3-030-21583-5 (eBook)
https://doi.org/10.1007/978-3-030-21583-5



This Springer imprint is published by the registered company Springer Nature Switzerland AG
The registered company address is: Gewerbestrasse 11, 6330 Cham, Switzerland

# Contents

# Contributors

**Parisa Abdi** Cornea Service, Farabi Eye Hospital, Tehran University of Medical Sciences, Tehran, Iran

**Loghman Alaei** Pharmaceutical Sciences Research Center, Health Institute, Kermanshah University of Medical Sciences, Kermanshah, Iran

**Abdolreza Ardeshirylajimi** Department of Tissue Engineering and Applied Cell Sciences, School of Advanced Technologies in Medicine, Shahid Beheshti University of Medical Sciences, Tehran, Iran

**Rizwan Bader** Marquette University School of Dentistry, Milwaukee, WI, USA

**Mohamadreza Baghaban Eslaminejad** Department of Stem Cells and Developmental Biology, Cell Science Research Center, Royan Institute for Stem Cell Biology and Technology, ACECR, Tehran, Iran

**Mahboubeh Bohlouli** Department of Tissue Engineering and Applied Cell Sciences, School of Advanced Technologies in Medicine, Shahid Beheshti University of Medical Sciences, Tehran, Iran

**Annamarie Ciancio** Marquette University School of Dentistry, Milwaukee, WI, USA

**Sara DeGrave** Marquette University School of Dentistry, Milwaukee, WI, USA

**Hossein Derakhshankhah** Pharmaceutical Sciences Research Center, Health Institute, Kermanshah University of Medical Sciences, Kermanshah, Iran

**Amin Ebrahimi** Department of Stem Cells and Developmental Biology, Cell Science Research Center, Royan Institute for Stem Cell Biology and Technology, ACECR, Tehran, Iran

**Noha A. El-Wassefy** Mansoura University, Faculty of Dentistry, Mansoura, Egypt

**Mina D. Fahmy** University of Tennessee Medical Center, Department of Oral & Maxillofacial Surgery, Knoxville, TN, USA

**Dina S. Farahat** Mansoura University, Faculty of Dentistry, Mansoura, Egypt

**Reza Fekrazad** International Network for Photo Medicine and Photo Dynamic Therapy (INPMPDT), Universal Scientific Education and Research Network (USERN), Tehran, Iran

**Hamed Ghassemi** Cornea Service, Farabi Eye Hospital, Tehran University of Medical Sciences, Tehran, Iran

**Mehrsima Ghavami-Lahiji** Department of Dental Biomaterials, School of Dentistry, Tehran University of Medical Sciences, Tehran, Iran

Research Center for Science and Technology in Medicine, Tehran University of Medical Sciences, Tehran, Iran

**Leila Gholami** Department of Periodontics, Dental Research Center, Hamadan University of Medical Sciences, Hamadan, Iran

**Ali Golchin** Department of Tissue Engineering and Applied Cell Sciences, Student Research Committee, School of Advanced Technologies in Medicine, Shahid Beheshti University of Medical Sciences, Tehran, Iran

**Arndt Guentsch** Marquette University School of Dentistry, Department of Surgical Sciences, Milwaukee, WI, USA

**Anish Gupta** Michigan Center for Oral Surgery, Southgate, MI, USA

**Majid Halvaei** Department of Cell Engineering, Cell Science Research Center, Royan Institute for Stem Cell Biology and Technology, ACECR, Tehran, Iran

**Samaneh Hosseini** Department of Stem Cells and Developmental Biology, Cell Science Research Center, Royan Institute for Stem Cell Biology and Technology, ACECR, Tehran, Iran

**Sepanta Hosseinpour** Department of Tissue Engineering and Applied Cell Sciences, School of Advanced Technologies in Medicine, Shahid Beheshti University of Medical Sciences, Tehran, Iran

School of Dentistry, The University of Queensland, Brisbane, Australia

**Mohamed S. Ibrahim** Marquette University, School of Dentistry, Milwaukee, WI, USA

Mansoura University, Faculty of Dentistry, Mansoura, Egypt

**Aysel Iranparvar** Tehran Dental Branch, Islamic Azad University, Tehran, Iran

**Zhila Izadi** Pharmaceutical Sciences Research Center, Health Institute, Kermanshah University of Medical Sciences, Kermanshah, Iran

**Samira Jafari** Pharmaceutical Sciences Research Center, Health Institute, Kermanshah University of Medical Sciences, Kermanshah, Iran

**Mohammad Reza Jamalpour** Dental Implants Research Center, Dental School, Hamadan University of Medical Sciences, Hamadan, Iran

**Alexander Karkazis** Marquette University School of Dentistry, Milwaukee, WI, USA

**Emelia Karkazis** Marquette University School of Dentistry, Milwaukee, WI, USA

**Zahra Khamverdi** Department of Operative Dentistry, Dental Research Center, Hamadan University of Medical Sciences, Hamadan, Iran

**Arash Khojasteh** Department of Tissue Engineering and Applied Cell Sciences, School of Advanced Technologies in Medicine, Shahid Beheshti University of Medical Sciences, Tehran, Iran

Department of Oral and Maxillofacial Surgery, Dental School, Shahid Beheshti University of Medical Sciences, Tehran, Iran

**Golshan Latifi** Cornea Service, Farabi Eye Hospital, Tehran University of Medical Sciences, Tehran, Iran

**Amanda Lindemuth** Marquette University School of Dentistry, Milwaukee, WI, USA

**Leila Mohammadi Amirabad** Marquette University School of Dentistry, Milwaukee, WI, USA

**Hanieh Nokhbatolfoghahaei** Dental Research Center, Research Institute of Dental Sciences, Shahid Beheshti University of Medical Sciences, Tehran, Iran

**Amin Nozariasbmarz** Department of Materials Science and Engineering, Pennsylvania State University, University Park, PA, USA

**Zahrasadat Paknejad** Medical Nanotechnology and Tissue Engineering Research Center, Shahid Beheshti University of Medical Sciences, Tehran, Iran

Department of Tissue Engineering and Applied Cell Sciences, School of Advanced Technologies in Medicine, Shahid Beheshti University of Medical Sciences, Tehran, Iran

**Andre Peisker** Department of Cranio-Maxillofacial and Plastic Surgery, Jena University Hospital, Jena, Germany

**Jamie Perugini** Marquette University School of Dentistry, Milwaukee, WI, USA

**Maryam Rezai Rad** Dental Research Center, Research Institute of Dental Sciences, Shahid Beheshti University of Medical Sciences, Tehran, Iran

**Kousar Ramezani** School of Dentistry, Hamadan Medical Sciences University, Hamadan, Iran

**Hassan Salehipour Masooleh** MEMS and NEMS Laboratory, School of Electrical and Computer Engineering, University of Tehran, Tehran, Iran

**Mohammad Amin Shamekhi** Department of Polymer Engineering, Islamic Azad University, Sarvestan Branch, Sarvestan, Iran

**Abbas Shokri** School of Dentistry, Hamadan Medical Sciences University, Hamadan, Iran

**Fahimeh Sadat Tabatabaei** Department of Dental Biomaterials, School of Dentistry, Shahid Beheshti University of Medical Sciences, Tehran, Iran

Marquette University School of Dentistry, Milwaukee, WI, USA

**Mohammadreza Tahriri** Marquette University School of Dentistry, Milwaukee, WI, USA

**Lobat Tayebi** Marquette University School of Dentistry, Milwaukee, WI, USA

**Parviz Torkzaban** Department of Periodontics, Dental Research Center, Hamadan University of Medical Sciences, Hamadan, Iran

**Regine Torres** Marquette University School of Dentistry, Milwaukee, WI, USA

**Farshid Vahdatinia** Dental Implants Research Center, Hamadan University of Medical Sciences, Hamadan, Iran

**Jessica Vargas** Marquette University School of Dentistry, Milwaukee, WI, USA

**Daryoosh Vashaee** Electrical and Computer Engineering Department, North Carolina State University, Raleigh, NC, USA

**Jonathan Wirth** Marquette University School of Dentistry, Milwaukee, WI, USA

**Payam Zarrintaj** Color and Polymer Research Center (CPRC), Amirkabir University of Technology, Tehran, Iran

Polymer Engineering Department, Faculty of Engineering, Urmia University, Urmia, Iran

# Chapter 1
# Introduction to Application of Biomedical Engineering in Dentistry

**Lobat Tayebi**

"Good fences make good neighbors" …"Why do they make good neighbors?"… "Something there is that doesn't love a wall"…."He says again, Good fences make good neighbors" [1].

These are scattered verses from an American poet Robert Frost (1874–1963) in his famous poem *Mending Wall* (published in 1914, North of Boston by David Nutt). In this poem, there is a stone wall between two farms. Farmer 1 asked his neighbor in the spring mending-time to reconstruct the wall. Farmer 2 wondered if he should. The dialogue continued between them with repeating the verse by Farmer 2 "Something there is that doesn't love a wall" followed by the insisting of Farmer 1 relying on the proverb of "Good fences make good neighbors!"

It is interesting that the story still continues between groups of Farmer 1 and Farmer 2 after more than a hundred years. Do we need a wall? "That is the question." We don't know who is right in farms and livestock grazing, but we do know that in today's dentistry. "Something there is that doesn't love a wall" [1].

More broadly, in today's science, technology, and medicine, each field is trying to touch the concept of interdisciplinary. Do we *need* the interdisciplinary approach to succeed? Perhaps not. Do we *need* the interdisciplinary approach to be modern, progressive, and advanced? Definitely yes.

Modern dentistry tries its best to take advantage of linking with other fields, especially biomedical engineering. This book aims to present some of these efforts. Biomedical engineering, itself, is known as an exceedingly multidisciplinary field spanning biology, material science, physics, chemistry, engineering, and medicine. The recent progress in biomedical engineering significantly impacts many relevant areas. Such impacts on dentistry are the focus of this book, in which an interdisciplinary document is presented, that relates biomedical engineering

L. Tayebi (✉)
Marquette University School of Dentistry, Milwaukee, WI, USA
e-mail: lobat.tayebi@marquette.edu



L. Tayebi (ed.), *Applications of Biomedical Engineering in Dentistry*,
https://doi.org/10.1007/978-3-030-21583-5_1

and dentistry by introducing the recent technological achievements in engineering with applications in dentistry.

The book will begin by studying the biomaterials in dentistry and materials used intraoperatively during oral and maxillofacial surgery procedures. Next, it will consider the subjects in which biomedical engineers can be influential, such as three-dimensional (3D) imaging, *laser and photobiomodulation,* surface modification of dental implants, and bioreactors. Hard and soft tissue engineering in dentistry will be discussed, and some specific and essential methods such as 3D printing will be elaborated. Presenting particular clinical functions of regenerative dentistry and tissue engineering in the treatment of oral and maxillofacial soft tissues is the subject of a separate chapter. Challenges in the rehabilitation handling of large and localized oral and maxillofacial defects are severe issues in dentistry, which will be considered to understand how bioengineers help with treatment methods in this regard.

Recent advances in nanodentistry will be discussed followed by a chapter on the applications of stem cell-encapsulated hydrogel in dentistry.

Periodontal regeneration is a challenging issue in dentistry and, thus, is going to be considered separately to understand the efforts and achievements of tissue engineers in this matter.

Oral mucosa grafting is a practical approach in engineering and treatment of tissues in ophthalmology, which is the subject of another chapter. Microfluidic approaches became more popular in biomedical engineering during the last decade; hence, one chapter will focus on the advanced topic of microfluidics technologies using oral factors as saliva-based studies. Injectable gels in endodontics is a new theme in dentistry that bioengineering skills can advance its development, specifically by producing clinically safe and effective gels with regeneration and antibacterial properties. Engineered products often need to be tested in vivo before being clinical in dentistry; thus, one chapter is dedicated to reviewing applicable animal models in dental research. The last chapter will cover the progress on the whole tooth bioengineering as a valuable and ultimate goal of many dental researchers.

## Reference

1. Frost, R. (1914). *North of Boston*. Henry Holt. New York

# Chapter 2
# Biomedical Materials in Dentistry

**Fahimeh Sadat Tabatabaei, Regine Torres, and Lobat Tayebi**

## 1 Introduction

Biomedical materials are biomaterials intended to be in long-term contact with biological tissues. Based on the American National Institute of Health definition, a biomaterial is "any substance or combination of substances, other than drugs, synthetic or natural in origin, which can be used for any period, which augments or replaces partially or totally any tissue, organ or function of the body, to maintain or improve the quality of life of the individual" [1]. This definition does not comprise materials such as orthodontic brackets, impression materials, gypsum, waxes, investment materials, finishing materials, irrigants, bleaching materials, or instruments.

The biomaterials used in dentistry can be classified into metals, ceramics, polymers, and composites (Fig. 2.1), which will be the focus of this chapter.

## 2 Metallic Biomaterials

Due to the inherent characteristic of metallic bonds, metals and alloys have high density, thermal and electrical conductivity, strength, and hardness.

F. S. Tabatabaei
Department of Dental Biomaterials, School of Dentistry, Shahid Beheshti University of Medical Sciences, Tehran, Iran

Marquette University School of Dentistry, Milwaukee, WI, USA

R. Torres · L. Tayebi (✉)
Marquette University School of Dentistry, Milwaukee, WI, USA
e-mail: lobat.tayebi@marquette.edu



L. Tayebi (ed.), *Applications of Biomedical Engineering in Dentistry*,
https://doi.org/10.1007/978-3-030-21583-5_2

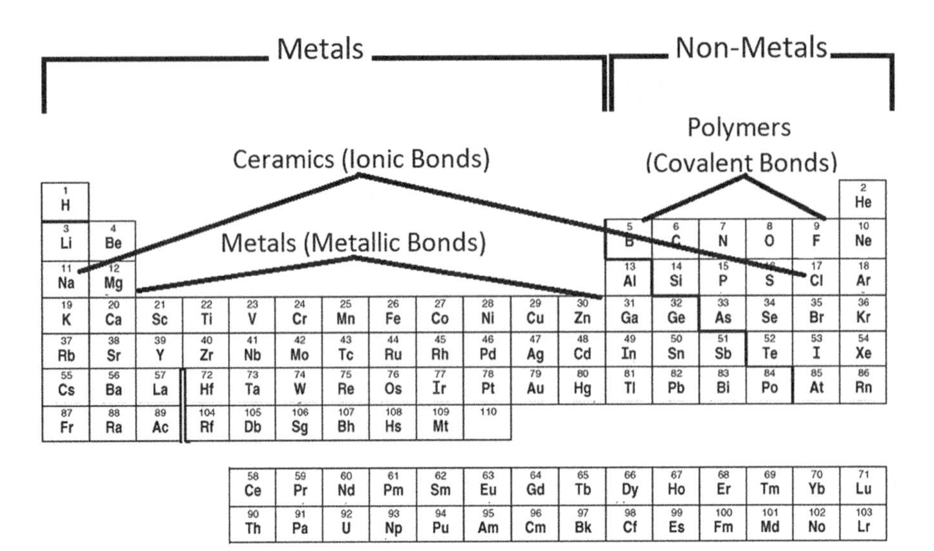


**Fig. 2.1** Metals, ceramics, and polymers in the periodic table

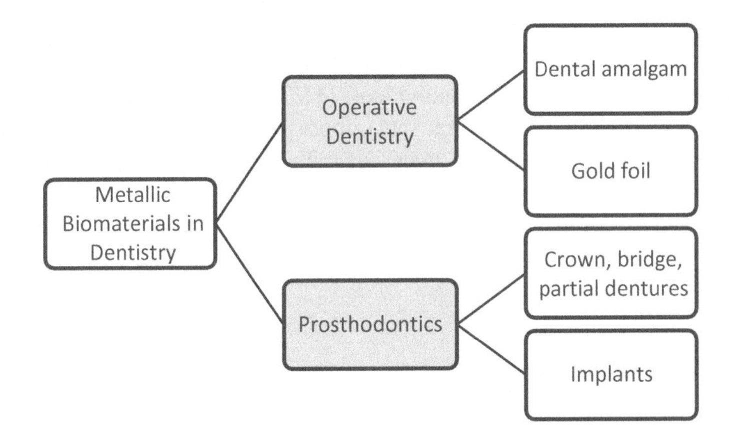


**Fig. 2.2** Metallic biomaterials used in operative dentistry and prosthodontics

In dentistry, metals and their alloys are used for direct restorations as dental amalgams or for indirect restorations as casting alloys or dental implants (Fig. 2.2).

## 2.1 *Dental Amalgam*

The primary goals of dental restorative treatment are to replace diseased or damaged tooth structure and to restore function. Interest in the use of amalgam for the restoration of teeth dates back to the 1800s onward. *Amalgam* is a *metal* alloy, of which one of the components is *mercury*. Dental amalgam is the result of mixture of liquid mercury with amalgam alloy powder composed *principally* of silver, tin, and copper. Amalgam alloy is derived from the intermetallic compound $Ag_3Sn$, and the powder can be lathe-cut (irregular-shaped) particles, spherical particles, or a combination of these. When the powder is mixed with mercury (about 40–50% by weight), it can be packed or condensed into a prepared tooth cavity. In the setting reactions of dental amalgam, a series of intermetallic compounds are formed. The reaction products of Hg with pure γ-phase ($Ag_3Sn$) alloy are $Ag_4Hg_5$ ($\gamma_1$) and $Sn_{7-8}Hg$ ($\gamma_2$). The γ-phase does not react completely with mercury, and some of the original $Ag_3Sn$ remains as unreacted particles, which is the source of strength in dental amalgam. The $\gamma_2$-phase is very weak, is prone to corrosion, deforms readily, and contributes to the static creep of amalgam. Because of these properties, extra copper (Cu) is incorporated either in the form of a second alloy powder mixed with the first (admixed alloy) or by coating of $Ag_3Sn$ alloy with Cu alloy (unicompositional alloy). These new generations are referred to as high-copper amalgams, in which the copper content of the alloy particles may be as high as 30% by weight. Increase in the copper content, which results in decrease of silver content, has a direct influence on the cost of product. It is of relevance to note that no $\gamma_2$-phase is present in these new generations. At the end of the amalgamation reaction, little or no unreacted mercury remains, and reacted mercury is not easily released from the amalgam. Dental amalgam restorations are easy to manipulate and place, are able to withstand normal occlusal forces, and have a low cost. Some disadvantages, however, are that the material is silver-colored, sensitive to mixing technique, and subject to corrosion and does not have bonding properties. Additionally, amalgam restorations usually require larger cavity preparation to provide sufficient mechanical retention, and there are regulatory concerns about amalgam disposal in the wastewater. Due to these disadvantages, especially the emerging concerns over its potential neurotoxic effects and environmental issues associated with waste amalgam disposal, clinical use of amalgam continues to decline [2, 3].

## 2.2 *Alloys for Metallic Restorations*

Besides dental amalgams, other alloys used in dentistry are casting dental alloys, wrought alloys, and solders. Cast alloys are melted and cast into the shape of a wax-up. These alloys could be in the form of noble metals, which are resistant to corrosion, or base–metal alloys like cobalt–chromium, nickel–chromium, stainless steel, titanium, and titanium alloys [4].

Wrought alloys—like those used in dental wire, endodontic posts and instruments, orthodontic brackets, and stainless steel crowns and implants—are alloys that have been worked or shaped after casting by mechanical force, compression, or tension into a serviceable form for an appliance. Cold working applied during the shaping process results in a fibrous microstructure, increase in tensile strength and hardness, and decrease in ductility and resistance to corrosion in comparison to corresponding cast structures. One of the promising biomaterials in this category is Ni–Ti, which has huge application in endodontics and orthodontics. This material possesses special characteristics, like shape-memory and superelasticity. Shape-memory permits shaping at a higher temperature, followed by deformation at a lower temperature, and a return to the original shape upon reheating. On the other hand, superelasticity is characterized by an extensive region of elastic activation and deactivation at a nearly constant bending moment [5–7].

Solders, which are used for joining metals together or repairing cast restorations, are gold-based or silver-based.

Alloys used as bases for porcelain have special formulations because they need to provide a firm bond to the applied porcelain via an oxide layer on the alloy surface. Another important property is the thermal expansion of ceramic and alloy. A high difference in the coefficient of thermal expansion results in more expansion on heating and more contraction on cooling, which could increase the risk of fracture of ceramic during service [8].

Metal and alloys used in different fields of dentistry include inlays, onlays, and crowns in operative dentistry; crowns, bridges, implants, clasp wires, and solders in prosthodontics; wires and brackets in orthodontics; and files and reamers in endodontics.

## 2.3 *Titanium in Implant Dentistry*

The use of titanium dental implants rather than dentures or fixed bridges has changed the rehabilitation of patients in modern dentistry. Dental implants protrude through the mucosa as a suitable structure for supporting a denture, crown, or bridge. The rigidity of the implant structure is related to its dimensions, and the modulus of elasticity has an important role in its function. In fact, we can use materials with a high modulus of elasticity with smaller cross-sectional bulk, but these materials also are at risk of stress shielding. Currently, most dental implants are fabricated from titanium and its alloys, which are light and have adequate strength. The interfacial condition when bone grows to within 100 Å of the titanium surface without any fibrous tissue in this space is called osseointegration. Osseointegration would result in non-mobility of the implant and should be maintained over the long term. Attempts have been made to improve the efficacy and rate of osseointegration by techniques such as different designs and microtextures on the surface of the implant, coating the surface with hydroxyapatite, as well as coating with a layer of protein-containing drugs. The degradation of coatings over time could jeopardize the stability of the interface in the long term [9, 10].

# 3 Polymeric Biomaterials

Polymers, which are long chain molecules consisting of many small repeating units (*monomers*), represent the largest class of biomaterials in dentistry and play a major role in most areas of dentistry. Covalent bonding along the backbone and the amount of cross-linking is responsible for the properties of polymers, such as low density, insulation, and flexibility. Figure 2.3 represents the polymeric biomaterials in different fields of dentistry.

## *3.1 Bonding Agents*

Bonding agents (adhesive systems) are used with composites to obtain a strong and durable bond to dentin and enamel. Three important components of bonding agents are etchant (conditioner), primer, and adhesive. Etchants are 30% to 40% phosphoric acid gels used for the demineralization of tooth structure. Primers are hydrophilic monomers, oligomers, or polymers and act to improve wetting and penetration of the treated dentin. Adhesives have hydrophobic groups that polymerize and form a bond with the composite; they also contain a small amount of a hydrophilic monomer to diffuse into the hydrophilic, primer-wetted dentin. These components can be combined to simplify the application of bonding agents. Bonding agents are classified as light-cured and dual-cured multi-bottle systems (fourth generation);

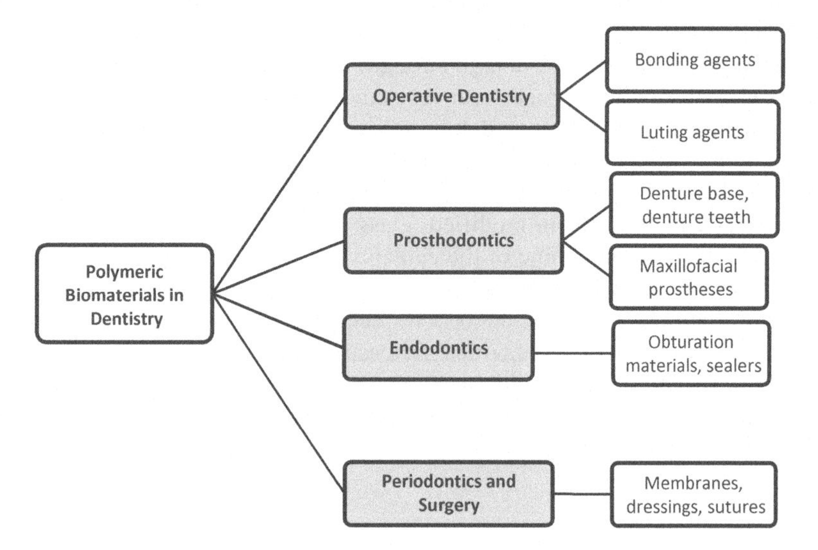


**Fig. 2.3** Polymeric biomaterials in different fields of dentistry

light-cured single-bottle systems (fifth generation); and self-etching systems (sixth and seventh generation). Fourth- and fifth-generation bonding agents are called total-etch (etch-and-rinse) systems. Universal bonding agents can be either total-etch or self-etch systems. Bonding agents may also contain fluoride to prevent secondary caries, chlorhexidine to prevent collagen degradation, antimicrobial ingredients like MDPB and paraben, or desensitizers such as glutaraldehyde [11, 12].

Bonding of resins to enamel involves its penetration into the porous surface of the etched enamel. This micromechanical bond results from adequate etching and drying of the surface. Composite resins may be applied directly to the etched enamel surface without using bonding agent. However, using unfilled resin may enhance the adhesive bond strength. Bonding to moist enamel could be achieved by using an enamel bonding resin containing primers and solvents. Bonding to dentin occurs through a complex mechanism involving wetting, penetration, and the formation of a layer of bound material at the interface between the restorative material and the substrate. Dentin bonding agents have an affinity for calcium or the organic collagenous component of dentin [13, 14].

## *3.2 Luting Agents*

Luting agents are either provisional or permanent. Provisional cements (like zinc oxide–eugenol and noneugenol cements or calcium hydroxide pastes) have a relatively low strength. Permanent cements should seal the tooth/restoration interface, have a low film thickness, be resistant to disintegration and dissolution, have good esthetics, have high strength (both static and fatigue) and fracture toughness, and have good wear resistance. These cements can be divided into those that set through an acid–base reaction (glass ionomer, resin-modified glass ionomer, zinc oxide–eugenol, zinc polycarboxylate, and zinc phosphate) and those that set by polymerization (resin cements, compomers, and self-adhesive resin cements). Resin-modified glass ionomers and compomers may undergo both reactions. Some of the cements (like glass ionomer cements) are self-adhesive materials that bond to tooth structure via micromechanical and chemical bonding; therefore, there is no need for the application of bonding agents when placing GICs in cavities. Release of fluoride from cements and the capacity to recharge them could inhibit the progression of initial proximal caries in adjacent teeth. Calcium aluminate/glass ionomer cement is a new cement which was shown to be bioactive due to its calcium content and high pH [15–17].

### 3.3 Prosthetic Polymers and Resins

The part of the denture that rests on the soft tissues is termed the acrylic denture base. Denture-based material should be capable of matching the appearance of the natural oral soft tissues, should have a value of glass transition temperature (Tg) to prevent softening and distortion during use, should have good dimensional stability, and should have a low value of specific gravity and high value of thermal conductivity. Polymeric denture-based materials can be heat-processing polymers, autopolymerized polymers, thermoplastic blank or powder, light-activated materials, or microwave-cured materials. The major component is polymethylmethacrylate (PMMA). The set material can be considered a composite system in which residual PMMA particles are bound in a matrix of freshly polymerized material. Resin or acrylic teeth have good bonding with acrylic denture-based material. Occasionally, hard reline materials, tissue conditioners, or soft lining materials may be applied to the fitting surface of the denture base in order to improve the fit of the denture or enable traumatized soft tissues to recover. These materials also contain polymethylmethacrylate in combination with some monomers and plasticizers to perform their functions. Silicone elastomers and polyphosphazine fluoroelastomers are also available for use as denture soft lining materials. Hydrogels, which are biopolymers containing poly(N-substituted methacrylamides), can also be used as soft tissue conditioners. Acrylic resins and other polymers and copolymers—like latex, polyurethane, and silicone—are used for maxillofacial prostheses. New-generation color-stable resins, incorporation of antimicrobial agents, and nanoparticle-reinforced PMMA are recent advances in prosthetic materials [18–20].

### 3.4 Endodontic Obturation Materials

Endodontic biomaterials obturate the root canal system of teeth when the pulp tissuehas been destroyed.

Bulk-filling materials are based on a modified natural rubber gutta-percha or a polyester resin-based material. Gutta-percha is derived from latex as an isomer of trans-polyisoprene and can be produced in two crystalline forms, which are interchangeable depending on the temperature of the material. Currently there are different forms of gutta-percha:

- Gutta-percha pellets or bars (e.g., Obtura system)
- Pre-coated core carrier gutta-percha (e.g., Thermafil)
- Syringe systems (use low viscosity gutta-percha) (e.g., Alpha Seal)
- Gutta flow: gutta-percha powder incorporated into a resin-based sealer
- Gutta-percha dissolved in chloroform/eucalyptol (e.g., Chloropersha and Eucopercha)
- Medicated gutta-percha (e.g., calcium hydroxide, iodoform, or chlorhexidine-containing GP points)

Polyester resin (Resilon) based on a thermoplastic synthetic polyester may contain bioactive glass fillers and claims to release calcium and phosphate ions from its surface, stimulating bone growth [21].

Sealer cement fills the spaces between increments of the bulk-fill material and maintains the seal around the root filling. The most commonly used sealers are zinc oxide–eugenol and calcium hydroxide-based cements. There are also resin-based products, such as AH26, which are based on epoxy resins, contain formaldehyde, have antimicrobial action, and provide a good seal. Photocuring resin sealers are also used as sealants with the polyester bulk-fill materials and are typically a mixture of hydrophilic difunctional methacrylates [22].

Castor oil polymer (COP) extracted from plants is a new material for use in dentistry as a biocompatible retrograde filling material. The chemical composition of this biopolymer consists of a chain of fatty acids. The body does not recognize it as a foreign body. In comparison to MTA and GIC, COP displays excellent sealing ability as a root-end filling material [23].

## *3.5 PEEK in Dentistry*

PEEK, or polyether ether ketone (-C6H4-OC6H4-O-C6H4-CO-)n, is a tooth-colored semi-crystalline linear polycyclic aromatic polymer with mechanical properties close to human bone, enamel, and dentin. This biomaterial has many potential uses in dentistry as fixed restorations, dental implants, individual abutments, and removable prostheses. Due to its low Young's (elastic) modulus, it may exhibit lower stress shielding than titanium dental implants although some literature reported nonhomogeneous stress distribution to the surrounding bone. Moreover, its poor wetting properties limit its osteoconductivity. Improving its bioactivity without compromising its mechanical properties is challenging [24, 25].

## *3.6 Membranes and Polymeric Periodontal Biomaterials*

Periodontitis can lead to the destruction of interfaces between the root cementum and alveolar bone, which constitute the periodontium. Isolation of periodontal defects through the use of a barrier to avoid epithelial and connective tissue migration into the defect led to the development of GTR/GBR membranes. The membrane must also support bone cell infiltration from the bone defect side. A GTR/GBR membrane should have proper physical properties and an acceptable degradation rate matching that of new tissue formation. According to degradation feature, GTR/GBR membranes can be divided into two groups: resorbable (such as polylactic acid (PLA) and its copolymers, in addition to tissue-derived collagen) and non-resorbable (like titanium membranes, polytetrafluoroethylene (PTFE) reinforced with or without a titanium framework). The most commonly used membranes are collagen-based or derived from the human skin, porcine skin, or bovine Achilles tendon. They are available in various forms, such as sheets, gels, tubes, powders, and sponges. Nevertheless, improvement of the biomechanical properties and matrix stability of native collagen is necessary. Research on new bioactive and multilayered membranes with the aim of biomolecule delivery (e.g., antimicrobials and growth factors) is underway. Polypeptide growth factors—such as platelet-derived growth factor (PDGF), enamel matrix proteins (Emdogain of porcine origin), and bone morphogenetic proteins (BMPs)—can mediate the periodontal regeneration. Nowadays, sustained drug delivery can be used in the periodontal regeneration process. Arestin (PLGA microspheres containing minocycline) and Periochip (gelatin chip containing 2.5 mg of chlorhexidine (CHX) gluconate) are two examples of these products [26, 27].

Periodontal pack or dressing is another biomaterial used for wound protection in periodontal surgery to facilitate healing. Wonder Pak is a eugenol dressing containing antiseptic additives, such as thymol or septol, whereas Coe-pack does not contain eugenol. Cyanoacrylates have also been used as periodontal dressings but are not very popular. Light-cured elastomeric resin is also available as a periodontal dressing material. Incorporation of antimicrobials into the unset gel is a method of delivering these agents in situ [28].

### *3.7 Sutures and Alternatives*

Suture materials should have good physical and biological properties. The source of suture material can be natural (silk, collagen fibers from the intestine of healthy sheep or cows) or synthetic (polyglactin, polyglecaprone, polydioxanone (PDS)). Based on degradability, the sutures are either absorbable (catgut, PDS) or nonabsorbable (silk). Hydrolysis of synthetic absorbable sutures does not cause any adverse tissue reactions. If hemostasis cannot be managed by sutures, fibrin glue can be used to arrest bleeding. It consists of fibrinogen and thrombin and acts faster than sutures. The fibrin sealant kit contains sealer protein concentrate (human) freeze-dried, fibrinolysis inhibitor solution, thrombin (human) freeze-dried, and calcium chloride solution. Liquid stitches, skin adhesives, or cyanoacrylates can be used as an alternative to sutures. Polymerization of the adhesive on contact with tissue fluids results in the formation of a thin layer that adheres to the underlying surface [29].

## 4 Ceramic Biomaterials

Ceramics are brittle, and inorganic/nonmetallic biomaterials, composed of metal–oxygen ionic bonds. As they have no free electrons to conduct heat or electricity, they are poor thermal conductors. They have also excellent biocompatibility.

## 4.1 Dental Ceramics

Due to their excellent *esthetic* value, ceramics have been used widely in restorations. Dental ceramics can be classified into four major types: (1) traditional feldspathic (glassy or porcelain), (2) predominantly glass (glass dominated), (3) particle-filled glass (crystalline dominated), and (4) polycrystalline, which has no glass phase. Feldspathic ceramics (dental porcelain) are the most esthetic but weakest of the ceramics. They are made by mixing kaolin (hydrated aluminosilicate), quartz (silica), and feldspars (potassium and sodium aluminosilicates) and composed principally of an amorphous phase with embedded leucite crystals. These ceramics are primarily used as veneers for porcelain fused-to-metal (PFM) and all-ceramic restorations. Ceramic–metal restorations (PFM) consist of several layers of ceramic (core [opaque], dentin [body], enamel) bonded to an alloy substructure. Figure 2.4 shows different techniques for fabrication of dental ceramics. In the dental laboratory, the physical process of fabrication of dental porcelains is sintering or stacking. In sintering, slurry of porcelain powder in water is applied to the alloy surface or ceramic core, and after condensation (the green state), the ceramic is fired (heating without melting). Glass-dominated ceramics (particle-filled glass) contain crystals like leucite or fluoroapatite. They have more strength than glassy ceramics and sufficient translucency, but they cannot be used for posterior crowns or bridges. Pressing techniques (heat-pressing) are used in the dental laboratory for fabrication of these ceramics. In this technique, after wax-up, investing, and lost-wax process, a viscous mass of molten ceramic will be forced into the mold to get the desired final form. The composition of crystalline-dominated ceramics is crystalline 70% by volume. They

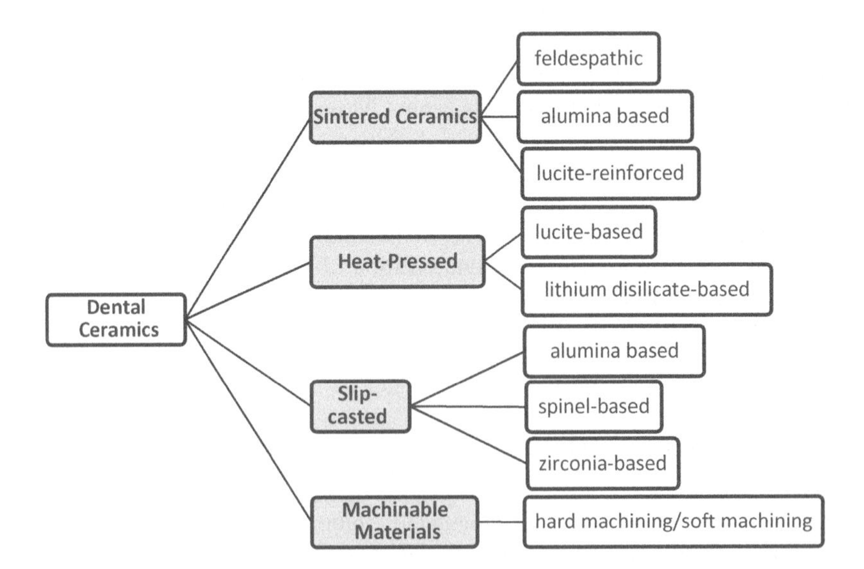


**Fig. 2.4** Different techniques used for fabrication of dental ceramics

contain crystals like spinel ($MgAl_2O_4$), zirconia ($ZrO_2$), alumina ($Al_2O_3$), or lithium disilicate. Although not highly esthetic, they can be used as cores for anterior or posterior all-ceramic crowns. The fabrication method of these ceramics is heat-pressing (for lithium disilicate) or infusion (slip casting). In slip casting, ceramic slurry is sintered, then a silica glass is infiltrated in the porous sintered ceramic, and the restoration is sintered again. Today, this technique has been replaced by machining. The newest and strongest ceramics are the polycrystalline ceramics (ceramic oxides), which are formed from alumina or zirconia (Procera). They cannot be used as esthetic veneers on alloys or teeth; however, because of their high strength, they can be used in posterior crowns and bridges. These ceramics are prepared from blocks by CAD/CAM. Ceramic blocks for CAD/CAM can be conventional feldspathic porcelains, glass ceramics, and heat-pressed or infiltrated with glass [30–34].

## 4.2 HA and Other Bioceramics

Hydroxyapatite (HA) [$Ca_{10}(PO_4)_6(OH)_2$], tricalcium phosphate (TCP) [$Ca_3(PO_4)_2$], and biphasic calcium phosphate (consisting of HA with TCP) are common brittle materials used for craniofacial defects. Although porosity in these ceramics allows faster bony ingrowth, it also weakens them. HA is a natural component of enamel, dentin, cementum, and bone. This non-resorbable material could be applied in different situations, like periodontal osseous defects, ridge augmentation/implant placement, sinus elevation surgeries, etc. Substitution of strontium, carbonate, zinc, or silicates in the structure of HA could favor its dissolution and bioactivity or increase the strength of porous ceramics. Tricalcium phosphate (TCP) is similar to HA, but it is not a natural component of hard tissues, as it is converted in part to crystalline HA in the body. The resorption period of TCP is 3–24 months. Cerasorb is a commercial product of TCP, but there are also some products that are prepared from combinations of HA and TCP. These materials, based on porosity, could be dense, macroporous, or microporous. Based on crystallinity, these materials are classified as crystalline, amorphous, granular, or molded. Calcium phosphate material, derived from calcium-encrusted sea algae, has the hexagonal structure of HA and high bioactivity. Interconnected microporosity in this material guides hard and soft tissue formation. Coraline is another ceramic material derived from the calcium carbonate skeleton of coral that has a three-dimensional structure similar to the bone. Calcium sulfate, or plaster of Paris, is a salt used for bone implantation. The resorption of calcium sulfate is rapid, and this drawback limits the application of the material in the oral and maxillofacial region. The addition of HA to this material provides osteoconductivity and sufficient strength. Cements based on calcium salts, phosphates, or sulfates have excellent biocompatibility and bone-repair properties without the need for delivery in prefabricated forms [35–37].

## 4.3 Bioactive Glass

Bioactive glasses are materials consisting of a three-dimensional network structure of *silica* that have the capacity to form chemical bonds with apatite crystals in bone tissue and teeth via formation of apatite crystals on their surface. This material has appropriate strength, stiffness, and hardness but—like other glasses—is brittle and cannot be used in load-bearing areas. However, it can be used in some areas as powder, particles, or small monoliths. There are three different types of bioactive glass: (1) glasses based on silicates ($SiO_2$), (2) glasses based on phosphates ($P_2O_5$), and (3) glasses based on borates ($B_2O_3$). Bioactive glass is a promising material in dentistry, since it has the ability to support bonding to biological tissue, to regenerate tissue, and to inhibit bacterial growth. Therefore, there are many studies on its ability to prevent loss of bone after tooth extraction, to regenerate tissue in periodontal disease (as PerioGlass), to induce bone regeneration before denture replacement, to reduce dental hypersensitivity, and to remineralize damaged dentin in combination with glass ionomer cement. Coating of titanium implants and fiber-reinforced polymer composites for dental prosthetic devices is also considered in some studies. In addition, the formulation of toothpastes with bioactive glass could be helpful in the release of antibacterial, remineralizing, or desensitizing agents. All of the commercial products available in dentistry are based on the 45S5 Bioglass formulation [38, 39].

## 4.4 Endodontic Obturation Materials: MTA and Others

Calcium hydroxide [$Ca(OH)_2$] is a strong base with a high pH that has been used in endodontics as an intracanal medication, sealer, and pulp-capping agent. This biomaterial is antibacterial, aids in the dissolution of necrotic pulp tissue, promotes dentinal bridge formation, and preserves the vitality of the pulp. Some of the $Ca(OH)_2$ formulations with lower pH values (9–10) produce a more uniform dentin bridge in comparison to higher pH (11–13) calcium hydroxide. As this material is used for a wide range of applications, it has various forms with different setting times: fast setting and controlled setting (light cure) as a liner, slow setting as a pediatric obturating material or sealer, and non-setting as an intracanal medicament [40].

Mineral trioxide aggregate (MTA), which is chemically identical to Portland cement, is a strongly alkaline material. In its set condition, it is biocompatible and antimicrobial, can induce cementogenesis, and can provide a good seal at the root–material interface. The effects of calcium hydroxide and MTA on stem cells are the subject of many studies. Other materials based on MTA include endo CPM sealer, viscosity enhanced root repair material (VERRM), and calcium-enriched mixture (CEM) cement. Bioaggregate, which is the modified version of MTA, is aluminum-free and contains ceramic nanoparticles. Biodentin is another material containing calcium chloride and hydrosoluble polymer to shorten setting time. In addition, calcium phosphate cement (CPC) is a mixture of two calcium phosphate compounds, one acidic and the other basic, and is under study as root-end filling and root repair material [41].

Minerals (ceramic in nature), like MTA, have good biocompatibility but also potentially contain toxic heavy metals. It seems that bioceramics (chemically bonded ceramic) are the future of root-end filling materials [42].

### *4.5 Zirconia in Dentistry*

Zirconia, or zirconium dioxide ($ZrO_2$), is a special ceramic that has been used in single-crowns, long-span fixed dentures, and root canal posts and as a subgingival implant material in dentistry. This ceramic is a white biomaterial, with reduced plaque affinity and resistance to chemical attacks. It is one of the best currently known biocompatible ceramic biomaterials. Zirconia consists of different crystallographic forms at different temperatures: monoclinic (M) phase, tetragonal (T) phase, and cubic (C) phase. Addition of some amount of metal oxide, like yttria (yttrium trioxide, $Y_2O_3$) and ceria (cerium trioxide, $Ce_2O_3$), to zirconia can transform pure zirconia into a partially stabilized zirconia called "tetragonal zirconia polycrystal (TZP)," which has high flexural strength and fracture toughness. Under stress, transformation of the tetragonal phase to the monoclinic phase, which is called transformation toughening, could inhibit crack propagation. However, it makes the implant susceptible to aging. Addition of higher amounts of yttrium oxide increases the amount of cubic phase, which results in zirconia ceramics with increased translucency. Restorations made of TZP are prepared by CAD/CAM (soft machining of pre-sintered blanks followed by sintering or hard machining of fully sintered blocks). Evidence shows that Y-TZP implants have osseointegration comparable to titanium implants and superior biocompatibility and esthetics. Nevertheless, high elastic modulus of zirconia (210 GPa) could result in even higher stress shielding than titanium implants. Moreover, there is not enough scientific clinical data for recommendation of ceramic implants for routine clinical use [43, 44].

## 5 Composite Biomaterials

Composites are biomaterials consisting of two or more constituents, which when combined leads to a material with properties different from those of its individual components. Enamel, dentin, and bone are some examples of composites in the body.

## 5.1 Resin-Based Composites

Resin composites are a mixture of resin phase and inorganic filler. The resins used are composed of methacrylate monomers. Depending on the resin matrix used, there are Bis-GMA-based, UDMA-based, and silorane-based dental composites. Fillers commonly used are quartz, fused silica, and many other types of glasses. Ormocers (organically modified ceramics) are fillers with molecule-sized hybrid structures that are used in the formulation of several commercial composites. Polyhedral oligomeric silsesquioxane (POSS) is another molecule-sized hybrid compound, which, like ormocer, provides a reinforcing function, but filler particles must also be included in the composite. Incorporation of fillers in resin composite materials will linearly affect the properties like coefficient of thermal expansion, setting contraction, and surface hardness. A coupling agent will enhance bonding between the filler and resin matrix. Polymerization in resin composites occurs through free radical addition or a ring-opening mechanism. The method used to activate polymerization can be chemical (in self-curing composites) or through a visible light source (in light-cured composites). Dual-cure materials have a self-curing mechanism but are also cured by light or heat. Based on the particle size distribution of fillers, there are different types of resin composites. Conventional composites contain 60–80% (by weight) of filler in the particle size range of 1–50 μm. Microfilled composites contain fillers in the range of 0.01–0.1 μm (30–60% by weight). Hybrid composites that contain a blend of both conventional filler (75% by weight, 1–50 μm) together with some submicron fillers (8%, 0.04 μm average) enable filler loading of up to 90% by weight to be achieved. There are also nanocomposites with particles of less than 1 μm average diameter and filler loading of up to 79.5%. Highly viscous resin composites are classified as "packable" composites, while more fluid products are referred to as "syringeable" composites. Laboratory composites may be used to indirectly prepare crowns, inlays, veneers bonded to metal substructures, and metal-free bridges. Pre-cured composites for in-office milling are also available. Low-viscosity composite materials with adjusted filler distribution can be used as resin cements [45, 46].

## 5.2 Modified Composites and GIOMERS

Modified composites are resin–matrix composites in which the usual filler has been replaced by a glass that exhibits fluoride release. Setting of these biomaterials is the same as usual composites (often light-activated). In polyacid-modified composites or compomers, there is also the possibility of an acid–base reaction with the filler component, which may help in liberating fluoride. In these materials, the first reaction is still a polymerization reaction. In GIOMERS, the acid–base reaction is completed before blending the filler with resin. Partially or fully reacted fillers are blended with resin to form a composite structure. GIOMERS are single paste materials that set through light-activated free radical addition polymerization [47, 48].

### *5.3 Bone Augmentation Materials*

Hard tissue grafts—such as autografts, allografts, xenografts, and alloplasts—are composite biomaterials used for bone regeneration. Allografts (like mineralized or demineralized freeze-dried bone allografts (FDBA)) refer to grafting between genetically dissimilar members of the same species. Generally, they are frozen, freeze-dried (lyophilized), demineralized freeze-dried, and irradiated. In contrast, xenografts (like Bio-Oss (bovine bone grafts)) are taken from a donor of another species. Studies show dentin as another composite biomaterial that could be used for bone augmentation [49].

A different composite of calcium hydroxide and polymer (like Bioplant) can be used for ridge preservation and augmentation [50].

## 6 Conclusion

Material science is an integral part of dentistry, and during the last decades, dental biomaterials have advanced rapidly. Some of these advances include biomimetic materials with the ability of mimicking nature; smart materials with the capability of showing different responses to change in temperature, pH, etc.; nanostructured materials with the capacity of modification of surface properties of different materials; and tissue engineering through the use of biomaterials and cells for tissue regeneration.

The common feature of first-generation dental biomaterials was biological inertness. The second generation intended to be bioactive and recruit specific interactions with surrounding tissue. But these two generations of biomaterials could not change with physiological load and biochemical stimuli. It seems that repair and regeneration of tissues require a more biologically based method, and the third generation of biomaterials are cell- and gene-activated materials designed to regrow, rather than replace, tissues.

Interaction between biomaterials and new technologies like biotechnology, nanotechnology, and tissue engineering will have a huge impact on the future of dentistry.

## References

1. *Clinical applications of biomaterials*. (1982). NIH Consens Statement.
2. Aaseth, J., Hilt, B., & Bjorklund, G. (2018). Mercury exposure and health impacts in dental personnel. *Environmental Research, 164*, 65–69.
3. Larson, T. D. (2015). Amalgam restorations: To bond or not. *Northwest Dentistry, 94*(5), 35–37.
4. Roach, M. (2007). Base metal alloys used for dental restorations and implants. *Dental Clinics of North America, 51*(3), 603–627, vi.
5. Shen, Y., et al. (2013). Current challenges and concepts of the thermomechanical treatment of nickel-titanium instruments. *Journal of Endodontia, 39*(2), 163–172.
6. Thompson, S. A. (2000). An overview of nickel-titanium alloys used in dentistry. *International Endodontic Journal, 33*(4), 297–310.
7. Wolcott, J. (2003). Nickel-titanium usage and breakage: An update. *Compendium of Continuing Education in Dentistry, 24*(11), 852, 854, 856 passim.
8. Roberts, H. W., et al. (2009). Metal-ceramic alloys in dentistry: A review. *Journal of Prosthodontics, 18*(2), 188–194.
9. Bosshardt, D. D., Chappuis, V., & Buser, D. (2017). Osseointegration of titanium, titanium alloy and zirconia dental implants: Current knowledge and open questions. *Periodontology 2000, 73*(1), 22–40.
10. Rupp, F., et al. (2018). Surface characteristics of dental implants: A review. *Dental Materials, 34*(1), 40–57.
11. Jafarzadeh Kashi, T. S., et al. (2011). An in vitro assessment of the effects of three surface treatments on repair bond strength of aged composites. *Operative Dentistry, 36*(6), 608–617.
12. Matos, A. B., et al. (2017). Bonding efficiency and durability: Current possibilities. *Brazilian Oral Research, 31*(suppl 1), e57.
13. Scotti, N., et al. (2017). New adhesives and bonding techniques. Why and when? *The International Journal of Esthetic Dentistry, 12*(4), 524–535.
14. Sofan, E., et al. (2017). Classification review of dental adhesive systems: From the IV generation to the universal type. *Annali di Stomatologia (Roma), 8*(1), 1–17.
15. Hill, E. E. (2007). Dental cements for definitive luting: A review and practical clinical considerations. *Dental Clinics of North America, 51*(3), 643–658, vi.
16. Lad, P. P., et al. (2014). Practical clinical considerations of luting cements: A review. *Journal of International Oral Health, 6*(1), 116–120.
17. Vahid Dastjerdie, E., et al. (2012). In-vitro comparison of the antimicrobial properties of glass ionomer cements with zinc phosphate cements. *Iranian Journal of Pharmaceutical Research, 11*(1), 77–82.
18. Patil, S. B., Naveen, B. H., & Patil, N. P. (2006). Bonding acrylic teeth to acrylic resin denture bases: A review. *Gerodontology, 23*(3), 131–139.
19. Rodrigues, S., Shenoy, V., & Shetty, T. (2013). Resilient liners: A review. *Journal Indian Prosthodontic Society, 13*(3), 155–164.
20. Takamata, T., & Setcos, J. C. (1989). Resin denture bases: Review of accuracy and methods of polymerization. *The International Journal of Prosthodontics, 2*(6), 555–562.
21. Shanahan, D. J., & Duncan, H. F. (2011). Root canal filling using Resilon: A review. *British Dental Journal, 211*(2), 81–88.
22. Gatewood, R. S. (2007). Endodontic materials. *Dental Clinics of North America, 51*(3), 695–712, vii.
23. Ma, X., et al. (2016). Materials for retrograde filling in root canal therapy. *Cochrane Database of Systematic Reviews, 12*, CD005517.
24. Najeeb, S., et al. (2016). Applications of polyetheretherketone (PEEK) in oral implantology and prosthodontics. *Journal of Prosthodontic Research, 60*(1), 12–19.

25. Schwitalla, A., & Muller, W. D. (2013). PEEK dental implants: A review of the literature. *The Journal of Oral Implantology, 39*(6), 743–749.
26. Tayebi, L., et al. (2018). 3D-printed membrane for guided tissue regeneration. *Materials Science and Engineering: C, 84*, 148–158.
27. Torshabi, M., Nojehdehian, H., & Tabatabaei, F. S. (2017). In vitro behavior of poly-lactic-co-glycolic acid microspheres containing minocycline, metronidazole, and ciprofloxacin. *Journal of Investigative and Clinical Dentistry, 8*(2), e12201.
28. Freedman, M., & Stassen, L. F. (2013). Commonly used topical oral wound dressing materials in dental and surgical practice--a literature review. *Journal of the Irish Dental Association, 59*(4), 190–195.
29. Selvi, F., et al. (2016). Effects of different suture materials on tissue healing. *Journal of Istanbul University Faculty of Dentistry, 50*(1), 35–42.
30. Hallmann, L., Ulmer, P., & Kern, M. (2018). Effect of microstructure on the mechanical properties of lithium disilicate glass-ceramics. *Journal of the Mechanical Behavior of Biomedical Materials, 82*, 355–370.
31. McLaren, E. A., & Figueira, J. (2015). Updating classifications of ceramic dental materials: A guide to material selection. *Compendium of Continuing Education in Dentistry, 36*(6), 400–405; quiz 406, 416.
32. Silva, L. H. D., et al. (2017). Dental ceramics: A review of new materials and processing methods. *Brazilian Oral Research, 31*(suppl 1), e58.
33. Turon-Vinas, M., & Anglada, M. (2018). Strength and fracture toughness of zirconia dental ceramics. *Dental Materials, 34*(3), 365–375.
34. Zhang, Y., & Kelly, J. R. (2017). Dental ceramics for restoration and metal veneering. *Dental Clinics of North America, 61*(4), 797–819.
35. Eliaz, N., & Metoki, N. (2017). Calcium phosphate bioceramics: A review of their history, structure, properties, coating technologies and biomedical applications. *Materials (Basel), 10*(4).
36. Prati, C., & Gandolfi, M. G. (2015). Calcium silicate bioactive cements: Biological perspectives and clinical applications. *Dental Materials, 31*(4), 351–370.
37. Xu, H. H., et al. (2017). Calcium phosphate cements for bone engineering and their biological properties. *Bone Research, 5*, 17056.
38. Ali, S., Farooq, I., & Iqbal, K. (2014). A review of the effect of various ions on the properties and the clinical applications of novel bioactive glasses in medicine and dentistry. *The Saudi Dental Journal, 26*(1), 1–5.
39. Chen, L., Shen, H., & Suh, B. I. (2013). Bioactive dental restorative materials: A review. *American Journal of Dentistry, 26*(4), 219–227.
40. Ahangari, Z., et al. (2017). Comparison of the antimicrobial efficacy of calcium hydroxide and photodynamic therapy against Enterococcus faecalis and Candida albicans in teeth with periapical lesions; an in vivo study. *Journal of Lasers in Medical Science, 8*(2), 72–78.
41. Torabinejad, M., Parirokh, M., & Dummer, P. M. H. (2018). Mineral trioxide aggregate and other bioactive endodontic cements: An updated overview – part II: Other clinical applications and complications. *International Endodontic Journal, 51*(3), 284–317.
42. Raghavendra, S. S., et al. (2017). Bioceramics in endodontics – A review. *Journal of Istanbul University Faculty of Dentistry, 51*(3 Suppl 1), S128–S137.
43. Cionca, N., Hashim, D., & Mombelli, A. (2017). Zirconia dental implants: Where are we now, and where are we heading? *Periodontology 2000, 73*(1), 241–258.
44. Kubasiewicz-Ross, P., et al. (2017). Zirconium: The material of the future in modern implantology. *Advances in Clinical and Experimental Medicine, 26*(3), 533–537.
45. Ilie, N., & Hickel, R. (2011). Resin composite restorative materials. *Australian Dental Journal, 56*(Suppl 1), 59–66.
46. Vaderhobli, R. M. (2011). Advances in dental materials. *Dental Clinics of North America, 55*(3), 619–25, x.

47. Ikemura, K., et al. (2008). A review of chemical-approach and ultramorphological studies on the development of fluoride-releasing dental adhesives comprising new pre-reacted glass ionomer (PRG) fillers. *Dental Materials Journal, 27*(3), 315–339.
48. Kramer, N., & Frankenberger, R. (2007). Compomers in restorative therapy of children: A literature review. *International Journal of Paediatric Dentistry, 17*(1), 2–9.
49. Tabatabaei, F. S., et al. (2016). Different methods of dentin processing for application in bone tissue engineering: A systematic review. *Journal of Biomedical Materials Research. Part A, 104*(10), 2616–2627.
50. Singh, J., et al. (2016). Bone Gaft materials: Dental aspects. *International Journal of Novel Research in Healhcare and Nursing, 3*(1), 99–103.

# Chapter 3
# Materials Used Intraoperatively During Oral and Maxillofacial Surgery Procedures

**Mina D. Fahmy, Anish Gupta, Arndt Guentsch, and Andre Peisker**

## 1 Introduction

The methods that currently exist for treating maxillofacial defects are not as robust as they could be. Moreover, large contributors to success are the surgeon's skill and the patient's own bodily reactions to materials used intraoperatively [1]. Often, patients are left with oral and maxillofacial defects or fractures, which range in size due to such things as congenital anomalies, acquired pathologies, and trauma. For instance, complete or partial resection in the midface or mandible due to oncologic surgery or following trauma requires the use of grafting materials, whether natural or synthetic, to resolve the void created. Further, bone graft materials are applied to congenital defects such as cleft palate, facial clefts, and facial asymmetries [2]. To enhance the effectiveness of such grafts, growth factors are used. Growth factors are steroid hormones or proteins that aid in cellular differentiation, proliferation, growth, and maturation. Growth factors may also have both inhibitory and stimulatory effects and have been shown to aid in the regeneration of bodily hard and soft tissues. Growth factors are also involved in a multitude of processes including mitogenesis, angiogenesis, metabolism, and wound healing [3]. In this chapter, we place

M. D. Fahmy (✉)
University of Tennessee Medical Center, Department of Oral & Maxillofacial Surgery, Knoxville, TN, USA
e-mail: mfahmy@utmck.edu

A. Gupta
Michigan Center for Oral Surgery, Southgate, MI, USA

A. Guentsch
Marquette University School of Dentistry, Department of Surgical Sciences, Milwaukee, WI, USA

A. Peisker
Department of Cranio-Maxillofacial and Plastic Surgery, Jena University Hospital, Jena, Germany



L. Tayebi (ed.), *Applications of Biomedical Engineering in Dentistry*,
https://doi.org/10.1007/978-3-030-21583-5_3

emphasis on BMP, TGF, FGF, and PDGF. Within the realm of oral and maxillofacial surgery, oral implantology is becoming more popular among patients hoping to bridge gaps within their dentition for improvement in form, function, and esthetics. As will be discussed later in the chapter, there are a multitude of different implant systems and numerous types of implant materials, shapes, and coatings that are used at the surgeon's preference and skill level [4]. This chapter will also explore different options concerning inter-maxillary and mandible fractures and how to fixate with plates, and screws, either biodegradable or permanent, in an effort to speed healing and recovery.

## 2 Grafting and Growth Factors

### *2.1 Grafting*

Recovery and maintenance of natural structures has been a great challenge within the realm of oral and maxillofacial surgery. For a number of years, autogenous bone has been the gold standard for grafting due to its osteogenic, osteoinductive, and osteoconductive properties. However, there are several drawbacks to using autogenous bone including morbidity, availability, and inability to customize shape and potential resorption [5–8]. To date, the perfect grafting material has not been identified, as this may be very patient specific. This section focuses on autografts; however, properties of various bone grafts and bone substitutes will be discussed later in this chapter.

Autogenous grafts may include cortical, cancellous, or cortico-cancellous bone with multiple factors determining successful incorporation. The healing process of these grafts requires both osteoconduction and osteoinduction. Embryonic origin, extent of revascularization, biomechanical features, type of fixation, and availability of growth factors are all factors of significant importance for incorporation of autogenous bone grafts [9]. Albrektsson and colleagues used a rabbit model to investigate the survivability of both cortical and cancellous bone grafts. It was found that trauma to the graft compromised cell viability in addition to a lag in the revascularization time, whereas the carefully handled graft revascularized and remodeled faster [10]. Furthermore, it was found that the cancellous bone grafts demonstrated a faster rate of revascularization than the cortical grafts [11–13]. More regarding grafting techniques will be discussed later in this chapter.

With regard to healing, it has been suggested that soft tissue pressure applied by the periosteum and/or the flap covering the graft may in fact increase the osteoclastic activity [14, 15]. As will be discussed in more detail later in the chapter, rigid fixation, a technique often used in the operating room, is important for healing. Several studies have concluded that rigid fixation (Figs. 3.1 and 3.2) increases the survival rate of the graft [16, 17].

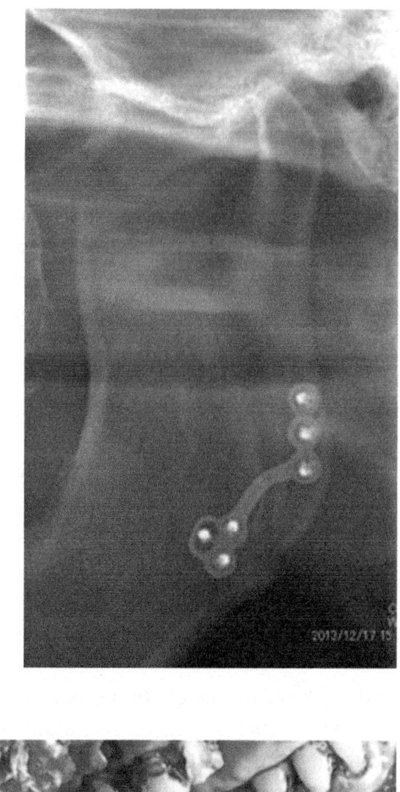

**Fig. 3.1** Mandibular angle fracture with rigid fixation [18]

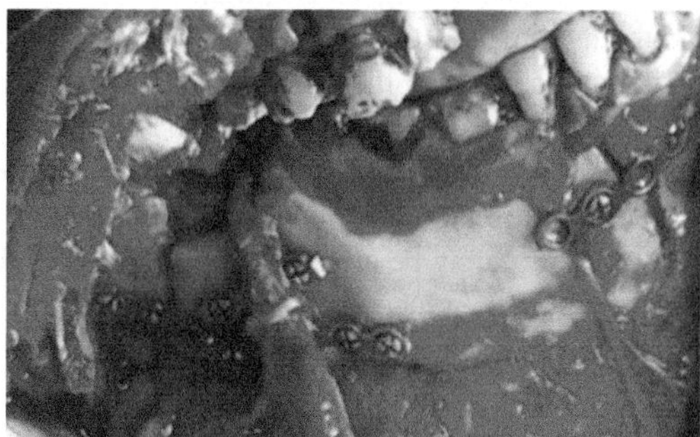

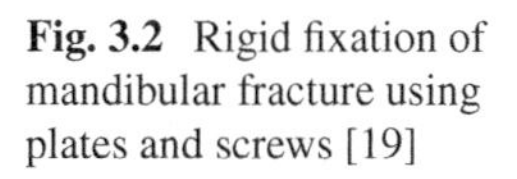

**Fig. 3.2** Rigid fixation of mandibular fracture using plates and screws [19]

## 2.2 *Growth Factors Relevant to Surgery*

Currently, researchers are investigating proteins and carriers for the delivery of growth factors (GFs): however, there are questions that exist with regard to the efficacy of these materials [20]. GFs are present in bone matrix and plasma, albeit in low concentrations [21]. GFs are biological mediators that have been shown to help in the regeneration of the natural periodontium. They are key factors in cellular differentiation, proliferation, and maturation. In addition, these GFs have been shown to have both stimulatory and inhibitory effects [3].

### 2.2.1 Bone Morphogenetic Protein

In 1971, it was shown that protein extracted from demineralized bone matrix induced the formation of the bone. This extracted protein was named BMP [22]. BMPs can provoke local immediate action, bind to extracellular antagonists, or interact with the extracellular matrix proteins and, subsequently, target cells. Interestingly, BMPs can regulate morphogenesis during development while also inducing bone and cartilage formation [23]. In their work, Karsenty and Kingsley describe how BMPs form a large group of proteins, which affect migration, differentiation, and cell growth. This protein group is the TGF-β superfamily [24, 25]. The TGF-β superfamily includes a number of proteins such as BMPs, osteogenic proteins, cartilage-derived morphogenic proteins, and growth differentiation factors [26]. Mesenchymal stem cells exhibit several BMP receptors [27] while also synthesizing the BMP antagonists noggin, gremlin, follistatin, and sclerostin. The osteoconductive biomaterial BMP/hydroxyapatite has been used in oral and maxillofacial surgery for contour augmentation by means of a macroporous delivery system [28].

### 2.2.2 Transforming Growth Factor

TGF-β increases the chemotaxis as well as the mitogenesis of the osteoblast precursors while also acting to stimulate osteoblast deposition of collagen matrix for wound healing and the regeneration of the bone [29]. TGF-β is produced by osteoblasts and is found at the highest concentration in platelets [30]. This growth factor stimulates the expression of bone matrix proteins [31] and moderates the breakdown activity of matrix metalloproteinases, among others [32]. The differentiation and proliferation of osteoblastic cells, along with the inhibition of osteoclast precursor formation, may be attributed to TGF-β [33]. Unlike BMP, TGF-β does not have the capacity to induce ectopic bone formation [34]. During the healing of bone fractures, the release of TGF-β, BMP 1–8, and growth differentiation factors (GDFs) 1, 5, 8, and 10 are plentiful [35]. Signaling molecules that are released after a bone fracture and during the progression of healing include pro-inflammatory cytokines, TGF-β superfamily, and other growth factors like PDGF, fibroblast growth factor, and insulin-like growth factors, as well as angiogenic factors such as vascular endothelial growth factor, angiopoietins 1 and 2, and matrix metalloproteinases [36]. TGF-β is found in high amounts in PRP which will be discussed in a later section.

### 2.2.3 Platelet-Derived Growth Factor

PDGF has the important biological activity of initiating connective tissue healing while also increasing mitogenesis and macrophage activation [29]. PDGF is produced by monocytes, macrophages, osteoblasts, endothelial cells, and platelets [37]. There are three types of PDGF, including PDGF AB, AA, and BB, with PDGF BB being the most biologically potent. In the early stages of fracture healing, PDGF plays a key role in acting as a chemotactic agent for inflammatory cells and as an inducer for osteoblasts and macrophages [34]. Hock and Canalis proposed that PDGF acts as a stimulant for osteoblasts, as well as osteoclast lineages, which may allow for decreased healing time [38]. As mentioned previously, PRP, which on its own will be discussed in a following section, is an autologous source of PDGF and TGF-β. Moreover, both of these growth factors play a primary role in the creation of platelet gels that, unlike fibrin glue, have a high concentration of platelets that release bioactive proteins necessary for tissue repair and regeneration .

### 2.2.4 Fibroblast Growth Factor

FGF may be produced by macrophages, mesenchymal cells, monocytes, chondrocytes, and osteoblasts. FGF is essential in the process of bone resorption and chondrogenesis [39]. Of the two isoforms that exist, α-FGF plays a key role in chondrocyte proliferation, while β-FGF is significant in the maturation of chondrocytes and bone resorption during the process of fracture healing, which often occurs after oral and maxillofacial surgery. Basic fibroblast growth factor (bFGF) is a growth factor that may be isolated from the pituitary glands of bovine [40]. bFGFs have also been isolated from a number of cells and tissues in tumors [3]. FGF-2 is considered a mitogen that has an effect on angiogenesis, thereby inducing a differentiation stimulus for mesodermal cells. In the short term, FGFs prevent the mineralization of the bone; however, in the long term, they act to speed and support bone development [41]. This was shown in a study by Takayama and colleagues where topical application of FGF-2 had a healing effect on bone fractures [42].

## 3 Growth Factor Enhancements

At the foundation of any surgical discipline is the science of wound healing. The oral and maxillofacial surgeon is usually blessed to work in an environment with rich vasculature; surgical and traumatic wounds tend to heal. But there will be compromised patients and ambitious reconstructive goals, and the surgeon will take any advantage given to assist his patient's natural healing process.

As discussed previously, growth factors with cytokine-mediated healing have been shown to assist in the biological healing process. Many of these growth factors can be resultant from platelets, including PDGF, TGF, VEGF, and EGF [43]. Platelet-derived products have been used as early as the 1970s, starting with fibrin glue [44]. Fibrin adhesives are still commercially available today (e.g., Tisseel from Baxter Healthcare) and are primarily used for hemostasis of diffuse microvascular bleeding. Its use is well documented in multiple surgical specialties, including oral and maxillofacial surgery [45]. Fibrin glue evolved into other autologous platelet concentrates including PRP [46], platelet gel, and platelet-rich fibrin (PRF) [47].

The literature reveals multiple studies with favorable treatment effects, not only in dentistry but also in orthopedics, dermatology, and ophthalmology [48]. Unfortunately, the literature has not come up with any consensus in terminology for platelet derivatives [49], and even less uniformity in their preparations, which likely accounts for inconsistencies in reported therapeutic effects.

## 3.1 The Biology of Wound Healing

Injury to tissue, whether surgical or traumatic, starts a cascade of events to allow wound healing. There are overlapping phases of inflammation, proliferation, and remodeling. The initial priority is to prevent hemorrhage, then prevent infection, and ultimately, restore the injured tissue [50]. The immediate reaction to injured tissue is vasoconstriction to limit bleeding. Coagulation factors are activated and multiple cascades are set into motion. A fibrin matrix is formed at the injured vasculature, and circulating platelets aggregate at the exposed subendothelium, creating a platelet plug. This plug functions not only for hemostasis but also orchestrates subsequent healing [51]. Activated platelets in the plug degranulate and create cellular signals through cytokines and growth factors.

Entire chapters can be devoted to each individual component of the wound healing process. We will limit and simplify our discussion to the roles of fibrin and platelets.

Platelets are anuclear structures arising from bone marrow precursors. The platelet membrane contains receptors for many molecules, including thrombin, and the cytoplasm contains granules that are released on activation [52]. Fibrin is a fibrous protein, which is activated by thrombin. Activated platelets and resulting thrombin allow fibrin to form a cross-linked mesh with the platelet plug to finalize a blood clot.

## 3.2 Collection and Preparation of Platelet Derivatives

Platelet derivatives have few contraindications, specifically in patients with platelet counts less than $10^5$/microliter, hemoglobin level less than 10 g/dL, or presence of active infections [53]. PRP has shown great variability in centrifugation protocol. Current PRP procedures start with the collection of whole blood in acid/citrate/dextrose, which are then centrifuged. The red blood cells are removed, and the PRP then undergoes a second centrifugation step to obtain a supernatant of platelet-poor plasma (PPP) and the pellet of platelets. Growth factor release of the PRP happens with platelet activation from thrombin, either bovine thrombin or autologous thrombin obtained by adding calcium gluconate to the PPP. Thrombin is combined to the PRP and allows handling as a gel [48].

PRF is considered a second-generation platelet concentrate, notably with a simplified preparation in comparison to PRP. Whole blood is collected without anticoagulants and centrifuged to form a fibrin clot, which contains the platelets. As opposed to PRP where the activation of the platelets is due to thrombin, the PRF activation is a result of the centrifugation process itself. The PRF clot is homogenous and is interpreted to have the cytokines incorporated into the fibrin mesh, allowing for an increased lifespan of these intrinsic growth factors and cell signaling molecules [52]. The inflammatory markers present also indicate degranulation of the leucocytes, which may play a role in the reduction of infection [54].

## 3.3 Applications in Oral and Maxillofacial Surgery

Both PRP and PRF continue to be used and reviewed in the literature. The therapeutic effects are not validated with multi-center randomized trials, and there still exists discrepancies in overall benefits. In the literature, benefits have been documented when platelet concentrates are used in multiple maxillofacial applications. In post-extraction sites, including third molars, healing times have been improved, with reduction of complications including alveolar osteitis [55–61]. However there are studies that show no significant benefit using scintigraphic evaluation [62]. Many studies discuss platelet concentrates used in combination with bone grafting for both reconstruction and for site preparations for dental implants. Studies showed accelerated healing, particularly of the soft tissue [63]. Reviews of the literature in regard to sinus augmentation show increased bone density [64] but no significant improvement in bone formation or implant survivability [65, 66]. In the setting of poor wound healing, we see applications of platelet derivatives in the setting of medication-related osteonecrosis of the jaws (MRONJ) and other oral mucosal lesions, with cautious interpretation of results suggesting benefits of their use [67–70]. Successful treatment of alveolar cleft bone grafting has been shown by multiple teams [71–73].

In the temporomandibular joint (TMJ), platelet concentrates have been hypothesized to help, given that the cartilage is avascular and has difficulty with self-repair. Bone growth was significantly improved in osteoarthritis in the rabbit model, with improved, but not significant, regeneration of the cartilage [74]. Injections of platelet concentrates into the TMJ have been shown to be effective for treatment of temporomandibular osteoarthritis [75–77] and better than arthrocentesis alone [78]. However, it has been pointed out that growth factors associated with PRP, including VEGF, may be detrimental to cartilaginous healing [79].

## 3.4 Future Applications

The common complaint in the systematic reviews of PRP and PRF therapy continues to be a large discrepancy in preparation and use of platelet concentrates. Good evidence is available that there is a quantifiable increase in growth factors when using platelet-rich products [80–83]. However, large multi-center trials need to be conducted to prove the efficacy of these treatments reliably and reproducibly.

# 4 Implantable Devices

## *4.1 Replacement of Teeth*

Oral implants have become the sought-after method of treatment, which is scientifically accepted and well documented in the literature [84–86]. Oral implants were introduced some 30–40 years ago [87–89]. Since then, implants have revolutionized the concept of replacing missing teeth and improved the quality of life for patients [90, 91]. Today, there are over 1300 different implant systems worldwide. They vary in shape, dimension, bulk, surface material, topography, surface chemistry, wettability, and surface modification [92]. Titanium is the material most commonly used for oral endosseous implants, due to its mechanical strength, excellent biocompatibility, and osseointegration [93]. Some studies have reported regarding the clinical disadvantages of titanium, such as host sensitivity to titanium, electrical conductivity, corrosive properties, and esthetic concerns as a result of their dark-grayish coloring [94–96]. Furthermore, elevated titanium concentrations have been found in close proximity to oral implants [97] and in regional lymph nodes [98]. However, the clinical relevance of these facts is still unclear [99]. Ceramic materials have been suggested as a substitute to titanium for oral implants because of their esthetic benefits and excellent biocompatibility in vitro and in vivo [100–102], great tissue integration, low affinity to plaque, and favorable biomechanical properties [103]. These ceramic materials have already been investigated and clinically used since approximately 30–40 years ago. The first ceramic material utilized was aluminum oxide [104, 105], and later, the Cerasand ceramic and the ceramic anchor implant were introduced [106, 107]. The physical and mechanical properties of alumina ceramics are high hardness and modulus of elasticity, which make the material brittle. In combination with the relatively low bending strength and fracture toughness, alumina ceramics are vulnerable to fractures. Based on these drawbacks, there are no alumina implant systems remaining on the market [86, 108]. Currently, the material of choice for ceramic oral implants is zirconia (ZrO2), containing tetragonal polycrystalline yttria (Y2O3) (Y-TZP). In comparison to alumina, Y-TZP has a higher bending strength, a lower modulus of elasticity, and a higher fracture toughness [86, 109, 110]. Through in vitro and in vivo studies, zirconia has become an attractive alternative to titanium for the fabrication of oral implants [103]. However, animal studies have indicated a better bone-to-implant contact with titanium implants than with Y-TZP implants [101, 111]. In addition, early failures were significantly higher for zirconia implants than for titanium implants [103].

Surface topography is one of the important parameters for the achievement of osseointegration and can be classified into macro-, micro-, and nanoscale [112]. The three major modifications of macrotopography are screw threads (tapped or self-tapping), solid body press-fit designs, and sintered bead technologies. Recently, studies were mainly focused on micro- and nanogeometry. The osteoblast activity is significantly increased at 1–100 μm of the surface roughness compared to a smooth surface [113]. Increased surface roughness of dental implants can be achieved by machining, plasma spray coating, grit blasting, acid etching, sandblasting, anodizing, and applying a biomimetic coating, or other combinations of the several mentioned techniques [114–117] resulted in greater bone apposition [118] and reduced healing time [119].

## 4.2 *Reconstruction of the Craniomaxillofacial Skeleton*

Reconstruction of the craniomaxillofacial skeleton, resulting from resection of benign and malignant tumor, osteomyelitis, or osteoradionecrosis, still remains a challenge for the surgeon [120].

### 4.2.1 Natural Bone Grafts

Since the nineteenth century, autologous bone has been successfully used as bone substitute [121]. Different donor sites are described in the current literature. Intraoral donor sites include the symphysis of the mandible, mandibular ramus, and maxillary tuberosity [122]. The common extraoral donor sites for non-vascularized bone grafts are the iliac crest and rib. The non-vascularized iliac crest graft is a treatment possibility for reconstruction of moderate mandibular defects [123], whereas the costochondral graft from the rib is used predominantly for condylar reconstruction [124, 125]. During the past decade, a variety of donor sites for vascular bone flaps and soft tissue have been recommended. The osteocutaneous radial forearm free flap [126, 127], fibular free flap [127, 128], scapula free flap [128], and iliac crest free flap [129] are the most commonly utilized donor sites for vascularized reconstruction.

Allogenic bone refers to the bone that is harvested from one individual and transplanted into another individual, both of the same species. Due to the limitations of autologous bone grafting, allogenic grafts are considered an effective alternative. Allografts, to a limited extent, can be customized by being machined and shaped to fit the defect. It can be available in a variety of forms, including cortical and cancellous. The disadvantage, however, is that compared to autografts, they have a higher failure rate due to their immunogenicity [130, 131].

Xenograft bone has been taken from a donor of another species [122], usually of bovine origin. Mineral xenograft has been applied in oral and maxillofacial surgery for several years [132]. Demineralized bone, harvested from human donors, has been frequently used in craniofacial reconstruction [133, 134]. The demineralization is achieved through the process of acidification, resulting in a matrix containing type I collagen and osteoinductive growth factors, predominantly BMP. Based on porosity, it can be easily formed and remodeled intraoperatively [135, 136].

### 4.2.2 Synthetic Bone Grafts

Craniofacial reconstruction using alloplastic implants has shown to be associated with low rates of infection and other types of morbidity [137]. Computer-aided designed and manufactured (CAD/CAM) titanium implants which are prefabricated are a reasonable option for secondary reconstruction [138]. The major disadvantages are the thermosensitivity and limited possibility of intraoperative customization [136]. Synthetically manufactured bioactive glass-ceramic is an option as a single CAD/CAM implant for craniofacial reconstruction with good clinical outcomes. As opposed to titanium implants, it allows intraoperative remodeling and adjustment without thermosensitivity [139]. Calcium phosphates belong to the group of bioactive synthetic materials. The most commonly used are hydroxyapatite, tricalcium phosphate, and biphasic calcium phosphate [140–142]. Calcium phosphates are osteoconductive, do not cause any foreign body response, and are nontoxic [136].

Hard tissue replacement (HTR)-sintered polymers consist of poly(methyl methacrylate (pMMA), poly(hydroxyethyl methacrylate) (pHEMA), and calcium hydroxide. The porosity of the plastic allows for the indwelling growth of blood vessels as well as connective tissue [136]. HTR implants can be used for the reconstruction of large defects of the cranio-orbital region when combined with simultaneous bone tumor resection [143]. The implants are fixated with titanium or resorbable plates and screws.

Polyetheretherketone (PEEK) is a synthetic material that has been used for a number of years in neurosurgery due to its excellent biocompatibility, good mechanical strength, and radiographic translucency. In recent years, studies of maxillofacial reconstructions have been reported using PEEK for the construction of patient-specific implants [144–146]. The major disadvantage of computer-designed PEEK is its high cost [147].

Porous polyethylene (PPE) or high-density polyethylene (HDPE) is a linear highly compressed (sintered) aliphatic hydrocarbon. It is a biocompatible, durable, and stable material. Furthermore, it shows rapid surrounding soft tissue ingrowth without capsule formation around it [137, 148, 149]. PPE has proven to be a reasonable alternative to PEEK as a material for craniofacial reconstructions. The use of this material seems to be safe and has minimal morbidity [149]. In summary, autografts are osteoconductive, osteoinductive, and osteogenic; however, they have limited availability and have donor-site morbidity. Allografts are osteoconductive and osteoinductive but are not osteogenic; they carry the same disadvantages as autografts with the addition of having disease transmission risk. Xenografts are osteoconductive, but not osteoinductive or osteogenic, and carry the potential for foreign body reaction. Alloplastic materials are osteoconductive but often costly [150].

# 5 Maintenance of Structural Integrity and Fixation

## 5.1 *Plates and Screws*

Today, nearly all the metal plates and screws for the fixation of the craniomaxillofacial skeleton consist of titanium and are stored in sets that can be re-sterilized. Titanium is the most biocompatible and corrosion-resistant metal and has an innate ability to fuse with human bone [151, 152]. Therefore, it has received much attention in the area of craniofacial reconstruction [153]. Prior to the use of titanium, several other materials were applied for craniofacial applications. These metals, which included stainless steel and vitallium, an alloy from cobalt, chrome, and molybdenum, have fallen out of favor because of their corrosion profile and/or lack of inertness [154, 155]. Furthermore, vitallium and stainless steel produce more artifacts on computed tomography scans and magnetic resonance imaging than titanium [156–158]. There exist miniplates of different shapes with corresponding osteosynthesis screws of different lengths (Fig. 3.3) [159].

### 5.1.1 Midface

Osteosynthesis screws are also based on different systems. For the midface, osteosynthesis is based on systems 1.0, 1.3, 1.5, and 2.0. The numbers refer to the outer screw thread diameter in mm. Low profile plates are recommended for the infraorbital rim because the structural forces are not significant in this region. In contrast, increased stability with stronger implants is needed for the zygomaticomaxillary buttress where high masticatory forces are transmitted [160, 161].

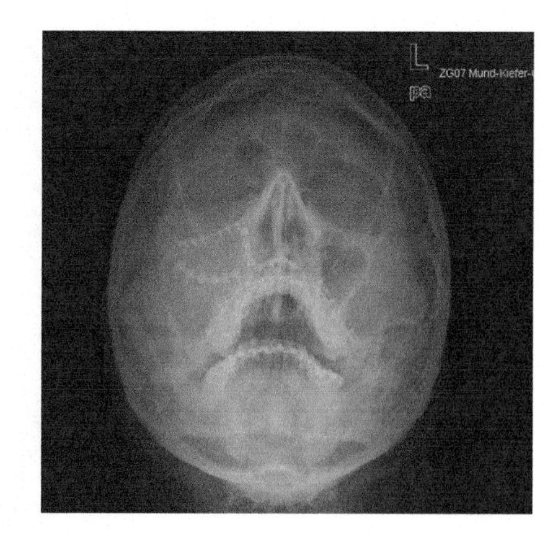

**Fig. 3.3** Postoperative x-ray of a complex midface fracture treated with several malleable fixation plates

Depending on the size and location of the orbital defect, reconstruction can be achieved by using implants of various materials with different benefits and disadvantages. Currently, the ideal implant material for orbital reconstruction still remains unclear [153]. The use of silastic implants, bioactive glass, and porous polyethylene to bridge the bony defect has been extensively documented in the literature [162–164]. In addition, titanium mesh (Fig. 3.4) or pre-shaped plates, such as the 3D titanium orbital plate, are applied in special cases [165, 166]. Biodegradable polyglycolic acid [167] and polydioxanone [168] are options as resorbable alloplastic materials. Alternatively, autogenous transplants can be used [169–172]. Considering donor-site morbidity of autologous transplants and infections with nonresorbable materials, resorbable implants for reconstruction could be recommended [168].

### 5.1.2 Mandible

Different osteosynthesis plating systems are in use for application to the mandible. According to Arbeitsgemeinschaft für Osteosynthesefragen (AO)/Association for the study of Internal Fixation (ASIF) principles, the types of plates include mandible plates 2.0, locking plates 2.0, (locking) reconstruction plates, dynamic compression plates, and universal fracture plates [173–176]. Mandibular miniplates are designed to be used with monocortical screws (Fig. 3.5). Bicortical screws can be used for additional stability in selected cases. In approaches with limited space (e.g., condylar and subcondylar regions), plates of modified design, such as the compression plate, the trapezoid plate, or the delta plate, are applied [177, 178]. Lag screw osteosynthesis of fractures of the mandibular condyle is a method to combine functional stability with simple removal of osteosynthesis materials, without re-exposure of the temporomandibular joint region [179, 180].

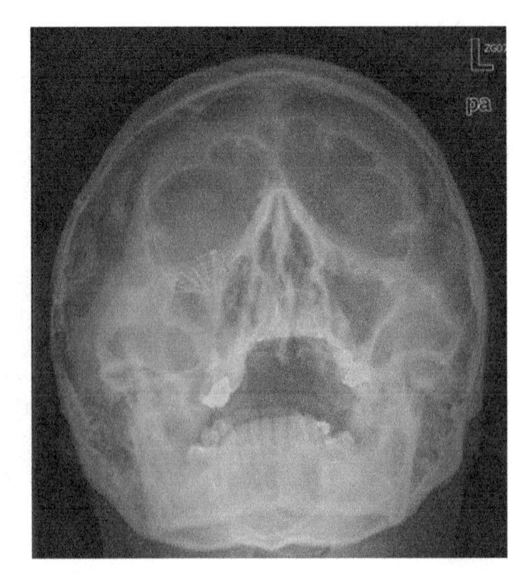


**Fig. 3.4** Postoperative x-ray of an orbital floor fracture treated with a titanium mesh

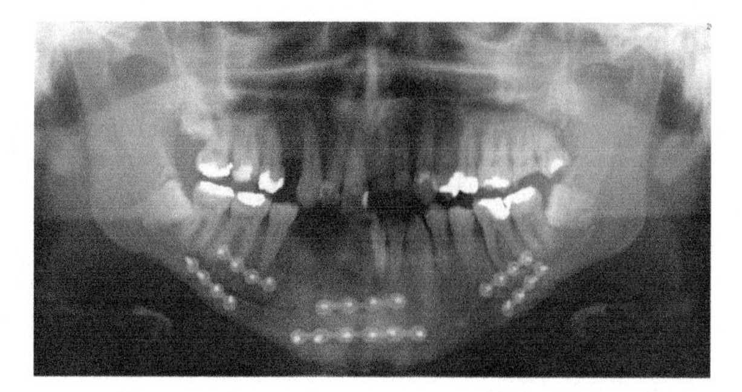

**Fig. 3.5** Postoperative x-rays shows fracture fixation with six mandibular miniplates 2.0

### 5.1.3 Absorbable Materials

Absorbable osteosynthetic material is an option to make metal removal unnecessary [181]. A complete resorption occurs approximately 1 year in experimental models [182]. Further advantages are the absence of thermal sensitivity and radiological artifacts [136]. Use of bioresorbable miniplates has been suggested in the pediatric population because of possible growth disturbances associated with titanium-based hardware [183]. A variety of biodegradable implants are commercially available in the field of oral and maxillofacial surgery. Polymers of α-hydroxy acids as glycolic acid (PGA), L-lactic and D, L-lactic acids (PLLA, PDLLA), and their copolymers are the substances largely used as osteosynthesis materials [184–188]. These materials have proven clinical success throughout the world; however, there are some arguments against biodegradable fixation. The complications of biodegradable fixation are infections, foreign body reactions, malocclusions, and malunions [188]. Furthermore, the duration of surgery is more challenging and costly [187, 189].

## 6 Summary

Oral and maxillofacial surgery is an incredible and evolving field. Injuries, defects, and pathologies to the head, neck, and face, as well as hard and soft tissues of the oral region, are often taken care of by specialists extensively trained as oral and maxillofacial surgeons. As further research is completed and scientists continue exploration of materials and methods, techniques and strategies are altered to benefit the patient in clinical settings. In this chapter, we focused on the use of different grafting materials, both natural and synthetic for bone regeneration and defect repair, growth factors that aid in healing and growth of tissues, as well as fixation devices used in the repair of maxillofacial bone fractures. The techniques discussed are effective; however, future work needs to be outlined in order to improve efficiency and efficacy, both inside and outside of the operating room.

## References

1. Fahmy, M. D., et al. (2016). Three-dimensional bioprinting materials with potential application in preprosthetic surgery. *Journal of Prosthodontics, 25*(4), 310–318.
2. Boyne, P. J. (2001). Application of bone morphogenetic proteins in the treatment of clinical oral and maxillofacial osseous defects. *JBJS, 83*(1_suppl_2), S146–S150.
3. Rifkin, D. B., & Moscatelli, D. (1989). Recent developments in the cell biology of basic fibroblast growth factor. *The Journal of Cell Biology, 109*(1), 1–6.
4. Sykaras, N., et al. (2000). Implant materials, designs, and surface topographies: Their effect on osseointegration. A literature review. *International Journal of Oral & Maxillofacial Implants, 15*(5).
5. Hjørting-Hansen, E. (2001). Bone grafting to the jaws with special reference to reconstructive preprosthetic surgery: A historical review (Übersicht). *Mund-, Kiefer-und Gesichtschirurgie, 6*(1), 6–14.
6. Hirsch, J. M. (2001). Volumetry of simulated bone grafts in the edentulous maxilla by computed tomography: An experimental study. *Dentomaxillofacial Radiology, 30*, 153–156.
7. Sjöström, M., On healing of titanium implants in iliac crest bone grafts. 2006.
8. Springer, I. N., et al. (2004). Particulated bone grafts–effectiveness of bone cell supply. *Clinical Oral Implants Research, 15*(2), 205–212.
9. Alberius, M. G. (1999). Per, *Some basic factors essential to autogeneic nonvascularized onlay bone grafting to the craniofacial skeleton. Scandinavian Journal of Plastic and Reconstructive Surgery and Hand Surgery, 33*(2), 129–146.
10. Albrektsson, T., & Albrektsson, B. (1978). Microcirculation in grafted bone: A chamber technique for vital microscopy of rabbit bone transplants. *Acta Orthopaedica Scandinavica, 49*(1), 1–7.
11. Chen, N. T., et al. (1994). The roles of revascularization and resorption on endurance of craniofacial onlay bone grafts in the rabbit. *Plastic and Reconstructive Surgery, 93*(4), 714–722; discussion 723-4.
12. Lin, K. Y., et al. (1990). The effect of rigid fixation on the survival of onlay bone grafts: An experimental study. *Plastic and Reconstructive Surgery, 86*(3), 449–456.
13. Pinholt, E. M., et al. (1994). Revascularization of calvarial, mandibular, tibial, and iliac bone grafts in rats. *Annals of Plastic Surgery, 33*(2), 193–197.
14. Goldstein, J., Mase, C., & Newman, M. H. (1993). Fixed membranous bone graft survival after recipient bed alteration. *Plastic and Reconstructive Surgery, 91*(4), 589–596.
15. Goldstein, J. A., Mase, C. A., & Newman, M. H. (1995). The influence of bony architecture on fixed membranous bone graft survival. *Annals of Plastic Surgery, 34*(2), 162–167.
16. Phillips, J. H., & Rahn, B. A. (1988). Fixation effects on membranous and endochondral onlay bone-graft resorption. *Plastic and Reconstructive Surgery, 82*(5), 872–877.
17. Phillips, J. H., & Rahn, B. A. (1990). Fixation effects on membranous and endochondral onlay bone graft revascularization and bone deposition. *Plastic and Reconstructive Surgery, 85*(6), 891–897.
18. Hara, S., Mitsugi, M., & Tatemoto, Y. (2017). Variation of plate fixation for mandibular advancement with intraoral vertical ramus osteotomy using endoscopically-assisted intraoral rigid or semi-rigid internal fixation: Postoperative condylar seating control for mandibular advancement. *International Journal of Oral and Maxillofacial Surgery, 46*, 158.
19. Rao, S. S., Baliga, S. D., & Bhatnagar, A. (2018). Management of extensive maxillofacial injury related to a Tyre Blast: A rare case report. *The Saudi Dental Journal, 30*(1), 97–101.
20. Esposito, M., et al. (2006). The efficacy of various bone augmentation procedures for dental implants: A Cochrane systematic review of randomized controlled clinical trials. *International Journal of Oral & Maxillofacial Implants, 21*(5).
21. Trippel, S. B. (1997). Growth factors as therapeutic agents. *Instructional Course Lectures-American Academy of Orthopaedic Surgeons, 46*, 473–476.

22. Urist, M. R., & Strates, B. S. (1971). Bone morphogenetic protein. *Journal of Dental Research, 50*(6), 1392–1406.
23. Wozney, J. M., et al. (1988). Novel regulators of bone formation: Molecular clones and activities. *Science, 242*(4885), 1528–1534.
24. Karsenty, G. (1998). Genetics of skeletogenesis. *Developmental Genetics, 22*(4), 301–313.
25. Kingsley, D. M. (1994). The TGF-beta superfamily: New members, new receptors, and new genetic tests of function in different organisms. *Genes & Development, 8*(2), 133–146.
26. Ducy, P., & Karsenty, G. (2000). The family of bone morphogenetic proteins. *Kidney International, 57*(6), 2207–2214.
27. Rosen, V. (2006). BMP and BMP inhibitors in bone. *Annals of the New York Academy of Sciences, 1068*(1), 19–25.
28. Hotz, G., & Herr, G. (1994). Bone substitute with osteoinductive biomaterials—Current and future clinical applications. *International Journal of Oral and Maxillofacial Surgery, 23*(6), 413–417.
29. Bhanot, S., & Alex, J. C. (2002). Current applications of platelet gels in facial plastic surgery. *Facial Plastic Surgery, 18*(1), 27–34.
30. Assoian, R. K., et al. (1983). Transforming growth factor-beta in human platelets. Identification of a major storage site, purification, and characterization. *Journal of Biological Chemistry, 258*(11), 7155–7160.
31. Wiltfang, J., et al. (2003). Sinus floor augmentation with β-tricalciumphosphate (β-TCP): Does platelet-rich plasma promote its osseous integration and degradation? *Clinical Oral Implants Research, 14*(2), 213–218.
32. Overall, C. M., Wrana, J., & Sodek, J. (1989). Independent regulation of collagenase, 72-kDa progelatinase, and metalloendoproteinase inhibitor expression in human fibroblasts by transforming growth factor-beta. *Journal of Biological Chemistry, 264*(3), 1860–1869.
33. Bonewald, L., & Mundy, G. (1990). Role of transforming growth factor-beta in bone remodeling. *Clinical Orthopaedics and Related Research*, (250), 261–276.
34. Lieberman, J. R., Daluiski, A., & Einhorn, T. A. (2002). The role of growth factors in the repair of bone: Biology and clinical applications. *JBJS, 84*(6), 1032–1044.
35. Cho, T. J., Gerstenfeld, L. C., & Einhorn, T. A. (2002). Differential temporal expression of members of the transforming growth factor β superfamily during murine fracture healing. *Journal of Bone and Mineral Research, 17*(3), 513–520.
36. Dimitriou, R., Tsiridis, E., & Giannoudis, P. V. (2005). Current concepts of molecular aspects of bone healing. *Injury, 36*(12), 1392–1404.
37. Andrew, J., et al. (1995). Platelet-derived growth factor expression in normally healing human fractures. *Bone, 16*(4), 455–460.
38. Hock, J. M., & Canalis, E. (1994). Platelet-derived growth factor enhances bone cell replication, but not differentiated function of osteoblasts. *Endocrinology, 134*(3), 1423–1428.
39. Hallman, M., & Thor, A. (2008). Bone substitutes and growth factors as an alternative/complement to autogenous bone for grafting in implant dentistry. *Periodontology 2000, 47*(1), 172–192.
40. Sonmez, A. B., & Castelnuovo, J. (2014). Applications of basic fibroblastic growth factor (FGF-2, bFGF) in dentistry. *Dental Traumatology, 30*(2), 107–111.
41. Hatch, N., & Franceschi, R. (2008). FGF2 induced expression of the pyrophosphate generating enzyme, PC-1, is mediated by Runx2 and Msx2. *Journal of Musculoskeletal & Neuronal Interactions, 8*(4), 318.
42. Takayama, S., et al. (2001). Periodontal regeneration by FGF-2 (bFGF) in primate models. *Journal of Dental Research, 80*(12), 2075–2079.
43. Marx, R. E. (2004). Platelet-rich plasma: Evidence to support its use. *Journal of Oral and Maxillofacial Surgery, 62*(4), 489–496.
44. Gibble, J. W., & Ness, P. M. (1990). Fibrin glue: The perfect operative sealant? *Transfusion, 30*(8), 741–747.

45. Matras, H. (1985). Fibrin sealant in maxillofacial surgery. Development and indications. A review of the past 12 years. *Facial Plastic Surgery, 2*(4), 297–313.
46. Whitman, D. H., Berry, R. L., & Green, D. M. (1997). Platelet gel: An autologous alternative to fibrin glue with applications in oral and maxillofacial surgery. *Journal of Oral and Maxillofacial Surgery, 55*(11), 1294–1299.
47. Dohan, D. M., et al. (2006). Platelet-rich fibrin (PRF): A second-generation platelet concentrate. Part I: Technological concepts and evolution. *Oral Surgery, Oral Medicine, Oral Pathology, Oral Radiology, and Endodontics, 101*(3), e37–e44.
48. De Pascale, M. R., et al. (2015). Platelet derivatives in regenerative medicine: An update. *Transfusion Medicine Reviews, 29*(1), 52–61.
49. Dohan Ehrenfest, D. M., Rasmusson, L., & Albrektsson, T. (2009). Classification of platelet concentrates: From pure platelet-rich plasma (P-PRP) to leucocyte- and platelet-rich fibrin (L-PRF). *Trends in Biotechnology, 27*(3), 158–167.
50. Miloro, M., et al. (2004). *Peterson's principles of oral and maxillofacial surgery* (2nd ed.). Hamilton, ON/London: B C Decker.
51. Singer, A. J., & Clark, R. A. (1999). Cutaneous wound healing. *The New England Journal of Medicine, 341*(10), 738–746.
52. Dohan, D. M., et al. (2006). Platelet-rich fibrin (PRF): A second-generation platelet concentrate. Part II: Platelet-related biologic features. *Oral Surgery, Oral Medicine, Oral Pathology, Oral Radiology, and Endodontics, 101*(3), e45–e50.
53. Dauendorffer, J. N., Fraitag, S., & Dupuy, A. (2013). Basal cell carcinoma following platelet-rich plasma injection for skin rejuvenation. *Annales de Dermatologie et de Vénéréologie, 140*(11), 723–724.
54. Dohan, D. M., et al. (2006). Platelet-rich fibrin (PRF): A second-generation platelet concentrate. Part III: Leucocyte activation: A new feature for platelet concentrates? *Oral Surgery, Oral Medicine, Oral Pathology, Oral Radiology, and Endodontics, 101*(3), e51–e55.
55. Del Fabbro, M., Bortolin, M., & Taschieri, S. (2011). Is autologous platelet concentrate beneficial for post-extraction socket healing? A systematic review. *International Journal of Oral and Maxillofacial Surgery, 40*(9), 891–900.
56. Del Fabbro, M., et al. (2017). Healing of Postextraction sockets preserved with autologous platelet concentrates. A systematic review and meta-analysis. *Journal of Oral and Maxillofacial Surgery, 75*(8), 1601–1615.
57. Eshghpour, M., et al. (2014). Effect of platelet-rich fibrin on frequency of alveolar Osteitis following mandibular third molar surgery: A double-blinded randomized clinical trial. *Journal of Oral and Maxillofacial Surgery, 72*(8), 1463–1467.
58. Al-Hamed, F. S., et al. (2017). Efficacy of platelet-rich fibrin after mandibular third molar extraction: A systematic review and meta-analysis. *Journal of Oral and Maxillofacial Surgery, 75*(6), 1124–1135.
59. Bilginaylar, K., & Uyanik, L. O. (2016). Evaluation of the effects of platelet-rich fibrin and piezosurgery on outcomes after removal of ımpacted mandibular third molars. *British Journal of Oral and Maxillofacial Surgery, 54*(6), 629–633.
60. Canellas, J., Ritto, F. G., & Medeiros, P. J. D. (2017). Evaluation of postoperative complications after mandibular third molar surgery with the use of platelet-rich fibrin: A systematic review and meta-analysis. *International Journal of Oral and Maxillofacial Surgery, 46*(9), 1138–1146.
61. Varghese, M. P., Manuel, S., Kumar, S., & K, L. (2017). Potential for osseous regeneration of platelet-rich fibrin—A comparative study in mandibular third molar impaction sockets. *Journal of Oral and Maxillofacial Surgery, 75*(7), 1322–1329.
62. Gürbüzer, B., et al. (2010). Scintigraphic evaluation of Osteoblastic activity in extraction sockets treated with platelet-rich fibrin. *Journal of Oral and Maxillofacial Surgery, 68*(5), 980–989.
63. Moraschini, V., & Barboza, E. S. P. (2015). Effect of autologous platelet concentrates for alveolar socket preservation: A systematic review. *International Journal of Oral and Maxillofacial Surgery, 44*(5), 632–641.

64. Khairy, N. M., et al. (2013). Effect of platelet rich plasma on bone regeneration in maxillary sinus augmentation (randomized clinical trial). *International Journal of Oral and Maxillofacial Surgery, 42*(2), 249–255.
65. Lemos, C. A. A., et al. (2016). Effects of platelet-rich plasma in association with bone grafts in maxillary sinus augmentation: A systematic review and meta-analysis. *International Journal of Oral and Maxillofacial Surgery, 45*(4), 517–525.
66. Pocaterra, A., et al. (2016). Effectiveness of platelet-rich plasma as an adjunctive material to bone graft: A systematic review and meta-analysis of randomized controlled clinical trials. *International Journal of Oral and Maxillofacial Surgery, 45*(8), 1027–1034.
67. Del Fabbro, M., Gallesio, G., & Mozzati, M. (2015). Autologous platelet concentrates for bisphosphonate-related osteonecrosis of the jaw treatment and prevention. A systematic review of the literature. *European Journal of Cancer, 51*(1), 62–74.
68. Kim, J.-W., Kim, S.-J., & Kim, M.-R. (2014). Leucocyte-rich and platelet-rich fibrin for the treatment of bisphosphonate-related osteonecrosis of the jaw: A prospective feasibility study. *British Journal of Oral and Maxillofacial Surgery, 52*(9), 854–859.
69. Lopez-Jornet, P., et al. (2016). Medication-related osteonecrosis of the jaw: Is autologous platelet concentrate application effective for prevention and treatment? A systematic review. *Journal of Cranio-Maxillofacial Surgery, 44*(8), 1067–1072.
70. Mohanty, S., Pathak, H., & Dabas, J. (2014). Platelet rich fibrin: A new covering material for oral mucosal defects. *Journal of Oral Biology and Craniofacial Research, 4*(2), 144–146.
71. Oyama, T., et al. (2004). Efficacy of platelet-rich plasma in alveolar bone grafting. *Journal of Oral and Maxillofacial Surgery, 62*(5), 555–558.
72. Marukawa, E., et al. (2011). Reduction of bone resorption by the application of platelet-rich plasma (PRP) in bone grafting of the alveolar cleft. *Journal of Cranio-Maxillofacial Surgery, 39*(4), 278–283.
73. Lee, C., et al. (2009). A quantitative radiological assessment of outcomes of autogenous bone graft combined with platelet-rich plasma in the alveolar cleft. *International Journal of Oral and Maxillofacial Surgery, 38*(2), 117–125.
74. Kütük, N., et al. (2014). Effect of platelet-rich plasma on fibrocartilage, cartilage, and bone repair in Temporomandibular joint. *Journal of Oral and Maxillofacial Surgery, 72*(2), 277–284.
75. Lin, S. L., et al. (2018). Effect of arthrocentesis plus platelet-rich plasma and platelet-rich plasma alone in the treatment of temporomandibular joint osteoarthritis: A retrospective matched cohort study (a STROBE-compliant article). *Medicine (Baltimore), 97*(16), e0477.
76. Hegab, A. F., et al. (2015). Platelet-rich plasma injection as an effective treatment for Temporomandibular joint osteoarthritis. *Journal of Oral and Maxillofacial Surgery, 73*(9), 1706–1713.
77. Bousnaki, M., Bakopoulou, A., & Koidis, P. (2018). Platelet-rich plasma for the therapeutic management of temporomandibular joint disorders: A systematic review. *International Journal of Oral and Maxillofacial Surgery, 47*(2), 188–198.
78. Cömert Kiliç, S., Güngörmüş, M., & Sümbüllü, M. A. (2015). Is arthrocentesis plus platelet-rich plasma superior to arthrocentesis alone in the treatment of Temporomandibular joint osteoarthritis? A randomized clinical trial. *Journal of Oral and Maxillofacial Surgery, 73*(8), 1473–1483.
79. Zhu, Y., et al. (2013). Basic science and clinical application of platelet-rich plasma for cartilage defects and osteoarthritis: A review. *Osteoarthritis and Cartilage, 21*(11), 1627–1637.
80. Kim, T.-H., et al. (2014). Comparison of platelet-rich plasma (PRP), platelet-rich fibrin (PRF), and concentrated growth factor (CGF) in rabbit-skull defect healing. *Archives of Oral Biology, 59*(5), 550–558.
81. Miron, R. J., et al. (2017). Injectable platelet rich fibrin (i-PRF): Opportunities in regenerative dentistry? *Clinical Oral Investigations, 21*(8), 2619–2627.
82. Kobayashi, E., et al. (2016). Comparative release of growth factors from PRP, PRF, and advanced-PRF. *Clinical Oral Investigations, 20*(9), 2353–2360.

83. Su, C. Y., et al. (2009). In vitro release of growth factors from platelet-rich fibrin (PRF): A proposal to optimize the clinical applications of PRF. *Oral Surgery, Oral Medicine, Oral Pathology, Oral Radiology, and Endodontics, 108*(1), 56–61.
84. Manzano, G., Herrero, L. R., & Montero, J. (2014). Comparison of clinical performance of zirconia implants and titanium implants in animal models: A systematic review. *The International Journal of Oral & Maxillofacial Implants, 29*(2), 311–320.
85. Shin, D., et al. (2011). Peripheral quantitative computer tomographic, histomorphometric, and removal torque analyses of two different non-coated implants in a rabbit model. *Clinical Oral Implants Research, 22*(3), 242–250.
86. Andreiotelli, M., Wenz, H. J., & Kohal, R. J. (2009). Are ceramic implants a viable alternative to titanium implants? A systematic literature review. *Clinical Oral Implants Research, 20*(Suppl 4), 32–47.
87. Branemark, P. I., et al. (1969). Intra-osseous anchorage of dental prostheses. I. Experimental studies. *Scandinavian Journal of Plastic and Reconstructive Surgery, 3*(2), 81–100.
88. Branemark, P. I., et al. (1977). Osseointegrated implants in the treatment of the edentulous jaw. Experience from a 10-year period. *Scandinavian Journal of Plastic and Reconstructive Surgery. Supplementum, 16*, 1–132.
89. Adell, R., et al. (1981). A 15-year study of osseointegrated implants in the treatment of the edentulous jaw. *International Journal of Oral Surgery, 10*(6), 387–416.
90. Heydecke, G., et al. (2003). Oral and general health-related quality of life with conventional and implant dentures. *Community Dentistry and Oral Epidemiology, 31*(3), 161–168.
91. Heydecke, G., et al. (2005). The impact of conventional and implant supported prostheses on social and sexual activities in edentulous adults results from a randomized trial 2 months after treatment. *Journal of Dentistry, 33*(8), 649–657.
92. Junker, R., et al. (2009). Effects of implant surface coatings and composition on bone integration: A systematic review. *Clinical Oral Implants Research, 20*(Suppl 4), 185–206.
93. Linkevicius, T., & Vaitelis, J. (2015). The effect of zirconia or titanium as abutment material on soft peri-implant tissues: A systematic review and meta-analysis. *Clinical Oral Implants Research, 26 Suppl 11*, 139–147.
94. Ozkurt, Z., & Kazazoglu, E. (2011). Zirconia dental implants: A literature review. *The Journal of Oral Implantology, 37*(3), 367–376.
95. Javed, F., et al. (2013). Is titanium sensitivity associated with allergic reactions in patients with dental implants? A systematic review. *Clinical Implant Dentistry and Related Research, 15*(1), 47–52.
96. Siddiqi, A., et al. (2011). Titanium allergy: Could it affect dental implant integration? *Clinical Oral Implants Research, 22*(7), 673–680.
97. Bianco, P. D., Ducheyne, P., & Cuckler, J. M. (1996). Titanium serum and urine levels in rabbits with a titanium implant in the absence of wear. *Biomaterials, 17*(20), 1937–1942.
98. Weingart, D., et al. (1994). Titanium deposition in regional lymph nodes after insertion of titanium screw implants in maxillofacial region. *International Journal of Oral and Maxillofacial Surgery, 23*(6 Pt 2), 450–452.
99. Meyer, U., et al. (2006). Fast element mapping of titanium wear around implants of different surface structures. *Clinical Oral Implants Research, 17*(2), 206–211.
100. Gahlert, M., et al. (2007). Biomechanical and histomorphometric comparison between zirconia implants with varying surface textures and a titanium implant in the maxilla of miniature pigs. *Clinical Oral Implants Research, 18*(5), 662–668.
101. Kohal, R. J., et al. (2009). Biomechanical and histological behavior of zirconia implants: An experiment in the rat. *Clinical Oral Implants Research, 20*(4), 333–339.
102. Kim, H. K., et al. (2015). Comparison of peri-implant bone formation around injection-molded and machined surface zirconia implants in rabbit tibiae. *Dental Materials Journal, 34*(4), 508–515.
103. Cionca, N., Hashim, D., & Mombelli, A. (2017). Zirconia dental implants: Where are we now, and where are we heading? *Periodontology 2000, 73*(1), 241–258.

104. Sandhaus, S. (1968). Technic and instrumentation of the implant C.B.S. (Cristalline Bone Screw). *Informatore Odonto-Stomatologico, 4*(3), 19–24.
105. Schulte, W., & Heimke, G. (1976). Das Tübinger Sofortimplantat. *Die Quintessenz, 27*(1), 17–23.
106. Sandhaus, S. (1991). Cerasand ceramic implants. *Attualità Dentale, 7*(12), 14–18.
107. Ehrl, P., & Frenkel, G. (1981). Klinische Ergebnisse mit einem enossalen Extensionsimplantat aus Al203-Keramik nach drei Jahren. *Die Quintessenz, 32*, 2007–2015.
108. Silva, N. R., et al. (2010). Performance of zirconia for dental healthcare. *Materials, 3*(2), 863–896.
109. Andreiotelli, M., & Kohal, R. J. (2009). Fracture strength of zirconia implants after artificial aging. *Clinical Implant Dentistry and Related Research, 11*(2), 158–166.
110. Silva, N. R., et al. (2009). Reliability of one-piece ceramic implant. *Journal of Biomedical Materials Research. Part B, Applied Biomaterials, 88*(2), 419–426.
111. Depprich, R., et al. (2008). Osseointegration of zirconia implants compared with titanium: An in vivo study. *Head & Face Medicine, 4*, 30.
112. Smeets, R., et al. (2016). Impact of dental implant surface modifications on Osseointegration. *BioMed Research International, 2016*, 6285620.
113. von Wilmowsky, C., et al. (2014). Implants in bone: Part I. A current overview about tissue response, surface modifications and future perspectives. *Oral and Maxillofacial Surgery, 18*(3), 243–257.
114. Jemat, A., et al. (2015). Surface modifications and their effects on titanium dental implants. *BioMed Research International, 2015*, 791725.
115. Oue, H., et al. (2015). Influence of implant surface topography on primary stability in a standardized osteoporosis rabbit model study. *Journal of Functional Biomaterials, 6*(1), 143–152.
116. Hong, D. G. K., & Oh, J. H. (2017). Recent advances in dental implants. *Maxillofacial Plastic and Reconstructive Surgery, 39*(1), 33.
117. Jung, U. W., et al. (2012). Surface characteristics of a novel hydroxyapatite-coated dental implant. *Journal of Periodontal & Implant Science, 42*(2), 59–63.
118. Buser, D., et al. (2004). Enhanced bone apposition to a chemically modified SLA titanium surface. *Journal of Dental Research, 83*(7), 529–533.
119. Cochran, D. L., et al. (2002). The use of reduced healing times on ITI implants with a sandblasted and acid-etched (SLA) surface: Early results from clinical trials on ITI SLA implants. *Clinical Oral Implants Research, 13*(2), 144–153.
120. Kumar, B. P., et al. (2016). Mandibular reconstruction: Overview. *Journal of Maxillofacial and Oral Surgery, 15*(4), 425–441.
121. Macewen, W. (1885). Cases illustrative of cerebral surgery. *The Lancet, 125*(3221), 934–936.
122. Simion, M., & Fontana, F. (2004). Autogenous and xenogeneic bone grafts for the bone regeneration. A literature review. *Minerva Stomatologica, 53*(5), 191–206.
123. Handschel, J., et al. (2011). Nonvascularized iliac bone grafts for mandibular reconstruction – Requirements and limitations. *In Vivo, 25*(5), 795–799.
124. Poswillo, D. (1974). Experimental reconstruction of the mandibular joint. *International Journal of Oral Surgery, 3*(6), 400–411.
125. El-Sayed, K. M. (2008). Temporomandibular joint reconstruction with costochondral graft using modified approach. *International Journal of Oral and Maxillofacial Surgery, 37*(10), 897–902.
126. Connolly, T. M., et al. (2017). Reconstruction of midface defects with the osteocutaneous radial forearm flap: Evaluation of long term outcomes including patient reported quality of life. *Microsurgery, 37*(7), 752–762.
127. Dean, N. R., et al. (2012). Free flap reconstruction of lateral mandibular defects: Indications and outcomes. *Otolaryngology and Head and Neck Surgery, 146*(4), 547–552.
128. Dowthwaite, S. A., et al. (2013). Comparison of fibular and scapular osseous free flaps for oromandibular reconstruction: A patient-centered approach to flap selection. *JAMA Otolaryngology. Head & Neck Surgery, 139*(3), 285–292.

129. Moscoso, J. F., & Urken, M. L. (1994). The iliac crest composite flap for oromandibular reconstruction. *Otolaryngologic Clinics of North America, 27*(6), 1097–1117.
130. Roberts, T. T., & Rosenbaum, A. J. (2012). Bone grafts, bone substitutes and orthobiologics: The bridge between basic science and clinical advancements in fracture healing. *Organogenesis, 8*(4), 114–124.
131. Goldberg, V. M., & Akhavan, S. (2005). Biology of bone grafts. In *Bone regeneration and repair* (pp. 57–65). Humana Press.
132. Aludden, H. C., et al. (2017). Lateral ridge augmentation with Bio-Oss alone or Bio-Oss mixed with particulate autogenous bone graft: A systematic review. *International Journal of Oral and Maxillofacial Surgery, 46*(8), 1030–1038.
133. Moss, S. D., et al. (1995). Transplanted demineralized bone graft in cranial reconstructive surgery. *Pediatric Neurosurgery, 23*(4), 199–204; discussion 204-5.
134. Elsalanty, M. E., & Genecov, D. G. (2009). Bone grafts in craniofacial surgery. *Craniomaxillofacial Trauma & Reconstruction, 2*(3), 125–134.
135. Salyer, K. E., et al. (1992). Demineralized perforated bone implants in craniofacial surgery. *The Journal of Craniofacial Surgery, 3*(2), 55–62.
136. Neumann, A., & Kevenhoerster, K. (2009). Biomaterials for craniofacial reconstruction. *GMS Current Topics in Otorhinolaryngology, Head and Neck Surgery, 8*, Doc08.
137. Menderes, A., et al. (2004). Craniofacial reconstruction with high-density porous polyethylene implants. *The Journal of Craniofacial Surgery, 15*(5), 719–724.
138. Eufinger, H., & Wehmoller, M. (2002). Microsurgical tissue transfer and individual computer-aided designed and manufactured prefabricated titanium implants for complex craniofacial reconstruction. *Scandinavian Journal of Plastic and Reconstructive Surgery and Hand Surgery, 36*(6), 326–331.
139. Siebert, H., et al. (2006). Evaluation of individual ceramic implants made of Bioverit with CAD/CAM technology to reconstruct multidimensional craniofacial defects of the human skull. *Mund-, Kiefer- und Gesichtschirurgie, 10*(3), 185–191.
140. Biskup, N. I., et al. (2010). Pediatric cranial vault defects: Early experience with beta-tricalcium phosphate bone graft substitute. *The Journal of Craniofacial Surgery, 21*(2), 358–362.
141. Verret, D. J., et al. (2005). Hydroxyapatite cement in craniofacial reconstruction. *Otolaryngology and Head and Neck Surgery, 133*(6), 897–899.
142. Rezaei, M., et al. (2018). Nano-biphasic calcium phosphate ceramic for the repair of bone defects. *The Journal of Craniofacial Surgery, 29*(6), e543–e548.
143. Eppley, B. L. (2002). Craniofacial reconstruction with computer-generated HTR patient-matched implants: Use in primary bony tumor excision. *The Journal of Craniofacial Surgery, 13*(5), 650–657.
144. Scolozzi, P., Martinez, A., & Jaques, B. (2007). Complex orbito-fronto-temporal reconstruction using computer-designed PEEK implant. *The Journal of Craniofacial Surgery, 18*(1), 224–228.
145. Ng, Z. Y., & Nawaz, I. (2014). Computer-designed PEEK implants: A peek into the future of cranioplasty? *The Journal of Craniofacial Surgery, 25*(1), e55–e58.
146. Nieminen, T., et al. (2008). Amorphous and crystalline polyetheretherketone: Mechanical properties and tissue reactions during a 3-year follow-up. *Journal of Biomedical Materials Research. Part A, 84*(2), 377–383.
147. Lethaus, B., et al. (2011). A treatment algorithm for patients with large skull bone defects and first results. *Journal of Cranio-Maxillo-Facial Surgery, 39*(6), 435–440.
148. Ridwan-Pramana, A., et al. (2015). Porous polyethylene implants in facial reconstruction: Outcome and complications. *Journal of Cranio-Maxillo-Facial Surgery, 43*(8), 1330–1334.
149. Eski, M., et al. (2007). Contour restoration of the secondary deformities of zygomaticoorbital fractures with porous polyethylene implant. *The Journal of Craniofacial Surgery, 18*(3), 520–525.
150. Wang, W., & Yeung, K. W. (2017). Bone grafts and biomaterials substitutes for bone defect repair: A review. *Bioactive Materials, 2*(4), 224–247.

151. Steinmann, S., et al. (1986). *Biological and biomechanical performance of biomaterials*. Amsterdam: Elsevier Science.
152. Actis, L., et al. (2013). Antimicrobial surfaces for craniofacial implants: State of the art. *Journal of the Korean Association of Oral and Maxillofacial Surgeons, 39*(2), 43–54.
153. Mok, D., et al. (2004). A review of materials currently used in orbital floor reconstruction. *The Canadian Journal of Plastic Surgery, 12*(3), 134–140.
154. Gross, P. P., & Gold, L. (1957). The compatibility of Vitallium and Austanium in completely buried implants in dogs. *Oral Surgery, Oral Medicine, Oral Pathology, 10*(7), 769–780.
155. Simpson, J. P., Geret, V., Brown, S. A., & Merrit, K. (1981). *Implant retrieval: Material and biologic analysis* (Vol. 601, pp. 395–422). NBS Spec Publ.
156. Barone, C. M., et al. (1994). Effects of rigid fixation device composition on three-dimensional computed axial tomography imaging: Direct measurements on a pig model. *Journal of Oral and Maxillofacial Surgery, 52*(7), 737–740; discussion 740-1.
157. Fiala, T. G., Novelline, R. A., & Yaremchuk, M. J. (1993). Comparison of CT imaging artifacts from craniomaxillofacial internal fixation devices. *Plastic and Reconstructive Surgery, 92*(7), 1227–1232.
158. Sullivan, P. K., Smith, J. F., & Rozzelle, A. A. (1994). Cranio-orbital reconstruction: Safety and image quality of metallic implants on CT and MRI scanning. *Plastic and Reconstructive Surgery, 94*(5), 589–596.
159. Meslemani, D., & Kellman, R. M. (2012). Recent advances in fixation of the craniomaxillofacial skeleton. *Current Opinion in Otolaryngology & Head and Neck Surgery, 20*(4), 304–309.
160. McRae, M., & Frodel, J. (2000). Midface fractures. *Facial Plastic Surgery, 16*(2), 107–113.
161. Nastri, A. L., & Gurney, B. (2016). Current concepts in midface fracture management. *Current Opinion in Otolaryngology & Head and Neck Surgery, 24*(4), 368–375.
162. Haug, R. H., Nuveen, E., & Bredbenner, T. (1999). An evaluation of the support provided by common internal orbital reconstruction materials. *Journal of Oral and Maxillofacial Surgery, 57*(5), 564–570.
163. Kinnunen, I., et al. (2000). Reconstruction of orbital floor fractures using bioactive glass. *Journal of Cranio-Maxillo-Facial Surgery, 28*(4), 229–234.
164. Romano, J. J., Iliff, N. T., & Manson, P. N. (1993). Use of Medpor porous polyethylene implants in 140 patients with facial fractures. *The Journal of Craniofacial Surgery, 4*(3), 142–147.
165. Metzger, M. C., et al. (2006). Anatomical 3-dimensional pre-bent titanium implant for orbital floor fractures. *Ophthalmology, 113*(10), 1863–1868.
166. Scolozzi, P., et al. (2009). Accuracy and predictability in use of AO three-dimensionally preformed titanium mesh plates for posttraumatic orbital reconstruction: A pilot study. *The Journal of Craniofacial Surgery, 20*(4), 1108–1113.
167. Balogh, C., et al. (2001). Lactic acid polymer implants in the repair of traumatic defects of the orbital floor. *Revue de Stomatologie et de Chirurgie Maxillo-Faciale, 102*(2), 109–114.
168. Gierloff, M., et al. (2012). Orbital floor reconstruction with resorbable polydioxanone implants. *The Journal of Craniofacial Surgery, 23*(1), 161–164.
169. Chowdhury, K., & Krause, G. E. (1998). Selection of materials for orbital floor reconstruction. *Archives of Otolaryngology – Head & Neck Surgery, 124*(12), 1398–1401.
170. Krishnan, V., & Johnson, J. V. (1997). Orbital floor reconstruction with autogenous mandibular symphyseal bone grafts. *Journal of Oral and Maxillofacial Surgery, 55*(4), 327–330; discussion 330-2.
171. Celikoz, B., Duman, H., & Selmanpakoglu, N. (1997). Reconstruction of the orbital floor with lyophilized tensor fascia lata. *Journal of Oral and Maxillofacial Surgery, 55*(3), 240–244.
172. Johnson, P. E., & Raftopoulos, I. (1999). In situ splitting of a rib graft for reconstruction of the orbital floor. *Plastic and Reconstructive Surgery, 103*(6), 1709–1711.
173. Ellis, E., 3rd. (1999). Treatment methods for fractures of the mandibular angle. *International Journal of Oral and Maxillofacial Surgery, 28*(4), 243–252.
174. Rastogi, S., et al. (2016). Assessment of bite force in patients treated with 2.0-mm traditional miniplates versus 2.0-mm locking plates for mandibular fracture. *Craniomaxillofacial Trauma & Reconstruction, 9*(1), 62–68.

175. Flores-Hidalgo, A., et al. (2015). Management of fractures of the atrophic mandible: A case series. *Oral Surgery, Oral Medicine, Oral Pathology, Oral Radiology, 119*(6), 619–627.
176. Sauerbier, S., et al. (2008). The development of plate osteosynthesis for the treatment of fractures of the mandibular body – a literature review. *Journal of Cranio-Maxillo-Facial Surgery, 36*(5), 251–259.
177. Chaudhary, M., et al. (2015). Evaluation of trapezoidal-shaped 3-D plates for internal fixation of mandibular subcondylar fractures in adults. *Journal of Oral Biology and Craniofacial Research, 5*(3), 134–139.
178. Kang, D. H. (2012). Surgical management of a mandible subcondylar fracture. *Archives of Plastic Surgery, 39*(4), 284–290.
179. Eckelt, U., & Hlawitschka, M. (1999). Clinical and radiological evaluation following surgical treatment of condylar neck fractures with lag screws. *Journal of Cranio-Maxillo-Facial Surgery, 27*(4), 235–242.
180. Luo, S., et al. (2011). Surgical treatment of sagittal fracture of mandibular condyle using long-screw osteosynthesis. *Journal of Oral and Maxillofacial Surgery, 69*(7), 1988–1994.
181. Gerlach, K. L. (2000). *Resorbable polymers as osteosynthesis material. Mund Kiefer Gesichtschir,* ***4 Suppl 1***, S91–S102.
182. Eppley, B. L., & Sadove, A. M. (1995). A comparison of resorbable and metallic fixation in healing of calvarial bone grafts. *Plastic and Reconstructive Surgery, 96*(2), 316–322.
183. Stanton, D. C., et al. (2014). Use of bioresorbable plating systems in paediatric mandible fractures. *Journal of Cranio-Maxillo-Facial Surgery, 42*(7), 1305–1309.
184. Suuronen, R., Kallela, I., & Lindqvist, C. (2000). Bioabsorbable plates and screws: Current state of the art in facial fracture repair. *The Journal of Cranio-Maxillofacial Trauma, 6*(1), 19–27; discussion 28–30.
185. Eppley, B. L. (2005). Use of resorbable plates and screws in pediatric facial fractures. *Journal of Oral and Maxillofacial Surgery, 63*(3), 385–391.
186. Pietrzak, W. S. (2012). Degradation of LactoSorb fixation devices in the craniofacial skeleton. *The Journal of Craniofacial Surgery, 23*(2), 578–581.
187. Ferretti, C. (2008). A prospective trial of poly-L-lactic/polyglycolic acid co-polymer plates and screws for internal fixation of mandibular fractures. *International Journal of Oral and Maxillofacial Surgery, 37*(3), 242–248.
188. Agarwal, S., et al. (2009). Use of resorbable implants for mandibular fixation: A systematic review. *The Journal of Craniofacial Surgery, 20*(2), 331–339.
189. Bell, R. B., & Kindsfater, C. S. (2006). The use of biodegradable plates and screws to stabilize facial fractures. *Journal of Oral and Maxillofacial Surgery, 64*(1), 31–39.

# Chapter 4
# 3D Imaging in Dentistry and Oral Tissue Engineering

**Abbas Shokri, Kousar Ramezani, Farshid Vahdatinia, Emelia Karkazis, and Lobat Tayebi**

## 1 Introduction

Tissue engineering is a multidisciplinary approach developed in response to the need for regeneration of the diseased or lost tissues. It employs the principles of biology and engineering to produce vital replacements for the lost tissues and functional organs. Soft and hard tissue may be defective or lost due to trauma, congenital defects, or acquired diseases, such as cancer, and need a replacement. Bio-artificial organs are produced in the laboratory and then transferred to the vital environment of human body.

Emersion of tissue engineering science and significant advances in this field, particularly after the introduction of 3D printing technology, opened a new gate for repair and regeneration of body organs and tissues. The progresses made in this field have led to a wide range of regenerative treatments and, combining it with 3D printing, have provided feasibility of several tissue regenerations, completely specified for each patient. Imaging is in the front line of this process (Fig. 4.1). However, advances in tissue engineering have highlighted the need for further in vitro and clinical studies on the mechanism and outcome of these approaches using advanced diagnostic tools and techniques. Imaging is an efficient diagnostic method in this field, which currently plays a fundamental role in promotion of regenerative medicine. Imaging is a commonly used diagnostic modality that aims to detect normal anatomy and disease symptoms, as well as scientific and research surveys. The medical imaging science has been awarded two Nobel Prizes thus far in physiology and medicine for introduction of CT and MRI, which have revolutionized medical imaging.

A. Shokri · K. Ramezani ·
School of Dentistry, Hamadan Medical Sciences University, Hamadan, Iran

F. Vahdatinia
Dental Implants Research Center, Hamadan University of Medical Sciences, Hamadan, Iran

E. Karkazis · L. Tayebi (✉)
Marquette University School of Dentistry, Milwaukee, WI, USA
e-mail: lobat.tayebi@marquette.edu



L. Tayebi (ed.), *Applications of Biomedical Engineering in Dentistry*,
https://doi.org/10.1007/978-3-030-21583-5_4

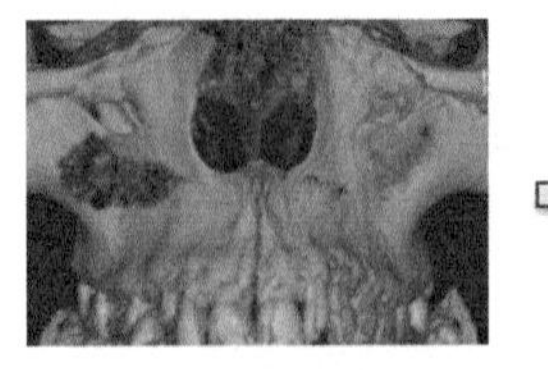


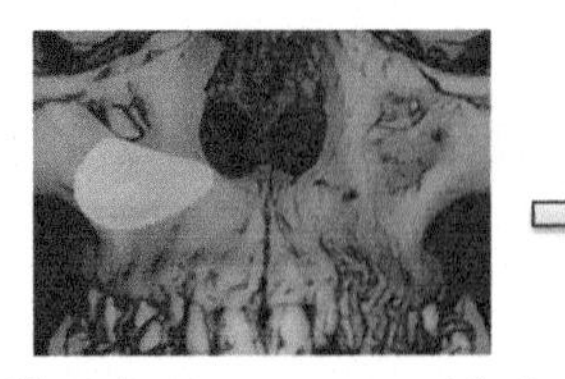


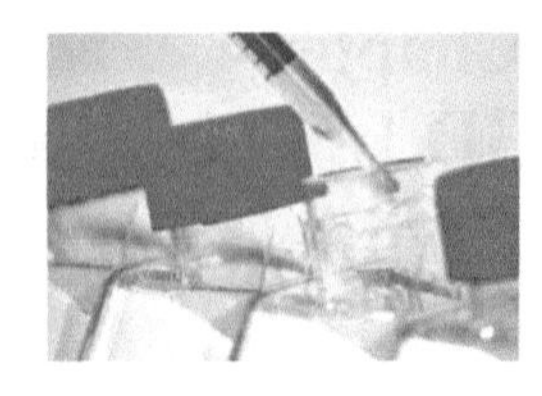

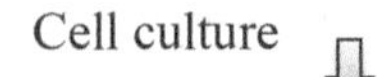


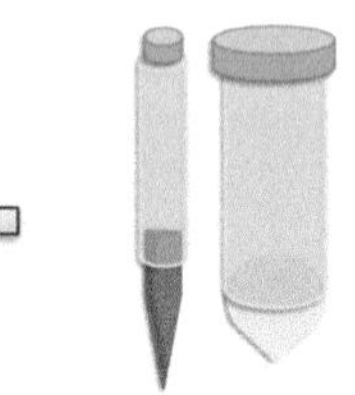


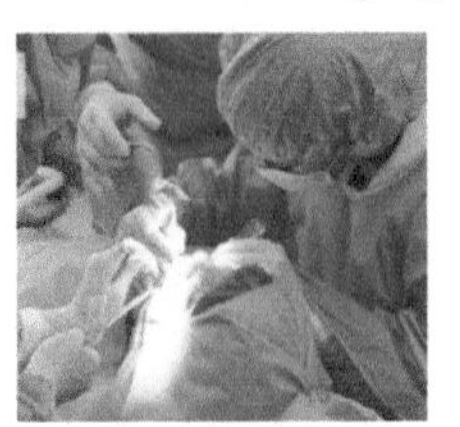


**Fig. 4.1** Imaging, first step in 3D printing tissue engineering

Despite the presence of complex imaging systems and techniques, the role of conventional imaging in provision of acceptable diagnostic information should not be underestimated. The conventional radiographic modalities are the premier diagnostic imaging techniques for many cases, which may be later accompanied by more complex, 3D imaging modalities, if required. Confirming the presence or absence of disease by 3D imaging is a basis for further molecular, immunologic, histologic, and genetic studies.

Several imaging techniques are employed in tissue engineering, such as CT, CBCT, micro-CT, MRI, ultrasound imaging, optical imaging, nuclear imaging (including positron-emission tomography and single-photon emission CT), multimodal imaging, photoacoustic microscopy, and other emerging technologies. Of all, the more popular modalities that have the highest application and are more easily accessible are discussed in this chapter. The basic knowledge acquired about the functional physics and application of these systems will be helpful in understanding the important terms used in imaging science and the function of other imaging modalities.

## 2 Computed Tomography (CT)

The basis of CT imaging is to record information obtained from the collimated, fan-shaped X-ray beams by the scintillation detectors in cross-sectional images. In fact, a CT image is a complex of transverse or trans-axial images captured perpendicular to the long axis of the body, and coronal and sagittal images are reconstructed by the combination of these transverse images. Efficient processing of all transverse projections by the computer and their superimposition yields a 3D reconstructed image of the scanned anatomical structures.

The CT scanner is a large, square-shaped apparatus known as the gantry, with a central circular hole. The patient lies on a bed that moves through the gantry for imaging. The X-ray tube and detectors are embedded inside the gantry. The gantry is the component of the CT machine that contains the X-ray tube, a row of detectors, a high-voltage generator, the patient bed, and mechanical components. These mechanical components support the afore-mentioned pieces, receive the orders sent from the console, and send the data to a computer after scanning to generate the image. The patient bed is made of materials with low atomic numbers, such as carbon fiber, in order to impede interference with the passage of the X-ray beam. It enables accurate positioning of the patient and smoothly moves through the gantry. In the first generations of CT machines, both the X-ray tube and detector simultaneously rotated around the patient, and this rotation combined with the mechanical movement of the gantry-generated CT images. The first generation of CT machines had pencil-shaped X-ray beams. From the second generation on, the X-ray beam type was changed to fan-shaped. The main advantage of second-generation CT scanners was enhanced speed and decreased scanning time, mainly as the result of using multiple rows of detectors.

In the third generation of CT scanners, the X-ray tube and detector both rotated around the patient; however, in the fourth generation, one row of detectors is stationary in circumference, and only the X-ray tube rotates around the patient. The fourth generation of CT scanners was introduced with the hope to resolve the ring artifact problem of the third generation. The image acquisition time in the third and fourth generations of CT scanners can be as rapid as a sub-second scale.

Irrespective of the geometric mechanism, detectors receive the attenuated radiations of an axial slice. The patient moves through the gantry, and the same is repeated for the next adjacent slice until the entire volume of the respective area is scanned. This stop-start process takes several minutes.

In helical CT scanners, which are the currently used standard CT scanners, the X-ray tube and detector both rotate around the patient in a helical path, while the patient continuously moves through the gantry. This decreases the overall scanning time. The volume thickness scanned in each shot varies from 0.5 to 6.0 mm and can be manipulated by adjusting the collimator and selecting different rows of detectors [1, 2].

Multi-detector CT (MDCT) is a type of helical scanner, benefitting from 16, 64, or 128 rows of detectors positioned next to each other in a helical path for image acquisition. Thus, in one rotation, images are obtained from several slices at the same time. As a result, the scanning time is significantly shorter than that of single-slice systems [3]. Tens of thousands of detectors are present in each row. In addition to several rows of detectors, the high-processing capability of computers utilized in these systems is another paramount aspect, which is mandatory to process these abundant volumes of data (Fig. 4.2).

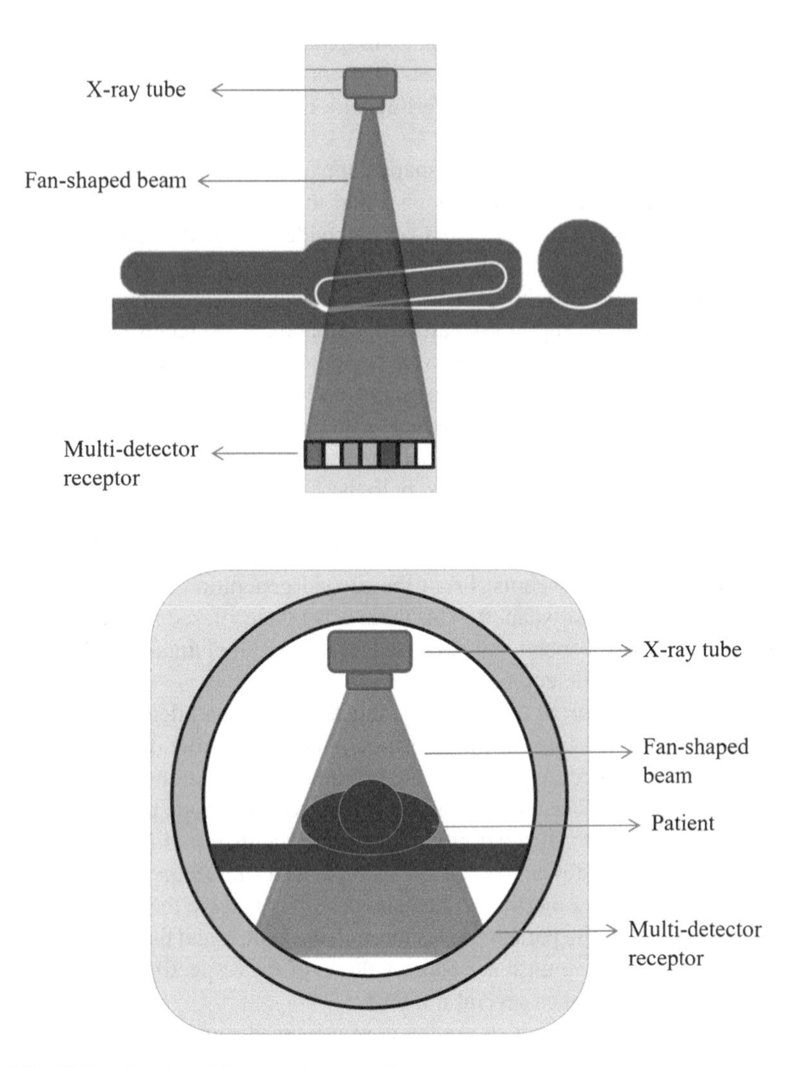


**Fig. 4.2** MDCT; fan-shaped beam and multi-detector rows

Pitch is defined as the ratio of movement of bed after a complete 360° rotation of the X-ray tube to the volume thickness scanned in each shot (or width of the X-ray beam). If the slice thickness in a scan is 1 mm, and the movement of the bed after one full rotation of X-ray beam is 2 mm, then the pitch would be 2:1. This means that half of the respective volume will be exposed at the time of scanning. As the result, the patient radiation dose will decrease by half, in addition to the spatial resolution also decreasing. In the case of pitch >1:1, the interpolation algorithm is used to enhance the quality of reconstructed coronal and sagittal sections. This algorithm estimates the un-scanned thickness according to the two adjacent scanned thicknesses. Pitch >1:1 allows scanning of a larger volume within the same time period. In practice, the overall scanning time will decrease, which is important in uncooperative patients or in angiography. Pitch <1:1 increases the patient radiation dose due to superimposition of the scanned adjacent thicknesses. Pitch 2:1 is an acceptable ratio. The pitch in multi-slice helical CTs is practically 1:1.

Decreased scanning time translates to decreased motion artifacts due to intentional movements of the patient or physiological movements, such as respiration and heartbeat. It is particularly substantial in children and trauma patients. However, the overall patient radiation dose increases in MDCT.

The X-ray beams are collimated twice in CT: once for the generation of fan-shaped beams prior to reaching the patient, which limits the exposed area and once after passing through the patient to decrease scattered radiation and improve image quality [1, 2].

The X-ray detectors collect the X-ray photons passed through the patient or object and convert them to an electric charge, which is later digitized. The CT detectors are often of solid-state type and can support 0.625 mm pixel size. The routine matrices used in detectors have 512 × 512 or 1024 × 1024 pixels [4].

Pixels are data cells that form digital two-dimensional (2D) images. Voxel is defined as a thickness that volumizes the 2D pixels and depends on the tomographic slice thickness. The volumetric data are composed of separate voxel blocks. The pixel size is determined by the detector and the image reconstruction software. However, as stated earlier, the voxel length is determined by the width of the X-ray beam, which is affected by pre- and post-patient collimation. Generation of isotropic cubic voxels enables image reconstruction in different planes, without losing resolution. Larger voxels require less X-ray dose and lower amperage (mA) but reduce image resolution. Although it has no effect on the general accuracy of measurements and structural relationships, fine details, such as fractures, require smaller voxels for more accurate diagnosis [2].

Field of view (FOV) is the observable area on a reconstructed image. Increasing the FOV in a matrix with a fixed size proportionally increases the pixel size as well. However, increasing the size of the matrix in a constant FOV decreases the pixel size. A CT number or Hounsfield unit (HU) is allocated to each voxel, which determines its grayness or optical density and enables observation of images on a monitor in the form of various shades of gray. CT number is determined by the coefficient of beam attenuation in the tissue and ranges from −1000 to +3000 for each pixel. The CT number of air is −1000, 0 for water, and + 3000 for dense bone. The HU usually ranges from −1000 to +1000 (Table 4.1).

**Table 4.1** Hounsfield units of tissues

| Tissue | Hounsfield units |
|---|---|
| Air | −1000 |
| Fat | −60 to −100 |
| Water | 0 |
| Soft tissue | +40 to +80 |
| Bone | +400 to +1000 |

Displaying such a wide range on a monitor is not feasible; showing part of this range by window and level adjustment allows for visualization of a suitable range for interpretation [1, 2]. The window level and window width are two variables that enable observation of the desired range and level of densities. The window level is the CT number selected at the center of the chosen range of densities, and its selection depends on the type of tissue intended to be evaluated (hard or soft tissue). The window width is the selected range of gray shades to display [4]. A narrow range enables observation of fine differences between tissues with similar density and better displays the gray shades close to each other. In this regard, bone window shows a range of +400 to +1000 Hus, and soft tissue window indicates a range of +40 to +80 HUs.

An important preponderance of computer-generated images is that they allow alteration and reconstruction of images in different dimensions and generation of new images of different views without the need to re-expose the patient to ionizing radiation. Data obtained from numerous axial sections can be used to reconstruct coronal and sagittal sections, or any other plane required as well as 3D integrated images, although these images do not have the same sharpness of axial views [5]. Higher-quality images are the result of thinner axial scans that are arranged consecutively or are superimposed, which consequently increases the patient radiation dose.

CT images visualize reconstructed 3D images in all three spatial planes and, in contrast to conventional radiography, do not have the limitation of superimposition of multiple structures. The contrast resolution of CT is much higher than that of plain radiography. To observe deep anatomical structures, outer layers of image can be removed by the software features. The reconstruction time is an important factor with regard to CT systems, which is defined as the time period from the end of imaging to image display and depends on the capabilities of the computer processor.

## 2.1 Image Reconstruction

### 2.1.1 Multiplanar Reformation (MPR)

MPR refers to 3D multiplanar reconstruction, which combines images of transverse sections to yield images in other different planes (Fig. 4.3).

### 2.1.2 Maximum Intensity Projection (MIP)

MIP is defined as selection of the highest pixel value along a hypothetical line and displaying only these pixels. The reconstruction is swift and yields the simplest shape of 3D images, enabling differentiation of vascular structures around tissues with high accuracy (Fig. 4.4).

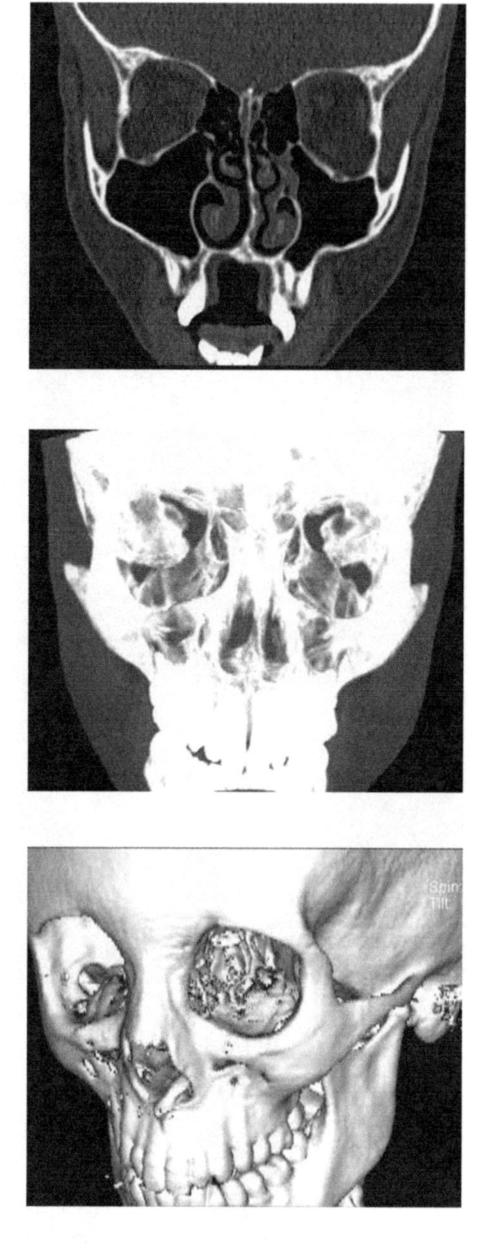

**Fig. 4.3** CT, coronal view in MPR range

**Fig. 4.4** MIP reconstruction of CT volume data

**Fig. 4.5** SSD reconstruction of CT volume data

### 2.1.3 Shaded Surface Display (SSD)

SSD is detection of a narrow range of values of an object and displaying the same range in the form of organ surface (Fig. 4.5).

### 2.1.4 Volume Rendered

The boundaries of the surface can be displayed clearly, and the image is rendered three-dimensional, which is referred to as volume-rendered image (Fig. 4.6) [1].

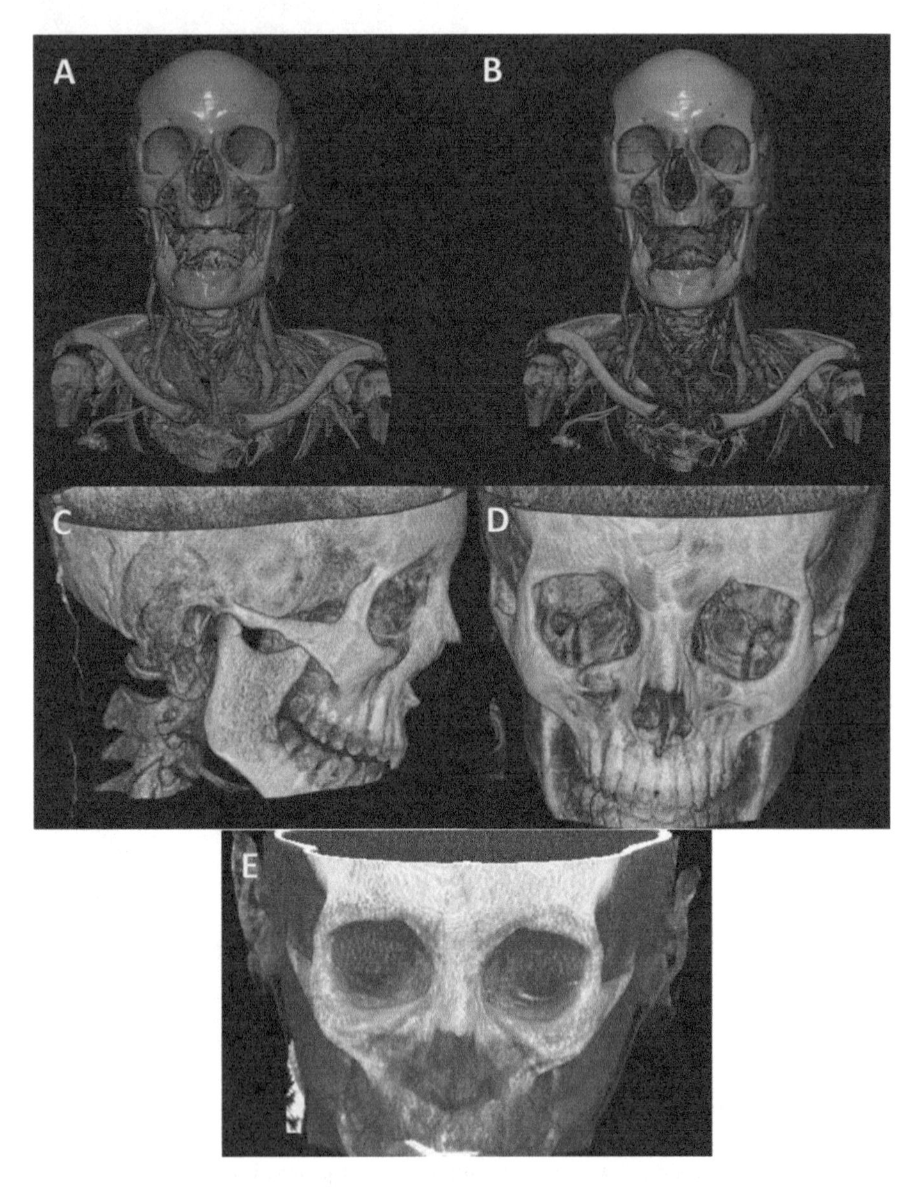


**Fig. 4.6** (**a**) [6]: SSD; (**b**) [6], (**c**–**e**) volume rendering reconstruction of CT volume data

## 2.2 Advantages of CT Compared to Conventional Radiography

Small differences in absorption of the X-ray beams could be detected in CT, which reveals the details of intracranial lesions and helps in better differentiation of the normal and diseased tissues.

The contrast resolution of CT imaging systems is excellent due to rejection of scattered X-ray beams by the pre-detector collimator. Both hard and soft tissues can be evaluated using CT, and images can be enhanced using intravenous contrast medium.

## 2.3 Advantages of MDCT Compared to Conventional Step-and-Shoot CT

MDCT has less motion blur and motion artifact, reduced overall scanning time, and decreased partial volume artifact. It also allows imaging of a larger volume of tissue.

## 2.4 Disadvantages of CT

CT imaging is costly. Consecutive slices and overlap highly increase the patient radiation dose. It has limited ability to visualize anatomical structures with low contrast due to noise of the system, and metal objects, such as metal dental restorations, cause streak or star artifacts. Contrast media are contraindicated in some patients. CT also has limited availability [1, 2, 4].

## 2.5 Applications of CT

CT is the modality of choice for assessment of lesions involving the bone, such as tumors, cysts, and intraosseous infections.

It also enables assessment of the location, size, and extension of interosseous lesions.

It allows evaluation of intracranial conditions such as tumors, hemorrhage, or stroke. Intracranial or spinal trauma and traumatic injuries to complex craniofacial structures can be evaluated using CT.

Treatment planning for reconstructive craniofacial surgeries and correction of craniofacial deformities, guiding the fabrication of surgical stents or reconstructed models of CT images, evaluation of paranasal sinuses, tumor staging for benign and malignant lesions, and evaluation of temporomandibular joint are among other applications of CT.

CT also enables assessment of the height and thickness of maxillary and mandibular alveolar bone prior to implant placement. However, considering the increased availability and unique advantages of CBCT imaging systems, application of CT for this particular purpose has recently decreased.

### 2.6 Rapid Prototyping

Rapid prototyping is a process through which data obtained from a 3D design by a software is converted to actual models. This process can be used for the fabrication of a model of an anatomical structure with its actual shape and dimensions. These models are used for treatment planning prior to maxillofacial surgeries. They also have applications in tumor resection, dental implant placement, distraction osteogenesis, and correction of deformities developed by trauma. They decrease the duration of surgery and anesthesia and increase the accuracy of procedures [2, 4, 5] (Fig. 4.7).

### 2.7 Tissue Engineering

Tissue engineering has promoted the applications of CT beyond diagnostic purposes for diseases. One major advantage of CT in tissue engineering is provision of 3D images. In anatomical maxillofacial defects, CT has been used to create a template for the mirror image of the normal side to correct the anatomic anomaly of the malformed side.

Reconstruction of bony and cartilaginous structures of the temporomandibular joint (TMJ) is a major challenge in maxillofacial surgery due to the complex geometric shape and function of the TMJ. CT has been used to design scaffolds for condylar reconstruction in animal models and has yielded promising results due to the combined use of 3D imaging, tissue engineering, and maxillofacial surgery [7]. CT has also been used to design scaffolds required for tissue regeneration in terms of morphological properties, external surface, and internal structure of the scaffold and porosities.

## 3 Cone Beam Computed Tomography (CBCT)

Since the use of the first generation of CBCT for angiography in 1982 (Mayo Clinic Biodynamics Research Laboratory), its applications in different fields of medicine have greatly increased. It has the highest application in dentistry and maxillofacial studies. Due to its numerous advantages, it is commonly used in dental clinical settings, even for pediatric patients. In the recent years, the use of CBCT for obtaining diagnostic images of the oral and maxillofacial region has greatly increased

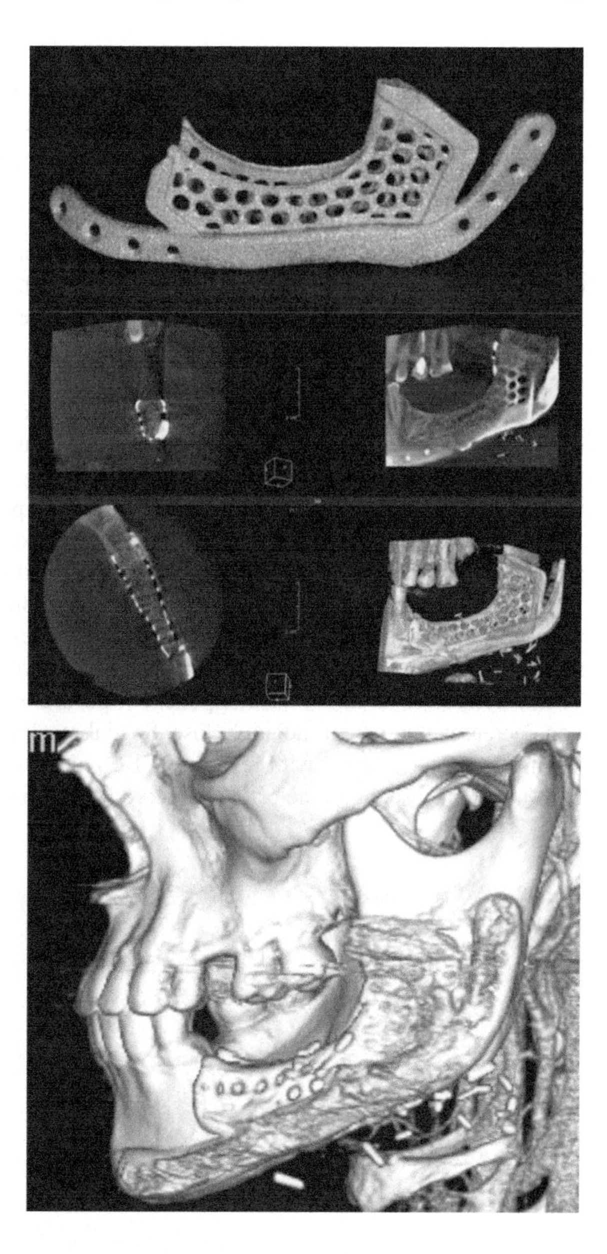

**Fig. 4.7** Rapid prototyped patient-specific implant for mandible reconstruction [8]

compared to conventional radiography. CBCT was introduced to dentistry aiming to replace the conventional CT and other 2D imaging modalities as an adjunct for diagnosis, treatment planning, and follow-up. Feasibility of imaging of hard tissue with high-resolution and low patient radiation dose led to great applicability of CBCT in orthodontics, maxillofacial surgery, dentoalveolar pathology, implantology, and endodontics. The mean X-ray radiation dose in CBCT is 60–1000 μSv[1]

[1] Sievert (Sv) is the unit of equivalent dose (the biological effect of ionizing radiation) in the International System of Units (SI).

(for imaging of the mandible) with 10–70 seconds of irradiation time, which is much lower than the radiation dose of CT, which is 1320–3324 μSv [9].

Evidence shows that CT and CBCT are suitable for imaging of hard and soft tissue surfaces to allow anthropometric measurements due to their optimal accuracy, reliability, and repeatability [10–12]. However, it should be noted that the patient radiation dose in CBCT is higher than that of other commonly requested radiographies of the jaws, such as panoramic and/or periapical radiography. This is especially important in children. Through advances in technology, attempts have been made to decrease the patient radiation dose by decreasing the size of field of view (FOV) and the tube current-time product (mAs), without affecting the image quality [13].

Although theoretically it has been approximately two decades since the introduction of CBCT for clinical applications, the use of commercially available devices was accomplished by the advances in affordable X-ray tubes; high-quality, exceptionally accurate detectors; and powerful personal computers.

CBCT is a compact, faster, and safer version of conventional CT. The CBCT system has a gantry that contains the X-ray tube and detector. Scanning is performed by one 360° rotation of a cone-shaped or pyramidal X-ray beam and detector against each other and around the object. The center of rotation is the center of region of interest, which is also the center of the final volumetric image (Fig. 4.8).

The detector is an important component of the scanning cycle, and its optimization decreases the patient radiation dose. Spatial resolution and contrast resolution are important parameters with regard to CBCT detectors affecting image quality. CBCT systems use digital detectors to record image data.

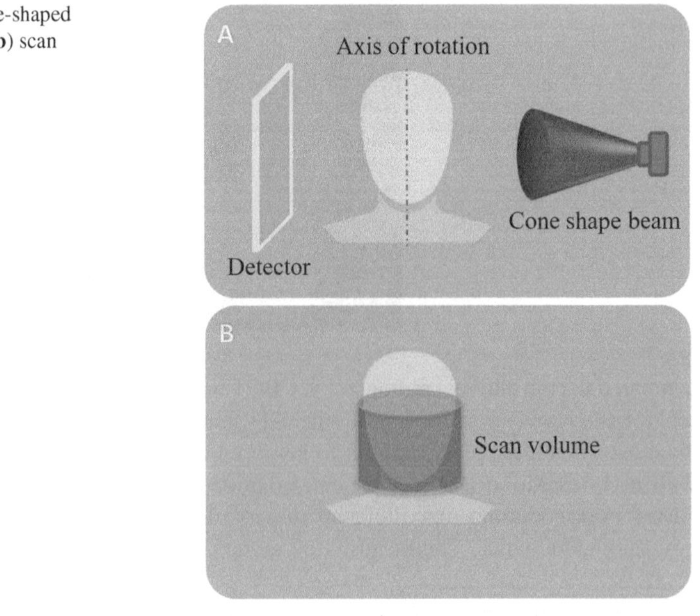


**Fig. 4.8** (**a**) Cone-shaped beam in CBCT; (**b**) scan volume

During scanning, the system creates a set of projection data, which is similar to a series of cephalometric radiographs taken from different angles. The total amount of the acquired projection data depends on the rotation time, frame rate (number of projections scanned per time unit), and completion of trajectory arc. Higher number of projections increases the patient radiation dose but provides higher spatial resolution and better contrast resolution. However, it has no significant effect on linear accuracy of CBCT images. Such raw data is converted to volumetric data by complex software algorithms such as filtered back projection, which can be evaluated in all three planes—axial, sagittal, and coronal. In contrast to CT, data reconstruction in CBCT can be implemented using personal computers.

The specific geometry of the radiation beam in CBCT increases the speed of image acquisition compared to MDCT; this results in saving time and decreasing motion artifact. In contrast to CT where axial sections are the most ideal images, all reconstructed CBCT images are equally sharp and show equivalent details of the scanned volume. CBCT scans can be obtained in seated, standing, or supine position, depending on the type of system. In all systems, immobilization of the head is more important than its positioning.

FOV is a cylindrical or spherical volume that can be scanned by the CBCT system, which is determined by the beam collimation ability, geometry of the radiation beam, and detector size and ranges from a few centimeters in width and height to complete reconstruction of the head and face. FOV is constant in some CBCT systems, while some others allow selection of the size of FOV. Larger FOVs enable observation of more structures but inflicts higher radiation dose to the patients. Limiting the FOV to the minimum size covering the region of interest minimizes the unnecessary patient radiation dose. Region of interest (ROI) is determined according to the reason for requesting imaging and personal characteristics [2, 3].

Voxels play a fundamental role in spatial resolution and details of image and are isotropic in CBCT systems. Smaller voxels yield images with higher spatial resolution but have a higher noise, since they receive smaller amounts of X-ray beam. In such cases, radiation dose should be increased to preserve the diagnostic quality of image. Different CBCT systems may vary in terms of voxel size; consequently, they have different spatial resolution and image quality as well [5].

The exposure parameters, such as the kVp and mA, must be adjusted in accordance with the diagnostic goals and size of patient; however, exposure parameters are constant in some CBCT systems. Motion artifact, which negatively affects the image quality, can be minimized by correct adjustment of these parameters in CBCT systems that allow adjustment of exposure parameters.

Aside from the voxel size, the size of focal spot, and geometric properties of the X-ray tube, object and detector relative to each other also affect the spatial resolution of imaging systems. However, due to a standard footprint of CBCT system, the distance from the detector to X-ray tube can be increased only to a limited extent.

The ability to show visible gray shadows is assessed with bit depth. A system with higher bit depth can show even the slightest differences in contrast. CBCT systems can show the difference in gray shadows by 12 bits and higher. In addition, contrast, brightness, sharpening, filtering, and marginal algorithm enhancements can be performed on images. The acceptable time for data reconstruction is less than 5 minutes.

Although CBCT has less radiation dose than CT, it is not used for routine diagnostic or screening purposes because of higher patient radiation dose than plain radiography. CBCT is essentially an adjunct diagnostic tool used as a supplement to conventional imaging modalities, and its use should have a logical justification based on clinical examination and patient history. The CBCT imaging dose may be decreased to 3 μSv depending on the required resolution and other modifying factors. This decreased dose is equal to the radiation dose of four bitewing radiographs. CBCT should not be avoided solely because of its higher radiation dose; in many cases for imaging of restricted volumes, the radiation dose of CBCT is equal to that of intraoral and panoramic radiographs.

## *3.1 CBCT Basic Formats for Image Reconstruction*

### 3.1.1 Multiplanar Reformation (MPR)

Due to CBCT image isotropic nature, volumetric data in non-orthogonal cuts can be reconstructed. Volumetric CBCT data by default is displayed in two-dimensional images on axial, sagittal, and coronal planes with a default thickness. By scrolling through the image volume, different cuts can be observed. Oblique sections of the mandibular condyle or automatic panoramic reconstruction and cross-sectional images are different types of MPR reconstructions. Cross-sectional or para-axial images are perpendicular to the plane of the reconstructed dental arch and enable the assessment of the dental arch in the third dimension. These images are obtained in 0.5–1 mm thicknesses and demonstrate well the relationship of dental arch and inferior alveolar canal. This provides valuable information for dental implant surgery (Fig. 4.9).

### 3.1.2 Ray Sum

The thickness of an orthogonal or MPR cut increases with accumulation of adjacent voxels. The simulated lateral cephalometric images are of this type, but their difference with the conventional type is in that they do not have magnification and parallax.

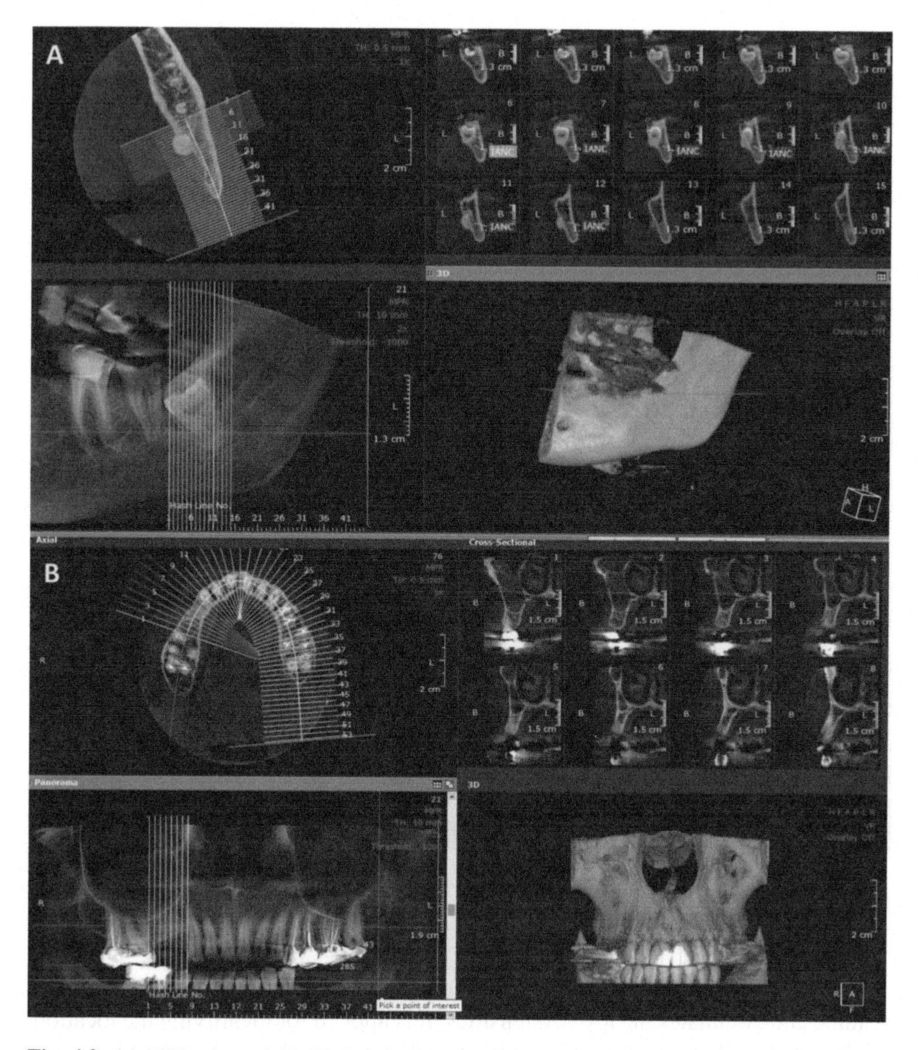


**Fig. 4.9** (**a**) MPR view of CBCT for mandibular left third molar evaluation; (**b**) MPR view of CBCT for right maxillary ridge evaluation prior to dental implant insertion

### 3.1.3 Volume Rendering

In its indirect form, volumetric reconstruction is performed from the surface and the depth and is suitable for overall evaluation of craniofacial structures and anatomical relations. Surface rendering yields a solid image of the surface of a 3D volume, while volume rendering has a transparent view (Fig. 4.10).

In direct type, a certain intensity of voxels is selected, and the gray shadows above and below it are eliminated. MIP is a type of direct volume rendering that

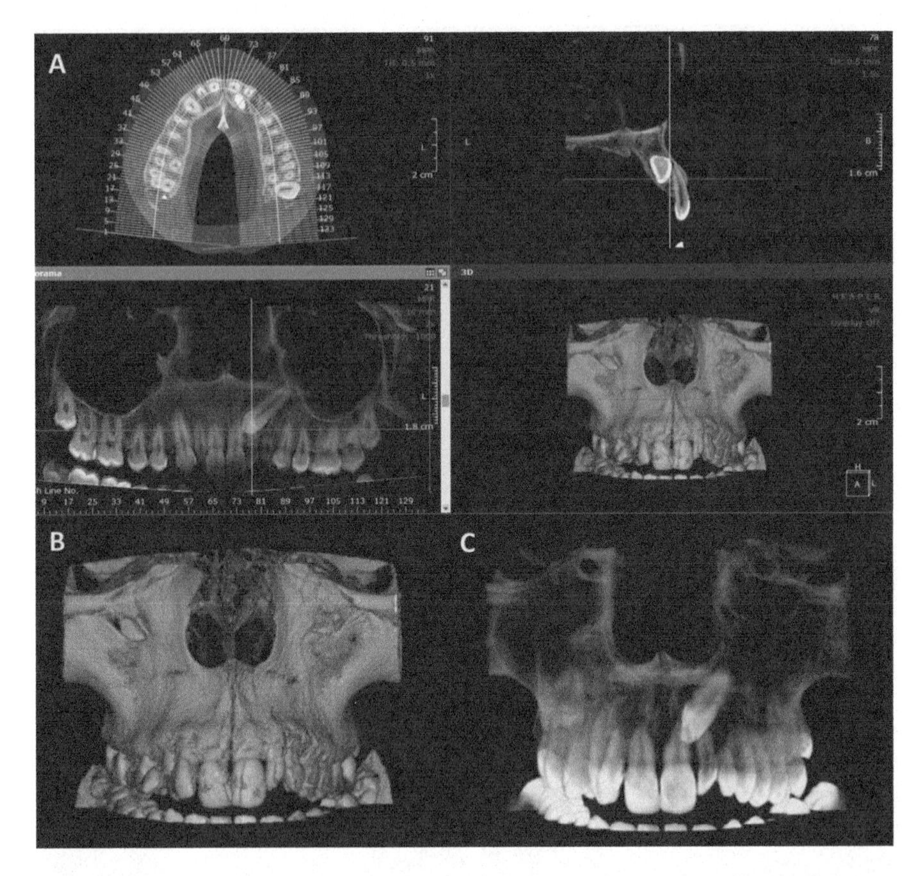


**Fig. 4.10** (**a**) MPR; (**b**, **c**) volume rendering CBCT image of an impacted maxillary canine

identifies the voxels with maximum intensity in a specific direction of scanned volume and eliminates the lower intensities. It is applied for identifying the location of impacted teeth, fractures, and soft tissue calcifications (Fig. 4.11).

## *3.2 Advantages of CBCT*

CBCT enables multiplanar reformatting and observation of anatomical and pathological structures in different planes. CBCT yields accurate geometric images, has high spatial resolution, is a smaller size, and has lower cost and faster scanning time than CT. CBCT does not have high technical sensitivity; if the patient is not accurately positioned, the orientation can be later corrected by the software programs given that the region of interest is within the FOV. CBCT has high spatial resolution, and its submillimeter voxel size provides detailed resolution and enables

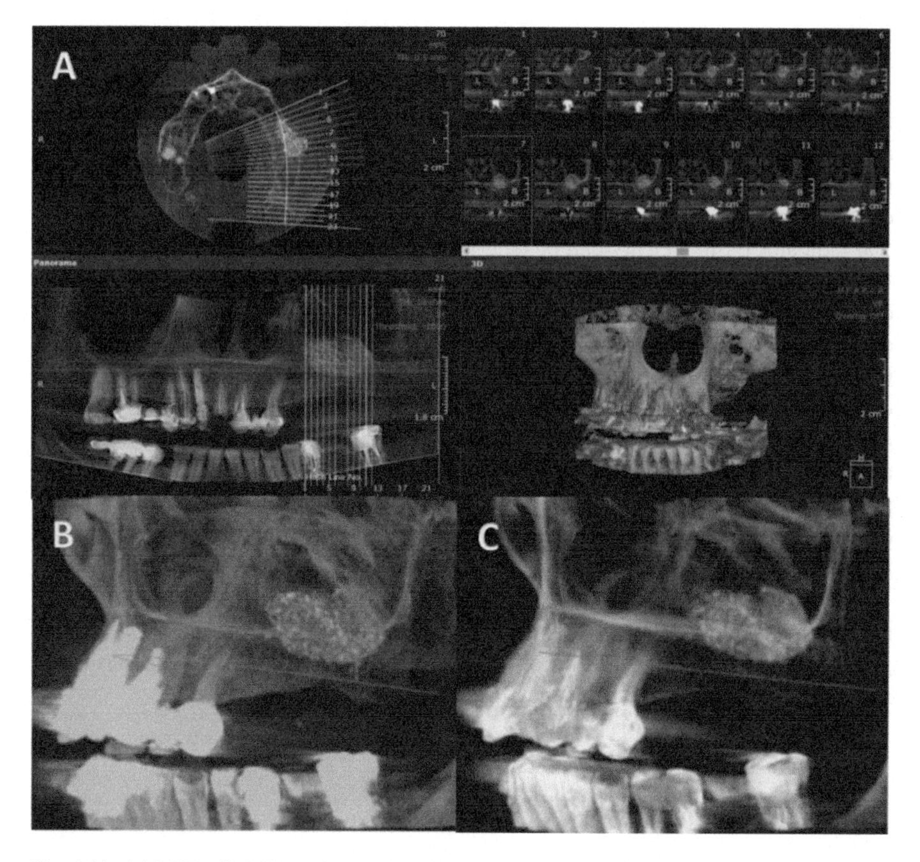


**Fig. 4.11** (**a**) MPR; (**b**) MIP; and (**c**) volume rendering view of a lifted sinus

observation of fine structures such as the periodontal ligament, root fractures, and root canals. In addition, CBCT has a considerably lower patient radiation dose compared to CT, allowing for a big step forward in 3D imaging.

Streak artifacts due to metals, such as metallic dental restorations, decrease the quality of CT images, especially the adjacent bone. CBCT has significantly lower metal streak artifacts compared to CT. CBCT images are less affected by beam hardening artifact generated by the presence of metal restorative materials and implants compared to MDCT. Also, CBCT has an easier application with the use of a personal computer. Furthermore, it is compatible with cephalometric planning and implant software programs. Although the soft tissue itself is not clearly visualized on CBCT images, its swelling or asymmetry, airways, and soft tissue calcifications can be evaluated and detected on CBCT scans.

## 3.3 Limitations of CBCT

A major limitation of CBCT is that patients must remain still during scanning. It also has higher noise compared to CT. Noise is defined as scattered radiation recorded by the detector that diminishes the quality of image. In contrast to CT, direct measurement of tissue density is not possible using CBCT. Although the HU that indicates tissue density can be determined using CBCT, it is actually a relative scale of density compared to other scanned tissues. However, in CT, this number can determine the nature of tissue. Soft tissue contrast of CBCT images is low, and compared to MDCT images, it illustrates soft tissues with lower quality. Thus, soft tissue tumors or extension of intraosseous tumors to soft tissue cannot be evaluated on CBCT scans. The temporomandibular joint disc cannot be determined precisely on CBCT scans either. For the latter, MRI is definitely a superior choice. However, airways and sinuses can be well observed on CBCT scans. Using cadmium telluride photon counting (CaTePC) sensors, the potential of soft tissue observation independently of the hard tissue on CBCT scans exists, and the provided HU would determine the nature of tissue, similar to CT.

The presence of artifacts due to restorations or metal prosthesis in the oral and maxillofacial region can affect the quality of CBCT and CT images [14, 15]. In general, radiodense objects produce beam hardening or streak or star artifacts. However, they have lower frequency in CBCT compared to CT [2–5].

## 3.4 Applications of CBCT

### 3.4.1 Determining the Proper Location for Dental Implants

CBCT not only provides accurate information about the width and height of the alveolar bone; it is also useful in determining the location and spatial relationship of vital structures, such as the mandibular canal, mental foramen, incisive foramen, maxillary sinuses, and nasal cavity. Cross-sectional images provide valuable information about the height and width of the alveolar bone and relationship to adjacent vital structures. Imaging of the dental arches, along with marked stents, provides an acceptable guide for correct dental implant placement. Quick measurement and 3D reconstruction enable confirmation of implant dimensions and angle of placement. Some software programs allow virtual implant placement and simulation of the final results displayed on the images. CBCT can also be used to predict the possible causes of failure and the need for bone grafting and post-implant assessments.

Implant placement adjacent to a pathologic lesion compromises implant prognosis; CBCT can detect these lesions. There are less metal artifacts due to dental implants on CBCT scans than CT. By downsizing the FOV, the patient radiation dose can be decreased. Due to these specifications, CBCT is now the imaging modality of choice for short-term assessments, such as evaluation of the accuracy of implant placement and the required bone volume for maxillary sinus floor augmentation before implant insertion. In addition to short-term assessments, CBCT is also used for long-term assessments to determine the success of treatment and the process of osseointegration.

### 3.4.2 Inflammatory and Degenerative Diseases

CBCT is an efficient tool for assessment of periodontal and endodontic conditions and associated periapical lesions. In periodontal disease, detection of primary changes in bone affects the outcome of treatment. The conventional 2D images used for periodontal disease appraisal cannot detect reduction in bone density in the primary stages of periodontitis, the extent of bone destruction, nor lesions located in the buccal and lingual surfaces of teeth. CBCT has relatively overcome these limitations. Periapical lesions with endodontic origin, root fracture, and extension of periapical lesion to the surrounding tissues, such as sinuses, can be well detected and localized on CBCT images. Periapical and/or panoramic radiography are conventionally used for diagnostic evaluation of marginal bone and periodontal space. Introduction of CBCT to dentistry enabled assessment of alveolar bone level and periodontal space in the buccolingual direction without image distortion and tissue superimposition. Thus, CBCT can be requested when conventional imaging cannot provide adequate diagnostic information [16–18].

### 3.4.3 Cysts and Tumors

CBCT provides valuable information about the extension of lesions and their proximity to vital anatomical structures. CBCT does not have the limitations of panoramic radiography, which provides 2D views with superimposition of multiple structures. MPR and 3D reconstruction enable more accurate assessment of the size of lesions in all three dimensions. Higher spatial resolution of CBCT images more accurately visualizes the bony margins of the lesions and better reveals the relationship of lesions with the adjacent vital structures. It is also applicable for postoperative follow-up.

### 3.4.4 Endodontics

Linear and curved measurements for efficient root canal therapy, identification of accessory canals and complex variations of the root canal system, detection of periapical lesions irrelevant to teeth, detection of dentoalveolar trauma and root fractures, detection of internal and external root resorption, and preoperative assessments of the apical region and evaluation of proximity to anatomical structures are among the applications of CBCT in this field [13, 19].

### 3.4.5 Orthodontics

Detection of dental anomalies, angulation of teeth, location of impacted teeth, and their relationship with adjacent teeth are important for biomechanical orthodontic treatment planning. Preoperative assessments prior to insertion of mini-implants, assessment of bone width available for tooth movement in the alveolar bone, evaluation of the temporomandibular joint, pharyngeal airways, 3D cephalometry, and 3D observation of the soft and hard tissue boundaries have simplified treatment planning, treatment, and follow-up of orthodontic patients [13, 19].

### 3.4.6 Surgery

Evaluation of alveolar ridge contour changes after tooth extraction over time is another capability of CBCT. This technique has currently replaced previous methods, such as obtaining different sections of study casts and manual measurement of the thickness of the alveolar ridge at different steps of treatment. Compared to CBCT, inaccuracy and unreliability were the main shortcomings of previous techniques for assessment of ridge contour before and after tooth extraction.

One of the most common applications of CBCT is to determine the exact location of impacted teeth, particularly mandibular third molars, to prevent nerve injuries and damage to adjacent structures. Localization of the mandibular canal is also imperative to decrease complications following maxillofacial surgery. MPR images can help in detecting the canal path and evaluating the presence of canals with two or more branches.

### 3.4.7 Dental Anomalies

Anomalies in size, shape, and location of teeth can be detected on CBCT images. Impaction of third molars and canine teeth is a type of dental anomaly that CBCT can aid in detecting and providing information about the accurate position, angulation, and relationship with adjacent anatomical structures.

### 3.4.8 Temporomandibular Joint

CBCT provides accurate information about pathological changes of the temporomandibular joint in both mandibular and temporal components. Although CBCT only visualizes the hard tissue of the joint, it would often suffice to detect most pathological conditions, such as osteophytes, erosion, traumatic bone injuries, and fractures.

### 3.4.9 Paranasal Sinuses

CBCT has been widely implemented for imaging of paranasal sinuses, since it shows fine anatomical details of the bone and it has high isotropic spatial resolution and lower dose of X-ray beam compared to CT.

The natural contrast of the nasal cavity and paranasal sinuses surrounded by bony walls on CBCT images can help in detection of airway diseases. Assessment of maxillary sinuses is important for implant placement, as well as sinus pathologies, qualitative and quantitative assessments, traumatic injuries, and extension of odontogenic lesions to the sinuses. CBCT can well reveal mucoperiosteal thickening and subsequent inflammatory changes, accumulation of calcifications, and sclerotic reactions.

## *3.5 Rapid Prototyping*

CBCT images can not only serve as a visual guide for surgery but also enable fabrication of actual models by providing visual data for the surgeons [2, 3, 5] (Fig. 4.12).

## *3.6 Tissue Regeneration*

Radiographic evaluation of bone regeneration must be able to accurately record bone formation and degradation of bioscaffolds. CBCT is a reliable and well-documented technique for bioengineered bone imaging. Its main advantage is lower X-ray radiation dose compared to conventional CT [20].

Aimetti et al. utilized three-dimensionally evaluated bone remodeling following ridge augmentation by the use of collagenated bovine-derived bone covered with a collagen membrane using CBCT. They evaluated postoperative changes in the test and control groups by linear and volumetric measurements made on superimposed pre- and postoperative CBCT images [21]. Araujo-Pires et al. used CBCT to study the efficacy of poly-DL-lactide-co-glycolide/calcium phosphate [22] scaffold for preservation of alveolar bone after tooth extraction. They also performed further histological assessments on the samples after CBCT, since the samples remained intact. Min et al. evaluated the performance of socket cap and socket cage for alveolar socket preservation after tooth extraction by linear analysis using CBCT [23]. Al-Fotawei selected CBCT to assess the regeneration of critical-size mandibular bone defects using beta-tricalcium phosphate scaffolds along with stem cells [20].

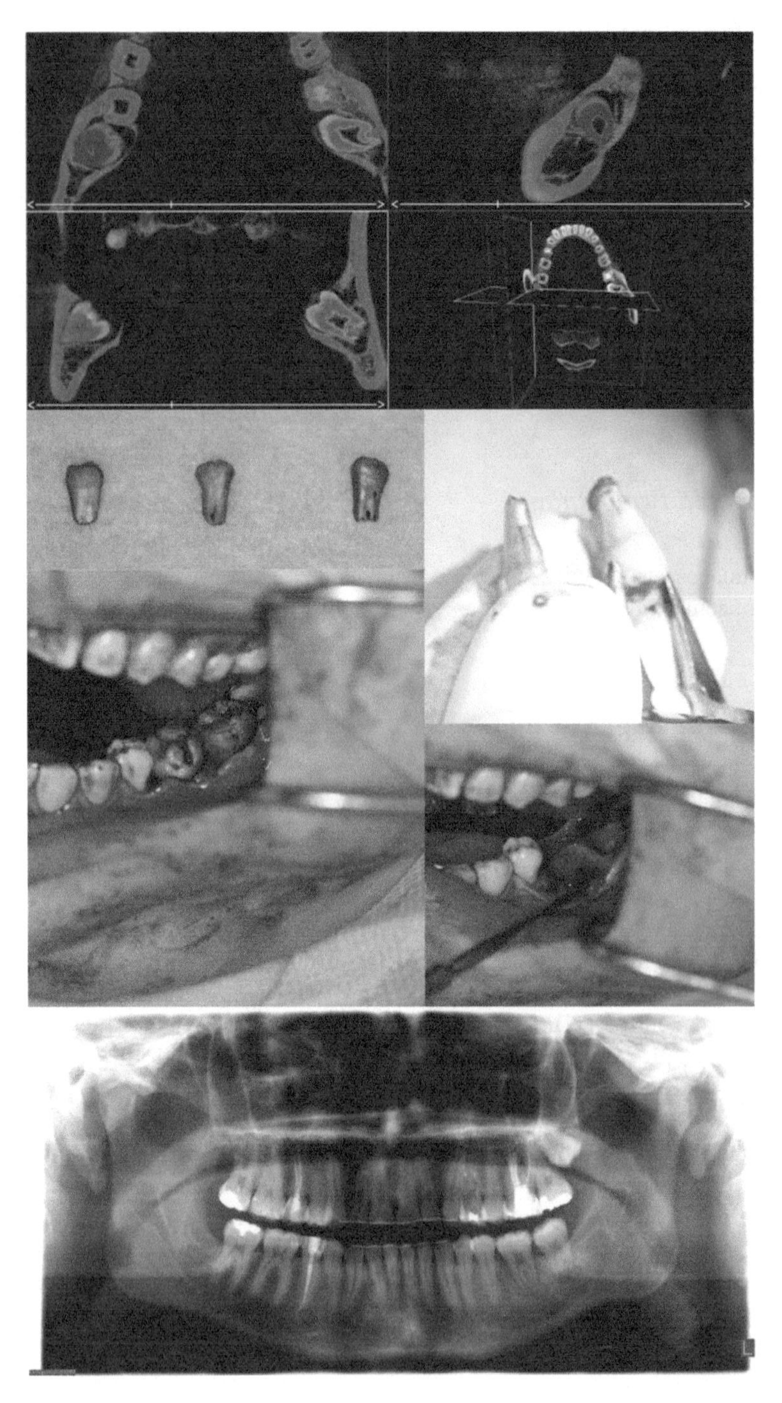

**Fig. 4.12** Rapid prototyping by CBCT. Sockets have been prepared in left edentulous ridge of mandible by rapid prototyped three-dimensional printed replica of the donor tooth for autotransplantation [24]

# 4 Microcomputed Tomography (Micro-CT)

Micro-CT is a noninvasive imaging modality that provides high-resolution 3D images of 2D projections or slices of the target sample.

The first micro-CT system was introduced in the early 1980s to assess structural defects of ceramic materials. It had cone-shaped beams, and the object was rotated for 360° during scanning. It was later used for evaluation of bone structure, osteoarthritis, and trabecular structure of bone [25]. Many samples have been directly evaluated by micro-CT such as tooth, bone, ceramics, polymers, and biomaterial scaffolds. Advanced generations enable imaging of small living animals. Micro-CT is not destructive; thus, the internal structure of sample can be evaluated repeatedly without physical sectioning or application of toxic chemicals. The intact sample can later undergo other mechanical and biological tests. Thus, there would be no issue with regard to shortage of samples for further studies or various tests. High resolution and the ability to three-dimensionally reconstruct the images have made it a suitable choice for noninvasive imaging of different organs in preclinical studies [26, 27].

Micro-CT is composed of an X-ray tube, a high-voltage power source, a collimator, a customized stage with customized sample holder, a charge-coupled device/phosphor detector, and a personal computer. The X-ray beam can be fan-shaped or cone-shaped. X-ray tube has a microfocal spot approximately 50 μm in size and benefits from high-resolution detectors. The intensity of X-ray beam depends on the voltage and current (amperage) of the tube. Recently, microfocused X-ray tubes have developed with the help of carbon nano-tubes for micro-CT, with a focal spot diameter of around 30 μm and high spatial-temporal resolution [25, 28]. At present, most micro-CT systems use third-generation scanning systems, in which both the X-ray tube and the detector simultaneously rotate around the object to scan it [28].

Three-dimensional imaging is performed in two ways:

1. Desktop system

The bed with the object placed on it rotates, while the X-ray tube and detector remain still. The X-ray tube continuously exposes the subject, which rotates step by step, and the receptor captures a 2D image of each step of exposure. In 2D map of the pixels, each pixel is coded by a threshold value for the coefficient of attenuation, and then 3D reconstruction is performed in a personal computer. The attenuation coefficient is related to the material density. Thus, 2D maps reveal the phases of the material [27, 29].

2. Live animal imaging.

The X-ray tube and detector both rotate. Noninvasive imaging provides valuable and practical information about the anatomy, pathology, and development of small laboratory animals, such as rodents [25, 28] (Fig. 4.13).

A noteworthy issue in application of micro-CT in vivo is the small animal radiation dose. Radiation-induced injuries, immune response, and apoptosis following

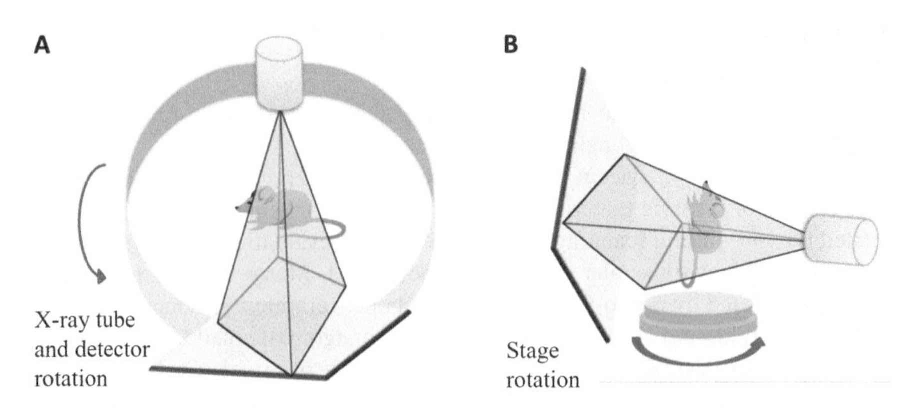


**Fig. 4.13** (**a**) Live animal imaging; (**b**) desktop system in micro-CT

X-ray radiation in micro-CT are observed in 0.1–0.5 Gy absorption doses. Unusual biological effects have also been reported in some cases, such as prevention of progression of type I diabetes in diabetic rats that received 0.5 Gy dose in one exposure. The important issue here is to consider the effects of radiation in longitudinal studies.

Most micro-CT systems use charge-coupled devices with phosphor screens and an optical or fiber optic lens to detect the X-ray beam that passes through the object. However, hydrogen amorphous silicon, amorphous selenium, and CMOS are still used. Currently, CMOS sensors are increasingly being used as an alternative to charge-coupled device detectors in micro-CT, because they have lower energy consumption and less fabrication cost and can be miniaturized. However, high noise, lower sensitivity, and narrower dynamic range limit their application [28]. Two-dimensional projections are converted to 3D images using the filtered back projection algorithm, which is the most commonly used algorithm in micro-CT [25].

Micro-CT has the ability to provide images with 1 μm voxel size, which has higher spatial resolution than other imaging modalities. Very high collimated and monochromatic X-ray beam provide a spatial resolution around 1 μm and do not have the beam hardening artifact of polychromatic X-ray tube in the conventional micro-CT system. This imaging system is also known as the nano-CT. CT number is a traditional unit for measurement of attenuation coefficient, which is used in micro-CT systems as well. The current devices are under constant development to increase their speed, resolution, and applications in non-mineralized tissues.

The attenuation map obtained by the micro-CT can be used to help other imaging modalities, such as micro positron-emission tomography and micro single-photon emission computed tomography. This is referred to as multimodality imaging and is desirable for biological studies. In functional imaging, a combination of modalities can be efficiently utilized.

Spectral micro-CT is a new technique that uses a spectrum of X-ray density instead of unifying the entire spectrum.

The use of dual-energy X-ray for imaging decreases the Compton scattering and photoelectric effect. Phase-contrast micro-CT is another technique that complements micro-CT and is based on image detection through refracted X-ray phase shift. This technique provides a high-resolution image, even for soft tissue without using a contrast medium. The X-ray phase shift is proportionate to the tissue mass density. This method provides high-contrast images of the hard and soft tissues using micro-CT.

## *4.1 Advantages and Limitations of Micro-CT*

Micro-CT has high spatial resolution and low cost and has various applications, making it a standard imaging modality for research purposes. However, low contrast of soft tissue and injuries caused by radiation limit its application to research imaging only. High-resolution demands high radiation dose and prolonged scanning time; this provides abundant volume of data. Micro-CT can also only be applied on small animals, such as small rodents. Another shortcoming of some micro-CT systems is that they still use polychromatic X-ray beam [27–29]. Lower energy beams are immediately attenuated; thus, the center of object is subjected to higher exposure. Difficult thresholding and beam hardening are among other shortcomings of these systems.

## *4.2 Applications of Micro-CT*

### 4.2.1 Evaluation of Enamel Thickness, Measurement of Dental Structures, and Assessment of Mineral Content

Evaluation of enamel thickness is often performed in anthropometric and human evolution studies, as well as studies on the effects of forces on teeth. CT does not provide accurate information about the enamel due to its low resolution for the enamel and dramatic effect on the enamel. Comparison of enamel thickness measurements made on micro-CT scans with the actual values obtained by conventional measurement methods confirms the accuracy and reliability of these measurements with high confidence interval. Aside from the total thickness, highly accurate surveys of slices from different areas of the enamel, dentin, and pulp are feasible. Micro-CT also enables 3D image reconstruction by the software. However, areas with very thin enamel thickness (100 μm) are difficult to detect and visualize.

Micro-CT enables quantitative measurement of the concentration of minerals in the bone, enamel, and dentin with >1% accuracy and 5–30 μm resolution. The advantages of micro-CT over other conventional techniques include noninvasiveness and constant slice thickness. It does not require physical sectioning of slices that causes irregularities. Moreover, the thinnest slice thickness obtained by micro-CT depends on the size of X-ray beam, which is much thinner than the slices prepared by mechanical methods. Changes in mineral tooth structure caused by caries, etching, bleaching, and remineralization can be more accurately studied using micro-CT with this method [26].

### 4.2.2 Evaluation of Root Canal Morphology

Micro-CT enables observation of narrow canals, communication between canals, accessory canals, and several foramina. The conventional method of assessment of root canal morphology requires irreversible destruction of samples. Data obtained by the use of this imaging modality can be converted to 3D images and can be analyzed qualitatively and quantitatively. Some studies have used certain methods to calculate the area and volume of each root canal. It is also possible to eliminate the hard tissue on the image and observe the pulp chamber and root canals as radiopaque structures. Furthermore, it also enables assessment of the internal structure and morphology of teeth [26] (Fig. 4.14).

### 4.2.3 Biomechanics

Finite element modeling is a commonly used method to analyze physical phenomena in terms of structure, liquid, and solid mechanics and biomechanics. The spatial shape of objects with a complex internal structure can be more accurately assessed in this method. Since teeth and bone have layered structure and anatomical shapes, CT reconstruction algorithms can be used efficiently for modeling of these complex structures. Foams, textiles, and nanofiber scaffolds can also be evaluated using this technique [27]. Micro-CT images can result in constructing finite element models with high accuracy. At present, micro-CT-based finite element method is commonly used due to optimal resolution and high accuracy.

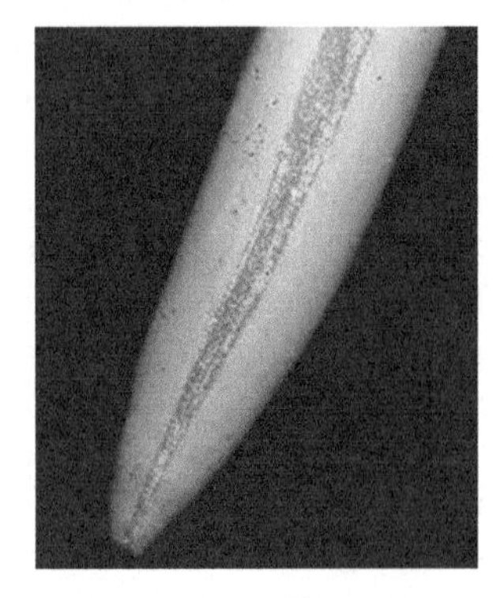

**Fig. 4.14** Root canal morphology evaluation by micro-CT

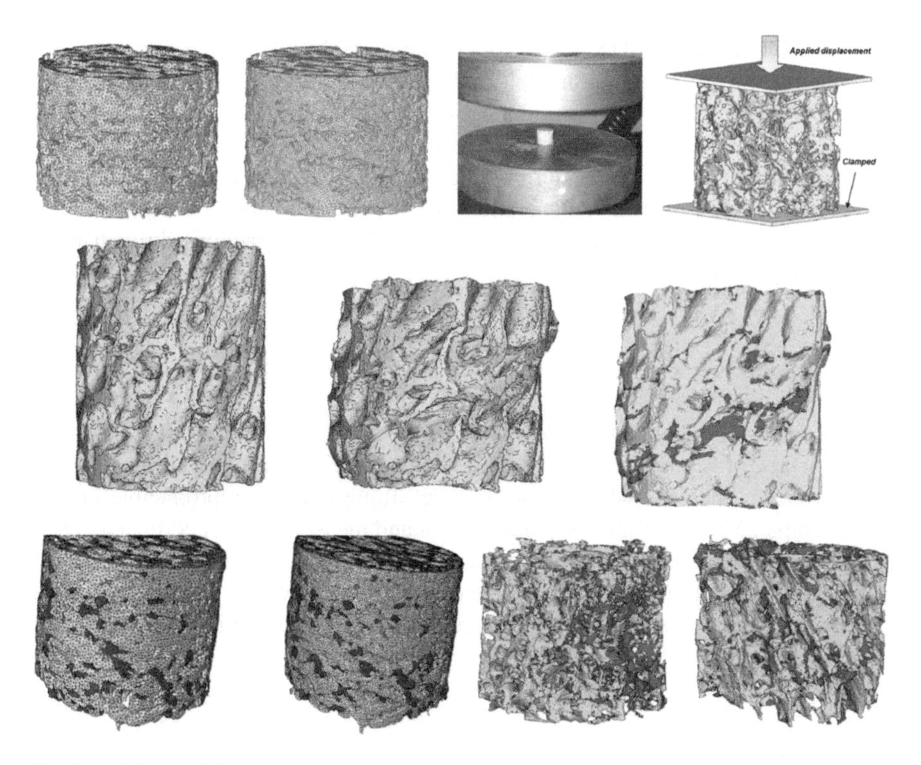


**Fig. 4.15** Micro-CT finite element model and experimental validation of trabecular bone damage and fracture [30]

After obtaining a micro-CT scan from the teeth, the enamel, dentin, and pulp can be segmented into different parts according to the pixel gray values or mineral density (Fig. 4.15).

### 4.2.4 Structure, Diseases, Development, and Adaptation of the Bone

Micro-CT enables noninvasive evaluation of bone geometry in several longitudinal studies on the same object. Skeletal diseases, such as osteoporosis, can be thoroughly evaluated using micro-CT. Micro-CT can also aid in assessment of models of disease emersion and consequences of various treatments. Additionally, skeletal micro-damage can be evaluated on micro-CT scans using a contrast medium. Micro-CT scans allow 3D evaluation of trabecular bone with 1–6 μm isotropic resolution including trabecular thickness, the number of trabeculae, distance and distribution pattern of trabeculae and trabecular spaces, the overall tissue volume, the trabecular bone score, the structure model index, trabecular relations, and bone density. It is superior to 2D histological assessment of bone. Micro-CT is the gold standard for quantitative evaluation of bone structure [29, 31].

Micro-CT is a standard technique for evaluation of the effects of genomic factors on bone phenotype in animal models and can be used to simulate biomechanical behaviors of sample structures under complicated loading conditions using finite element analysis. Finite element models reconstructed using micro-CT enable evaluation of bone quality and micron-scale damage, evaluation of the effects of mechanical stimuli on bone regeneration, mechanical regulation of differentiation and remodeling, and detection of bone marrow liquid interactions through bone trabeculae [25, 26].

### 4.2.5 Implants

The success of implant depends on the quality of osseointegration between the titanium surface of implant and the adjacent bone. Studies conventionally use histomorphometric analysis, which is destructive, limited, and unreproducible on the same sample. Micro-CT allows quantification and measurement of cortical and trabecular bone without these limitations and visualizes the quality and quantity of bone integrated with implant with excellent resolution. However, further studies are required to increase the accuracy and decrease the inherent metallic halation artifact caused by titanium [26].

### 4.2.6 Vascular Imaging

Vascular system studies using micro-CT with a spatial resolution smaller than 50 μm and evaluation of 3D vascular connections are easier and more accurate than the conventional methods, such as the use of opaque polymers injected into the vessels.

The use of contrast medium enables observation of cardiovascular structures on a micron scale using micro-CT in vivo and ex vivo. Analysis of the vascular structures of animal models using micro-CT was first performed on the renal vascular system. At present, ex vivo angiography is used for 3D assessment of vascularization in ischemic tissues. It also enables observation of major biological processes in the vasculature. The viscosity and radiopacity of the contrast medium used in micro-CT should be chosen precisely, because small size of the vessels and permeability of the arterioles and venules may allow perfusion of the contrast medium out of the vascular system.

Micro-CT can evaluate a 3D region of interest of the vascular system independently of the other parts of the vasculature. In other words, it enables independent analysis of the upper extremities where arteriogenesis is dominant during revascularization and lower extremities where angiogenesis is dominant.

Recent advances in contrast media for the micro-CT have enabled imaging of cardiovascular structures in vivo. However, it has lower contrast resolution and quantitative functionality than micro-CT angiography ex vivo.

### 4.2.7 Imaging with Contrast Medium

Radiopaque contrast media enables imaging of non-mineralized cartilaginous tissues using micro-CT. The extracellular matrix of the sound cartilage has a high charge, which makes it capable of imaging. Sound articular cartilage has a high negative charge, while the interstitial fluid is positively charged. Thus, this complex has a neutral charge. In initial phases of osteoarthritis, the negative charge of the cartilage decreases. A negatively charged radiopaque contrast medium is used to balance the charge of cartilage, which enables assessment of the morphology and composition of cartilage using micro-CT. This technique is known as the equilibrium partitioning of ionic contrast agent via micro-CT or EPIC-μCT and is used for noninvasive longitudinal evaluation of cartilage degeneration [25]. The X-ray micro- and nano-focus CT can also be used for soft tissue imaging, accompanied by an opaque contrast medium. A large number of studies have focused on this topic recently. Opaque contrast media utilization is not confined to soft tissue diagnoses adjacent to the bone, such as bone marrow, adipocytes, and blood vessels, but can also be used for detection of tissue components, such as extracellular matrix, cartilage, adipocytes, and connective tissue. Osmium tetroxide, iodine potassium iodide ($I_2KI$), and phosphotungstic acid (PTA) are among the most important opaque contrast agents [32–36].

### 4.2.8 Drug Delivery

Micro-CT has been utilized to design and evaluate the structure of materials, playing the role of carriers in drug delivery (Fig. 4.16).

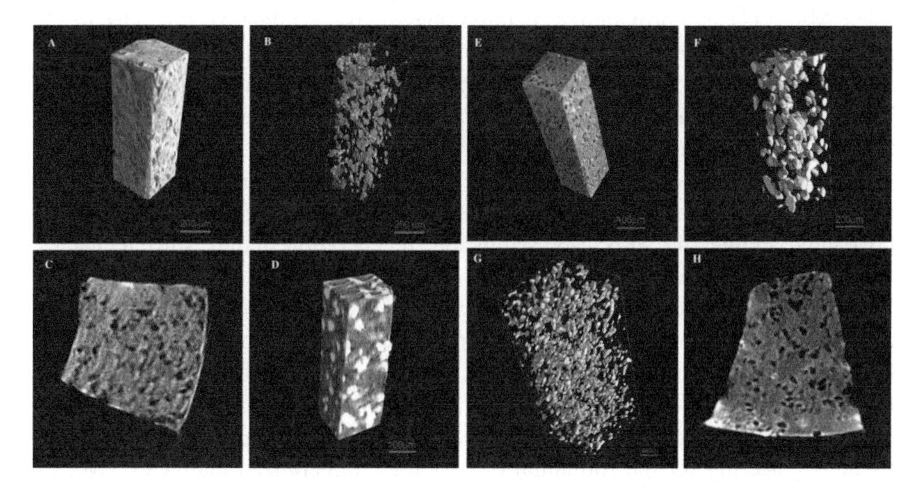


**Fig. 4.16** Internal microtomographs of matrices before and after drug release [37]

### 4.3 Rapid Prototyping

Micro-CT is a computational method, and different parameters can be calculated considering its hardware and software capabilities. Rapid prototyping is the result of such capabilities [38].

Evaluation of microstructure of materials in other fields of research is other applications of micro-CT, such as geosciences, medical device and pharmaceutical packaging, developmental biology, and toxicology. The type and origin of structures evaluated may vary and include tissue engineering scaffolds, human tissues, small laboratory animals (e.g., mouse and rabbit), goat, non-human primates, fish, shrimp, insects, human kidney stones, and fossils.

### 4.4 Tissue Engineering

Micro-CT meets the tissue engineering imaging requirements, which include non-invasiveness, quantitative nature, and 3D design. The biomaterials used in tissue engineering must be able to meet the biomechanical and biological requirements of tissues and complex organs.

Scaffolds play an important role in tissue engineering and provide a supportive environment for other components. Scaffolds used in tissue engineering should be evaluated in terms of production of by-products, presence of adequate porosities with ideal size enabling distribution of cells and blood vessels, and optimal mechanical properties. Quantitative assessment of scaffolds in micron-scale is imperative in terms of volume, surface area, strut width, porosity, surface area to volume ratio, inter-structural relations, and anisotropy for designing and fabrication of ideal scaffolds. Micro-CT can provide the required quantitative 3D data for this purpose. It allows meticulous evaluation of the internal structure of scaffolds, their mechanical and structural behavior, and their rate and mechanism of degradation over time. However, micro-CT is not appropriate for assessment of metal-containing scaffolds, because light and dark grainy artifacts mask the valuable details of image [27].

Micro-CT enables precise quantitative evaluation of the morphometry of mineralized tissues. This technique can provide high-resolution images for assessment of bone microarchitecture. It is also used in bone regeneration studies, since it enables volumetric assessment of complex tissue structures with different densities. Wongsupa et al. benefitted utilization of micro-CT to evaluate the tissues they had engineered. They appraised bone regeneration process with poly(ε-caprolactone) biphasic calcium phosphate scaffold accompanied by human dental pulp stem cells using micro-CT [39].

Micro-CT can be used to evaluate the efficacy of bone structures produced by tissue engineering for the formation of a biologic mineralized matrix ex vivo. In contrast to other methods of evaluation of bone formation, micro-CT quantifies mineralization over time in a 3D fashion, without damaging the samples. Moreover, it enables assessment of bone formation by tissue engineering in animal models using micro-CT. Micro-CT systems with a fixed container and a rotating X-ray tube and detector are used for in vivo evaluation of small animals. Small animals are scanned under general anesthesia. Correct positioning of the animal, selection of the volume of interest, and radiation dose should be performed accurately [27, 38, 40].

# 5 Magnetic Resonance Imaging (MRI)

MRI is a non-ionizing and noninvasive modality with excellent capabilities for structural and functional imaging of the human body. In the oral cavity, it can be used for structural assessment of the tongue and vocal tract [41, 42].

To put it simply, what occurs in MRI is that radio waves are transmitted to a patient in a strong magnetic field. By discontinuing the transmission of radio waves, the human body emits electromagnetic signals, which are detected by the internal coil of the MRI device and converted to image according to the dissemination pattern of hydrogen atoms (Fig. 4.17).

Protons, which have positive electrical charge, rotate diagonally around an axis, known as "spin," and generate a magnetic field. Protons can be imagined as small dipolar magnets with a magnetic field. They are randomly oriented in space, but when placed in a strong, external magnetic field, they are aligned in parallel and non-parallel fashions referred to as the parallel or spin-up and antiparallel or spin-down fashion, respectively. The parallel protons have a lower state of energy, and higher number of protons are arranged in parallel compared to antiparallel fashion; however, this difference is low (Fig. 4.18).

In addition to diagonal spin, protons in an external magnetic field have precession movement, which is the oscillating movement of a proton along the external magnetic field in a conical path (Fig. 4.19). The higher the intensity of the external magnetic field, the higher the speed of oscillation and the frequency of this movement, known as the precessional frequency or Larmor frequency. Parallel protons

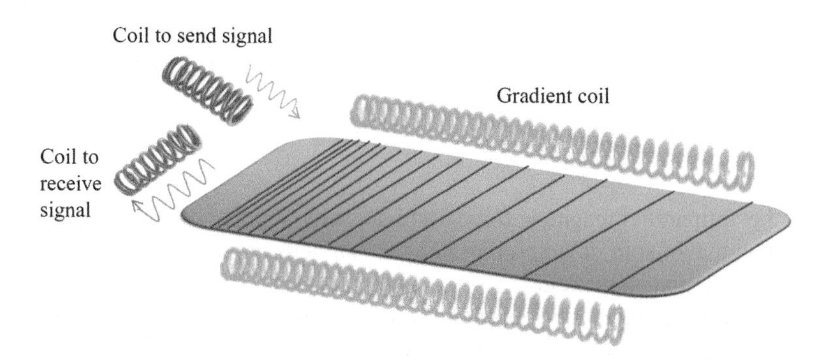


**Fig. 4.17** Gradient magnetic field and coils to send and receive signals in the MRI device

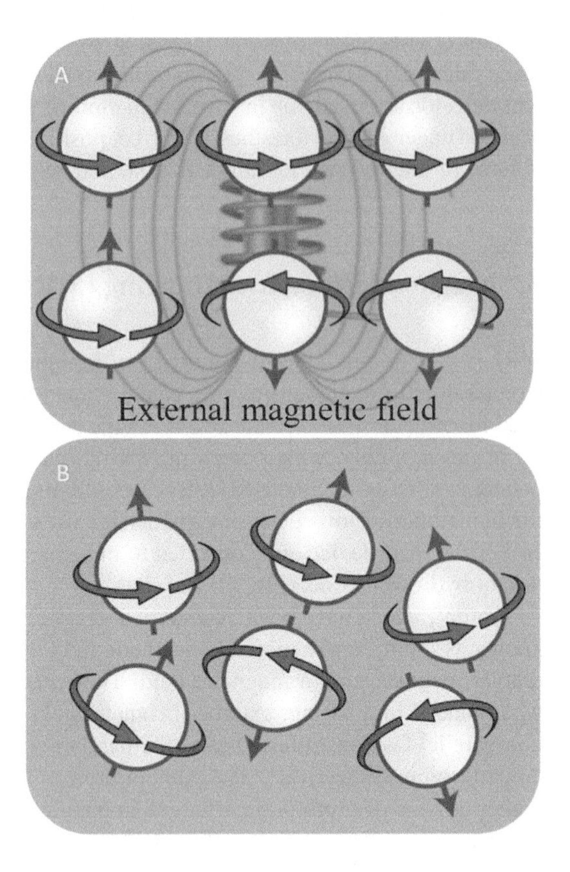


**Fig. 4.18** (**a**) Protons aligned in magnetic field (**b**) and randomly orientated in the absence of magnetic field

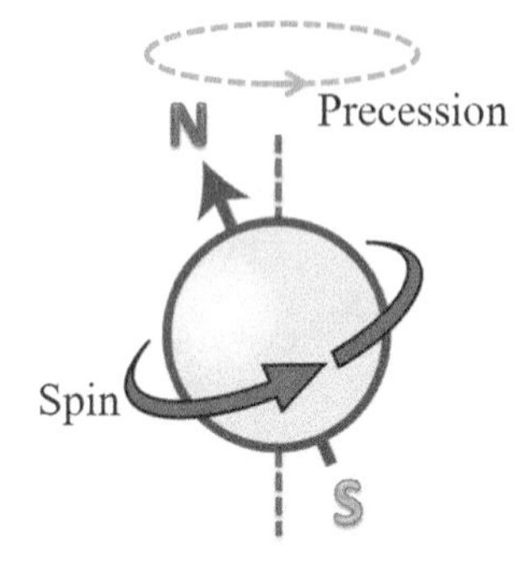


**Fig. 4.19** Spin and precessional movement of proton

cancel the antiparallel magnetic forces, and since the number of spin-up protons is higher than that of spin-down protons, the net magnetization vector would be in the direction of the magnetic field.

If the magnetic force of a spin-up proton is divided into two components in the z and y or z and x axes, the components in the x and y axes of protons cancel each other, but the components aligned in the z axis collect and form a magnetization

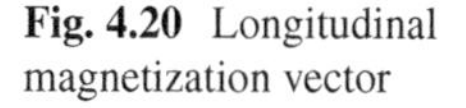

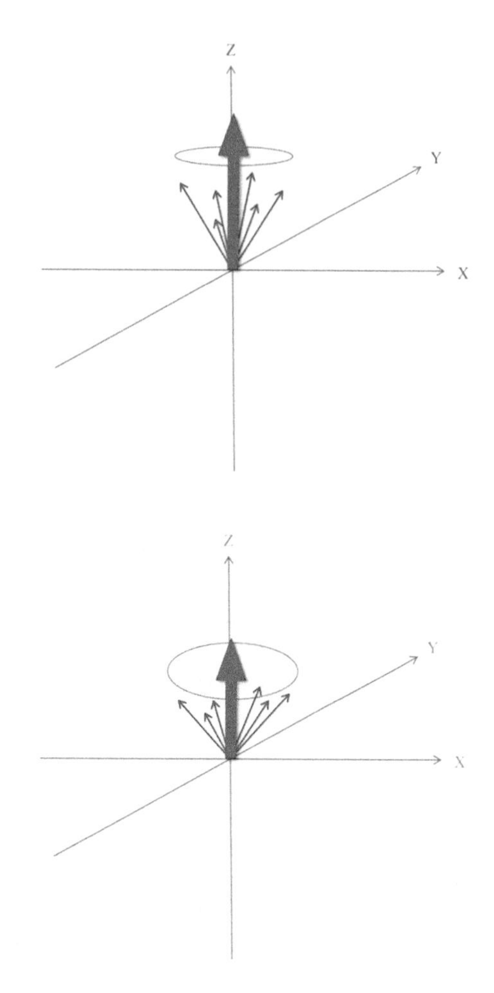


**Fig. 4.20** Longitudinal magnetization vector

**Fig. 4.21** Decreased magnetization in longitudinal direction

vector along the external magnetic field, which is known as the longitudinal magnetization vector (Fig. 4.20). This vector is aligned in the external magnetic field direction, and in order to be detectable and measurable, it should change its direction in the external magnetic field. In other words, to measure the rate of magnetization, magnetization should be perpendicular to the external magnetic field direction, which is accomplished by radiofrequency (RF) pulses that should have a speed and frequency similar to the speed and frequency of protons. Given that the RF pulse frequency emitted from the coil of MRI system is similar to the Larmor frequency of protons, protons can receive energy from radio waves, which is referred to as resonance. This energy is spent to raise the level of energy of protons such that some of the spin-up protons become spin-down, and thus, the magnetization in longitudinal direction decreases (Fig. 4.21). Moreover, the absorbed energy causes in-phase and in-step movement of protons. Resultantly, all transverse magnetization vectors are collected in x–y plane and result in the creation of a net

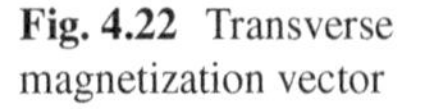

**Fig. 4.22** Transverse magnetization vector

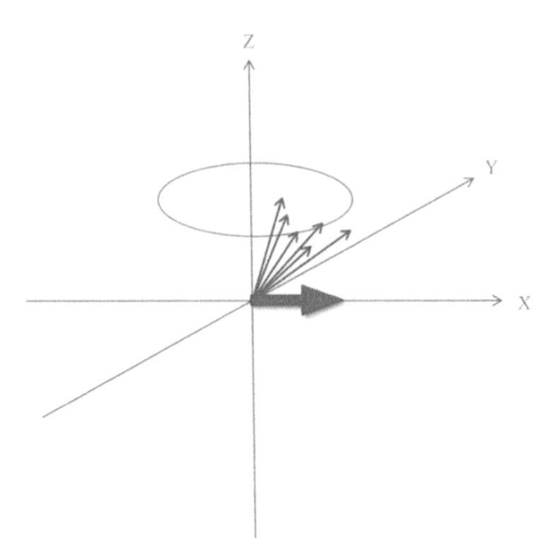


transverse magnetization vector (Fig. 4.22). Continuous movement of transverse magnetization vector induces an electric current in the receptor coil, which is the MRI signal. The magnitude of this signal is proportionate to the overall concentration of hydrogen nuclei (proton density) in a tissue and the degree to which hydrogen is bound within a molecule. Higher concentration of weakly bound hydrogen nuclei creates a stronger signal and a brighter image.

When the RF pulse is off, transverse magnetization starts to decay, which is known as transverse relaxation. Also, longitudinal magnetization increases again and gradually returns to its baseline state, referred to as longitudinal relaxation. The relationship of longitudinal magnetization with time after the RF pulse is switched off is known as the T1 curve, which indicates the energy emitted to the surrounding lattice from protons. However, with regard to transverse magnetization, protons that are in-phase and in-step become out of phase and random when the RF pulse is switched off. Thus, transverse magnetization gradually decreases. Reduction in longitudinal magnetization per unit of time is shown in T2 curve, which indicates spin-spin relaxation. T2 relaxation occurs five to ten times faster than T1 recovery. T1 and T2 are inherent characteristics of the tissue and are constant for a specific tissue in a certain magnetic field.

Due to difficulty in determining the exact time of return of longitudinal magnetization to baseline state and elimination of transverse magnetization, T1 and T2 are defined as follows:

T1: Time required for the longitudinal magnetization to reach 63% of its baseline value.

T2: Time required for the transverse magnetization to decrease to 37% of its baseline value.

Water and tissues, containing high amounts of water, such as cerebrospinal fluid, have long T1 and T2, while fat and tissues containing high amounts of fat, such as bone marrow, have a short T1 and shorter T2 in comparison to water. Pathological tissues have higher water content than the adjacent healthy tissues, which enhances their detection on images. If molecules comprising the tissue are small and quickly movable, T1 would be long because energy transfer to lattice would be more difficult due to fast movement of small molecules. Impure liquids containing larger molecules have a shorter T2 because they have more discrepancies in internal magnetic fields of the material, which would cause greater differences in oscillation frequencies. This difference results in faster diphase of protons and shorter T2.

Some other terms need to be defined here:

Time to repeat (TR) is the time between sending two consecutive RF pulses. We set an example here to explain its significance. If two tissues have the same transverse magnetization after sending the RF pulse, and adequate time is allowed for both tissues for decay of transverse magnetization and recovery of longitudinal magnetization until sending the second RF pulse, the signals generated by the two tissues would be equal. Thus, they could not be differentiated. However, due to the difference in nature of the tissues, the speed of decay of transverse magnetization in the two tissues would not be the same. Therefore, if the second RF pulse is sent in a shorter time, the longitudinal magnetization of the two tissues would be different from the baseline values; consequently, different signals are generated, and they could be differentiable. TR is the parameter indicative of longitudinal magnetization.

Echo time (TE) is the time period between the moment of sending the RF pulse and the moment of receiving the signal. The TE is the time after the application of the RF pulse when the MR signal is read. The shorter the TE time, the stronger the received signal from tissue would be. However, adequate time should be allowed for signal transmission, because if the TE is too short, the difference in the signals sent from two tissues would be too small to differentiate between them (Fig. 4.23).

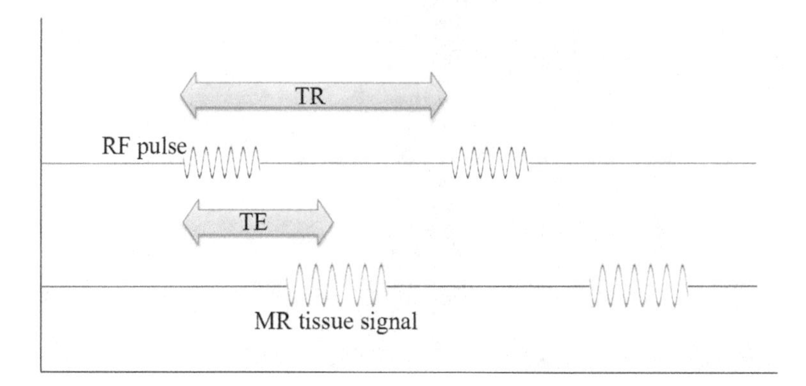


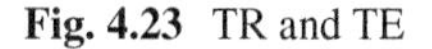
**Fig. 4.23** TR and TE

TR determines the T1 relaxation, and TE controls the T2 relaxation at the time of signal collection. In other words, TE is responsible for T2-weighted images, while TR is responsible for T1-weighted images.

In signal-time curve, if the T1 and T2 curves of a specific tissue are combined, the longitudinal magnetization is tilted toward the horizontal plane during TR. It is the point at which, transverse magnetization decreases and the T2 curve initiates.

Since in long TR all tissues recover their longitudinal magnetization, if TR is long and TE is short, they produce equal or close signals, and difference in T1 of tissues would have no effect on signal intensity. Thus, they could not be differentiable. Moreover, if TE is short, the difference in T2 of tissues would not have adequate time to be revealed. Consequently, the obtained signal is neither T1-weighted nor T2-weighted; instead, it is affected by proton density of tissue. The tissue with greater protons would create a stronger signal.

With that same concept, in long TR and long TE, T2-weighted images would be obtained. On these images, tissues with long T2, such as cerebrospinal fluid and water, appear bright, while tissues with short T2, such as fat, are seen darker than water-containing tissues. T2-weighted images are used for detection of pathologies (Fig. 4.24).

In short TR and short TE, T1-weighted images are obtained. On these images, tissues with short T1 appear bright, while tissues with long T1 appear dark. T1-weighted images are often used for evaluation of anatomical structures.

Image contrast between different tissues depends on the internal tissue characteristics, such as proton density, and T1 and T2 and external parameters, such as TE and TR.

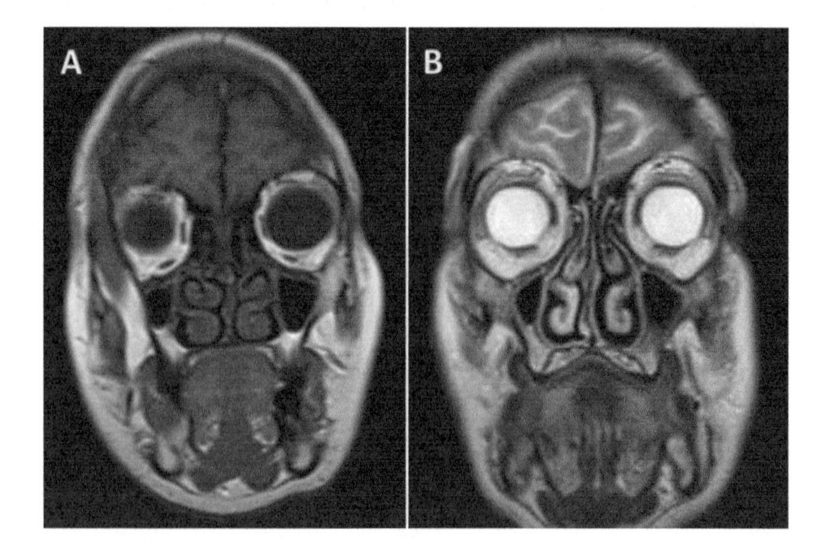


**Fig. 4.24** (**a**) T1; (**b**) T2 MR images in a coronal section

Several sequences of change in strength or timing of RF pulses can be applied to tissues, which can suppress or emphasize the signals of different tissues [2, 43, 44].

## 5.1 Contrast Media

Contrast media in MRI are paramagnetic materials that shorten the T1 and T2 times and enhance proton relaxation. In other words, in a constant TR, higher signals are produced, and in a constant TE, lower signals are produced. In other words, the signal is enhanced in T1-weighted images, while the signal decreases in T2-weighted images. Thus, T1-weighted images are the imaging technique of choice after injection of contrast medium. Diffusion of contrast medium is not the same in different tissues. Thus, the signals obtained from different tissues are not equally affected. Normal tissues such as the vasculature with slow blood flow, sinus mucosa, and muscles are enhanced. The signal of tumoral tissues, infections, inflammations, and posttraumatic defects are further enhanced. Thus, they become brighter on post-contrast T1 images, and their differentiation from the adjacent normal tissues becomes easier. Using the contrast medium, tumoral tissues can be differentiated from the adjacent edema, which would be impossible to differentiate without contrast injection. Gadolinium compounds are the most commonly used contrast media. Another advantage of using contrast medium is that it decreases the TR and, thus, decreases the overall imaging time [2, 43, 44] (Fig. 4.25).

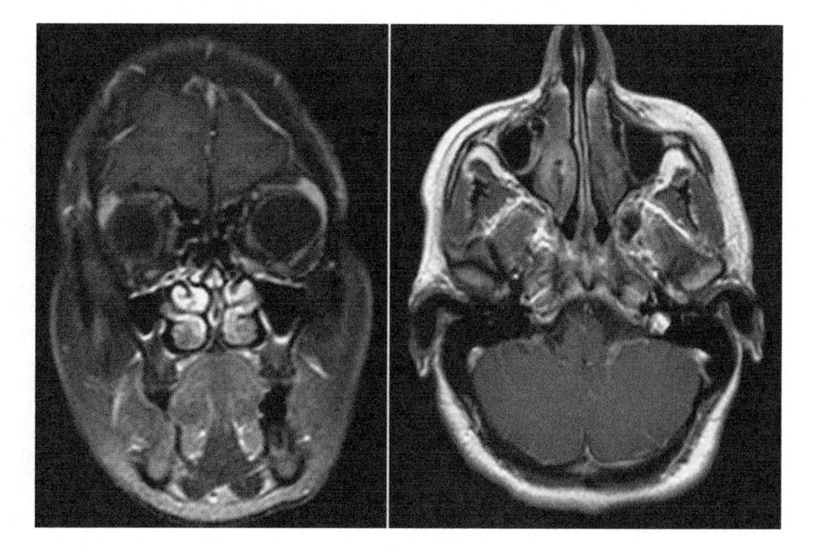

**Fig. 4.25** T1, post-contrast MR images

## 5.2 Spin Echo

If a 180° pulse is sent after a 90° RF pulse in TE/2 time, protons oscillate in a clockwise direction, and those with faster oscillation are positioned behind those with slower oscillation. When they reach each other, they become in-phase and produce a stronger magnetization and signal. This strong signal is referred to as spin echo. A 180° pulse has twice the power or duration of a 90° pulse [43, 44].

## 5.3 Short Tau Inversion Recovery (STIR) and Fluid-Attenuated Inversion Recovery (FLAIR)

One benefit of MRI is imaging of the part of the body, while the signal emitted from another tissue in that specific region can be suppressed. This would eliminate the disturbances created by the specific tissue and its effect on the adjacent structures and results in a consequently stronger signal from the target tissue. Water and adipose tissue are commonly suppressed tissues in clinical applications. Several techniques are available for this purpose. However, their visual outcome is eventually the same. STIR minimizes the fat signals and enables better observation of adjacent structures. FLAIR minimizes the signal of fluids and makes better observation of tissues or pathologies adjacent to fluids, such as the cerebrospinal fluid possible [2, 43, 44] (Fig. 4.26).

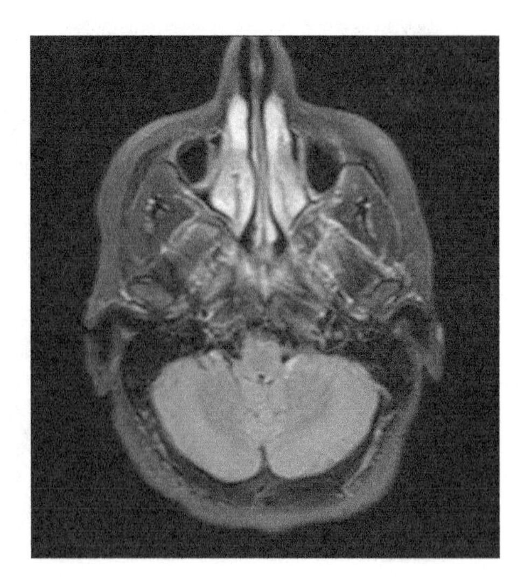

**Fig. 4.26** Fluid-attenuated inversion recovery

## 5.4 Flow

Flow of liquids, such as blood flow in the human body, is another factor affecting the MR images. When the RF pulse is sent to one slice of the human body, transverse magnetization is produced in the blood in that specific slice. However, by the time of receipt of the signal, the blood flow has moved the transverse magnetization in that slice, which may lead to no signal receipt and creation of a void on the image or signal reinforcement in the slice.

## 5.5 Determining the Section of Imaging

An external magnetic field is used for selection of the respective section for examination, which has different magnetic intensities at different parts, referred to as the gradient field. It is created by a gradient coil. Due to different intensities of the magnetic field, protons in different parts oscillate at different frequencies. Thus, to receive signal from each slice, the RF pulse suitable for that specific slice is used. The signal of this slice is received, and the location sending the signal is detected. Using a steep magnetic field gradient, signals can be received from different slices in the desired plane. The narrower the frequency domain of the RF pulse, the lower thickness of the imaged slice is. A steeper magnetic field gradient is used to decrease the slice thickness. By doing so, a narrower slice can be imaged with a constant RF.

Hydrogen, carbon-13, nitrogen-15, and oxygen-17 have active nuclei in terms of magnetic resonance. However, hydrogen nucleus is used for MRI because:

1. It is abundantly found in the human body.
2. It sends a stronger signal than other nuclei.
3. It contains one proton and no neutron. Thus, considering the odd number of protons, the magnetic torque of protons is not neutralized [43, 44].

MRI is composed of several hardware components:

1. A strong superconducting magnet. Its intensity and power are expressed in tesla (T). The intensity used in MRI is often 0.5–1.5 T, but it can range from 0.1 to 4 T. Systems with stronger magnetic fields have a higher SR but are more expensive.
2. A Faraday cage to block interference of external radio waves.
3. A coil for sending RF pulse and a coil to receive tissue signal. Some coils do both.

## 5.6 Advantages of MRI

MRI does not have ionizing radiation and does not have the risks of X-ray-based imaging systems.

It is a noninvasive method of imaging and provides the best soft tissue images with the highest quality and resolution.

Also, direct multiplanar imaging is possible without the need to change the patient's position.

## 5.7 *Limitations of MRI*

Limitations of MRI include that it is costly, has limited availability, has long scanning time, and is difficult to perform in claustrophobic patients.

Additionally, there is a risk of dislocation and increased heat and damage in patients who have metals with ferromagnetic properties in their body, when placed in the strong magnetic field of MRI.

It has image distortion in the presence of metals, and the contrast medium used in MRI is contraindicated in some individuals, as there is a risk of adverse consequences, such as nephrogenic cystic fibrosis in some patients with impaired renal function.

## 5.8 *Applications of MRI*

### 5.8.1 Imaging and Evaluation of Soft Tissue

Evaluation of component position and structure of the temporomandibular joint is an important application of MRI in the maxillofacial region. Chan et al. utilized this remarkable application of MRI in their study. They employed contrast-enhanced MRI method for the follow-up and determination of the regeneration rate of temporomandibular joint disc following implantation of a reconstructed collagen template in an animal model [45].

MRI can also aid in locating the mandibular nerve in cases where conventional imaging modalities cannot accurately determine its location.

### 5.8.2 Pathologies Involving the Soft Tissues

MRI can be used for assessment of lymph node involvement and perineural involvement in malignancies. It also plays a fundamental role in the diagnosis of peripheral nerve lesions. Bendszus et al. highlighted the positive role of this technique in primary diagnosis of acute axonal nerve lesions and monitoring of nerve regeneration [46]. MRI can be helpful for detection of areas of ischemic tissues with regenerative ability for targeting of treatments supporting tissue recovery. Accordingly, Laakso et al. evaluated different MRI relaxation and diffusion tensor imaging parameters for detection of areas with signs of regeneration in ischemic mouse skeletal muscles. Last but not least, MRI is used for evaluating invasion of intraosseous lesions to the adjacent soft tissues [47].

### 5.8.3 MR Spectroscopy

Superconducting magnets with higher field strengths (4–7 T) are used for magnetic resonance spectroscopy. Magnetic resonance spectroscopy evaluates the chemical composition of specific elements in a noninvasive manner. Spectroscopy combined with imaging can be used to assess the chemical and metabolic activity of specific areas. It provides valuable information about cellular physiology in vivo. Also, the course of specific diseases and the efficacy of some therapeutic procedures can be evaluated as such.

### 5.8.4 Cardiac Magnetic Resonance Imaging

Cardiac MRI is one of the most complex MRI techniques, which should not only compensate for the respiratory movements but must also consider unstoppable heartbeats. It provides information about the physiological function and anatomy of the heart [48].

### 5.8.5 Magnetic Resonance Angiography

It is a noninvasive method of blood vessels imaging to visualize and detect vascular abnormalities (Fig. 4.27).

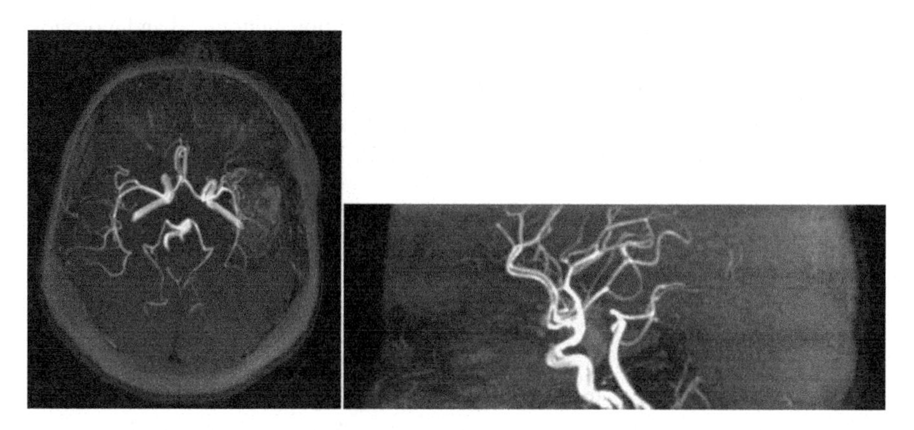

**Fig. 4.27** Magnetic resonance angiography

### 5.9 Tissue Regeneration Appraisal

Kamei et al. evaluated the regeneration process of focal articular cartilage defect in the knee following injection of mesenchymal stem cells using MRI T2 mapping as an adjunct diagnostic tool [49].

Ribot et al. evaluated high spatial and temporal resolution 3D MR images to follow the bone regeneration and vascularization in femoral bone defects of rats. They implanted three different biomaterials and compared the progress of healing in MR images with μCT and histologic observations. Findings of MR images were confirmed by μCT and histology, and it was concluded that MRI presents great potential for evaluation of tissue-engineered bone and even an alternative for μCT and histology in preclinical bone tissue engineering studies [43, 44].

Superparamagnetic iron oxide nanoparticle-labeled scaffolds have been developed, which make in vivo monitoring of location and function of implanted scaffolds more feasible by MRI. These MRI-visible scaffolds can be tracked in situ.

## 6 Summary

The use of 3D imaging technology plays a pivotal role in promoting the quality of different steps of tissue engineering from the fabrication of scaffold and biomaterials to long-term assessment of the success of used materials and adopted procedures.

The spatial scale of the obtained data varies from as small as micrometers to as large as the overall evaluation of a living creature, in addition to having applications both in vivo and in vitro; hence, the spectrum of 3D imaging is quite expansive. Although advanced imaging modalities are superior to conventional imaging in many ways, a specific imaging modality alone cannot provide all the required information. For instance, CT can provide high-resolution anatomical and morphological information; however, it imposes the patient a high radiation dose. CBCT has a much lower radiation dose than CT, but it has limited ability in visualizing soft tissue. The imaging modality of choice must be selected according to its applicability and the required information (Table 4.2). The nondestructive nature of

**Table 4.2** Summary of 3D imaging in dental and oral tissue engineering

| | Soft tissue illustration | Hard tissue illustration | Imaging time | Radiation dose | Cost |
|---|---|---|---|---|---|
| CT | Moderate | Good | High | High | High |
| CBCT | Weak | Good | Low | Lower than CT | Lower than CT |
| μCT | Moderate | Excellent | High | High | Lower than CT |
| MRI | Good | Weak | High | None | High |

imaging systems is a great advantage in longitudinal studies, which allows evaluation of changes in engineered tissues or materials used in tissue engineering in viable biological systems, which paves the way for further clinical applications. CT, CBCT, MRI, and micro-CT can be used in vivo. Due to higher applicability and availability, they are more commonly used for morphological assessments, and after imaging, samples remain intact for further studies. Some imaging systems have applications in functional and molecular assessments, and their use in tissue engineering of the maxillofacial region is on the rise.

## References


1. Bushong, S. C. (2016). *Radiologic science for technologists-E-book: Physics, biology, and protection*. St. Louis, MO: Elsevier Health Sciences.
2. White, S. C., & Pharoah, M. J. (2014). *Oral radiology-E-book: Principles and interpretation*. St. Louis, MO: Elsevier Health Sciences.
3. Caruso, P., Silvestri, E., & Sconfienza, L. M. (2013). *Cone beam CT and 3D imaging: A practical guide*. Milan: Springer.
4. Whaites, E., & Drage, N. (2016). *Essentials of dental radiography and radiology*. St. Louis, MO: Elsevier Health Sciences.
5. Langlais, R. P. (2016). *Exercises in oral radiology and interpretation*. St. Louis, MO: WB Saunders Company.
6. Glemser, P. A., Engel, K., Simons, D., Steffens, J., Schlemmer, H. P., & Orakcioglu, B. (2018). A new approach for photorealistic visualization of rendered computed tomography images. *World Neurosurgery, 114*, e283–ee92.
7. Smith, M. H., Flanagan, C. L., Kemppainen, J. M., Sack, J. A., Chung, H., Das, S., et al. (2007). Computed tomography-based tissue-engineered scaffolds in craniomaxillofacial surgery. *The International Journal of Medical Robotics, 3*(3), 207–216.
8. Stoor, P., Suomalainen, A., Mesimaki, K., & Kontio, R. (2017). Rapid prototyped patient specific guiding implants in critical mandibular reconstruction. *Journal of Cranio-Maxillo-Facial Surgery, 45*(1), 63–70.
9. Lincoln, K. P., Sun, A. Y., Prihoda, T. J., & Sutton, A. J. (2016). Comparative accuracy of facial models fabricated using traditional and 3D imaging techniques. *Journal of Prosthodontics, 25*(3), 207–215.
10. Damstra, J., Fourie, Z., Huddleston Slater, J. J., & Ren, Y. (2010). Accuracy of linear measurements from cone-beam computed tomography-derived surface models of different voxel sizes. *American Journal of Orthodontics and Dentofacial Orthopedics, 137*(1), 16.e1–16.e6; discussion -7.
11. Mischkowski, R. A., Pulsfort, R., Ritter, L., Neugebauer, J., Brochhagen, H. G., Keeve, E., et al. (2007). Geometric accuracy of a newly developed cone-beam device for maxillofacial imaging. *Oral Surgery, Oral Medicine, Oral Pathology, Oral Radiology, and Endodontics, 104*(4), 551–559.
12. Stratemann, S. A., Huang, J. C., Maki, K., Miller, A. J., & Hatcher, D. C. (2008). Comparison of cone beam computed tomography imaging with physical measures. *Dento Maxillo Facial Radiology, 37*(2), 80–93.
13. Al-Okshi, A., Theodorakou, C., & Lindh, C. (2017). Dose optimization for assessment of periodontal structures in cone beam CT examinations. *Dento Maxillo Facial Radiology, 46*(3), 20160311.
14. Katsumata, A., Hirukawa, A., Okumura, S., Naitoh, M., Fujishita, M., Ariji, E., et al. (2007). Effects of image artifacts on gray-value density in limited-volume cone-beam computerized

tomography. *Oral Surgery, Oral Medicine, Oral Pathology, Oral Radiology, and Endodontics, 104*(6), 829–836.
15. Schulze, R. K., Berndt, D., & d'Hoedt, B. (2010). On cone-beam computed tomography artifacts induced by titanium implants. *Clinical Oral Implants Research, 21*(1), 100–107.
16. Mol, A., & Balasundaram, A. (2008). In vitro cone beam computed tomography imaging of periodontal bone. *Dento Maxillo Facial Radiology, 37*(6), 319–324.
17. Noujeim, M., Prihoda, T., Langlais, R., & Nummikoski, P. (2009). Evaluation of high-resolution cone beam computed tomography in the detection of simulated interradicular bone lesions. *Dento Maxillo Facial Radiology, 38*(3), 156–162.
18. Prakash, N., Karjodkar, F. R., Sansare, K., Sonawane, H. V., Bansal, N., & Arwade, R. (2015). Visibility of lamina dura and periodontal space on periapical radiographs and its comparison with cone beam computed tomography. *Contemporary Clinical Dentistry, 6*(1), 21–25.
19. Yuan, F., Chen, L., Wang, X., Wang, Y., Lyu, P., & Sun, Y. (2016). Comparative evaluation of the artefacts index of dental materials on two-dimensional cone-beam computed tomography. *Scientific Reports, 6*, 26107.
20. Al-Fotawei, R., Ayoub, A. F., Heath, N., Naudi, K. B., Tanner, K. E., Dalby, M. J., et al. (2014). Radiological assessment of bioengineered bone in a muscle flap for the reconstruction of critical-size mandibular defect. *PLoS One, 9*(9), e107403.
21. Aimetti, M., Manavella, V., Corano, L., Ercoli, E., Bignardi, C., & Romano, F. (2018). Three-dimensional analysis of bone remodeling following ridge augmentation of compromised extraction sockets in periodontitis patients: A randomized controlled study. *Clinical Oral Implants Research, 29*(2), 202–214.
22. Araujo-Pires, A. C., Mendes, V. C., Ferreira-Junior, O., Carvalho, P. S., Guan, L., & Davies, J. E. (2016). Investigation of a novel PLGA/CaP scaffold in the healing of tooth extraction sockets to alveolar bone preservation in humans. *Clinical Implant Dentistry and Related Research, 18*(3), 559–570.
23. Min, S., Liu, Y., Tang, J., Xie, Y., Xiong, J., You, H. K., et al. (2016). Alveolar ridge dimensional changes following ridge preservation procedure with novel devices: Part 1--CBCT linear analysis in non-human primate model. *Clinical Oral Implants Research, 27*(1), 97–105.
24. Verweij, J. P., Anssari Moin, D., Wismeijer, D., & van Merkesteyn, J. P. R. (2017). Replacing heavily damaged teeth by third molar autotransplantation with the use of cone-beam computed tomography and rapid prototyping. *Journal of Oral and Maxillofacial Surgery, 75*(9), 1809–1816.
25. Boerckel, J. D., Mason, D. E., McDermott, A. M., & Alsberg, E. (2014). Microcomputed tomography: Approaches and applications in bioengineering. *Stem Cell Research & Therapy, 5*(6), 144.
26. Swain, M. V., & Xue, J. (2009). State of the art of Micro-CT applications in dental research. *International Journal of Oral Science, 1*(4), 177–188.
27. Ho, S. T., & Hutmacher, D. W. (2006). A comparison of micro CT with other techniques used in the characterization of scaffolds. *Biomaterials, 27*(8), 1362–1376.
28. Li, H., Zhang, H., Tang, Z., & Hu, G. (2008). Micro-computed tomography for small animal imaging: Technological details. *Progress in Natural Science, 18*(5), 513–521.
29. Donnelly, E. (2011). Methods for assessing bone quality: A review. *Clinical Orthopaedics and Related Research, 469*(8), 2128–2138.
30. Hambli, R. (2013). Micro-CT finite element model and experimental validation of trabecular bone damage and fracture. *Bone, 56*(2), 363–374.
31. Kothari, M., Keaveny, T. M., Lin, J. C., Newitt, D. C., Genant, H. K., & Majumdar, S. (1998). Impact of spatial resolution on the prediction of trabecular architecture parameters. *Bone, 22*(5), 437–443.
32. Buytaert, J., Goyens, J., De Greef, D., Aerts, P., & Dirckx, J. (2014). Volume shrinkage of bone, brain and muscle tissue in sample preparation for micro-CT and light sheet fluorescence microscopy (LSFM). *Microscopy and Microanalysis, 20*(4), 1208–1217.

33. Kallai, I., Mizrahi, O., Tawackoli, W., Gazit, Z., Pelled, G., & Gazit, D. (2011). Microcomputed tomography-based structural analysis of various bone tissue regeneration models. *Nature Protocols, 6*(1), 105–110.
34. Kerckhofs, G., Chai, Y. C., Luyten, F. P., & Geris, L. (2016). Combining microCT-based characterization with empirical modelling as a robust screening approach for the design of optimized CaP-containing scaffolds for progenitor cell-mediated bone formation. *Acta Biomaterialia, 35*, 330–340.
35. Kerckhofs, G., Stegen, S., van Gastel, N., Sap, A., Falgayrac, G., Penel, G., et al. (2018). Simultaneous three-dimensional visualization of mineralized and soft skeletal tissues by a novel microCT contrast agent with polyoxometalate structure. *Biomaterials, 159*, 1–12.
36. Vickerton, P., Jarvis, J., & Jeffery, N. (2013). Concentration-dependent specimen shrinkage in iodine-enhanced microCT. *Journal of Anatomy, 223*(2), 185–193.
37. Wang, Y., Wertheim, D. F., Jones, A. S., & Coombes, A. G. A. (2010). Micro-CT in drug delivery. *European Journal of Pharmaceutics and Biopharmaceutics, 74*(1), 41–49.
38. Cengiz, I. F., Oliveira, J. M., & Reis, R. L. (2017). Micro-computed tomography characterization of tissue engineering scaffolds: Effects of pixel size and rotation step. *Journal of Materials Science Materials in Medicine, 28*(8), 129.
39. Wongsupa, N., Nuntanaranont, T., Kamolmattayakul, S., & Thuaksuban, N. (2017). Assessment of bone regeneration of a tissue-engineered bone complex using human dental pulp stem cells/poly(epsilon-caprolactone)-biphasic calcium phosphate scaffold constructs in rabbit calvarial defects. *Journal of Materials Science Materials in Medicine, 28*(5), 77.
40. Mizutani, R., & Suzuki, Y. (2012). X-ray microtomography in biology. *Micron (Oxford, England: 1993), 43*(2–3), 104–115.
41. Abe, S., Kida, I., Esaki, M., Akasaka, T., Uo, M., Hosono, T., et al. (2009). Biodistribution imaging of magnetic particles in mice: X-ray scanning analytical microscopy and magnetic resonance imaging. *Bio-Medical Materials and Engineering, 19*(2–3), 213–220.
42. Lee, J., Woo, J., Xing, F., Murano, E. Z., Stone, M., & Prince, J. L. (2014). Semi-automatic segmentation for 3D motion analysis of the tongue with dynamic MRI. *Computerized Medical Imaging and Graphics, 38*(8), 714–724.
43. Hashemi, R. H., Bradley, W. G., & Lisanti, C. J. M. R. I. (2017). *The basics*. Philadelphia: Lippincott Williams & Wilkins.
44. Schild, H. H. (1992). *MRI made easy:(–well almost)*. Wayne, NJ: Berlex Laboratories.
45. Chan, W. P., Lin, M. F., Fang, C. L., & Lai, W. F. (2004). MRI and histology of collagen template disc implantation and regeneration in rabbit temporomandibular joint: Preliminary report. *Transplantation Proceedings, 36*(5), 1610–1612.
46. Laakso, H., Wirth, G., Korpisalo, P., Yla-Herttuala, E., Michaeli, S., Yla-Herttuala, S., et al. (2018). T2, T1rho and TRAFF4 detect early regenerative changes in mouse ischemic skeletal muscle. *NMR in Biomedicine, 31*(5), e3909.
47. Bendszus, M., Wessig, C., Solymosi, L., Reiners, K., & Koltzenburg, M. (2004). MRI of peripheral nerve degeneration and regeneration: Correlation with electrophysiology and histology. *Experimental Neurology, 188*(1), 171–177.
48. Ribot, E. J., Tournier, C., Aid-Launais, R., Koonjoo, N., Oliveira, H., Trotier, A. J., et al. (2017). 3D anatomical and perfusion MRI for longitudinal evaluation of biomaterials for bone regeneration of femoral bone defect in rats. *Scientific Reports, 7*(1), 6100.
49. Kamei, N., Ochi, M., Adachi, N., Ishikawa, M., Yanada, S., Levin, L. S., et al. (2018). The safety and efficacy of magnetic targeting using autologous mesenchymal stem cells for cartilage repair. *Knee Surgery, Sports Traumatology, Arthroscopy, 26*(12), 3626–3635.

# Chapter 5
# Application of Bioreactors in Dental and Oral Tissue Engineering

**Leila Mohammadi Amirabad, Jamie Perugini, and Lobat Tayebi**

## 1 Introduction

Increased rate of tooth loss and craniofacial trauma necessitate development of novel methods for regeneration of oral and dental tissues, including dentine-pulp complex, salivary glands, oral mucosa, connective tissues, temporomandibular joints (TMJ), periodontium, vascular, bone, cartilage tissues, and nerves. Scaffolds in tissue engineering can offer biomedical cues to the stem cells and thereby provide a new approach to tissue-engineered grafts.

In the engineering of oral tissues, the cells cannot penetrate into the center of three-dimensional scaffolds that are thicker than 100–200 μm. Even if the cells penetrate to the depth and spread homogeneously, after long periods in the cell culture, extracellular matrix (ECM) will accumulate throughout the scaffolds. In static culture, since the only way for transferring materials is diffusion, the nutrients and oxygen cannot penetrate sufficiently into the center of the scaffolds. Therefore, some cells move from the center to the peripheral region through chemotaxis. Accumulated cells at peripheral region secrete more ECM, which further impedes the diffusion of nutrients to the center region. This phenomenon causes cell necrosis and lack of tissue regeneration at the center of the scaffolds. To overcome this problem and make a larger homogenous engineered construct, fluid transport should be applied.

Bioreactors are engineered systems developed to provide a biologically active environment that delivers the nutrients and oxygen to the cells in the depth. The early systems of bioreactors were rotating wall, spinner flasks, and rocker bioreactors, which provide mass transport of medium to the scaffolds and development of homogenous engineered tissues.

L. Mohammadi Amirabad · J. Perugini · L. Tayebi (✉)
Marquette University School of Dentistry, Milwaukee, WI, USA
e-mail: lobat.tayebi@marquette.edu



L. Tayebi (ed.), *Applications of Biomedical Engineering in Dentistry*,
https://doi.org/10.1007/978-3-030-21583-5_5

In addition to homogenous distribution of cells and chemical factors, recapitulating the mechanical and electrical stimulation should also be established to make the fully functional engineered tissues. The next generation of bioreactors can impart such mechanical or electrical stimulations to the cells for developing engineered construct with more similarity to their native counterparts. The cells respond to these biophysical cues through modification of gene expression, production of ECM, etc. Each type of tissue requires specific stimulation on the basis of comprehensive recognition of its biological aspect. For example, shear stress enhanced regeneration of bone, cartilage, and blood vessels; torsional and tensile forces improved ligament differentiation; compressive forces increased chondrogenesis; and electrical impulses enhanced efficiency of nerve, cardiac, and skeletal muscle differentiation. Therefore, tissue-specific bioreactors should be applied according to biological cues of each kind of tissue.

Another important application of bioreactors is in vitro investigation of cellular interaction in tissue development by providing a specific microenvironment. The bioreactors should be designed to cover the microenvironment properties of target tissue we want to engineer.

In this chapter, first we focus on the key principles required for bioreactor designing used in oral and dental tissue engineering. Here, we discuss the structural, mechanical, and electrical properties in the microenvironment of dental and oral tissues. Moreover, we will illustrate the materials and structural design, which are important in manufacturing the bioreactors to recapitulate the tissue microenvironment. Subsequently, the different kinds of bioreactors with their different designs will be described. Eventually, an overview of bioreactors used in engineering of different dental and oral tissues is provided.

## 2 Bioreactor Design Requirements in Dental/Oral Tissue Engineering

Designed bioreactors can improve uniform distribution of the cells, delivering the nutrients and gases. Moreover, according to target tissue, they can provide controllable chemical and physical stimuli and, hence, information about the evolution of the tissues. Although the requirements for designing a bioreactor depend on its application, there are some universal principles.

Materials used to manufacture the bioreactors are very important factors. They should be sterilizable, bioinert, and biocompatible in 37 °C and humid atmosphere and have proper mechanical strength, chemical, and physical characteristics and structure.

Parts of the bioreactors that are in contact with culture medium should be sterilizable by autoclaving and soaking in disinfectant, such as 70% ethanol, gamma, UV, and X-rays. Hence, the materials should be resistant in aforementioned sterilization methods. Furthermore, the materials should be bioinert without any leakage in the medium after sterilization. For example, among metals, stainless steel with chromium ions is a bioinert material and easily autoclavable.

The other characteristics of materials used in the bioreactors are opaque and transparent. To monitor the events which are happening in the bioreactor, the material to create chambers should be transparent. Glass is a good candidate for this reason, but the difficulty of carving and manufacturing it to make specific shapes of chambers limits its usage. Plexiglass is another transparent material which can be carved easily into different shapes. But, the low stability of plexiglass against numerous cycles of sterilization limits its application.

Another characteristic of materials for making the components of bioreactors is flexibility. The pipes that transfer the medium between different chambers and O-rings, which prevent water leakage, should be flexible.

To transfer electrical stimulation and impulses to the cells and constructs in the bioreactors, some electrodes should be incorporated in the chambers. These electrodes should be electrically conductive as well as biocompatible, bioinert, and serializable. Stainless steel 316, with its high resistance against acids and corrosion, is an electroconductive metal with good biocompatible trait. Aluminum, gold, and carbon rod electrodes are the other conductive materials used for electrical stimulation.

The bioreactors also should be designed to be easily and quickly assembled without any contaminations. The sensor should be incorporated for monitoring oxygen and nutrient concentration, pH level, etc. For applying the mechanical and electrical forces, the motors, pumps, and devices should be designed to make stimulations with low intensity range, fit in an incubator, and work in humidified atmosphere and 37 °C temperature. Moreover, bioreactors should have multiple chambers to repeat the experiments simultaneously and achieve statistically true results. In tissue engineering using bioreactors, scaffolds are the usual constructs, which accelerate differentiation and tissue engineering. Therefore, some elements should be designed in the bioreactor to restrain the scaffolds and constructs in an appropriate place.

Despite abovementioned parameters in designing bioreactors, detailed design parameters depend on the target tissue and our goal of study. For example, to make neural or muscular tissue, electrical stimulation can enhance making functional tissues, whereas electrical stimulation does not affect significantly bone regeneration. Furthermore, for example, for investigation of hydrostatic pressure on the engineering of a specific tissue, flow perfusion should not be applied even with positive effect.

Although bioreactors can make some similar stimuli in the body, it is technically difficult to design and manipulate bioreactor systems that can recapitulate the physical/biological situation in tissues or organs due to the complexity of the structure of tissues and organs in the body. In the next section, we explain the structure, requirements, and work mechanisms of different types of bioreactors used in dental and oral tissue engineering.

## 3 Types of Bioreactors

A functional tissue construct is ordinarily achieved by applying some specific biological stimulation and cues, which recapitulate the crucial elements of the microenvironment of cell niche. These stimulations could be shear stress, dynamic compressive and torsional loads, flow-induced pressure, electrical impulses, etc. (Fig. 5.1). Each of this stimulation can be applied in vitro by designing specific tissue bioreactor according to the target tissue. Here, we will describe the different bioreactor models that have ever been used in oral and dental tissue engineering.

## 3.1 Spinner Flask Bioreactors

In this kind of bioreactor, the engineered constructs are suspended or placed in the moving fluid through microcarriers or different holders (Fig. 5.2a, b) [1, 2], which is produced by a magnetic rod stirrer. The convective and turbulent flow in the media makes eddies and shear forces in the pores of scaffolds, and, thereby, diffusion of the nutrients, gases, and wastes between the cells seeded at the center of the scaffolds and the surrounded bulk media. This diffusion of nutrients to the depths of the scaffolds allow uniform growth of the cells throughout the scaffolds. The volume of the spinner (or stirred-tank) flask bioreactor is between 100 and 8000 ml, and the speed of the stirrer runs at 40–80 RPM.

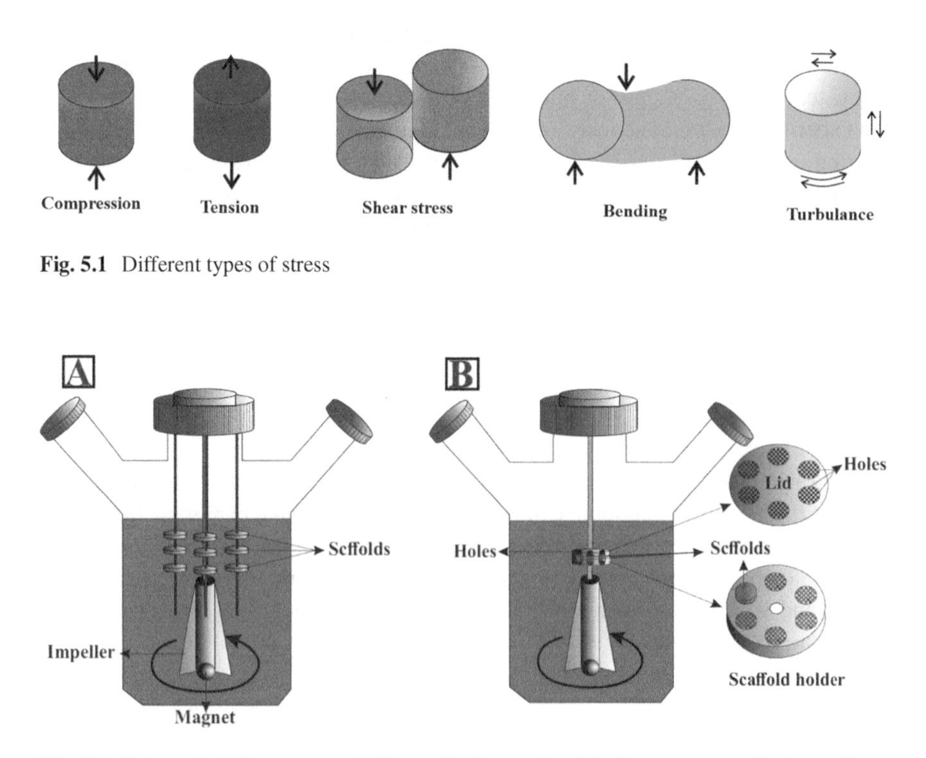


**Fig. 5.1** Different types of stress

**Fig. 5.2** Spinner flask bioreactors. (**a**) The scaffolds are placed in direct contact with the medium. (**b**) The scaffolds are placed in a holder where the scaffolds contact with media throughout the embedded holes in the lid and holder

The rotation flow in the spinner flasks cannot recapitulate the natural niche of tissues. Moreover, the difficulties in handling and scaling limit the spinner flask bioreactor in the tissue engineering.

## 3.2 *Rotating Wall Vessel Bioreactors*

Like spinner flask bioreactors, this kind of bioreactor is used for transferring the nutrients, gases, and wastes between the engineered construct and bulk of the fluid. These bioreactors induce shear stress with fewer turbulence, which provided a better controlled nutrient supply. In the rotating well vessel bioreactors, the cells, scaffolds, and other constructs are free to move in media between two concentric cylinders. The outer wall rotation (15–30 RPM) produces centrifugal force (Fc) and hydrodynamic drag force (Fd), which are in balance with gravitational force (Fg) (Fig. 5.3). As the cells in the scaffolds proliferate and the construct becomes heavier, the rotational speed of outer wall should be enhanced to counteract the force of gravity. Otherwise, the scaffolds lose their suspension and deposit at the bottom of the outer wall. Hence, a dynamic culture with mass transferring and low shear stress are made with this rotation. These bioreactors provide more homogenous cell distribution in the scaffolds than static culture. In this kind of bioreactor, gas exchange occurs through a semipermeable membrane on the inner cylinder or a filter. The size of engineered constructs in this kind of bioreactor is small, which negatively affects their clinical usage.

## 3.3 *Rocker Bioreactors*

The rocker or wave bioreactors consist of a heavy-duty base unit, rocker tray, bag, and sensors (Fig. 5.4). The tray is mounted underneath the bag and applies rocking motion using a smooth waveform motion to help gas transferring, bubble-free aeration, and minimize shear stress. Trays also include a heater and thermocouple. Bags are disposable and sterile chambers. The oxygen, pH, and temperature sensors are submerged in the bag of this bioreactor. Rocking angle and rate, bag volume, type, and geometry affect fluid flow and oxygen transfer efficiency. Indeed, the efficiency of mixing is directly related to rocking angle, rocking rate, and filling level. Moreover, with enhanced volume of the bag, the efficiency of mixing decreases [3]. The power input is another factor that is directly proportional to the angle and rate of rocking. The hydrodynamic cell stress is decreased by rocking rate. On the other hand, increasing the rocker rate causes effective transfer of the nutrient and oxygen, therefore enhancing cell growth. Some of bioreactors that are categorized in this kind of bioreactor group apply low-magnitude high-frequency motion to the construct. Numerous studies have shown that this mechanical vibration influences regeneration of some tissue like bone through ERK1/2 activation [3, 4]. The

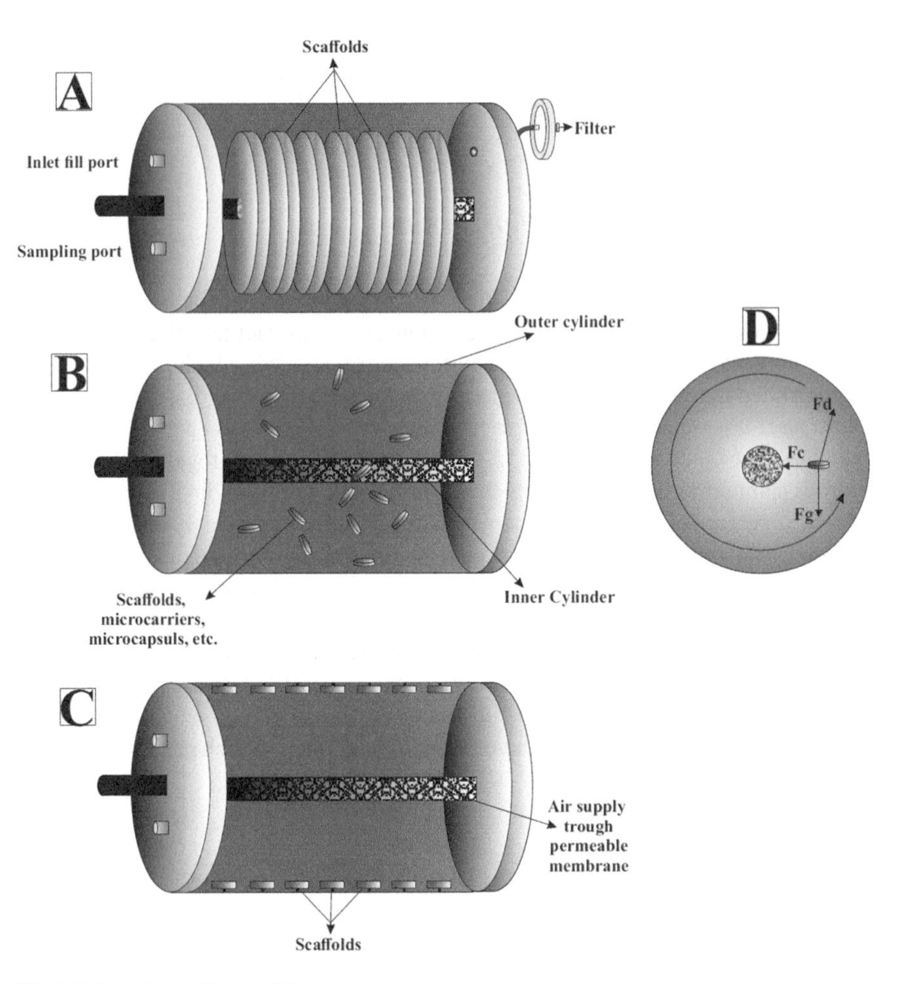


**Fig. 5.3** Rotating wall vessel bioreactors

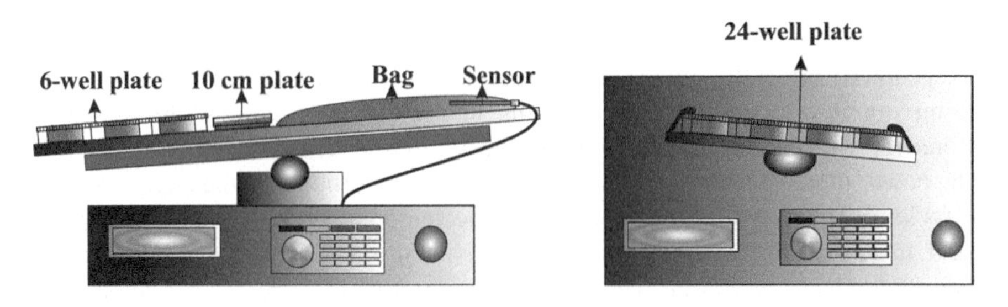


**Fig. 5.4** Rocker bioreactors. Two kinds of rocker bioreactor designed for applying vibration with different intension

vibration with low amplitude and low frequency recapitulates physiological processes such as walking and the pulsatile flow of blood. The vibration with a specific frequency and magnitude can induce bone and musculoskeletal regeneration [5, 6]. Accordingly, nano−/microvibrational bioreactors are designed for this purpose. However, this bioreactor cannot mimic appropriately the milieu of tissue, which limits their use in engineering of different tissues.

### *3.4 Flow Perfusion Bioreactors*

Although the previous described bioreactors can enhance the mass transferring at the center of the scaffolds, they still cannot mimic the microenvironment of tissues. Perfusion bioreactor systems may be more complicated to operate than the previous bioreactors by providing more controlled flow patterns. Flow perfusion bioreactors typically consist of a scaffold chamber, which connects to a reservoir thorough input and output tubes. A peristaltic pump can apply perfused flow in the chamber, recapitulating the releasing of nutrients and collecting of wastes throughout the blood vessels in the tissues. By using peristaltic pumps, since the medium does not contact with the pump elements, it is easy to maintain sterility.

Flow perfusion bioreactors are categorized into indirect or direct bioreactor. In the direct perfusion bioreactor, the scaffolds or constructs fit in the chambers and are kept in the path of media flow. This prevents the medium from flowing around the periphery, and, thereby, the medium perfuses into the interstices of the scaffolds and transfers shear stress to the cells. If the indirect perfusion bioreactor of the scaffolds or constructs does not fit in the chamber, the media pass around the scaffolds, causing a reduction in mass-transfer efficiency throughout the scaffolds. Among the rotating wall, spinner, rocker, and perfusion bioreactors, it has been proven that flow perfusion bioreactor provides the best biological fluid transport and homogenous cell distribution throughout the scaffolds in long-term cell culturing [3]. The peristaltic pumps make it possible to cultivate the large-sized engineered construct by enhancing mass transport.

Since perfusion systems need a large amount of cell culture medium to accelerate circulating flow between chamber and reservoir, the secreted factors from the cells may be remarkably diluted and a large volume of growth factors is required. To surmount this problem, the medium can be exchanged partially to maintain the advantage of the conditional medium (Fig. 5.5a).

In indirect perfusion bioreactors, the medium pass easily preferentially around the constructs. While, in direct perfusion bioreactors, the medium is perfused throughout the cell/scaffold constructs because the constructs are fitted in the chamber placed in a path of flow (Fig. 5.5b).

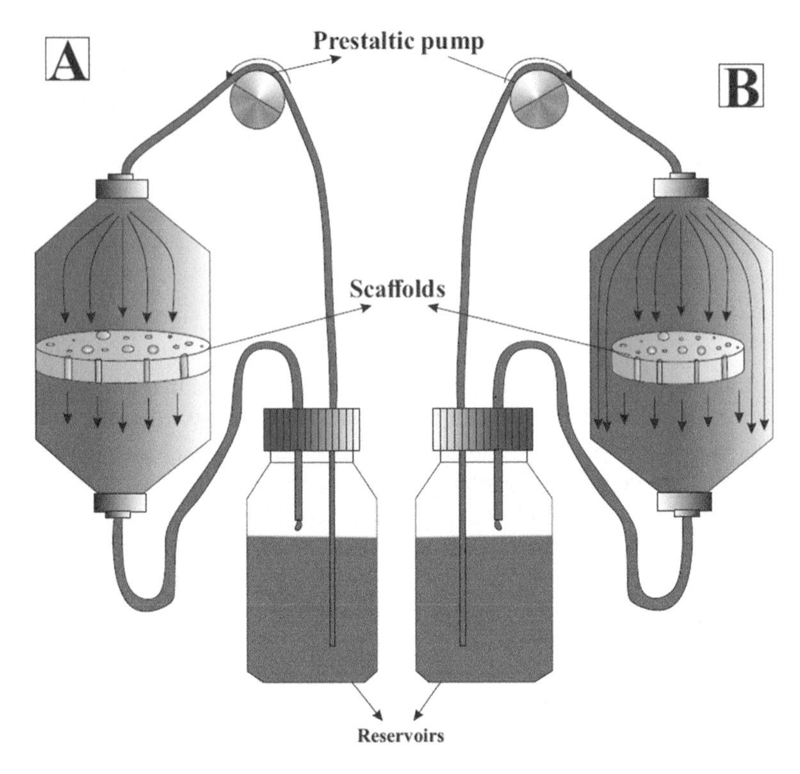


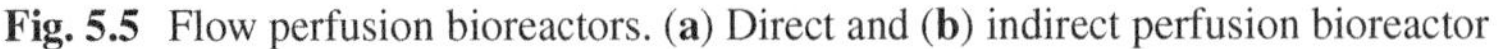

**Fig. 5.5** Flow perfusion bioreactors. (**a**) Direct and (**b**) indirect perfusion bioreactor

## *3.5 Hydrostatic Pressure Bioreactors*

In this kind of bioreactor, the cells are seeded on the scaffolds in static cell culture, then the cell-seeded scaffolds transfer to a hydrostatic chamber. A hydrostatic pressure bioreactor includes various parts such as the chamber where the scaffolds are located, a piston that is controlled by an actuator, and a sterile impermeable flexible membrane which is placed between piston and media in the chamber (Fig. 5.6). Design diversity of hydrostatic pressure bioreactors includes a pressure piston, which pressurizes the chamber containing medium through a flexible and impermeable film and is controlled by a variable back pressure valve and an actuator.

## *3.6 Strain Bioreactors*

This kind of bioreactor usually has been used in connective tissue and cardiac tissue engineering. In strain bioreactors, the way through which the strain force is transferred to engineered construct differs compared with compression bioreactor. The strain bioreactor system is composed of an actuator and a chamber where two anchors, including an actuating and fixed anchor, are located. The opposite ends of

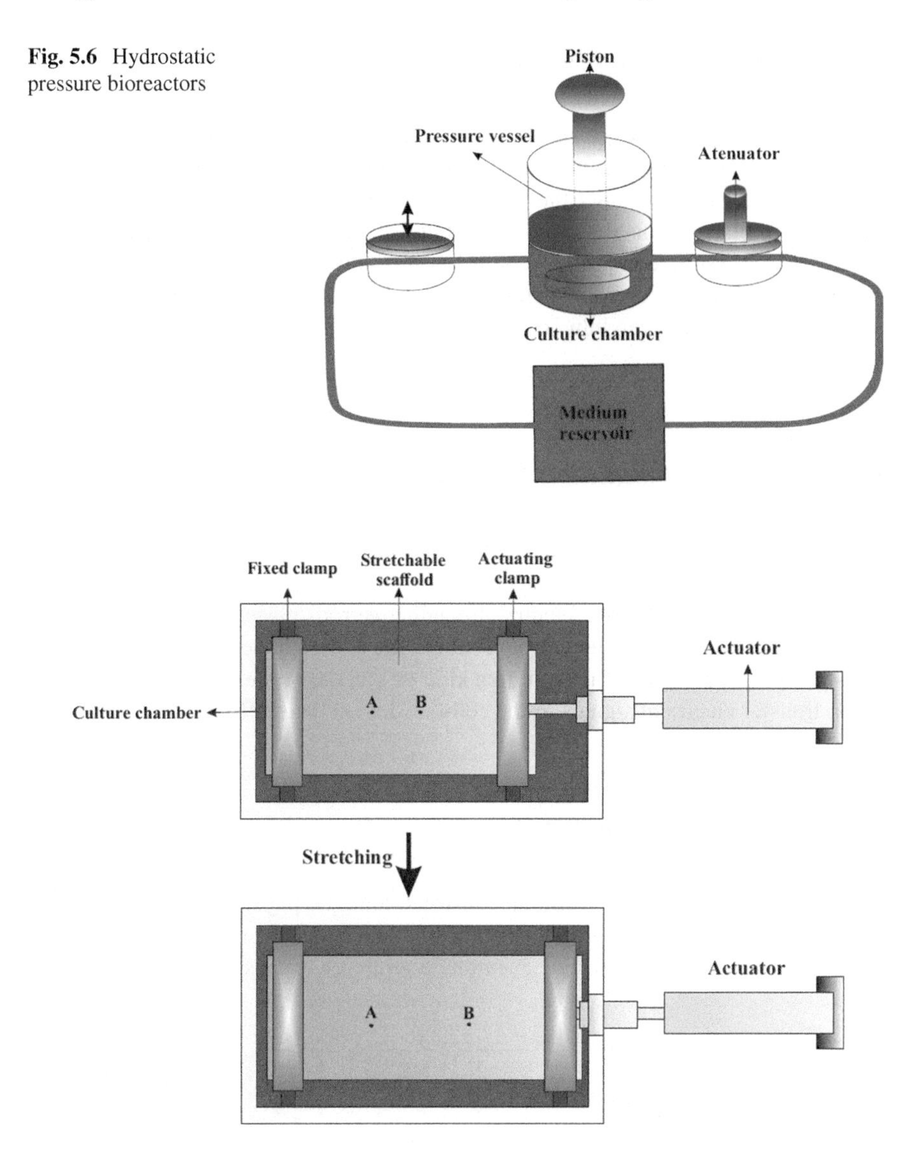


**Fig. 5.6** Hydrostatic pressure bioreactors

**Fig. 5.7** Strain bioreactor before and after stretching

scaffolds are held by fixed and actuating anchors. When stretching starts, the actuating anchor starts moving outward, whereas the fixed anchor remains in place (Fig. 5.7). The scaffolds used in these bioreactors should be a flexible material, such as PDMS membrane. In piezoelectric scaffolds two electrically conductive and flexible rods were placed on the two sides of scaffolds in a chamber. Whenever an electrical field is applied on these piezoelectric scaffolds, the scaffolds start stretching. This system could increase the Young's modulus of the construct in cartilage, ligament, and tendon tissue engineering.

## 3.7 Compression Bioreactors

Compression bioreactors are the other commonly used bioreactors for applying static and dynamic loadings. The static compression bioreactor consists of a system supplying linear motion and a flat platen placed on the lid of a chamber, in which scaffolds are placed. This flat platen distributes the load on the cells seeded on the scaffolds. In dynamic compression bioreactors, the mass transfer applies the compression load on the scaffold using the fluid flow. Compression bioreactor can enhance the aggregate modulus of cartilage and other connective tissue-like constructs [7].

## 3.8 Electrical Stimulation Bioreactors

Electrical stimuli are the other physical stimuli that are important for neural, skeletal muscle, and cardiac tissue engineering. The electrical field can be harnessed in a chamber of bioreactor by two electrical conductive rods placed at the two sides of the chamber, while a pulse generator produces the electrical field between two rods (Fig. 5.8) [8]. The scaffolds used in this kind of bioreactor are electrically conductive to transfer electrical signals to the cells seeded on the scaffolds.

## 3.9 Combined Bioreactors

Sometimes to make a fully functional construct, multiple physical stimuli should be applied on the engineering construct to recapitulate better the native microenvironment of the tissue (Fig. 5.9). For example, a strain or hydrostatic bioreactor with

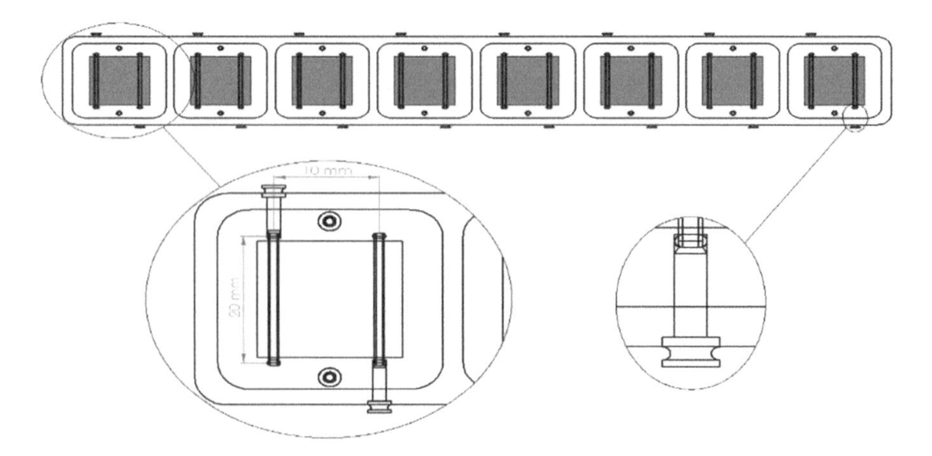


**Fig. 5.8** An eight-electrical stimulation bioreactor with two electrodes placed at the two ends of each chamber [8]

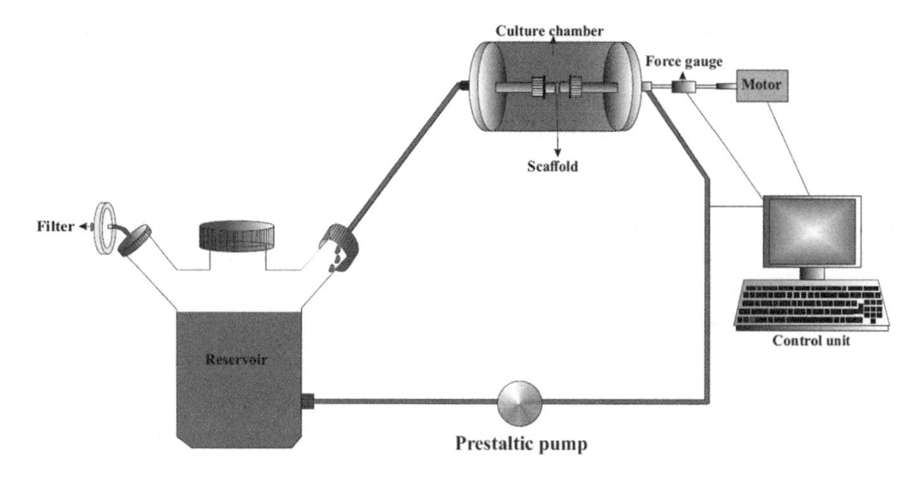


**Fig. 5.9** Perfusion bioreactor combined with compression one

added perfusion can deliver nutrients effectively along with applying mechanical stimuli [8–10]. Some bioreactors can also be designed for engineering of a specific tissue. For example, for vocal fold tissue, a combined tensile and vibrational bioreactor was designed with similar vibrations and amplitude in human [11].

## *3.10 In Vivo Bioreactors*

The previous described bioreactors are in vitro and provide some electrical and mechanical stimuli for the cells ex vivo. Nevertheless, in vitro recapitulating all local biophysical cues in the microenvironment of the natural tissue and vascularization are difficult. The body of organisms could be utilized as an in vivo bioreactor, where multiple biophysical cues, even those unknown factors which could enhance regeneration, can be applied on the engineering construct. The history of using this kind of bioreactor dates back to the 1960s when the scientists implanted silicon molds in the rat as in vivo bioreactors to generate vascularized bone construct [7]. Many small and large animal models can be used as in vivo bioreactors, such as rats, mice, and rabbits as small animals and sheep, mini pigs, and nonhuman primates as large animals. Using small animal is more common because their price and cost of maintenance are affordable. Moreover, this model requires only a small amount of materials, such as scaffolds and chemical. However, diffusional challenges in defects of the human cannot be simulated in small models, which make large animals more suitable in vivo bioreactors for therapeutic goals in human. In some defects, the defect position itself can be used as an in vivo bioreactor.

There are several important factors in using in vivo bioreactors such as prefabrication site, time, and geometry. Each site in an organism has different progenitor cells, signaling molecules, vascularization capacity, and nerves. For implantation, a site that most closely resembles the target tissue environment should be chosen. Moreover, the site should be accessible to the harness where less pain is felt and less inflammatory responses are produced. Time of implantation, when the development of the target tissue is at peak quality and quantity, is another important factor in using in vivo bioreactor. In tissue engineering of some constructs, the shape of the site of implantation is another prefabrication factor that can be designed to resemble the geometry of defect. For example, because geometric precision is a critical factor in facial bone tissue engineering, the site of in vivo bioreactor is considered the defect site in a patient, and, thereby, the scaffolds used are designed geometrically similar to defect site.

# 4 Applied Bioreactors in Dental/Oral Tissue Engineering

Engineering of 3D tissues needs transferring the materials throughout the engineering construct to make homogenous tissues. Hence, there is a requirement for bioreactors in tissue engineering of different constructs. Oral and dental tissues include a large range of tissues, such as dentine-pulp complex, salivary glands, oral mucosa, connective tissues, temporomandibular joints (TMJ), periodontium, vascular, bone, cartilage tissues, and nerves. The engineering of this tissue in vitro requires nutrients and gas delivery to the center of the construct, which could be achieved with the bioreactors. Here, the different bioreactors used in oral and dental tissue engineering will be described, and the efficiency of each bioreactor in engineering of each tissue will be discussed.

## *4.1 Bone Tissue*

In bone tissue engineering, the nutrients and gases should be transferred to recapitulate blood vessels in vitro using bioreactors that make flow fluid in the constructs. Spinner flask bioreactor, rotating wall vessels, rocker bioreactor, and flow perfusion bioreactor can make such fluid flow for the constructs with different efficiencies. Moreover, mechanical loads on the bone apply shear stress on the osteoblasts and osteoclasts, which cause enhancement in differentiation (gene expression of *ALP*, *BMP2, RUNX2, ColI*, *osteocalcin*, *fibronectin*, *osteonectin*) and $Ca^{2+}$ deposition. Perfusion bioreactors have more effective flow fluid perfusion and fewer turbulence in comparison to spinner flask and rotating wall bioreactors. The studies showed that rotating wall vessels bioreactors with applying more effective flow fluid and less turbulence compared with spinner flasks induce bone formation more effectively [12]. However, routine rocker bioreactors making high turbulence in the fluid are not good candidates for bone tissue engineering, yet rocker bioreactors with micro- and nano-vibration could be a useful instrument to enhance bone regeneration [13, 14]. Moreover, the studies show that hydrostatic pressure resembling the forces on the bones in the joints could enhance bone formation [15, 16]. Strain bioreactor is another type of bioreactor which could influence bone formation. Compression bioreactors are suitable bioreactors for bone reconstruction in vitro by recapitulating the compression forces on the bones of body. The studies showed that compression bioreactors could affect bone formation in vitro [17, 18]. Electrical stimulation is another factor that can affect bone formation [19, 20]. This electrical stimulation can resemble the electrical stimulation produced by neuron cells to induce bone regeneration. In the body, the progenitor cells of the bones and osteocytes are exposed to different forces and conditions produced by previous described bioreactors. By combination of aforementioned bioreactors, the condition of tissues in the body could be fully recapitulated, and therefore the bone formation could be effectively improved. It has been shown that there are different unknown factors which could influence bone regeneration. To achieve such a situation with all known and unknown factors, in vivo bioreactors could be used. The studies show that these bioreactors could augment bone regeneration in constructs produced in the aforementioned bioreactors [21, 22]. The different kinds of bioreactors and cell source are listed in Table 5.1.

## *4.2 Oral Cartilage, Tendon, and Ligament Tissue*

Cartilage tissues in different places, such as between the mandibular condyle and fossa-eminence, spread loads, absorb hits, and lubricate and facilitate bony surface. Cartilage injuries due to traumas and tumors at temporomandibular joint (TMJ) result in quality reduction of life. Lack of vascular and neural tissues in such cartilage tissues causes minimal capacity to repair. The advancement in tissue engineering using bioreactors confers a promising approach for cartilage regeneration.

The cartilage tissue, for example, at TMJ disk, primarily consists of fibrochondrocytes. The meniscus in TMJ is one of fibrocartilaginous cartilage tissues, which disperses loads in the joint and therefore decreases bone friction. These kind of stratified cartilage tissues are composed of different layers with different types and amount of extracellular matrix. This structure is created due to biomechanical forces in microenvironment of the cells. Calcified layers at deeper sites are exposed to the lowest oxygen levels and highest hydrostatic pressures. Compressive loads at the center of disk cause chondrocyte accumulation, whereas the middle layer is exposed to compression loads, hydrostatic pressure, and higher oxygen levels. Compression loads cause radial expansion of the disk, and hence the peripheral sites of disk are exposed to tensile hoop stresses, leading to fibroblast aggregation [79]. Previous studies have shown that mechanic stimuli could induce cell proliferation and chondrogenic differentiation [80]. Bioreactors that can provide these mechanical and oxygen stimuli in vitro are suitable for cartilage and other similar mechanosensitive tissues. The compression-tension/relaxation bioreactors can provide desirable mechanical stimuli and perfusion on the engineering construct. Some bioreactors used in tissue engineering of cartilage tissues are listed in Table 5.2.

**Table 5.1** Different kinds of bioreactors used in bone tissue engineering

| Bioreactor | Bioreactor (material and company) | Scaffolds (material, shape, and dimension) | Chemical factors | Cells/tissue | Condition | Results | Mechanical stimulation | Authors |
|---|---|---|---|---|---|---|---|---|
| Spinner flask | Bellco Glass, Vineland, NJ, USA | PET 3D-fibrous cylindric D: 6 mm × Fiber diameter: 22 μm | Ascorbic acid (50 μg/mL), dexamethasone (10 nM), and β-glycerophosphate (10 mM) | A-hMSCs ($10^6$ cells/ scaffold) | 21 days in differentiation medium; rotation rate: 50 RPM | Proliferation: ↑ Differentiation: ALP↓ | Shear stress Hydrodynamic pressure | Yasuda et al. [9] |
| | NA | Collagen films (cylindric, 11 × 1.5 mm); silk scaffolds (cylindric, 6 × 1.5 mm) | DMEM supplemented with 10% FBS, ascorbic acid 2-phosphate (50 μg/ml), dexamethasone (10 mM), β-glycerol phosphate (7 mM), and BMP-2 (1 μg/ ml) | BM-hMSCs (5 × $10^6$/ scaffold | 35 days in differentiation medium; rotation rate: 50 RPM | Differentiation: ALP↑, $Ca^{2+}$ ↑ | Shear stress Hydrodynamic pressure | Meinel et al. [23] |
| | Bellco Glass, Vineland, NJ, USA | Silk loaded with BMP-2 (cylindric 4 × 2 mm) | DMEM supplemented with 10% FBS, Pen-Strep, and Fungizone, ascorbic acid 2-phosphate (50 g/ mL), dexamethasone (10 nM), and β-glycerol phosphate (7 mM) | BM-hMSCs (Clonetics) 5 × $10^6$/ scaffold | 28 days in differentiation medium; rotation rate: 50 RPM | NA | Shear stress Hydrodynamic pressure | Karageorgiou et al. [24] |

| | | | | | | | | |
|---|---|---|---|---|---|---|---|---|
| | NA | Aqueous-derived fibroin silk scaffolds (cylindric, 15 × 5 mm) | α-MEM supplemented with 10% FBS, nonessential amino acids ($10^{-4}$ M), ascorbic acid 2-phosphate (50 mg/mL), dexamethasone ($10^{-8}$ M), β-glycerol phosphate (10 $10^{-3}$ M), and BMP-2 (1 $mg.ml^{-1}$) | BM-hMSCs (Cambrex) $10^6$/scaffold | 84 days in differentiation medium; rotation rate: 50 RPM | Proliferation: ↑ Differentiation: ALP↑, $Ca^{2+}$ ↑; gene expression of ALP/OP/BSP/Col1↑; compressive modulus and strength ↑ | Shear stress Hydrodynamic pressure | Kim et al. [25] |
| | Bellco Glass, Vineland NJ, USA | Silk fibroin disk (8 × 2 mm) small pores (112–224 μm) large pores (400–500 μm) mixed pores | DMEM, 10% FBS, Pen-Strep, Fungizone, L-ascorbic, 2-phosphate (0.5 mg/mL), dexamethasone (10 nM), β-glycerophosphate (10 mM), BMP-2 (1 mg/mL) | BM-hMSCs (Clonetics) 5 × $10^6$/scaffold | 35 days in differentiation and standard medium; rotation rate: 60 RPM | Proliferation: ↓; cell viability and cell activity: ↔; death cell deposition↓ | Shear stress Hydrodynamic pressure | Hofmann et al. [26] |

(continued)

**Table 5.1** (continued)

| Bioreactor | Bioreactor (material and company) | Scaffolds (material, shape, and dimension) | Chemical factors | Cells/tissue | Condition | Results | Mechanical stimulation | Authors |
|---|---|---|---|---|---|---|---|---|
| | Bellco Glass, Vineland NJ, USA | Coralline hydroxyapatite disk (10 × 2 mm) pores (200–500 μm) | MEM containing 10% FBS, and 1,25-(OH)2-vitamin D3 ($10^8$ M) | BM-hMSCs-TERT 2 × 106/ scaffold | 21 days in differentiation medium; rotation rate: 30 RPM | Proliferation: P200 = P500 Five differentiation: P200 ↑ ALP ↑; gene expression of ALP, COL1, RUNX2, BMP-2, BSP, Osterix, ON, OP ↑, P500 = ALP | Shear stress Hydrodynamic pressure | Mygind et al. [10] |
| | Bellco Glass, Vineland, NJ, USA | PLGA (cubic, 8 × 8 × 5 mm) | MEM containing 10% FBS, Penicillin (100 U/mL), and streptomycin (100 μg/mL); dexamethasone (100 nM), ascorbic acid (290 nM L), and β-glycerophosphate (5 mM) or with calcitriol (10 nM) | BM-hMSCs-TERT $2 \times 10^6$/ scaffold | 21 days in differentiation medium; rotation rate: 30 RPM | Proliferation: ↔ Differentiation: ↑ ALP, $Ca^{2+}$ ↑; gene expression of COL1, BMP-2, RUNX2, ON↑ | Shear stress Hydrodynamic pressure | Stiehler et al. [27] |

|  |  |  |  |  |  |  |  |  |
|---|---|---|---|---|---|---|---|---|
|  | Custom-made [11] | Gelatin-hyaluronic acid film (1.5 × 1.5 mm) | α-MEM medium supplemented with ascorbic acid (60 μM), β-glycerophosphate (10 mM), and dexamethasone (0.1 μM) | BM-hMSCs na/scaffold | 21 days in differentiation medium; rotation rate: 60 RPM | Proliferation: ↑<br>Differentiation: ALP, OC, COL1↑ | Shear stress<br>Hydrodynamic pressure | Wang et al. [28] |
|  | Bellco Glass, Vineland, NJ, USA | Disc-shaped scaffolds with copolymerization of LLA and LLA-co-DXO (1.3 × 12 mm) | α-MEM supplemented with FCS mixed with GM containing BBE, 2 mL; hEGF, 0.5 mL; hydrocortisone, 0.5 mL; FBS, 10 mL; GA-1000, 0.5 mL | HUVECs ($1–2.5 \times 10^6$/scaffold; osteoblast-like cells ($5 \times 10^6$/scaffold) | 25 days in differentiation medium | NA | Shear stress<br>Hydrodynamic pressure | Xing [29] |
|  | Bellco Glass, Vineland, NJ, USA | Chitosan disk (4 × 3 mm) | Low-glucose DMEM supplemented with 10% FBS, 1% Pen/Strep, dexamethasone (100 nM), β-glycerophosphate (10 mM), and 2-phospho-L-ascorbic acid (0.05 mM) | hMSCs; (Lonza) $5 \times 10^5$/scaffold | 14 days in differentiation and standard medium; rotation rate: 50 RPM | Proliferation: ↑<br>Differentiation: ALP, von Kossa ↑ | Shear stress<br>Hydrodynamic pressure | Teixeira et al. [1] |

(continued)

**Table 5.1** (continued)

| Bioreactor | Bioreactor (material and company) | Scaffolds (material, shape, and dimension) | Chemical factors | Cells/tissue | Condition | Results | Mechanical stimulation | Authors |
|---|---|---|---|---|---|---|---|---|
| | Custom-made [30] | Decellularized porcine bone (5 × 10 mm) | High-glucose DMEM, 10% FBS, ascorbic acid (50 mg/L), dexamethasone (1 mmol/L), β-sodium glycerophosphate (216 mg/L), penicillin (100 U/mL), and streptomycin (100 mg/mL) | BM-hMSCs AD-hMSCs $2.5 \times 10^5$/scaffold | 7 and 21 days in differentiation medium; rotation rate: 20 RPM | In AD-hMSCs »7 days: proliferation↑; gene expression of *COL1*↔, *OPN*↔, *RUNX2*↑, *OCN*↑, ALP activity↔; in 21 days: proliferation↑; COL1↔, OPN↔, RUNX2↔, OCN↔, ALP activity↑; In BM-hMSCs »7 days: proliferation↑; gene expression of *COL1*↔, *OPN*↓, *RUNX2*↔, *OCN*↑, ALP activity↔; in 21 days: proliferation↑; *COL1*↔, *OPN*↑, RUNX2↑, *OCN*↑, ALP activity↑↑-$Ca^{2+}$ deposition in AD-hMSCs ↑ << BM-hMSCs↑↑ | Shear stress Hydrodynamic pressure | Wei Wu et al. [30] |

| | | | | | | | | |
|---|---|---|---|---|---|---|---|---|
| | A custom-made spinner flask bioreactor system | 3D printed scaffolds (composite of PCL, PLGA, and β-TCP and mineralized ECM) (20 × 5.3× 0.6 mm) | DMEM 10% FBS, dexamethasone (10 nM), L-ascorbic acid (50 mg/mL), and β-glycerophosphate (10 mM) | hTMSCs[1] 2 × $10^5$/ scaffold | 14 days in differentiation medium; rotation rate: 50 RPM | NA | | |
| | Siliconized spinner flasks (Corning) | CultiSpher S microcarriers; beads with a diameter of 130–380 μm; pore size: ~10 μm | DMEM supplemented with 10% FBS, dexamethasone (2 μM), sodium β-glycerophosphate (0.5 mM), and ascorbic acid 2-phosphate (50 mg/L) (1 mL/24 well) | BM-hMSCs and HUVECs 1 × $10^5$ cells/ mL with 1:1 ratio | 4 weeks in differentiation and standard medium; rotation rate: 50 RPM | NA | Shear stress Hydrodynamic pressure | Zang et al. [2] |
| Rotating wall vessel | The Synthecon rotating wall bioreactor (TX, USA) | PLGA disk (4 × 2.5 mm) | M199 (GIBCO BRL, Grand Island, NY) culture medium supplemented with 10% FBS, and L-glutamine (2.5 mM) and β-glycerol phosphate (3 mM) | SAOS-2 (ATCC) ~2.22 × $10^5$/ scaffold | 7 days in differentiation medium; rotation rate: 25 RPM | Proliferation: ↓ Differentiation: ↑ ALP, Ca | Shear stress: <3.9 dynes/$cm^2$; hydrodynamic and mechanical forces | Botchwey et al. [31] |

(continued)

**Table 5.1** (continued)

| Bioreactor | Bioreactor (material and company) | Scaffolds (material, shape, and dimension) | Chemical factors | Cells/tissue | Condition | Results | Mechanical stimulation | Authors |
|---|---|---|---|---|---|---|---|---|
| | The Synthecon rotating wall bioreactor (TX, USA) | No scaffold | DMEM media treated with β-glycerophosphate (5 mM) and ascorbate (50 μg/mL) | HEPM (ATCC) $10 \times 10^6$/suspension | 28 days in differentiation and standard medium; rotation rate: 15 RPM; after aggregates formed this speed was increased | ↑ cell aggregation; ↑ Ca and P deposition | Shear stress: 0.5 dynes/$cm^3$ Gravity force: $10^{-2}$ g hydrodynamic pressure | Facer et al. [32] |
| | The Synthecon rotating wall bioreactor (TX, USA) | Alginate (containing TGF-β3 (10 ng/mL)/chitosan microcapsules (spheric, diameter = 5 mm) | α-MEM supplemented with 10% FCS and ascorbate-2-phosphate (100 μm) | Human MSC, human chondrocytes | 28 days in differentiation and standard medium; rotation rate: na | Proliferation↔, OC↑ | Shear stress Gravity force hydrodynamic pressure | Pound et al. [33] |
| | The Synthecon rotating wall bioreactor (TX, USA) | Gelatin-hyaluronic acid film (1.5 × 1.5 cm) | α-MEM medium supplemented with ascorbic acid (60 μM), β-glycerophosphate (10 mM), and dexamethasone (0.1 μM) | BM-hMSCs na/scaffold | 21 days in differentiation medium; rotation rate: 30 RPM | Proliferation: ↑ Differentiation: ↓ ALP, OC, COL1 | Shear stress Gravity force Hydrodynamic pressure | Wang et al. [28] |

| | | | | | | | | |
|---|---|---|---|---|---|---|---|---|
| | ZRP® system | ZrO2-based ceramic (Sponceram®) disk natural HA-coated (65 × 3 mm) | DMEM 10% FCS, 1% penicillin/streptomycin, dexamethasone (10 nM), ascorbic acid (0.3 mM), β-glycerol phosphate (10 mM) | AT-hMSCs $14 \times 10^6$/scaffold | 47 days in differentiation medium; rotation rate: 1 RPM | Proliferation: ↑<br>Differentiation: ↑ bone specific ECM; ↑ mineralization | Shear stress<br>Gravity force<br>Hydrodynamic pressure | Diederichs et al. [34] |
| | Rotating wall bioreactor (Cellon, Strassen, Luxembourg) | BCP-PCL nano-mesh PCL nano-mesh (10 × 10 × 0.06 mm) | DMEM 10% FBS, 1% antibiotic-antimycotic solution | MG63 (ATCC) $1.5 \times 10^5$/cm$^2$ | First 7- day in static; then 7 days in bioreactor; rotation rate: 16 RPM | Proliferation: ↔<br>Differentiation: ↑ protein amount | Shear stress<br>Gravity force<br>Hydrodynamic pressure | Araujo et al. [35] |
| | Pelco R2 rotary mixer | Gelatin-coral/HA (Pro-Osteon™) particles (0.5–1 mm) | α-MEM supplemented with 10% FCS, L-glutamine (2 mM), Pen-–Strep (both 100 U/ml), ascorbic acid (100 μg/mL), and dexamethasone (10–8 M) | BM-hMSCs; $5 \times 10^5$/scaffold | 21 days in differentiation medium; rotation rate: 7.5 RPM | Na | Shear stress<br>Gravity force<br>Hydrodynamic pressure | Ben-David et al. [36] |

(continued)

**Table 5.1** (continued)

| Bioreactor | Bioreactor (material and company) | Scaffolds (material, shape, and dimension) | Chemical factors | Cells/tissue | Condition | Results | Mechanical stimulation | Authors |
|---|---|---|---|---|---|---|---|---|
| | The Synthecon rotating wall bioreactor (TX, USA) | No scaffold | 1–3 days: osteoblast basal medium (10% FCS. OBM; Lonza, Allendale, NJ) supplemented with 10% (FCS), human recombinant M-CSF (50 ng/ml), and human recombinant RANKL (50 ng ml) 7–21 days: (mineralization medium) adding 200 μM hydrocortisone-21-hemisuccinate and 10 mm β-glycerol phosphate | Primary normal HOb cells (Lonza, Allendale, NJ); PromoCell (Heidelberg, Germany) $4.5–9 \times 10^6$ starting ratio of the HOb:HOcP cells in the initial seeding mixture (i.e., 2:1, 4:1 and 10:1) | Rotating speed: the initial rotation (first 4 hours for the construct formation) considered 15, 8, 4 and 1 rpm; 2–21 days ranging from 6 rpm to 25 RPM | NA | Shear stress<br>Gravity force<br>Hydrodynamic pressure | Clarke [37] |
| | High-aspect ratio vessel | PLAGA/n-HA and PLAGA (4 × 2.5 mm) | Osteogenic media (Lonza) | BM-hMSCs $5 \times 10^5$/scaffold | 28 days in differentiation medium; rotation rate: 35 RPM | NA | Shear stress<br>Gravity force<br>Hydrodynamic pressure | Lv et al. [38] |

| | | | | | | | | |
|---|---|---|---|---|---|---|---|---|
| | Biaxial rotating bioreactor (custom-made) | PolyActive™ 300/55/45 (PEOT[2]/PBT[3] scaffolds; PolyVation, the Netherlands) (8 × 3 mm) | α-MEM supplemented with 10% FBS, l-ascorbic acid 2-phosphate magnesium salt (0.2 mM), l-glutamine (2 mM), penicillin (100 U/mL), streptomycin (100 μg/mL), and bFGF (1 ng/mL) | hfMSCs; 7.5 × $10^5$/scaffold | 3 days in static culture; then 6 days in bioreactor; arm rotation rate: 2 RPM; chamber rotation speed: 3 RPM | Proliferation: ↑ Homogenous distribution of cells and ECM↑; Differentiation: gene expression of *F-actin*↑, *ALP*↔; *ColI*↑, *Runx2*↑ | Shear stress Gravity force Hydrodynamic pressure | Leferink [39] |
| Rocker bioreactor | The panel of GJX-5 vibration sensor (Beijing Sending Technology, Beijing, China) | Acellular human bone (tibias and femurs) derived scaffold; cubic, 13.4 × 8 × 5 mm; pore size: 90–700 μm; porosity: 88% | DMEM, 10% FBS, dexamethasone ($10^{-6}$ M), β-glycerol phosphate ($10^{-2}$ M), and ascorbic acid (50 μg/mL) | BM-MSCs $10^6$/scaffold | 26 days in differentiation medium at microvibration magnitude: 0.3 × g, frequency: 40 Hz, amplitude: ± 50 μm for 30 min every 12 h | Proliferation: ↓; Cbfa1, ALP, Col1, and osteocalcin↑ | Hydrodynamic pressure | Zhou et al. [13] |

(continued)

**Table 5.1** (continued)

| Bioreactor | Bioreactor (material and company) | Scaffolds (material, shape, and dimension) | Chemical factors | Cells/tissue | Condition | Results | Mechanical stimulation | Authors |
|---|---|---|---|---|---|---|---|---|
| | Custom-made; nanovibrational bioreactor with piezo-driven vibrational plate | Collagen (I) gel; cylindrical (7 × 33 mm) | DMEM supplemented with 10% FBS, ascorbic acid (100 μmol), and dexamethasone (50 nmol) | BM-MSCs $4 \times 10^4$ cells $ml^{-1}$ gel | 46 days in differentiation medium at (1000 Hz, 20 nm,) on the vibrational bioreactor | Proliferation: ↔; cell activity↑ Differentiation: gene expression of RUNX2, collagen I, ALP, OPN, osteocalcin (OCN), BMP2↑; mineralization↑ | Shear stress and strain | Tsimbouri [14] |
| Flow perfusion | Direct perfusion bioreactor | Cancellous human bone HA (Endobon®) (7.5 × 10 mm) | DMEM/F-12 (1:1) supplemented with 10% FCS | Human osteoblasts 12,500 cells/$cm^2$ | 10 days in standard medium; flow rate: 1 mL/h | NA | Hydrodynamic–/fluid-induced shear stress | Hofmann et al. [40] |
| | Perfusion cartridges (polycarbonate) | Collagen (film and cylindric, 11× 1.5 mm), silk (cylindric, 6 × 1.5 mm) | Osteogenic medium: control medium (DMEM supplemented with 10% FBS, Pen-Strep, and Fungizone) supplemented with ascorbic acid 2-phosphate (50 μg/ml), dexamethasone (10 mM), β-glycerol phosphate (7 mM), and BMP-2 (1 μg/ml) | Human MSC; passage 2 ($n = 2$ donors); $5 \times 10^6$ cells/scaffold | 35 days in osteogenic medium; flow rate: 0.2 mL/min | $Ca^{2+}$↓; individual bone rods oriented in the direction of fluid flow; biodegradation of the collagen scaffold↑ | Hydrodynamic–/fluid-induced shear stress | Meinel et al. [23] |

| | | | | | | | | |
|---|---|---|---|---|---|---|---|---|
| | Direct perfusion bioreactor | HA (Engipore®) (8 × 4 mm) | α-MEM containing 10% FBS, FGF-2 (5 ng/ml), dexamethasone (10 nM), and L-ascorbic acid 2-phosphate (0.1 mM) | hBMNCs; ~18 × $10^6$/ scaffold | 19 days in differentiation medium; flow rate: 100 μL/s | NA | Hydrodynamic–/ fluid-induced shear stress | Braccini et al. [41] |
| | Indirect perfusion bioreactor; custom-made, divergent, and convergent perfusion (cell culture flask) | ß-TCP cylinder (14 × 33 mm) | (DMEM) with high glucose (4.5 g /L) supplemented with 10% FBS, penicillin (100 U/ mL), streptomycin (100 μg/ mL), and 1% L-glutamine (200 mM) | h-MG63 osteoblast-like cells (10 × $10^6$/ scaffold) | 28 days in standard medium; flow rate: 3 mL/ min convergent and divergent flow setup | Proliferation: ↑; glucose consumption ↑; Homogeneous cell distribution: convergent > divergent > static | Hydrodynamic–/ fluid-induced shear stress | Olivier et al. [42] |

(continued)

**Table 5.1** (continued)

| Bioreactor | Bioreactor (material and company) | Scaffolds (material, shape, and dimension) | Chemical factors | Cells/tissue | Condition | Results | Mechanical stimulation | Authors |
|---|---|---|---|---|---|---|---|---|
| | Indirect perfusion bioreactor; perfusion containers (MINUCELLS and MINUTISSUE Vertriebs GmbH, Bad Abbach, Germany) | COL1-nanocrystalline HA tape (12 × 0.2 mm) | 1.Standard medium = $OS^-$: DMEM supplemented with 10% FCS, penicillin (10 U/mL) and streptomycin (100 μg/mL); osteogenic medium = $OS^+$ dexamethasone ($10^{-7}$ M), β-glycerophosphate (10 mM), and ascorbic acid 2-phosphate (0.05 mM) | BM-hMSCs (0.015 × $10^6$/scaffold) | 35 days in standard medium; 35 days in differentiation medium; flow rate: 1 mL/h | Proliferation: ↔ $OS^-$; ↔ Os+; differentiation: ↔ ALP in OS−; ↓ ALP in Os+ | Hydrodynamic−/fluid-induced shear stress | Bernhardt et al. [43] |
| | Custom-made, press-fit (PMMA) | 67% Si-TCP/33% HA/ß-TCP (SkeliteTM) (cylindric, 10 × 5 mm) | DMEM supplemented with 10% FBS | BM-hMSC-TERT 2 × $10^6$/scaffold | 21 days in standard medium; flow rate: 0.1 mL/min | Proliferation: ↑; Differentiation: gene expression of ALP, OPN, bone sialoprotein II, BMP2↑; gene expression of Col1, RUNX2, OC↓ homogenous distribution of cells and matrix↑ | Hydrodynamic−/fluid-induced shear stress | Bjerre et al. [44] |

| | | | | | | | | |
|---|---|---|---|---|---|---|---|---|
| | Custom-made (polycarbonate with PDMA) | Bovine cancellous bone (cylindric, 4 × 4 mm) | DMEM supplemented with 10% FBS and 1% penicillin-streptomycin, dexamethasone (10 nM), sodium β-glycerophosphate (10 mM), and ascorbic acid 2-phosphate (0.05 mM) | Human MSC Low density: $1.5\times 10^6$/scaffold High density: $3\times 10^6$/scaffold | 1 day in static, 7 days in osteogenic medium; flow rate: 10 μm/s; Then for 4 weeks the flow rate was increased to 1. 100 μm/s and 2. 400 μm/s | Increased perfusion rate from 100 mm/s to 400 mm/s: uniform cell distribution↑ Gene expression of Col, OP, BSP2↑ | Hydrodynamic−/fluid-induced shear stress | Grayson et al. [45] |
| | Direct perfusion bioreactor | $CaCO_3$ (Biocoral®) mineralized collagen TCP (Cerasorb®) (5 × 3 mm) | ZKT-1 medium, 15% FBS | hTBCs $5\times 10^6$ cells/$cm^3$ | 1 day in static condition,14 days in bioreactor with flow rate: at a speed to preserve freely suspention of the cell agregations mL/min | Osteocalcin (OC) expression↑; bone formation↑; VEGF expression↔; | Hydrodynamic−/fluid-induced shear stress | Schliephake et al. [46] |

(continued)

**Table 5.1** (continued)

| Bioreactor | Bioreactor (material and company) | Scaffolds (material, shape, and dimension) | Chemical factors | Cells/tissue | Condition | Results | Mechanical stimulation | Authors |
|---|---|---|---|---|---|---|---|---|
| | Indirect perfusion bioreactor | BCP particles (OsSatura™) (2–6 mm) | α-MEM supplemented with 10% FBS, antibiotics, L-ascorbic acid 2-phosphate (0.1 mM), L-glutamine (2 mM), dexamethasone ($1 \times 10^5$ mM), and bFGF (1 ng/ml) | BM-hMSCs (1–12) × $10^6$/all scaffolds | 20 days in differentiation medium; flow rate: 4 mL/s | Differentiation: ↔ ALP, CBFA1, COL1, OC, ON, S100A4, BMP-2 | Hydrodynamic−/fluid-induced shear stress | Janssen et al. [47] |
| | Direct perfusion bioreactor | Decellularized cow bone hTMJ-shaped (~15 × 15 × 5 mm) | High-glucose DMEM supplemented with 10% FBS, dexamethasone (10 nM), sodium β-glycerophosphate (10 mM), and ascorbic acid 2-phosphate (0.05 mM) | BM-hMSCs (Cambrex) 3.4 × $10^6$/scaffold | 35 days in differentiation medium; flow rate: 1.8 mL/s | Proliferation: ↑; Differentiation: ↑ bone volume | Hydrodynamic−/fluid-induced shear stress | Grayson et al. [47] |

| | | | | | | | | |
|---|---|---|---|---|---|---|---|---|
| | Direct perfusion bioreactor; custom-made (acrylic and polyetherimide plastics) | Decellularized cow bone plugs (4 × 4 mm) | High-glucose DMEM supplemented with 10% FBS, bFGF (1 ng/mL), and penicillin-streptomycin (1%) | A-hMSCs $1.5 \times 10^6$/ scaffold | 35 days in standard medium; 35 days in differentiation medium; flow rate: 1.8 mL/s | Proliferation: ↔ OS− ↔ OS+; Differentiation: bone specific ECM↑, COL, OP, BSP2↑; homogenous cell distribution↑ | Shear stress: ~0.01 Pa | Fröhlich et al. [48] |
| | Indirect perfusion bioreactor | B-TCP (Cerasorb®) (12 × 6 mm) 750 and 1400 μm pore size | Low-glucose DMEM containing 10% and 2% FCS, penicillin (10 U/ml), and streptomycin (100 μg/ml) | BM-hMSCs $0.2 \times 10^6$/ scaffold | 21 days in differentiation medium with 10% serum or 2% serum; flow rate: 1.5 mL/min | Proliferation: ↑ OS+ medium with 10% serum; ↔ OS+ medium with 2% serum; differentiation: ↔ OS+ medium with 10% serum; ↑ OS+ medium with 2% serum | Hydrodynamic−/ fluid-induced shear stress | Bernhardt et al. [49] |

(continued)

**Table 5.1** (continued)

| Bioreactor | Bioreactor (material and company) | Scaffolds (material, shape, and dimension) | Chemical factors | Cells/tissue | Condition | Results | Mechanical stimulation | Authors |
|---|---|---|---|---|---|---|---|---|
| | Direct perfusion bioreactor | Decellularized cow bone plugs ($4 \times 4$ mm) | DMEM supplemented with 10% FBS, nonessential amino acids (0.1 mM), 1% Pen-–Strep and 0.2% Fungizone, dexamethasone (10 nM), sodium β-glycerophosphate (7 mM), and ascorbic acid 2-phosphate (50 mg/mL) | BM-hMSCs (Cambrex) $1.2 \times 106$/scaffold | 35 days in differentiation medium; flow rate: 80, 400, 800, 1200, or 1800 μm/s | Flow velocities ranging from 400 to 800 μm/s: osteogenic responses↑ | Shear stress: 0.0006–0.02 Pa | Grayson et al. [50] |
| | Direct perfusion bioreactor | Porcine gelatin microcarrier (CultiSpher S) ($20 \times 10$ mm) | a-MEM supplemented with 10% FBS, ascorbic acid 2-phosphate (0.05 mg/mL), and mercaptoethanol ($5 \times 10^5$ M) | AM-hMSCs $5 \times 10^4$ cells/mg microcarriers | 28 days in standard medium; 7 days in differentiation medium; flow rate: 2 mL/min | NA | Hydrodynamic–/fluid-induced shear stress | Chen et al. [51] |

| | | | | | | | | |
|---|---|---|---|---|---|---|---|---|
| | Indirect perfusion bioreactor | PLLA disk (4 × 5 mm) 100, 250, and 500 μm pore size | High-glucose DMEM, with L-glutamine (4 mM), nonessential amino acids (0.1 mM), penicillin/streptomycin (1.0% v/v), 10% mesenchymal stem cells qualified FBS, β-dexamethasone (100 nM), β-glycerophosphate (10 mM), and ascorbic acid (50 mg/L) | BM-hMSCs (Lonza) $0.12 \times 10^6$/scaffold | 24 days in differentiation medium; flow rate: 0.3 mL/min | Differentiation: ↑ ALP, BMP-2 | Hydrodynamic−/fluid-induced shear stress | Pisanti et al. [52] |
| | A modified perfusion bioreactor introduced by Bader | Collagen meniscus implants (CMI, Menacell™, ReGen® Biologics Inc., Hackensack, NJ, USA) 5.5 mm (with hole: 4.5 mm) | DMEM/HAM's F-12 (1:1) with L-glutamine, 10% FCS, 5 μg/mL ascorbic acid, 3 ng/L FGF-2 | BM-hMSCs $10^6$/scaffold | 14 days in differentiation medium and continuous perfusion with flow rate: 10 mL/min (indirect) | Proliferation: ↑ Differentiation: procollagen I propeptide, ↑, procollagen III propeptide ↑, equilibrium modulus of the constructs↑ | Hydrodynamic−/fluid-induced shear stress | Petri et al. [17] |

(continued)

**Table 5.1** (continued)

| Bioreactor | Bioreactor (material and company) | Scaffolds (material, shape, and dimension) | Chemical factors | Cells/tissue | Condition | Results | Mechanical stimulation | Authors |
|---|---|---|---|---|---|---|---|---|
| | Direct perfusion bioreactor | Decellularized cow bone plugs (d 4 × h 4 mm) | DMEM supplemented with 10% (vol/vol) HyClone FBS and 1% (vol/vol) Pen-Strep, dexamethasone (1 μM), β-glycerophosphate (10 mM), ascorbic acid 2-phosphate (50 μM) | hESC-MPs $1.5 \times 10^6$/scaffold | 35 days in differentiation medium; flow rate: 3.6 mL/min | Proliferation: ↑; Differentiation: ↑ ALP, OP; ↑ bone specific ECM | Hydrodynamic−/fluid-induced shear stress | Marolt et al. [53] |
| | Indirect perfusion bioreactor | Decellularized cow bone plugs (4 × 4 mm) | DMEM-LG supplemented with HEPES (25 mM), 1% penicillin-streptomycin-amphotericin, L-glutamine (2 mM), 10% FBS, L-ascorbic acid ($4.5 \times 10^{-5}$ M), dexamethasone ($10^{-6}$ M), and β-glycerophosphate ($2 \times 10^2$ M; Calbiochem) | hiPSC-MPs $1.5 \times 10^6$/scaffold | 35 days in differentiation medium; flow rate: 3.6 mL/min | Differentiation: ↑ OP; ↑ bone specific ECM | Hydrodynamic−/fluid-induced shear stress | de Peppo et al. [54] |

|  |  |  |  |  |  |  |  |  |
|---|---|---|---|---|---|---|---|---|
|  | Indirect perfusion bioreactor | $CaCO_3$ cube (Biocoral®) (3 mm) | DMEM supplemented with 10% (vol/vol) HyClone FBS, penicillin/ streptomycin (100 U/mL), dexamethasone (1 μM), β-glycerophosphate (10 mM), and ascorbic acid 2-phosphate (50 μM) | BM-hMSCs hESC-MPs $0.1 \times 10^6$/ scaffold | 35 days in differentiation medium; flow rate: 10 mL/min | Proliferation: ↑ hESC-MPs > BM-hMSCs Differentiation: ↑ COL1, ALP, RUNX2, OP, ON; hESC-MPs > BM-hMSCs | Shear stress: 0.001 Pa | de Peppo et al. [21] |
|  | Direct perfusion bioreactor | PLGA-PCL (3 × 3 mm | DMEM supplemented with 10% FBS, penicillin/ streptomycin (1.0% v/v), nonessential amino acids (0.1 mM), and L-glutamine (4 mM), dexamethasone (100 nM), β-glycerophosphate (10 mM), and ascorbic acid (173 mM) | BM-hMSCs (Lonza) $0.25 \times 10^6$/ scaffold | 10 days in differentiation medium; flow rate: 1 mL/min | New bone area↑ | Hydrodynamic−/ fluid-induced shear stress | Yeatts et al. [22] |

(continued)

**Table 5.1** (continued)

| Bioreactor | Bioreactor (material and company) | Scaffolds (material, shape, and dimension) | Chemical factors | Cells/tissue | Condition | Results | Mechanical stimulation | Authors |
|---|---|---|---|---|---|---|---|---|
| | Custom-made [30] | Decellularized porcine bone (5 × 10 mm) | High-glucose DMEM supplemented with 10% FBS, ascorbic acid (50 mg/L), dexamethasone (1 mmol/L), β-sodium glycerophosphate (216 mg/L), penicillin (100 U/mL), and streptomycin (100 mg/mL) | BM-hMSCs AD-hMSCs $2.5 \times 10^5$/scaffold | 7 and 21 days in differentiation medium with flow rate: 1 mL/min | In AD-hMSCs »7 days: proliferation↑; gene expression of *COL1*↑, *OPN*↔, *RUNX2*↔, *OCN*↔, ALP activity↔; in 21 days: proliferation↑; gene expression of COL1↔, OPN↔, RUNX2↔, OCN↑, ALP activity↑; In BM-hMSCs »7 days: proliferation↑; gene expression of *COL1*↑, *OPN*↔, *RUNX2*↑, *OCN*↔, ALP activity↔; in 21 days: proliferation↑, *COL1*↔, *OPN*↑, RUNX2↑, *OCN*↑, ALP activity↑↑-$Ca^{2+}$ deposition in AD-hMSCs ↑ < < BM-hMSCs↑↑ | Shear stress Hydrodynamic pressure | Wu et al. [30] |

| | | | | | | | | |
|---|---|---|---|---|---|---|---|---|
| | Custom-made [55] | Polyurethane (PU) scaffold ($30 \times 5$ mm) | α-MEM supplemented with 10% FBS, L-glutamine (2 mM), penicillin/streptomycin (100 mg/mL), ascorbic acid (50 μg/mL), β-glycerol phosphate (5 mM), and dexamethasone (100 nM) | h-ES-MP cells $5 \times 10^5$/scaffold | 10 days in differentiation medium (3 days in static condition and 7 days in perfusion bioreactor with flow rate: 3.47 mL/min) | Proliferation: ↑ Differentiation: ALP activity↑ | Shear stress Hydrodynamic pressure | Bhaskar et al. [55] |
| Hydrostatic pressure | TEP-P02 bioprocessor (Takagi Industrial) | Hydroxyapatite scaffold (Pentax),cylindric ($5 \times 3$ mm), 80% porosity, and a pore size of 50–200 μm | DMEM/HAM's F-12, 10% FBS, 1% antibiotic-antimycotic, dexamethasone ($2 \times 10^{-7}$ mol/L), L-ascorbic acid 2-phosphate sesquimagnesium salt hydrate ($10^{-4}$ mol/L), β-glycerol 2-phosphate disodium salt n-hydrate ($2 \times 10^{-2}$ mol/L), and 5% ITS Premix | hMSCs; (Lonza) P2; $2.45 \times 10^5$ cells/scaffold | 1. 20% O2 in air for 3 weeks with cyclic HP at 0.5 Hz, 0–0.5 MPa (3750 mmHg, 4.93 atm) in a sinusoidal waveform, and with a medium replenishment rate of 50 mL/min | Differentiation: gene expression of *ON*, *COL1A1*, *ALPL*, *Cbfa1*, and *ITGB5*↑↑; PCNA↓ Protein expression of OC, OP, ON, and Col1↑ | Shear stress Hydrostatic pressure | Huang et al. [56] |

(continued)

**Table 5.1** (continued)

| Bioreactor | Bioreactor (material and company) | Scaffolds (material, shape, and dimension) | Chemical factors | Cells/tissue | Condition | Results | Mechanical stimulation | Authors |
|---|---|---|---|---|---|---|---|---|
| | Custom-made bioreactor (anodized aluminum vessel) | Alginate hydrogels with fluorescein; (10 × na mm) | (α-MEM) containing 1% penicillin-streptomycin and ascorbic acid (150 μg/ml); sodium β-glycerophosphate (2 mM) and dexamethasone ($10^{-7}$ M) | Chick fetal femurs | 1 hour per day, 5 days per week for 14 days; sinusoidal waveform (0–279 kPa at 0.005–2 Hz) | Mineralized portion ↑; gene expression *Col2*, osteonectin, osteopontin, CD44 ↑ | Shear stress Hydrostatic pressure | Henstock et al. [15] |
| | Hydrostatic pressure bioreactor (TGT/Instron, USA) | Aligned and random nanofibrous PCL scaffold | DMEM supplemented with penicillin (100 U/mL), streptomycin (0.1 mg/mL), dexamethasone (100 nM), L-ascorbic acid 2-phosphate (0.05 mM), β-glycerol phosphate (10 mM) | BM-hMSCs (Lonza); $2 \times 10^4$ cells (passage 2) | Hydrostatic pressure at 270 kPa, 1 Hz for 60 min/day over 21 days in differentiation medium | Differentiation: Col-I, ALP, and Runx-2↑; metabolic activity ↑<br>The differentiation in the groups with hydrostatic pressure and random nanofibrous scaffolds was more than non-stimulated and aligned ones | Shear stress Hydrostatic pressure | Reinwald et al. [16] |

| | | | | | | | | |
|---|---|---|---|---|---|---|---|---|
| Strain bioreactor | Rectangular, elastic silicone dishes (Wacker Chemie, Munich, Germany); eccentric motor (DC motor, 28 DT 12-222P; Portescap, Pforzheim, Germany) | Silicone dish, (cubic, 10 × 3.5 × 1.75 cm) | DMEM supplemented with 10–2% FCS, penicillin (100 U/ml), streptomycin (100 mg/ml), and 1-glutamine (0.5%) | Human osteoblasts | 3 days in medium with 10% FCS, 4 days in medium with 2% FCS (with 15 minutes of strain stimulation in days 4, 5, and 6), then cells were cultured in medium with 10% FCS for 5 days | Proliferation: ↑; LDH4 and ALP4↔ | Cyclic stretching (1.0, 2.4, 5.3 8.8% surface strains) | Neidlinger-Wilke [57] |
| | Custom-made, mechanical loading of bioreactor is controlled with an Instron Model 8511 Material Tester | Partially demineralized bovine cancellous bone (cubic, 63 × 6 × 6 mm) | α-MEM supplemented with 10% FCS, penicillin (100 u/mL), streptomycin (100 lg/mL), Fungizone (0.25 lg/mL), β-glycerophosphate (10 mM), and ascorbic acid 2-phosphate (0.05 mM), dexamethasone (0, 10, 100 nM) | h-MSC | 8 and 16 days in osteogenic medium with different concentration of dexamethasone Loading was applied in a triangular waveform at a rate of 5 mm/minute with a maximum external displacement of 0.2 mm for 250 cycles every 24 hours | ALP↑, gene expression of ALP↑, OC↔, OP↑, $Ca^{2+}$↑ | Four-point bending (max displacement of 0.2 mm for 250 cycles every 24 h) | Mauney [58] |

(continued)

**Table 5.1** (continued)

| Bioreactor | Bioreactor (material and company) | Scaffolds (material, shape, and dimension) | Chemical factors | Cells/tissue | Condition | Results | Mechanical stimulation | Authors |
|---|---|---|---|---|---|---|---|---|
| | Rectangular elastic silicone dishes (Wacker Chemie, Munich, Germany); eccentric motor (DC motor, 28 DT 12-222P; Portescap, Pforzheim, Germany) | Collagen type I gel (cubic, 3 × 3 × 0.4 cm) | DMEM/HAM's F-12 supplemented with 2% FBS, 1% glutamine, and 1% antibiotics | Human osteoblastic cell line (hFOB1.19) $4.5 \times 10^5$ cells/scaffold | Cells were cultured in standard medium stretched cyclically in the long axis every day for 30 min over a period of 3 weeks | Proliferation ↑, gene expression of RUNX2, ALP, OC, OP, and Col1↑ | Uniaxial stretching (1 Hz at a magnitude of 10,000 m strain (equivalent to 1%) and 1800 cycles | Ignatius [59] |
| | A base stage (clear plastic material acrylic or polycarbonate) with an acrylic piston with a model 31 load cell (Honeywell Sensotec, Inc., Columbus, OH) attached to M-227.10 DC-Mike actuators Physik Instrument, Inc., Auburn, MA) | Collagen type I scaffold (cubic, 10 × 20 × 1.5 mm) | DMEM supplemented with 10% FBS and antibiotic/ antimycotic | BM-hMSCs; $6.9 \times 10^6$ cells/scaffold | 4 weeks in static cell culture then displacement was applied twice daily for 1 h each with 1 h between each cycle and 2 h rest before the second set for a total of four consecutive days of testing | Proteoglycan ↑, matrix deposition ↑ | Biaxial; cyclic compression and tension (5% offset with a triangular waveform of 5% cyclic compression at a rate of 0.1 mm/s, and tension was set for a 3.8% offset with a triangular waveform of 3.8% cyclic tension at a rate of 0.875 mm/s | Wartella et al. [60] |

| | | | | | | | | |
|---|---|---|---|---|---|---|---|---|
| | Flexcell® [61] | Collagen type I (cubic, 15 × 4 × 2 mm) | α-MEM supplemented with 10% FBS, 1% penicillin/ streptomycin | Murine osteoblasts; 1 × $10^6$ cells/ ml | 3 days cyclic loading using the uniaxial tensile strain bioreactor at an applied load equivalent to 2% strain with 0.1 Hz loading frequency for 1 h/ day | Proliferation↑, cell viability↑, and matrix organization↑ | Loading strains (0–12%) and frequencies (0.01–1 Hz) | Subramanian et al. [61] |
| Compression bioreactor | Custom-made compression bioreactor | Human cancellous bone-fibrin composite (15 × 4 mm) | DMEM supplemented with 10% FCS, penicillin (100 U/ mL), streptomycin (100 μg/ml), 2.4% aprotinin | BM-hMSCs 1 × $10^6$/ scaffold | 1 day in standard medium; cyclic compression rate: 4 kPa 25% strain 0.05 Hz | Differentiation: gene expression of *osteopontin*↑, *integrin-β-1*↑, *TGF-βR1*↑, *SMAD5*↑, *PDGFα*↑, *annexin-V*↑ | Cyclically compression: 4 kPa 25% strain 0.05 Hz | Matziolis et al. [62] |

(continued)

**Table 5.1** (continued)

| Bioreactor | Bioreactor (material and company) | Scaffolds (material, shape, and dimension) | Chemical factors | Cells/tissue | Condition | Results | Mechanical stimulation | Authors |
|---|---|---|---|---|---|---|---|---|
| | A modified perfusion bioreactor introduced by Bader | Collagen meniscus implants (CMI, Menacell™, ReGen® Biologics Inc., Hackensack, NJ, USA) 5.5 mm (with hole: 4.5 mm) | DMEM/HAM's F-12 (1:1) with L-glutamine, 10% FCS, 5 μg/mL ascorbic acid, 3 ng/L FGF-2 | BM-hMSCs $10^6$/scaffold | 14 days in differentiation medium and compression: 8 h/day of 10% cyclic compression at 0.5 Hz or | 1. Proliferation: ↑↑ Differentiation: procollagen I propeptide ↑↑, procollagen III propeptide ↑↑, ↔ ALP; mechanical strength↑↑ (compression more effectively enhance differentiation than perfusion) | Compression | Petri et al. [17] |
| | Custom-made multichamber compression bioreactor system [63] | PCL/β-TCP; cylindrical scaffold with a lumen (3.2 mm diameter), 5 mm height, 8 mm outer diameter, and 3.2 mm inner diameter | DMEM-GlutaMAX supplemented with 10% FBS, penicillin and streptomycin (50 U/mL), ascorbic acid (0.2 mM), β-glycerophosphate (10 mM), and dexamethasone ($10^{-8}$ M) | BM-hMSCs; $6.9 \times 10^6$ cells/scaffold | 4 weeks in differentiation medium; cyclic compression rate: 0.22% strain 1 Hz 4 h/day | Proliferation: 14 days↑, 28 days↓ Differentiation: gene expression of *osteonectin*↑, *osteocalcin*↑, *COL1A1*↔; ALP activity↑; $Ca^{2+}$↑ | Cyclically compressed at 1 Hz and physiological strain value of 0.22% | Ravichandran et al. [18] |

| | | | | | | | | |
|---|---|---|---|---|---|---|---|---|
| Electrical/ Electromagnetic stimulation | Electromagnetic bioreactor consisting of a carrying structure custom-machined and Biostim SPT pulse generator (Igea, Carpi, Italy) | Polyurethane porous scaffold (cylindric, 15 × 2 mm) | McCoy's 5A modified medium with L-glutamine and HEPES supplemented with 15% FBS, 2% sodium pyruvate, 1% antibiotics, dexamethasone ($10^{-8}$ M), and β-glycerophosphate (10 mM) | Human osteosarcoma SAOS-2 cell line $10^6$ cells/ scaffold | 1 day in static cell culture, 24 days Electromagnetic stimulation (ES) 24 h/day with 75 Hz, 2 mT, 1.3 ms | $Ca^{2+}$↑, gene expression of DCN, OC, OPN, TGF-ß, and Col1↑ | Electromagnetic stimulation, IMF[4]: 2 ± 0.2 mT, AIET[5]: 5 ± 1 mV, 75 ± 2 Hz, 1.3 ms | Fassina et al. [64] |
| | Identical Helmholtz coils (Biomet, Parsippany, NJ) | Calcium phosphate (cylindric, 12.7 × 0.6 mm) | 10% FBS supplemented with dexamethasone ($10^{-7}$ M) β-glycerophosphate (5 mM), ascorbic acid, and antibiotics, BMP-2 (0, 10, 40, 70, 100 ng/mL) | hMSC (Cambrex Corp. (NJ)) | 24 days with ES of 4.5 ms bursts of 20 pulses repeating at 15 Hz. During each pulse, the field increased from 0 to 16 gauss in 200 ms and then decayed back to 0 in 25 ms for 8 h/day | Proliferation↓, in combination with BMP-2: ALP↑, OC↑, TGF-β1↑ | Electrical stimulation: 4.5 ms bursts of 20 pulses repeating, 15 Hz | Schwartz et al. [65] |

(continued)

**Table 5.1** (continued)

| Bioreactor | Bioreactor (material and company) | Scaffolds (material, shape, and dimension) | Chemical factors | Cells/tissue | Condition | Results | Mechanical stimulation | Authors |
|---|---|---|---|---|---|---|---|---|
| | Homemade electrical cell culture system | PPy[6]/PLLA membranes (cubic, $0.5 \times 20 \times 25$ mm) | DMEM supplemented with 10% FCS, penicillin G (100 UI/mL), gentamicin (25 mg/mL) | Human cutaneous fibroblasts $3 \times 10^5$ cells/scaffold | 1 day on the membrane in standard medium; then 1 day small DC potential gradient ES of 50 mV/mm was applied; 2–4 days membrane in standard medium without ES | Proliferation↑, cell viability↑, cell activity: gene expression of IL-6↑, *IL-8*↑ | DC potential gradient ES: 50 mV/mm | Shi et al. [66] |
| | Custom-made biphasic electric current system [67] | No scaffold | High-glucose DMEM with 10% HIFBS supplemented with ascorbic acid (50 mg/ mL), β-glycerophosphate (10 mM), and dexamethasone (10 nM) | BM-hMSCs $1.7 \times 10^4$ cells/cm$^2$ | 7 days in differentiation medium with ES of 1.5 or 15 μA/cm$^2$ biphasic current 250/25 μs at 100 Hz and 100 pulses/s | Proliferation↑ Differentiation: ALP activity↑ and calcium deposition↑, expression gene of VEGF↑, BMP-2↑ | Biphasic electric current: 250 ms duration and 1.5 μA/cm$^2$ amplitude, or 25 ms duration and 15 μA/cm$^2$ of amplitude | Kim et al. [68] |

| | | | | | | | | |
|---|---|---|---|---|---|---|---|---|
| | Custom-made PEMF device | 2D, tissue culture polystyrene | High-glucose DMEM supplemented with 10% FBS dexamethasone (0.1 mM), β-glycerol phosphate (10 mM), ascorbic acid (0.2 mM), penicillin (100 U), streptomycin (1000 U), L-glutamine, (2 mM) | BM-hMSCs $1.7 \times 10^4$ cells/cm$^2$ | 7 days in differentiation medium with pulsed electromagnetic fields of 15 Hz, 4.5 ms, 1.8 mT of 8 h/day during | Proliferation↑ Differentiation: gene expression of OC↑, ALP↑, Cbfa1↓, PTH-R1↓ COL1↓, BMP-2↑, ALP activity↑ | Pulsed electromagnetic fields: 15 Hz, 4.5 ms, 1.8 mT | Sun et al. [69] |
| | Custom-made electrical cell culture system | Collagen sponge | NA | hMSCs | 7 days in biphasic electric current (BEC) stimulation (20/40 uA, 100 us, 100 Hz). Then, 7 days without electrical stimulation | Proliferation↑ Differentiation: gene expression of *COLI*↑ | Biphasic electrical stimulation: 20/40uA, 100us, 100 Hz | Kim et al. [19] |

(continued)

**Table 5.1** (continued)

| Bioreactor | Bioreactor (material and company) | Scaffolds (material, shape, and dimension) | Chemical factors | Cells/tissue | Condition | Results | Mechanical stimulation | Authors |
|---|---|---|---|---|---|---|---|---|
| | Electromagnetic bioreactor consisting of a carrying structure custom-machined and Biostim SPT pulse generator (Igea, Carpi, Italy) | Gelatin-based Cryogel | McCoy's 5A modified medium with L-glutamine and HEPES supplemented with 15% FBS, 2% sodium pyruvate, 1% antibiotics, dexamethasone ($10^{-8}$ M), and β-glycerophosphate (10 mM) | Human osteosarcoma SAOS-2 cell line $4 \times 10^5$ cells/scaffold | 1 day in static cell culture, 24 days Electromagnetic stimulation (ES) 24 h/day with 75 Hz, 2 mT, 1.3 ms | Differentiation: DCN↔, ALP↔, OC[7]↑, OPN[8]↑, ColI↑, ColIII↑, human fibronectin↑, Osteonectin↑ | Electromagnetic stimulation, IMF[9]: 2 ± 0.2 mT, AIET[10]: 5 ± 1 mV, 75 ± 2 Hz, 1.3 ms | Fassina et al. [20] |
| Combined bioreactor | Custom-made perfusion bioreactor system according to Bader [70] was equipped with a linear servomotor (Linmots Inc., Delavan, WI) | Decellularized cow bone (Tutobone®) (d 20 × h 4 mm | DMEM/HAM's F-12 1:1 supplemented with 10% FCS, penicillin/ streptomycin (100 U/ml), amphotericin B (0.5 mg/ml), ascorbic acid (5 mg/ml), FGF-2 (3 ng/ml) buffered with HEPES buffer | BM-hMSCs $1 \times 10^6$/ scaffold | 1. 21 days in differentiation medium and flow rate: 0.1 mL/ min mL/min 2. 21 days in differentiation medium and flow rate: 10 mL/min; 10% strain, 0.5 Hz | Proliferation: ↑ Differentiation: ↔ OC Proliferation: ↑ Differentiation: ↑ OC; also > to perfusion only | Perfusion Compression/ perfusion | Jagodzinski et al. [71] |

| | | | | | | | | |
|---|---|---|---|---|---|---|---|---|
| | Compression bioreactor (BioDynamic ELF5110; Bose) | HEMA-lactate-dextran ($8 \times 4$ mm) | Low-glucose DMEM supplemented with 10% FBS, 1% antibiotics/antimycotics, and 1% L-glutamine | MG63 (ATTC) $1 \times 10^6$/scaffold | 1. 10 days in differentiation medium and flow rate: 0.1 mL/min<br>2. 21 days in differentiation medium and flow rate: 0.1 mL/min; 1.5% strain, 1 Hz, 1 h/day | 1. Differentiation: ALP↔<br>2. Differentiation: ↑ ALP | 1. Compression<br>2. Compression/perfusion | Bölgen et al. [72] |
| | Custom-made Perfusion/biaxial rotating bioreactor | PCL-TCP ($6 \times 6 \times 4$ mm) | DMEM-GlutaMAX supplemented with 10% FBS, penicillin (50 U/mL), and streptomycin (50 mg/mL) | hfMSCs $0.5 \times 10^6$/scaffold | 1. 28 days in differentiation medium and flow rate: 3.8 mL/min; rotation rate: 5 RPM | 1. Proliferation: ↑<br>2. Differentiation: ↑ ALP, $Ca^{2+}$ | Perfusion/rotation | Zhang et al. [73] |

(continued)

**Table 5.1** (continued)

| Bioreactor | Bioreactor (material and company) | Scaffolds (material, shape, and dimension) | Chemical factors | Cells/tissue | Condition | Results | Mechanical stimulation | Authors |
|---|---|---|---|---|---|---|---|---|
| | Modified perfusion bioreactor | PU-BDI shape of human meniscus (size NA) | NA | BM-hMSCs $6 \times 10^6$/scaffold | 1. 14 days in differentiation medium and flow rate: 10 mL/min<br>2. 14 days in differentiation medium and flow rate: 10 mL/min; 10% strain, 0.5 Hz, 1 time/day, 8 h/time<br>3. 14 days in differentiation medium and flow rate: 10 mL/min; 10% strain, 0.5 Hz, 4 times/day, 2 h/time, 4 h of rest | 1. Proliferation: ↑ Differentiation: ↔ ALP; ↔ mechanical strength<br>2. Proliferation: ↔ Differentiation: ↔ ALP; ↔ mechanical strength<br>3. Proliferation: ↑ Differentiation: ALP↑; mechanical strength↑ | 1. Perfusion<br>2. Compression/perfusion | Liu et al. [74] |

| | | | | | | | | |
|---|---|---|---|---|---|---|---|---|
| | Siliconized spinner flasks (Corning) + cylindrical perfusion chamber (2 cm in diameter), peristaltic pump (Masterflex L/S, Cole Parmer, USA) | Porcine gelatin microcarriers (8 × 4 mm) | DMEM supplemented with 10% FBS, dexamethasone (100 nM), sodium β-glycerophosphate (10 mM), ascorbic acid 2-phosphate (0.1 mg/mL), and mercaptoethanol ($5 \times 10^{-5}$ M) | AD-hMSCs $5 \times 10^4$/scaffold | 28 days in spinner flask: 8 days in standard medium and 20 days in differentiation medium. Then 7 and 14 days in differentiation medium in perfusion bioreactor | Proliferation↑, metabolic activity↑, cell viability↑ Differentiation: ALP activity↑, $Ca^2$ + ↑ | 1. Spinner flask/ perfusion (1 week) 2. Spinner flask/ perfusion (2 week) | Chen et al. [75] |
| | Custom-made PEMF device | PCL/PLGA/TCP (4 × 1 mm) | DMEM containing 10% (v/v) FBS, penicillin (100 U/mL), and streptomycin (100 mg/mL), dexamethasone (10 nM), β-glycerol phosphate (10 mM), and ascorbic acid 2-phosphate (50 mg/mL) | AD-hMSCs $2 \times 10^4$/scaffold | Cyclic strain: 1 Hz and 0.3%, Ultrasound: 20 min per day at a 1.5 MHz frequency and 30 mW/cm$^2$ intensity. Electromagnetic: 45 Hz was applied at 1 mT for 8 h per day | CEU: the highest expression of osteogenic markers (ALP, RUNX-2) in CEU group was the highest. E and CE: the largest volume of bone tissue, the most matured bone tissue. CEU: the lowest lamin A/C expression and degree of bone formation among C, E, and CE groups | Cyclic Strain (C) electromagnetic field (E) Ultrasound (U) Groups: 1.C 2.E 3.U 4.CE 5.CU 6.EU 7.CEU | Kang et al. [76] |

(continued)

**Table 5.1** (continued)

| Bioreactor | Bioreactor (material and company) | Scaffolds (material, shape, and dimension) | Chemical factors | Cells/tissue | Condition | Results | Mechanical stimulation | Authors |
|---|---|---|---|---|---|---|---|---|
| | A bioreactor (Bose ElectroForce 5210 Test Instrument, Electro Force Systems Group, Sissach, Switzerland) perfused by a peristaltic pump (Ismatec IPC, Glattbrugg, Switzerland) | PLGA/a-CaP disk (10 × 0.5–0.6 mm) | α-MEM medium with 20% of FBS and gentamicin (50 mg/mL) | AD-hMSCs $5 \times 10^5$/scaffold | 5 or 9 days in standard medium with flow rate: 0.3, 0.5, or 2.0 mL/ min (direct); compression: 0.2 mm displacement at 1 Hz once per day for 10 min | Stiffness of the cell free constructs↑, stiffness of AdSC-seeded constructs↔ Roundish of stem cells at higher flow rates↑ | 1. Perfusion/ comparison | Baumgartner [77] |
| | Custom-made bioreactor together with a tailor-made incubator system | The decellularized cancellous bone matrix Tutoplast (Tutogen Medical GmbH, Neunkirchen, Germany) (4–10 mm; 42–93 mg) | A-MEM supplemented with 0.5% gentamicin, 2.5% human platelet lysate (PL BioScience, Aachen, Germany), and 1 U/mL heparin β-glycerophosphate (5 m M), dexamethasone (0.1 μ M), and L- ascorbate-2-phosphate (200 μM) | AD-hMSCs $10^5$/scaffold | 4 days in standard medium and static condition, 21 days in perfusion bioreactor with standard/ differentiation medium (flow rate: 1.5 mL/ min); 3 h pressure/3 h pause was applied throughout the entire cultivation period of 6 days | Differentiation: Alp activity↑; calcein AM↑ | 1. Perfusion/ hydrostatic pressure (shear stress: 10 mPa) | Egger et al. [78] |

| | | | | | | | | |
|---|---|---|---|---|---|---|---|---|
| In vivo bioreactor | Nude mice; subcutaneous site | Hydroxyapatite (8 × 4 mm) | α-MEM containing 10% fetal bovine serum, FGF-2 (5 ng/ml), dexamethasone (10 nM), and L-ascorbic acid 2-phosphate (0.1 mM) | BM-hMSCs | Pre-culture period: direct perfusion bioreactor 19 days<br>In vivo bioreactor: 8 weeks | Differentiation: dynamic > static; mature laminar bone filled 52% vs. 9.6% of available pore space | Shear stress, hydrodynamic pressure, neural stimulation | Braccini et al. [78] |
| | Mice; cranial 4 mm defect | Silk loaded with BMP-2 (4 × 2 mm) | DMEM supplemented with 10% FBS, Pen-Strep, and Fungizone, ascorbic acid 2-phosphate (50 g/mL), dexamethasone (10 nM), and β-glycerol phosphate (7 mM) | BM-hMSCs (Clonetics) $5 \times 10^6$/scaffold | Pre-culture period: spinner flask 28 days<br>In vivo bioreactor: 5 weeks | Differentiation: dynamic ↔ static; mature laminar bone filled 0.28 vs. 0.11 $mm^2$ | Shear stress, hydrodynamic | Karageorgiou et al. [24] |
| | Nude rat; intramuscular site | $CaCO_3$ (Biocoral®) (d 5 × h 3 mm) | | hTBCs | Pre-culture period: direct perfusion bioreactor 14 days<br>In vivo bioreactor: 6 weeks | Dynamic ↔ static 22% vs. 16% of area | | Schliephake et al. [46] |

(continued)

**Table 5.1** (continued)

| Bioreactor | Bioreactor (material and company) | Scaffolds (material, shape, and dimension) | Chemical factors | Cells/tissue | Condition | Results | Mechanical stimulation | Authors |
|---|---|---|---|---|---|---|---|---|
| | Nude rats; mandibular; 5 mm defect | $CaCO_3$ (Biocoral®) mineralized collagen TCP (Cerasorb®) (5 × 3 mm) | ZKT-1 medium, 15% FBS | hTBCs $5 \times 10^6$ cells/cm$^3$ | Pre-culture period: direct perfusion bioreactor 14 days In vivo bioreactor: 6 weeks | Dynamic ↔ static $CaCO_3$: 7.2 vs. 8.7% of area Mineralized collagen: 10.3% vs. 12.5% of area; TCP: 14.6% vs. 22.8% of area | Hydrodynamic−/fluid-induced shear stress | Schliephake et al. [49] |
| | NOD/SCID mice; subcutaneous site | PCL-TCP (6 × 6 × 4 mm) | DMEM-GlutaMAX supplemented with 10% FBS, penicillin (50 U/mL), and streptomycin (50 mg/mL) | hfMSCs $0.5 \times 10^6$/scaffold | Pre-culture period: biaxial rotating bioreactor 14 days In vivo bioreactor: 12 weeks | Dynamic > static Dynamic: 3.2× fold increase | Perfusion/rotation | Zhang et al. [73] |
| | Nude mouse; subcutaneous site | Gelatin-coral/HA (Pro-Osteon™) particles (0.5–1 mm) | α-MEM medium containing 10% FCS, L-glutamine (2 mM), Pen–-Strep (both 100 U/ml), ascorbic acid (100 μg/mL), and dexamethasone (10–8 M) | BM-hMSCs; $5 \times 10^5$/scaffold | Pre-culture period: rotating wall vessel 21 days In vivo bioreactor: 8 weeks | Bone formation; no static group | Shear stress gravity force hydrodynamic pressure | Ben-David et al. [36] |

| | | | | | | | | |
|---|---|---|---|---|---|---|---|---|
| | Nude mice; subcutaneous site | BCP particles (OsSatura™) (2–6 mm) | α-MEM supplemented with 10% FBS, antibiotics, L-ascorbic acid 2-phosphate (0.1 mM), L-glutamine (2 mM), dexamethasone ($1 \times 10^5$ mM), and bFGF (1 ng/ml) | BM-hMSCs (1–12) × $10^6$/ all scaffolds | Pre-culture period: indirect perfusion bioreactor 7; 20; 40 days<br>In vivo bioreactor: 6 weeks | Dynamic ↔ static: gene expression of *ALP, CBFA1, COL1, OC, ON, S100A4, BMP-2* | | Janssen et al. [47] |
| | SCID-beige mice; subcutaneous site | Decellularized cow bone (4 × 4 mm) | DMEM supplemented with 10% (vol/vol) HyClone FBS and 1% (vol/vol) Pen-Strep, dexamethasone (1 μM), β-glycerophosphate (10 mM), ascorbic acid 2-phosphate (50 μM) | hESC-MPs 1.5 × $10^6$/ scaffold | Pre-culture period: direct perfusion bioreactor 35 days<br>In vivo bioreactor: 8 weeks | Dynamic > CSBI[11]; 7% vs. 2% of area | Hydrodynamic−/ fluid-induced shear stress | Marolt et al. [53] |

(continued)

**Table 5.1** (continued)

| Bioreactor | Bioreactor (material and company) | Scaffolds (material, shape, and dimension) | Chemical factors | Cells/tissue | Condition | Results | Mechanical stimulation | Authors |
|---|---|---|---|---|---|---|---|---|
| | SCID-beige mice; subcutaneous site | Decellularized cow bone (d 4 × h 4 mm | DMEM-LG supplemented with HEPES (25 mM), 1% penicillin-streptomycin-amphotericin, L-glutamine (2 mM), 10% FBS, L-ascorbic acid ($4.5 \times 10^{-5}$ M), dexamethasone ($10^{-6}$ M), and β-glycerophosphate ($2 \times 10^{2}$ M; Calbiochem) | hiPSC-MPs $1.5 \times 10^{6}$/scaffold | Pre-culture period: direct perfusion bioreactor 35 days In vivo bioreactor: 12 weeks | Bone-like tissue formation No static group | Hydrodynamic–/fluid-induced shear stress | de Peppo et al. [54] |

| | | | | | | | | |
|---|---|---|---|---|---|---|---|---|
| | Nude rats; femoral condyle; 2.5 mm defect | PLGA-PCL ($3 \times 3$ mm) | DMEM supplemented with 10% FBS, penicillin/ streptomycin (1.0% v/v), nonessential amino acids (0.1 mM), and L-glutamine (4 mM), dexamethasone (100 nM), β-glycerophosphate (10 mM), and ascorbic acid (173 mM) | BM-hMSCs (Lonza) $0.25 \times 10^6$/ scaffold | Pre-culture period: indirect perfusion bioreactor<br>10 days<br>In vivo bioreactor: 3 and 6 weeks | Dynamic > static (6 weeks only) 1.72 vs. 1.26 mm2 | Hydrodynamic–/ fluid-induced shear stress | Yeatts et al. [22] |

[1]Human nasal inferior turbinate tissue-derived mesenchymal stromal cells
[2]Poly (ethylene oxide terephthalate)
[3]Poly (butylene terephthalate)
[4]Intensity of the magnetic field
[5]Amplitude of the induced electric tension
[6]Polypyrrole nanoparticles
[7]Osteocalcin
[8]Osteopontin
[9]Intensity of the magnetic field
[10]Amplitude of the induced electric tension
[11]Cell-seeded scaffolds before implantation without pre-culturing

**Table 5.2** Different kinds of bioreactors used in cartilage tissue engineering

| Bioreactor | Bioreactor (material and company) | Scaffolds (material, shape, and dimension) | Chemical factors | Cells | Condition | Results | | Authors |
|---|---|---|---|---|---|---|---|---|
| Rotating wall vessel | RCCS-4 system with 50 mL disposable vessels, Synthecon Incorporated, Houston, Texas, USA | pC-HAp/ChS (porous material consisted of collagen, hydroxyapatite, and chondroitin sulfate) | D-MEM/F-12 containing 10% FBS, 1% AMS, L-ascorbic acid 2-phosphate, dexamethasone, insulin-like growth factor-1, and FGF-2 | Human cartilage progenitor cells, $2.5 \times 10^4$ cells/cm$^2$ | 6 weeks in differentiation medium; rotation rate: at a speed to preserve freely suspention of the cell agregations | Differentiation: ↑ type II collagen production | Shear Force | Takebe et al. [81] |
| | Synthecon, RCCS Model, Bereldange, Luxembourg | 2% alginate hydrogel | DMEM +20% FCS | Human cartilage progenitor cells, $10 \times 10^6$ cells/mL of hydrogel | 19 days in standard medium; rotation rate: 6–8 RPM | Proliferation: ↑ Differentiation: GAG↑, hydroxyproline↑, cells formed elastic cartilage-like tissue | Shear Force | Akmal et al. [82] |
| | High-aspect rotating vessel (HARV) was used (Synthecon, Inc., Houston, TX, USA) | Without any scaffold | DMEM with 450 mg/dl supplemented with 10% FBS, 2 g/l HEPES, 1% L-glutamine, 100 μg/ml streptomycin and 2.5 μg/ml Fungizone, and 50 mg/l ascorbic acid | Human articular chondrocytes; $5 \times 10^5$ cells/m | 12 weeks in controlled oxygenation and low shear stress in a rotating wall vessel (initiated at 10 rpm and increased daily as required to keep the cells and the tissue constructs in suspension) | Proliferation: ↑ Differentiation: COLII↑, extracellular matrix of the cartilage-like regions ↑ | Shear Force | Marlovits et al. [83] |

| | | | | | | | | |
|---|---|---|---|---|---|---|---|---|
| Spinner flask | Spinner flasks were siliconized with Sigmacote (Sigma, St. Louis, MO) | Fibrin Gel | DMEM, ascorbic acid (50 mg/mL), dexamethasone (100 nM) supplemented either with or without 10 ng/mL of TGF-β3 | Ad-hMSCs, $10^6$ cells/mL of hydrogel | 28 days in differentiation medium; rotation rate: 40 RPM | Chondrogenic differentiation of ASCs | Shear Force | Yoon et al. [84] |

## 5 Conclusion

To make the fully functional engineered oral and dental tissues, other factors should also be established, including homogenous distribution of cells, chemical factors, and recapitulating the mechanical and electrical stimulation. Bioreactors can improve uniform distribution of the cells, delivering the nutrients and gases, and apply different kinds of mechanical stimuli on the engineering constructs. However, oral and dental tissues are exposed to different kinds of unknown stimuli simultaneously that need to be discovered and investigated. This therefore requires designing more complex bioreactors based on geometry, different mechanical and physical stimulation in target tissue. Further studies are needed to discover the physical and mechanical factors affecting engineering oral and dental tissues and based on which suitable bioreactors will be manufactured.

## References

1. Teixeira, G. Q., et al. (2014). A multicompartment holder for spinner flasks improves expansion and osteogenic differentiation of mesenchymal stem cells in three-dimensional scaffolds. *Tissue Engineering Part C: Methods, 20*(12), 984–993.
2. Zhang, S., et al. (2017). Fabrication of viable and functional pre-vascularized modular bone tissues by coculturing MSCs and HUVECs on microcarriers in spinner flasks. *Biotechnology Journal, 12*(8).
3. Lau, E., et al. (2010). Effect of low-magnitude, high-frequency vibration on osteocytes in the regulation of osteoclasts. *Bone, 46*(6), 1508–1515.
4. Hess, R., et al. (2010). Hydrostatic pressure stimulation of human mesenchymal stem cells seeded on collagen-based artificial extracellular matrices. *Journal of Biomechanical Engineering, 132*(2), 021001.
5. Rubin, C., et al. (2004). Prevention of postmenopausal bone loss by a low-magnitude, high-frequency mechanical stimuli: A clinical trial assessing compliance, efficacy, and safety. *Journal of Bone and Mineral Research, 19*(3), 343–351.
6. Rubin, C., et al. (2007). Adipogenesis is inhibited by brief, daily exposure to high-frequency, extremely low-magnitude mechanical signals. *Proceedings of the National Academy of Sciences, 104*(45), 17879–17884.
7. Khouri, R. K., Koudsi, B., & Reddi, H. (1991). Tissue transformation into bone in vivo: a potential practical application. *JAMA, 266*(14), 1953–1955.
8. Mohammadi Amirabad, L., et al. (2017). Enhanced cardiac differentiation of human cardiovascular disease patient-specific induced pluripotent stem cells by applying unidirectional electrical pulses using aligned electroactive nanofibrous scaffolds. *ACS Applied Materials & Interfaces, 9*(8), 6849–6864.
9. Yasuda, K., Inoue, S., & Tabata, Y. (2004). Influence of culture method on the proliferation and osteogenic differentiation of human adipo-stromal cells in nonwoven fabrics. *Tissue Engineering, 10*(9–10), 1587–1596.
10. Mygind, T., et al. (2007). Mesenchymal stem cell ingrowth and differentiation on coralline hydroxyapatite scaffolds. *Biomaterials, 28*(6), 1036–1047.
11. Wang, T. W., et al. (2006). Biomimetic bilayered gelatin-chondroitin 6 sulfate-hyaluronic acid biopolymer as a scaffold for skin equivalent tissue engineering. *Artificial Organs, 30*(3), 141–149.

12. Song, K., et al. (2007). Three-dimensional expansion: In suspension culture of SD rat's osteoblasts in a rotating wall vessel bioreactor. *Biomedical and Environmental Sciences, 20*(2), 91.
13. Zhou, Y., et al. (2011). Osteogenic differentiation of bone marrow-derived mesenchymal stromal cells on bone-derived scaffolds: Effect of microvibration and role of ERK1/2 activation. *European Cells & Materials, 22*, 12–25.
14. Tsimbouri, P. M., et al. (2017). Stimulation of 3D osteogenesis by mesenchymal stem cells using a nanovibrational bioreactor. *Nature Biomedical Engineering, 1*(9), 758.
15. Henstock, J., et al. (2013). Cyclic hydrostatic pressure stimulates enhanced bone development in the foetal chick femur in vitro. *Bone, 53*(2), 468–477.
16. Reinwald, Y., & El Haj, A. J. (2018). Hydrostatic pressure in combination with topographical cues affects the fate of bone marrow-derived human mesenchymal stem cells for bone tissue regeneration. *Journal of Biomedical Materials Research Part A, 106*(3), 629–640.
17. Petri, M., et al. (2012). Effects of perfusion and cyclic compression on in vitro tissue engineered meniscus implants. *Knee Surgery, Sports Traumatology, Arthroscopy, 20*(2), 223–231.
18. Ravichandran, A., et al. (2017). In vitro cyclic compressive loads potentiate early osteogenic events in engineered bone tissue. *Journal of Biomedical Materials Research Part B: Applied Biomaterials, 105*(8), 2366–2375.
19. Kim, J. H., et al. 2011). An implantable electrical bioreactor for enhancement of cell viability. In *Engineering in Medicine and Biology Society, EMBC, 2011 Annual International Conference of the IEEE*. IEEE.
20. Fassina, L., et al. (2012). Electromagnetic stimulation to optimize the bone regeneration capacity of gelatin-based cryogels. *International Journal of Immunopathology and Pharmacology, 25*(1), 165–174.
21. de Peppo, G. M., et al. (2013). Engineering bone tissue substitutes from human induced pluripotent stem cells. *Proceedings of the National Academy of Sciences, 110*(21), 8680–8685.
22. Yeatts, A. B., et al. (2013). In vivo bone regeneration using tubular perfusion system bioreactor cultured nanofibrous scaffolds. *Tissue Engineering Part A, 20*(1–2), 139–146.
23. Meinel, L., et al. (2004). Bone tissue engineering using human mesenchymal stem cells: Effects of scaffold material and medium flow. *Annals of Biomedical Engineering, 32*(1), 112–122.
24. Karageorgiou, V., et al. (2006). Porous silk fibroin 3-D scaffolds for delivery of bone morphogenetic protein-2 in vitro and in vivo. *Journal of Biomedical Materials Research Part A, 78*(2), 324–334.
25. Kim, H. J., et al. (2007). Bone regeneration on macroporous aqueous-derived silk 3-D scaffolds. *Macromolecular Bioscience, 7*(5), 643–655.
26. Hofmann, S., et al. (2007). Control of in vitro tissue-engineered bone-like structures using human mesenchymal stem cells and porous silk scaffolds. *Biomaterials, 28*(6), 1152–1162.
27. Stiehler, M., et al. (2009). Effect of dynamic 3-D culture on proliferation, distribution, and osteogenic differentiation of human mesenchymal stem cells. *Journal of Biomedical Materials Research Part A, 89*(1), 96–107.
28. Wang, T. W., et al. (2009). Regulation of adult human mesenchymal stem cells into osteogenic and chondrogenic lineages by different bioreactor systems. *Journal of Biomedical Materials Research Part A, 88*(4), 935–946.
29. Xing, Z., et al. (2013). Copolymer cell/scaffold constructs for bone tissue engineering: Co-culture of low ratios of human endothelial and osteoblast-like cells in a dynamic culture system. *Journal of Biomedical Materials Research Part A, 101*(4), 1113–1120.
30. Wu, W., et al. (2015). Osteogenic performance of donor-matched human adipose and bone marrow mesenchymal cells under dynamic culture. *Tissue Engineering Part A, 21*(9–10), 1621–1632.
31. Botchwey, E., et al. (2001). Bone tissue engineering in a rotating bioreactor using a microcarrier matrix system. *Journal of Biomedical Materials Research Part A, 55*(2), 242–253.
32. Facer, S., et al. (2005). Rotary culture enhances pre-osteoblast aggregation and mineralization. *Journal of Dental Research, 84*(6), 542–547.

33. Pound, J. C., et al. (2007). An ex vivo model for chondrogenesis and osteogenesis. *Biomaterials, 28*(18), 2839–2849.
34. Diederichs, S., et al. (2009). Dynamic cultivation of human mesenchymal stem cells in a rotating bed bioreactor system based on the Z® RP platform. *Biotechnology Progress, 25*(6), 1762–1771.
35. Araujo, J. V., et al. (2009). Dynamic culture of osteogenic cells in biomimetically coated poly (caprolactone) nanofibre mesh constructs. *Tissue Engineering Part A, 16*(2), 557–563.
36. Ben-David, D., et al. (2010). A tissue-like construct of human bone marrow MSCs composite scaffold support in vivo ectopic bone formation. *Journal of Tissue Engineering and Regenerative Medicine, 4*(1), 30–37.
37. Clarke, M. S., et al. (2013). A three-dimensional tissue culture model of bone formation utilizing rotational co-culture of human adult osteoblasts and osteoclasts. *Acta Biomaterialia, 9*(8), 7908–7916.
38. Lv, Q., et al. (2013). Nano-ceramic composite scaffolds for bioreactor-based bone engineering. *Clinical Orthopaedics and Related Research, 471*(8), 2422–2433.
39. Leferink, A. M., et al. (2015). Distribution and viability of fetal and adult human bone marrow stromal cells in a biaxial rotating vessel bioreactor after seeding on polymeric 3D additive manufactured scaffolds. *Frontiers in Bioengineering and Biotechnology, 3*, 169.
40. Hofmann, A., et al. (2003). Bioengineered human bone tissue using autogenous osteoblasts cultured on different biomatrices. *Journal of Biomedical Materials Research Part A, 67*(1), 191–199.
41. Braccini, A., et al. (2005). Three-dimensional perfusion culture of human bone marrow cells and generation of osteoinductive grafts. *Stem Cells, 23*(8), 1066–1072.
42. Olivier, V., et al. (2007). In vitro culture of large bone substitutes in a new bioreactor: Importance of the flow direction. *Biomedical Materials, 2*(3), 174.
43. Bernhardt, A., et al. (2008). Mineralised collagen—An artificial, extracellular bone matrix—Improves osteogenic differentiation of bone marrow stromal cells. *Journal of Materials Science: Materials in Medicine, 19*(1), 269–275.
44. Bjerre, L., et al. (2008). Flow perfusion culture of human mesenchymal stem cells on silicate-substituted tricalcium phosphate scaffolds. *Biomaterials, 29*(17), 2616–2627.
45. Grayson, W. L., et al. (2008). Effects of initial seeding density and fluid perfusion rate on formation of tissue-engineered bone. *Tissue Engineering Part A, 14*(11), 1809–1820.
46. Schliephake, H., et al. (2009). Effect of seeding technique and scaffold material on bone formation in tissue-engineered constructs. *Journal of Biomedical Materials Research Part A, 90*(2), 429–437.
47. Janssen, F., et al. (2010). Human tissue-engineered bone produced in clinically relevant amounts using a semi-automated perfusion bioreactor system: A preliminary study. *Journal of Tissue Engineering and Regenerative Medicine, 4*(1), 12–24.
48. Fröhlich, M., et al. (2009). Bone grafts engineered from human adipose-derived stem cells in perfusion bioreactor culture. *Tissue Engineering Part A, 16*(1), 179–189.
49. Bernhardt, A., et al. (2011). Optimization of culture conditions for osteogenically-induced mesenchymal stem cells in β-tricalcium phosphate ceramics with large interconnected channels. *Journal of Tissue Engineering and Regenerative Medicine, 5*(6), 444–453.
50. Grayson, W. L., et al. (2011). Optimizing the medium perfusion rate in bone tissue engineering bioreactors. *Biotechnology and Bioengineering, 108*(5), 1159–1170.
51. Chen, M., et al. (2011). A modular approach to the engineering of a centimeter-sized bone tissue construct with human amniotic mesenchymal stem cells-laden microcarriers. *Biomaterials, 32*(30), 7532–7542.
52. Pisanti, P., et al. (2012). Tubular perfusion system culture of human mesenchymal stem cells on poly-L-lactic acid scaffolds produced using a supercritical carbon dioxide-assisted process. *Journal of Biomedical Materials Research Part A, 100*(10), 2563–2572.
53. Marolt, D., et al. (2012). Engineering bone tissue from human embryonic stem cells. *Proceedings of the National Academy of Sciences, 109*(22), 8705–8709.

54. de Peppo, G. M., et al. (2012). Human embryonic stem cell-derived mesodermal progenitors display substantially increased tissue formation compared to human mesenchymal stem cells under dynamic culture conditions in a packed bed/column bioreactor. *Tissue Engineering Part A, 19*(1–2), 175–187.
55. Bhaskar, B., et al. (2018). Design and assessment of a dynamic perfusion bioreactor for large bone tissue engineering scaffolds. *Applied Biochemistry and Biotechnology, 185*(2), 555–563.
56. Huang, C., & Ogawa, R. (2012). Effect of hydrostatic pressure on bone regeneration using human mesenchymal stem cells. *Tissue Engineering Part A, 18*(19–20), 2106–2113.
57. Neidlinger-Wilke, C., Wilke, H. J., & Claes, L. (1994). Cyclic stretching of human osteoblasts affects proliferation and metabolism: A new experimental method and its application. *Journal of Orthopaedic Research, 12*(1), 70–78.
58. Mauney, J., et al. (2004). Mechanical stimulation promotes osteogenic differentiation of human bone marrow stromal cells on 3-D partially demineralized bone scaffolds in vitro. *Calcified Tissue International, 74*(5), 458–468.
59. Ignatius, A., et al. (2005). Tissue engineering of bone: Effects of mechanical strain on osteoblastic cells in type I collagen matrices. *Biomaterials, 26*(3), 311–318.
60. Wartella, K. A., & Wayne, J. S. (2009). Bioreactor for biaxial mechanical stimulation to tissue engineered constructs. *Journal of Biomechanical Engineering, 131*(4), 044501.
61. Subramanian, G., et al. (2017). Creating homogenous strain distribution within 3D cell-encapsulated constructs using a simple and cost-effective uniaxial tensile bioreactor: Design and validation study. *Biotechnology and Bioengineering, 114*(8), 1878–1887.
62. Matziolis, D., et al. (2011). Osteogenic predifferentiation of human bone marrow-derived stem cells by short-term mechanical stimulation. *The Open Orthopaedics Journal, 5*, 1.
63. Matziolis, G., et al. (2006). Simulation of cell differentiation in fracture healing: Mechanically loaded composite scaffolds in a novel bioreactor system. *Tissue Engineering, 12*(1), 201–208.
64. Fassina, L., et al. (2006). Effects of electromagnetic stimulation on calcified matrix production by SAOS-2 cells over a polyurethane porous scaffold. *Tissue Engineering, 12*(7), 1985–1999.
65. Schwartz, Z., et al. (2008). Pulsed electromagnetic fields enhance BMP-2 dependent osteoblastic differentiation of human mesenchymal stem cells. *Journal of Orthopaedic Research, 26*(9), 1250–1255.
66. Shi, G., Zhang, Z., & Rouabhia, M. (2008). The regulation of cell functions electrically using biodegradable polypyrrole–polylactide conductors. *Biomaterials, 29*(28), 3792–3798.
67. Kim, I. S., et al. (2006). Biphasic electric current stimulates proliferation and induces VEGF production in osteoblasts. *Biochimica et Biophysica Acta (BBA)-Molecular Cell Research, 1763*(9), 907–916.
68. Kim, I. S., et al. (2009). Novel effect of biphasic electric current on in vitro osteogenesis and cytokine production in human mesenchymal stromal cells. *Tissue Engineering Part A, 15*(9), 2411–2422.
69. Sun, L. Y., et al. (2010). Pulsed electromagnetic fields accelerate proliferation and osteogenic gene expression in human bone marrow mesenchymal stem cells during osteogenic differentiation. *Bioelectromagnetics, 31*(3), 209–219.
70. Jasmund, I., & Bader, A. (2002). Bioreactor developments for tissue engineering applications by the example of the bioartificial liver. In *Tools and applications of biochemical engineering science* (pp. 99–109). Berlin: Springer.
71. Jagodzinski, M., et al. (2008). Influence of perfusion and cyclic compression on proliferation and differentiation of bone marrow stromal cells in 3-dimensional culture. *Journal of Biomechanics, 41*(9), 1885–1891.
72. Bölgen, N., et al. (2008). Three-dimensional ingrowth of bone cells within biodegradable cryogel scaffolds in bioreactors at different regimes. *Tissue Engineering Part A, 14*(10), 1743–1750.
73. Zhang, Z.-Y., et al. (2009). A biaxial rotating bioreactor for the culture of fetal mesenchymal stem cells for bone tissue engineering. *Biomaterials, 30*(14), 2694–2704.

74. Liu, C., et al. (2012). Influence of perfusion and compression on the proliferation and differentiation of bone mesenchymal stromal cells seeded on polyurethane scaffolds. *Biomaterials, 33*(4), 1052–1064.
75. Chen, M., et al. (2014). Ectopic osteogenesis of macroscopic tissue constructs assembled from human mesenchymal stem cell-laden microcarriers through in vitro perfusion culture. *PLoS One, 9*(10), e109214.
76. Kang, K. S., et al. (2014). Combined effect of three types of biophysical stimuli for bone regeneration. *Tissue Engineering Part A, 20*(11–12), 1767–1777.
77. Birmingham, E., et al. (2016). An experimental and computational investigation of bone formation in mechanically loaded trabecular bone explants. *Annals of Biomedical Engineering, 44*(4), 1191–1203.
78. Egger, D., et al. (2017). Application of a parallelizable perfusion bioreactor for physiologic 3D cell culture. *Cells, Tissues, Organs, 203*(5), 316–326.
79. Mauck, R., et al. (2007). Regulation of cartilaginous ECM gene transcription by chondrocytes and MSCs in 3D culture in response to dynamic loading. *Biomechanics and Modeling in Mechanobiology, 6*(1–2), 113–125.
80. Guo, T., et al. (2016). Effect of dynamic culture and periodic compression on human mesenchymal stem cell proliferation and chondrogenesis. *Annals of Biomedical Engineering, 44*(7), 2103–2113.
81. Takebe, T., et al. (2012). Human elastic cartilage engineering from cartilage progenitor cells using rotating wall vessel bioreactor. In *Transplantation proceedings*, *44*(4), 1158–1161.
82. Akmal, M., et al. (2006). The culture of articular chondrocytes in hydrogel constructs within a bioreactor enhances cell proliferation and matrix synthesis. *Bone & Joint Journal, 88*(4), 544–553.
83. Marlovits, S., et al. (2003). Collagen expression in tissue engineered cartilage of aged human articular chondrocytes in a rotating bioreactor. *The International Journal of Artificial Organs, 26*(4), 319–330.
84. Yoon, H. H., et al. (2012). Enhanced cartilage formation via three-dimensional cell engineering of human adipose-derived stem cells. *Tissue Engineering Part A, 18*(19–20), 1949–1956.

# Chapter 6
# Engineering of Dental Titanium Implants and Their Coating Techniques

**Jonathan Wirth and Lobat Tayebi**

## 1 Introduction

Implants provide a functional restoration of edentulous regions along the alveolar crest; thus, material selection should be durable for functional loading and biocompatible to achieve osseointegration. Long-term implant success is predicated on successful osseointegration, which provides the secondary retention for the span of the implant. Osseointegration is defined as a functional ankylosis of a load-bearing artificial implant [1].

Titanium is a favorable biomaterial for dental implants because of its rigidity, biocompatibility, and hydrophilicity properties. It induces bioactivity via electronegative potential [2]. It is resistant to a variety of forces and maintains a similar coefficient of expansion to bone, making it an ideal post material for load bearing in dental implantology. Innate properties of titanium can be bolstered with use of coating techniques, manipulating the microenvironment of the surgical site upon placement and through healing [3].

A controlled immune response, high rate of angiogenesis, and bioactivity are conducive to osseointegration; furthermore, the intimacy in which bone apatite is formed to the implant surface determines the seal of the implant, thus reducing incidence of bacterial adhesion [4]. A multitude of clinical presentations provide challenges to favorable wound healing conditions. Functionalization of titanium implant surfaces allows further control over osseointegration of the implant, providing wider patient selection for the restoration of function [4].

Surface modification is subdivided into two methodologies: additive and subtractive [5]. Additive modifications include coating or impregnation of a material on

J. Wirth · L. Tayebi (✉)
Marquette University School of Dentistry, Milwaukee, WI, USA
e-mail: lobat.tayebi@marquette.edu



L. Tayebi (ed.), *Applications of Biomedical Engineering in Dentistry*,
https://doi.org/10.1007/978-3-030-21583-5_6

the titanium surface. Subtractive methods remove material to roughen the surface, increasing porosity. Grit blasting, etching, and ablation are some examples. These methods can be combined to adjust the interface of titanium, leaving a wide range of possibilities for functionalization and more dimension planning an implant design. This article will focus on additive surface modifications of titanium, their biomechanics, and schema.

The chapter will also discuss the benefits and limitations of coating techniques and coating substrates, both conventional and prospective. The article is organized by substrate, as coating techniques may be used for a variety of materials; thus, a brief overview of the scheme and application of coating methods is included, with explanation of the advantages and limitations of these methods. Prospective studies are compared with conventional techniques to emphasize the future study.

## 2 Overview

Surface coating may be organic, inorganic, or a combination of both [5]. Organic coats consist of polymeric or biomimetic films deposed at the surface. Inorganic coats in implantology often consist of metals or ceramics. These coats can be assembled at a molecular level, forming highly organized surface topographies at a nanoscale. Many of these materials, both organic and inorganic, accept nanoparticles sterically or chemically, adding more control to a surface coating scheme. Furthermore, assembly of these coats may be implemented to be more inclusive, offering a multitude of alteration to the biochemistry at the implant surface.

Surface coats ideally adhere to the titanium implant surface in a stable and predictable manner after processing, exhibiting minimization of cytotoxicity and genotoxicity, efficacy of pharmaceutical reagent with optimal, sustained diffusion of incorporated pharmacy [4, 6]. Defects during processing may lead to premature, bulk fracturing of coat material in commercially used coating methods, such as plasma spraying, inducing undesired inflammation. Increased bond strength between the coat and implant reduces incidence of these unwanted outcomes. Ultimately, an ideal coat is conducive to apatite formation intimately adhering to the surface. Schematics for implant coats ideally allow intercalation of forming apatite or factor in metabolism of the coating material to reorganize the bone–implant interface for optimal osseointegration [7].

Peri-implantitis in the first year of implant placement constitutes 10% of premature failures, rendering it the leading cause of implant failure [8]. Reinforcing implants with antimicrobial potential is accomplished with the sustained release of antimicrobial medications for long-term healing or weigh the competitive adherence to the implant surface in favor of osteoblastic activity [9]. Antimicrobial medications can be bactericidal, bacteriostatic, or primers for immune response. Chemotaxis and the provision of an adherent media promote cell adhesion. These factors may be intrinsic properties of surface coating materials; however, nanoparticles localized at the implant surface allow the opportunity to introduce reagents to the surgical site. Because these nanoparticles are readily metabolized, they are often impregnated within a slowly metabolized matrix for sustained release overtime, lest they be exhausted prematurely. Materials such as hydroxyapatite (HA), graphene oxide, and chitosan offer the capacity to be impregnated by these nanoparticles [10–12].

## 3 Implant Coating Materials and Techniques

Biochemical substrates are biomimetic materials at the implant surface, creating a microenvironment that is primed for osseointegration. In conceiving these materials, there is a focus in mimicry of pre-existing compositions for optimal biocompatibility [13]. This can include the localization of plasma proteins and extracellular matrix (ECM) proteins to expedite wound healing, as well mimicry of bony architecture, which is accomplished by HA coating [14]. The challenge is in immobilizing and localizing these biochemical agents so that they aid in osseointegration reliably over time [15].

HA constitutes the inorganic matrix of bone, rendering a biomimetic environment on the surface of the implant. Localization of HA promotes bone morphogenic protein (BMP) in the area. Thus, HA is osteoinductive and improves the outcome of peri-implant osteogenesis. Clinical trials of full zirconia implants demonstrated failure due to its brittleness and inferior electronegative potential when compared to titanium [4].

Ideal coating methods for HA yield a high adhesion strength to the implant surface HA in a thin, uniform layer [16]. Furthermore, HA's capacity for drug delivery has prompted the investigation of coating mechanisms conducive to processing particles that would otherwise be disintegrated or denatured in processing. HA has multiple phases but is optimal in its crystalline phase; therefore, sintering is required for coating techniques that apply high heat and subject HA to phase changes [3].

Quercitrin is a naturally occurring flavonoid, demonstrating improved soft tissue integration, as well as anti-inflammatory and antioxidant properties, mimicking interleukin-1-beta. Excessive inflammation delays healing time; thus, optimized quercitrin-nanocoated titanium surfaces demonstrate enhanced mesenchymal stem cell recruitment and increased rate of osteoblast differentiation. This is supplemented by the inhibition of COX2 expression locally, decreasing PGE2. It also resolves inflammation through the reduction of oxidative stress at the surgical site. Furthermore, enhanced population of cellular activity at the implant site competes with bacteria, decreasing incidence of peri-implantitis [19]. Quercitrin demonstrates positive effects on cells, encouraging expression of hard and soft tissues, and may be used in conjunction with other biomaterials to enhance the rate of osseointegration.

Chitosan is a stable, naturally occurring polysaccharide that promotes the expression of extracellular matrix proteins in osteoblasts and chondrocytes [12]. It is found in normal mammalian tissue, rendering it biocompatible. It contains a primary amino group at the 2-position of each polymer subunit, allowing it to be easily conjugated [20]; thus, it may readily be used to deliver nanoparticles in conjunction with its intrinsic properties. In particular, conjugation with silver bolsters the chitosan with the beneficial antimicrobial effects of silver. Chitosan is also compatible with various matrices, including HA and graphene [11, 20, 21].

Chlorhexidine (CHX) is widely used in dentistry as an effective, broad-spectrum antiseptic agent. While CHX readily adsorbs to the implant surface, it is rapidly depleted—acting as a short-term, localized antimicrobial. Modification of this agent to CHX hexametaphosphate (HMP) demonstrates aggregation to a porous implant surface that provides a more sustained release [9].

Inorganic substrates, especially metals, have intrinsic properties providing antimicrobial effects. They also retain electronegative potential, promoting chemotaxis. Many of these materials can be conjugated onto a coating matrix to supplement it with these unique properties.

Niobium (Nb) is a biocompatible, anti-erosive element [22, 23] and can be applied to titanium in a single-phased subniobium with a conjugate atom. In this manner, a variety of Nb-based films may be produced with oxide, carbide, and nitride conjugates. Of these, NbC proves to be most optimal in vitro, forming a nanocomposite film with great protective efficiency [24], high corrosion resistance, and low coefficient of friction conducive to tribological performance when compared to other Nb film types [25].

Magnetron sputtering (see Table 6.1) of Nb thin films results in amorphous, crack-free coats with good adherence [26].

Graphene oxide demonstrates good mechanical properties with high biocompatibility and antibacterial properties. Its capacity for drug delivery and biosensing has garnered it recent attention in tissue engineering [27].

Graphene may be incorporated in HA coats to reinforce HA. This reinforced GO/HA coat exhibits enhanced physical properties when compared to HA alone [28]. It is also recipient to further addition of osteogenic materials [29].

PMMA transfer is used to coat graphene oxide in a uniform, minimally defective manner. A graphene sheet is seeded on polished Cu foil and treated with coated with a layer of PMMA. This sample is etched to clear the copper, and the unreacted PMMA/graphene is fished with a hexagonal boron nitride and silicon dioxide chip. The PMMA is removed with an organic solvent and $Ar/H_2$ environment. This new sample can be annealed to a target in an ultrahigh-vacuum chamber [30].

## 4 Immobilization

Immobilization describes the processes by which a biomolecular or nanoparticle substrate is arrested at a target surface. This can be accomplished via adsorption, covalent coupling, and physical entrapment. While whole growth factor proteins immobilized at the titanium surface demonstrate improved healing, research is focusing on the production of select GF peptide sequences, such as those that

**Table 6.1** HA deposition methods

| Deposition methods | Description | Adhesion strength (MPa) | Advantages | Disadvantages | References |
|---|---|---|---|---|---|
| Plasma spraying | Coating particle is heated into a molten state in a plasma flame and accelerated to the surface of the implant | 25 | Simple and efficient<br>Low cost<br>Rapid deposition | Highly permeable<br>Environmentally sensitive<br>High temperature processing<br>Sintering required | [3, 4, 10, 13, 17] |
| Sol-gel technique | Coating particle added to solvent, which is hydrolyzed, condensing the particle into a thin layer. This is applied to the surface. Gel is heat treated and melts away, leaving coating particle | 26 | High uniformity<br>Thin coating at a low temperature<br>Low cost | | [3, 4, 10, 17] |
| Electrophoretic deposition | Implant is placed in electrophoretic bath, acting as anode upon which electrolytes can be deposited | 18 | Simple set-up<br>High deposition rate<br>Low cost | Prone to bulk fracture<br>Sintering required | [4, 8, 10, 18] |
| Micro-arc oxidation | Pulsed DC field applied to Ti in an aqueous solution with the addition of electrolytes that deposit during MAO | 44 | Economical<br>Environmentally friendly<br>Increased corrosion resistance | | [8, 10, 17, 18] |
| Magnetron sputtering | Magnetic field of trapped particles is brought near a target electrode target. Particles are emitted and coat target in a thin, uniform layer | 80 | Dense and uniform<br>Low temperature processing<br>High purity and adhesion strength | Time-consuming<br>Low deposition rate<br>Not yet conducive to complex structures, like threaded implants | [8, 10, 18] |

promote growth [31, 32]. Nanoparticles, on the other hand, maintain well-researched, intrinsic properties which can contribute to chemistry of the coat. They can also be impregnated into implant surfaces and their coats to add additional chemical properties to the surface with negligible alteration to the surface topography [33].

Adsorption is the simplest method—the target is coated in a solution of proteins. This yields low surface loading; furthermore, immobilized substrate is easily exhausted.

Covalent coupling offers superior surface loading and improved control over the outcome of immobilization. Overall, nanocomposites, quercitrin, chitosan, and HA are all capable of covalent coupling. The substrate to be immobilized is limited by its interaction with the biomolecule to be linked.

Physical entrapment places the substrate in a physical barrier, such as a synthetic lacuna. HA provides a matrix in which physical entrapment of proteins and nanoparticles can be planned. This process is less predictable, but the range of substrate is extensive, since immobilization is not dependent on chemical interaction.

## *4.1 Peptide Immobilization*

Peptide utility in biomaterials provides accelerated synthesis with supplement of the specific peptide sequences conducive to desired osteoconductive effects. Antimicrobial peptides offer broad-spectrum potency against bacteria with lowered chance of resistance when compared to conventional antibiotics [34]. It is well documented that introduction of growth factors improves osteogenic effects.

Silanes are widely used cross-linkers for immobilizing bioactive peptide sequences. They also have the added effect of expressing osteogenic properties intrinsically [35].

## *4.2 Nanoparticles*

**Silver (Ag)** is one of the most well-researched antimicrobials. In all metallic, silver nitrate and silver sulfadiazine configurations, this element demonstrates stable and broad antimicrobial properties, with low toxicity to patients [36].

**Zinc oxide (ZnO)** is a biocompatible material that demonstrates antimicrobial properties, with wide commercial use. Its proposed mechanism is adherence to the microbes surface, attracting hydrogen peroxides due to electrostatic forces [9, 37].

**Copper oxide (CuO)** demonstrates a low cost solution to providing an antibacterial and antifungal nanocoat. They can be covalently localized to nanocomposites [38].

**$Al_2O_3$ $TiO_2$ nanotubes:** One study found that osteoblast adhesion increases on nanophase metals when compared to conventionally sized particles [39]. $TiO_2$ is intrinsically more electronegative when compared to HA and can be arranged in nanotubes, which exhibit high surface-to-volume ratio when compared conventional roughening modifications. $TiO_2$ also exhibits a more intimate bond than when compared to conventional HA coats. Because apatite arranges itself at a nanoscale, combined with the properties of the metal itself, uniform apatite precipitation is observed on the surface of nanofibrous surfaces, comparable to the intimacy of biointegration demonstrated in HA-coated biomaterials. Furthermore, the surface area to volume ratio is significantly improved over conventional grit blasting, improving bone bonding in vivo [40].

*Positive template-assisted fabrication* utilizes sol-gel deposition to deposit $TiO_2$ on a ZnO-nanorod template. This structure can be deposited to the implant surface and the ZnO selectively removed with chemical etchants, leaving the surface with the nanotubes only. This approach yields asymmetrical tubes with open ends [41].

*Negative template-assisted fabrication* utilizes an anodic aluminum oxide membrane that consists of monodisperse cylindrical pores through which nanotubes are deposited via sol-gel deposition. The resulting nanotubes are even [41].

In *anodization* method, the implant is anodized in an aqueous solution containing 0.5–3.5 wt% hydrofluoric acid; the nanotubes arrange themselves in varying lengths, resulting in an amorphous matrix. The nanotubes are annealed to return them to their crystalline state, which can cause sintering of the nanotubes and thus the collapse of the nanotubular structure. Therefore, this method is sensitive to the annealing process [41].

*Hydrothermal treatment* is the process by which $TiO_2$ particles are synthesized into nanotubes. Hydrothermal treatment of nanoparticles with NaOH breaks their bonds so they can reform as sheets. An HCL wash removes the electrostatic charge of the sheets, causing them to roll up into nanotubes. These nanotubes may then be used to coat implant surfaces. This method reports long reaction times with nanotubes of random alignment due to excessive intercalation from NaOH [41].

**Nanocrystalline diamond particles** are hard, inert, and highly thermally conductive. Corrosion resistance and biotolerance lends it to providing a selective protective barrier, preventing the release of metals to the body. Nanocrystalline coats may provide osteoconductivity, antimicrobial properties, and corrosion resistance [42]. An animal study in the mandibles of pigs demonstrated immobilized BMP-2 on nanocrystalline coats that were unaffected when exposed to radiation, which may preserve osteoinductive potential in irradiated bone [43]. They are also wear resistant, making them potential coats for load-bearing implants [44].

## 5 Discussion and Future Trends

Additive surface modifications are beneficial in that they offer control of localized chemistry while maintaining the properties that make titanium a favorable implant post-material [17]. The goal is to enhance the capacity for secondary retention, ultimately leading to long-term implant success. To this end, adoption of wound-healing elements, especially in the form of fibroblast adoption and differentiation, and antimicrobial activity are favorable [7]. Furthermore, reduction of inflammation at the surgical site expedites wound healing [19].

To this, the composition of surface coating is designed to enhance these properties. Research on surface coating lends itself to the capacity in which these materials may be combined for strategic enhancement of favorable local biochemistry overtime [7]. Ideal coats are biomimetic matrices capable of releasing beneficial particles to the surgical site, promoting healing, and reducing incidence of inflammation and peri-implantitis.

The challenges of surface coating are derived from mechanical properties between the implant and coat interface. Alternatives to HA coating are being investigated due to its poor adherence to titanium. Because of this, $TiO_2$ nanotubes present as a prospective surface modification [41, 45].

Nanoparticles are unique in that their properties are intrinsic and may be incorporated to supplement a coating material. While they can readily impregnate the implant surface, a slowly dissolving matrix is preferable for sustained release. Optimization of this strategy drives research in supplementing coating materials, such as HA, $TiO_2$, and graphene. Chemical conjugation and mechanical retention in synthetic lacunae are the approaches that facilitate this action.

***Prospective Coating Materials*** The interaction of titanium with a variety of novel biomaterials is being investigated. Nanocomposites and their unique properties are influencing new schemes for additive surface modifications. Graphene demonstrates unique approach to drug delivery—its high surface area to volume ratio offers functionalized capacity to surfaces to which it is applied [46]. This significant increase in surface area could have a multitude of implications for the future of surface modification. Graphene may be hybridized with metals and metal oxides. One study demonstrated graphene/zinc oxide nanocomposite films offer profound antimicrobial properties [47]. Research in hybridization of various other nanoparticles may offer more insight on the utility of this material. Currently, graphene lacks an efficient method to be applied to three-dimensional, complex objects, such as a dental screw-retained implant. Nb as a surface coating has garnered interest in bioengineering due to its biocompatibility and increased mitochondrial activity in comparison to cells cultured on titanium [48]. Furthermore, it has the capacity to form nanocomposites. Another study demonstrated intrinsic capacity of crystalline NbN and amorphous $Nb_2O_5$ coatings for cementoblast attachment [49]. Overall, graphene forms as a monolayer with considerably more corrosive resistance than Nb nanocomposites. A comparison of graphene and Nb's tribology may offer insight on the long-term properties of these materials in function [50]. $TiO_2$ nanotubes can form a high surface area to volume ratio that increases at the surface of the implant, but not in the organization with which graphene coats are capable. However, the efficacy of $TiO_2$ nanotubes as a surface treatment is well documented. Nanocrystalline diamond also has properties comparable to nanocomposites with similar capacity for covalent immobilization.

*Prospects in coating schematics* can be seen in the formulation of coats with multifunctionality [51]. Co-immobilization of a multitude of beneficial peptides and nanoparticles allows a wide range of osteogenic and antimicrobial potential. Furthermore, coating materials can reinforce the mechanical properties of one another. One study successfully coated titanium implants with a HA/chitosan/graphene coat [11]. Graphene reinforces the brittle nature of HA, while chitosan, along with its intrinsic properties, may be conjugated with nanoparticles for drug delivery. Delivery of this coating complex indicates the dimension with which additive modifications can enhance titanium implant success. The integrity of these materials in coexistence is not well documented. While graphene may reinforce the integrity of HA, stress testing with a multitude of these materials has little evidence. Nanocrystalline diamond demonstrates potential as a nanofiller in biopolymeric matrices [52]. Optimization and cross reactions between immobilized nanoparticles and peptides require further investigation. Histocompatibility of these materials should also be investigated. Further testing should be performed on the integrity of these materials in vivo. Both Nb and graphene can be deposited with similar methodologies. It has been suggested that hybridization is possible, compounding their anticorrosive and osteoconductive properties [26]. Overall, the future of additive surface coating is focused on optimization of multifactorial coats that demonstrate antimicrobial and osteoconductive properties.

## 6 Summary

HA has continually been the most important material in coating of titanium implants. HA is being developed in new ways to adapt more dimensions for its applications. A more reliable, commercial method of coating dental implants with HA is underway. Ion magnetron sputtering is a promising delivery of a controlled, even coat with significantly improved bond strength when compared to conventional HA coating mechanisms. This coating method is still in development.

Research in nanocomposites and their unique properties will play a key role in the development of prospective coating schematics. Based on enhanced tribology and osteoconductive potential of Nb and graphene-based nanocomposites, they are worth investigating. These materials also offer many advantages to formulating drug delivery strategies in more organized manner. Currently, stress testing and animal studies have little evidence in these multifunctional coating schemes. Understanding how the materials interact with each other needs to be better understood.

## References

1. Schroeder, A., et al. (1981). The reactions of bone, connective tissue, and epithelium to endosteal implants with titanium-sprayed surfaces. *Journal of Maxillofacial Surgery, 9*, 15–25.
2. Tagliareni, J. M., & Clarkson, E. (2015). Basic concepts and techniques of dental implants. *Dental Clinics, 59*(2), 255–264.
3. Ripamonti, U. (2018). Functionalized surface geometries induce:"*Bone: Formation by Autoinduction*". *Frontiers in Physiology, 8*, 1084.

4. Ong, J. L., & Chan, D. C. (2000). Hydroxyapatite and their use as coatings in dental implants: a review. *Critical Reviews™ in Biomedical Engineering, 28*(5&6), 667.
5. Chouirfa, H., et al. (2019). Review of titanium surface modification techniques and coatings for antibacterial applications. *Acta Biomaterialia, 83*, 37–54.
6. Ota-Tsuzuki, C., et al. (2011). Influence of titanium surface treatments on formation of the blood clot extension. *Journal of Oral Implantology, 37*(6), 641–647.
7. Shibata, Y., & Tanimoto, Y. (2015). A review of improved fixation methods for dental implants. Part I: Surface optimization for rapid osseointegration. *Journal of Prosthodontic Research, 59*(1), 20–33.
8. Damiati, L., et al. (2018). Impact of surface topography and coating on osteogenesis and bacterial attachment on titanium implants. *Journal of Tissue Engineering, 9*, 2041731418790694.
9. Parnia, F., et al. (2017). Overview of nanoparticle coating of dental implants for enhanced osseointegration and antimicrobial purposes. *Journal of Pharmacy & Pharmaceutical Sciences, 20*, 148–160.
10. Graziani, G., et al. (2017). Ion-substituted calcium phosphate coatings deposited by plasma-assisted techniques: A review. *Materials Science and Engineering: C, 74*, 219–229.
11. Yu, P., et al. (2017). Self-assembled high-strength hydroxyapatite/graphene oxide/chitosan composite hydrogel for bone tissue engineering. *Carbohydrate Polymers, 155*, 507–515.
12. Norowski, P. A., et al. (2011). Chitosan coatings deliver antimicrobials from titanium implants: a preliminary study. *Implant Dentistry, 20*(1), 56–67.
13. Kubasiewicz-Ross, P., et al. (2017). Zirconium: The material of the future in modern implantology. *Advances in Clinical and Experimental Medicine: Official Organ Wroclaw Medical University, 26*(3), 533–537.
14. La, W.-G., et al. (2014). Delivery of bone morphogenetic protein-2 and substance P using graphene oxide for bone regeneration. *International Journal of Nanomedicine, 9*(Suppl 1), 107.
15. Panayotov, I. V., et al. (2015). Strategies for immobilization of bioactive organic molecules on titanium implant surfaces–a review. *Folia Medica, 57*(1), 11–18.
16. Meng, H.-W., Chien, E. Y., & Chien, H.-H. (2016). Dental implant bioactive surface modifications and their effects on osseointegration: a review. *Biomarker Research, 4*(1), 24.
17. Zafar, M. S., et al. (2019). Bioactive surface coatings for enhancing osseointegration of dental implants. In *Biomedical, therapeutic and clinical applications of bioactive glasses* (pp. 313–329). Amsterdam, Netherlands: Elsevier.
18. Goldman, M., Juodzbalys, G., & Vilkinis, V. (2014). Titanium surfaces with nanostructures influence on osteoblasts proliferation: a systematic review. *Journal of Oral & Maxillofacial Research, 5*(3), e1.
19. Gomez-Florit, M., et al. (2016). Quercitrin-nanocoated titanium surfaces favour gingival cells against oral bacteria. *Scientific Reports, 6*, 22444.
20. Satheeshababu, B., & Shivakumar, K. (2013). Synthesis of conjugated chitosan and its effect on drug permeation from transdermal patches. *Indian Journal of Pharmaceutical Sciences, 75*(2), 162.
21. Shi, Y., et al. (2016). Electrophoretic deposition of graphene oxide reinforced chitosan–hydroxyapatite nanocomposite coatings on Ti substrate. *Journal of Materials Science: Materials in Medicine, 27*(3), 48.
22. Eisenbarth, E., et al. (2004). Biocompatibility of β-stabilizing elements of titanium alloys. *Biomaterials, 25*(26), 5705–5713.
23. Matsuno, H., et al. (2001). Biocompatibility and osteogenesis of refractory metal implants, titanium, hafnium, niobium, tantalum and rhenium. *Biomaterials, 22*(11), 1253–1262.
24. Braic, M., et al. (2011). Preparation and characterization of biocompatible Nb–C coatings. *Thin Solid Films, 519*(12), 4064–4068.
25. Xu, Z., et al. (2019). Potential of niobium-based thin films as a protective and osteogenic coating for dental implants: The role of the nonmetal elements. *Materials Science and Engineering: C, 96*, 166–175.
26. Kalisz, M., et al. (2015). Comparison of mechanical and corrosion properties of graphene monolayer on Ti–Al–V and nanometric Nb2O5 layer on Ti–Al–V alloy for dental implants applications. *Thin Solid Films, 589*, 356–363.

27. He, J., et al. (2015). Killing dental pathogens using antibacterial graphene oxide. *ACS Applied Materials & Interfaces, 7*(9), 5605–5611.
28. Li, M., et al. (2014). Graphene oxide/hydroxyapatite composite coatings fabricated by electrophoretic nanotechnology for biological applications. *Carbon, 67*, 185–197.
29. La, W. G., et al. (2013). Delivery of a therapeutic protein for bone regeneration from a substrate coated with graphene oxide. *Small, 9*(23), 4051–4060.
30. Jung, H. S., et al. (2015). Fabrication of gate-tunable graphene devices for scanning tunneling microscopy studies with Coulomb impurities. *JoVE (Journal of Visualized Experiments)*, (101), e52711.
31. Schliephake, H., et al. (2005). Effect of immobilized bone morphogenic protein 2 coating of titanium implants on peri-implant bone formation. *Clinical Oral Implants Research, 16*(5), 563–569.
32. Youn, Y. H., et al. (2019). Simple and facile preparation of recombinant human bone morphogenetic protein-2 immobilized titanium implant via initiated chemical vapor deposition technique to promote osteogenesis for bone tissue engineering application. *Materials Science and Engineering: C, 100*, 949.
33. de Jonge, L. T., et al. (2008). Organic–inorganic surface modifications for titanium implant surfaces. *Pharmaceutical Research, 25*(10), 2357–2369.
34. Ageitos, J., et al. (2017). Antimicrobial peptides (AMPs): Ancient compounds that represent novel weapons in the fight against bacteria. *Biochemical Pharmacology, 133*, 117–138.
35. Godoy-Gallardo, M., et al. (2016). Anhydride-functional silane immobilized onto titanium surfaces induces osteoblast cell differentiation and reduces bacterial adhesion and biofilm formation. *Materials Science and Engineering: C, 59*, 524–532.
36. Sharonova, A., et al. (2019). Surface functionalization of titanium with silver nanoparticles. *Journal of Physics: Conference Series*. IOP Publishing.
37. Zhao, Q., et al. (2019). Surface functionalization of titanium with zinc/strontium-doped titanium dioxide microporous coating via microarc oxidation. *Nanomedicine: Nanotechnology, Biology and Medicine, 16*, 149–161.
38. Ahmad, Z., et al. (2012). Antimicrobial properties of electrically formed elastomeric polyurethane–copper oxide nanocomposites for medical and dental applications. In *Methods in enzymology* (pp. 87–99). Amsterdam, Netherlands: Elsevier.
39. Webster, T. J., & Ejiofor, J. U. (2004). Increased osteoblast adhesion on nanophase metals: Ti, Ti6Al4V, and CoCrMo. *Biomaterials, 25*(19), 4731–4739.
40. Bjursten, L. M., et al. (2010). Titanium dioxide nanotubes enhance bone bonding in vivo. *Journal of Biomedical Materials Research Part A: An Official Journal of The Society for Biomaterials, The Japanese Society for Biomaterials, and The Australian Society for Biomaterials and the Korean Society for Biomaterials, 92*(3), 1218–1224.
41. Tan, A., et al. (2012). Review of titania nanotubes: Fabrication and cellular response. *Ceramics International, 38*(6), 4421–4435.
42. Goloshchapov, D., et al. (2019). Importance of defect nanocrystalline calcium hydroxyapatite characteristics for developing the dental biomimetic composites. In *Results in Physics* (p. 102158).
43. Braga, N., et al. (2008). From micro to nanocrystalline transition in the diamond formation on porous pure titanium. *Diamond and Related Materials, 17*(11), 1891–1896.
44. Cui, W., Cheng, J., & Liu, Z. (2019). Bio-tribocorrosion behavior of a nanocrystalline TiZrN coating on biomedical titanium alloy. *Surface and Coatings Technology, 369*, 79.
45. Louarn, G., et al. (2019). Nanostructured surface coatings for titanium alloy implants. *Journal of Materials Research, 34*, 1–8.
46. McCallion, C., et al. (2016). Graphene in therapeutics delivery: Problems, solutions and future opportunities. *European Journal of Pharmaceutics and Biopharmaceutics, 104*, 235–250.
47. Kulshrestha, S., et al. (2014). A graphene/zinc oxide nanocomposite film protects dental implant surfaces against cariogenic Streptococcus mutans. *Biofouling, 30*(10), 1281–1294.
48. Olivares-Navarrete, R., et al. (2011). Biocompatibility of niobium coatings. *Coatings, 1*(1), 72–87.

49. Ramírez, G., et al. (2011). Niobium based coatings for dental implants. *Applied Surface Science, 257*(7), 2555–2559.
50. Manini, N., et al. (2017). Current trends in the physics of nanoscale friction. *Advances in Physics: X, 2*(3), 569–590.
51. Mas-Moruno, C., Su, B., & Dalby, M. J. (2019). Multifunctional coatings and nanotopographies: Toward cell instructive and antibacterial implants. *Advanced Healthcare Materials, 8*(1), 1801103.
52. Das, D. (2019). Nanocrystalline diamond: a high-impact carbon nanomaterial for multifunctional applications including as nanofiller in biopolymeric matrices. In *Carbon-based nanofillers and their rubber nanocomposites* (pp. 123–181). Amsterdam, Netherlands: Elsevier.

# Chapter 7
# Applications of Laser in Dentistry

**Reza Fekrazad, Farshid Vahdatinia, Leila Gholami, Zahra Khamverdi, Parviz Torkzaban, Alexander Karkazis, and Lobat Tayebi**

## 1 Introduction

The word "laser" indicates "light amplification by stimulated emission of radiation," which was first introduced by Gordon Gould in 1959. The output light from the laser device is in fact a beam of coherent, collimated, monochromatic, and high-density beams that stay narrow over great distances and well-focused on surfaces. The laser light can be absorbed, reflected, transmitted, or scattered in accordance with the output wavelength and tissue properties after contact with the surfaces [1, 2].

Clinical application of the laser was first introduced in 1960 by Maiman [2]. With this, the three most relevant properties that should be considered for clinical application include wavelength, power density, and application mode (pulse or continuous, contact or noncontact).

Generally, classification of laser types is based on the physical nature (such as gas, liquid, solid, or semiconductor), the type of active media (such as erbium:

R. Fekrazad
International Network for Photo Medicine and Photo Dynamic Therapy (INPMPDT), Universal Scientific Education and Research Network (USERN), Tehran, Iran

F. Vahdatinia
Dental Implants Research Center, Hamadan University of Medical Sciences, Hamadan, Iran

L. Gholami · P. Torkzaban
Department of Periodontics, Dental Research Center, Hamadan University of Medical Sciences, Hamadan, Iran

Z. Khamverdi
Department of Operative Dentistry, Dental Research Center, Hamadan University of Medical Sciences, Hamadan, Iran

A. Karkazis · L. Tayebi (✉)
Marquette University School of Dentistry, Milwaukee, WI, USA
e-mail: lobat.tayebi@marquette.edu



L. Tayebi (ed.), *Applications of Biomedical Engineering in Dentistry*,
https://doi.org/10.1007/978-3-030-21583-5_7

yttrium aluminum garnet (Er: YAG)), and lastly, the degree of skin or eye injury [3]. Another common classification is the division of lasers into low-intensity and high-intensity groups. High-intensity lasers are known as surgical knives; their most important application is in tissue cutting. However, low-intensity lasers have wider therapeutic applications.

The first studies on low-intensity lasers indicate a positive effect of low-intensity radiation on hair growth and wound healing. Low-intensity lasers can cause both stimulatory and inhibitory responses, depending on the beam parameters. Today, the term "photobiomodulation (PBM)" is used rather than "low-intensity" lasers, which has a more precise and comprehensive meaning in the application of the therapeutic effects of electromagnetic waves [4].

The most commonly used laser systems in dentistry are presented in Fig. 7.1 and Table 7.1.

This chapter will first review the applications of PBM in regenerative dentistry including bone regeneration, wound healing, anti-inflammatory, pain therapy, nerve regeneration, and stem cells. Next, the chapter will focus on combination of laser

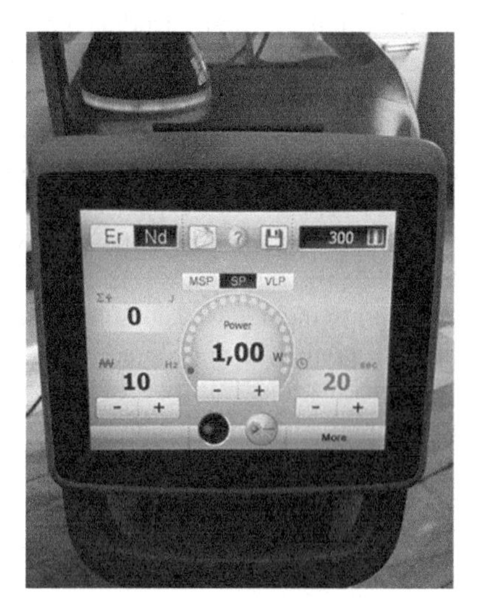


**Fig. 7.1** Two complementary laser wavelength (Er:YAG and Nd:YAG) in a single system

**Table 7.1** Most commonly used laser systems in dentistry

| Laser | Nature of active media | Wavelength |
|---|---|---|
| Argon | Gas | 488, 515 nm |
| KTP | Solid | 532 nm |
| Helium-neon | Gas | 633 nm |
| Diode | Semiconductor | 635, 670, 810, 830, 980 nm |
| Nd:YAG | Solid | 1064 nm |
| Er,Cr:YSGG | Solid | 2780 nm |
| Er:YAG | Solid | 2940 nm |
| $CO_2$ | Gas | 9600, 10,600 nm |

therapy and nanotechnology in dentistry such as oral cancer therapy, laser-assisted antimicrobial photodynamic therapy using nanoparticles, and nanophotodynamic therapy in dental caries, periodontitis, and peri-implantitis.

# 2 Photobiomodulation in Regenerative Dentistry

PBM is a noninvasive and painless method, which has known stimulatory effects on growth and tissue regeneration, reduces inflammation and pain, heals wounds and aides in the proliferation of fibroblasts and chondrocytes, collagen synthesis, and neuronal regeneration [5, 6].

Phototherapy (including coherent and noncoherent light sources) is a type of interaction between light with low energy density and tissue cells without thermal effects. Hence, this category of laser radiation is called "soft therapy" or "cold laser." PBM therapy (including low-level laser therapy/low-level laser irradiation) involves electromagnetic waves within the visible spectrum (or optical window 380–700 nm) or near-infrared region (700–1070 nm) and a radiation power between 10 and 500 mW or less than 250 mW. PBM therapy leads to the biomodulation of photophysical, photochemical, and photobiological reactions by affecting photoreceptors. Photochemical reactions can be produced as a result ATP synthesis and by exposure to visible light radiation or near infrared (NIR) on mitochondrial optical receptors. Additionally, photophysical reactions are caused by light radiation on calcium channels in the cell membrane.

Light absorption by the components of the respiratory chain produces short-term activation of the respiratory chain and oxidation of the NADH pool. Stimulation of oxidative phosphorylation subsequently leads to changes in the mitochondrial redox status, as well as the cytoplasm of the cell. The electron transfer chain provides increased levels of stimulatory forces to the cell by increasing the storage of ATP, thus increasing the electrical potential of the mitochondrial membrane and cytoplasmic alkalization, activating the synthesis of nucleic acids. Since ATP is a common form of energy for the cell, LLLT has the potential for stimulating normal cell function. By rising the respiratory metabolism of the cell, LLLT can also influence electrical-physiological properties of the cell, as demonstrated in Fig. 7.2 [7, 8].

## 2.1 *Photobiomodulation and Bone Regeneration*

PBM stimulates bone formation and regeneration by activating the proliferation and differentiation of osteoblasts and decreasing the activity of osteoclasts; furthermore, it increases the thickness of trabeculae and increases mineral deposition. In this regard, studies have shown that laser therapy can even affect orthodontic tooth movement or bone tissue repair around implants by stimulating bone remodeling. Based on bone cell biology findings, the expression of cytokines—such as the

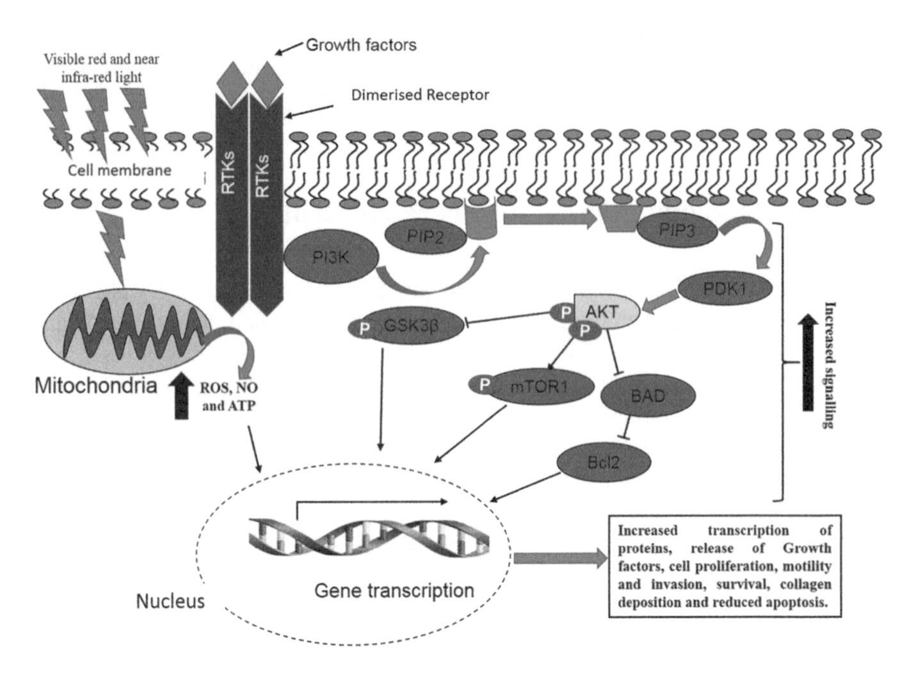


**Fig. 7.2** The photobiomodulation effects on cellular metabolism. (Reuse with permission) [9]

receptor activator of nuclear factor-kappa-β (RANK)/RANK ligand (RANKL)/ osteoprotegerin (OPG)—following laser radiation can affect osteoclastogenesis. Both RANKL and OPG are cytokines from the tumor necrosis factor family and are produced through osteoblasts and bone marrow cells. RANKL and OPG stimulate and inhibit, respectively, the specific RANK receptors present on the surface of osteoclast progenitor cells and hence play a vital role in the regulation of bone resorption [10]. It should be noted that, basically, infrared lasers have a greater effect on bone regeneration than visible light lasers due to increased depth of penetration within the bone tissue [11].

## 2.2 *Wound Healing Effects of Photobiomodulation*

PBM also plays a positive role in improving the speed of wound healing and scar tissue quality [12]. The ulcers can be classified into two categories based on the duration of repair: acute and chronic. Acute ulcers are caused by surgery or trauma—the reparation process occurs within the expected timeframe and is uncomplicated. Conversely, chronic ulcers are not repaired in an optimal timeframe and are commonly associated with secondary complications.

The process of wound healing in the craniofacial region is based on a central physiological process that maintains tissue integrity. Proper healing process requires successful coordination of multiple phases, such as hemostasis, inflammation, cell migration, matrix synthesis, and remodeling [13]. The wound healing process begins at the onset of an injury. Infiltration of blood components and inflammatory cells (such as neutrophils) occurs in the early stages of wound healing. Lymphocytes and plasma cells infiltrate later on, beginning the important action of phagocytosis to remove foreign bodies, bacteria, and damaged tissue. Subsequently, wound re-epithelialization occurs through the migration and reproduction of epithelial cells with the origin of margins and center of the lesion. Also, fibroblasts migrate to damaged areas and begin to produce extracellular matrix. The final repair or final remodeling process is also accomplished through cross-linking and organized interconnections within the new collagen matrix [14].

Simultaneously, the presence of factors can interfere with wound healing, such as inadequate nutrition, necrotic tissue, foreign body, bacterial infection, interference in blood circulation, lymphatic artery obstruction, systemic diseases, diabetes, and physiological factors [15, 16]. Also, mitogenic factors, such as TGF-β (transforming growth factor beta), and cytokines, such as IL-6 (interleukin 6) and TNF-α (tumor necrosis factor alpha), play an important role in the process of wound healing [17].

Despite the inadequate understanding of the exact mechanism of PBM in wound healing, numerous laboratory and clinical studies have consistently pointed to the positive effect of laser irradiation on wound healing. The findings indicate that PBM stimulates cell proliferation and migration, induces the production of growth factors through keratinocytes and stromal cells, inhibits cell death, promotes/inhibits collagen synthesis, helps to restore metabolism, and increases the expression of mediators—such as TGF-β1, PDGF-BB, and IL-8—in the wound fluid. However, in terms of the PBM's harmful potential in wound healing, controlling factors, like wavelength and radiation dosage, are critical for the success of PBM therapies. For example, some studies recommend a wavelength of 600–700 nm for treating superficial tissues, while 780 and 950 nm are recommended for deep tissue treatment.

## *2.3 Anti-inflammatory and Pain Therapy of Photobiomodulation*

As previously noted, one of the capabilities of PBM is its anti-inflammatory and analgesic effects, which can be used to reduce the oxidative stress in cases of chronic pain, diabetes, spinal cord injury, and also in the treatment of oral mucositis, especially those caused by chemotherapeutic complications.

Pain is a displeasing sensory and emotional experience resulting from actual tissue injury or damage to another type of tissue. According to the definition by the Association for the Study of Pain, neuropathic pain is defined as "pain caused by a lesion or a disease of the somatosensory system" (www.iasp-pain.org).

Based on physiotherapy sources, the use of low-intensity lasers is widely considered an effective method to treat pain. This therapeutic technique has advantages such as being noninvasive, low cost, and containing minimal side effects [18]. Although the exact mechanism of LLLT is unclear in pain reduction, several studies have indicated the treatment does in fact reduce pain. The effects of LLLT on pain relief are similar to NSAIDs (celecoxib, meloxicam, diclofenac) or corticosteroid (dexamethasone) application. Therefore, the most important theories related to the analgesic effect of LLLT are reduction of inflammatory mediators (such as prostaglandin E2, interleukin 1β, and tumor necrosis factor α), increased levels of endogenous opioids, and reduction of nerve cell permeation and ATP production. Inhibition of the signal transduction in the neuromuscular junction is another mechanism for reducing both myofascial pain and trigger points. Additionally, stimulating the neural regeneration process reduces pain after surgery and other inflammatory processes.

## 2.4 Nerve Regeneration and Photobiomodulation Therapy

The first studies on LLLT's effect on damaged peripheral nerve regeneration date back to the late 1970s. Researchers continue to study the spinal cord and sciatic and crushed peroneal nerves using LLLT. The results of these studies indicate the positive effect of axonotmesis and neurotmesis, increased axonal metabolism, and decreased pain and inflammation. Today, the use of LLLT for the repair of postoperative neurological damage, such as lower alveolar nerve injury after wisdom tooth extraction or after orthogonal surgery of sagittal osteotomy, is also recommended [19].

In addition to the effect of LLLT on cellular function, the production of nerve growth factor can also be regulated by laser radiation. Nerve growth factor is important for the spread of sympathetic and sensory neurons and inhibition of apoptosis, especially in cases of damage to neural fibers [20, 21]. Also, the most important effects of PBM therapy on the nervous system include improving post-injury function, increasing the axonal diameter, increasing the thickness of the myelin sheath, reducing the infiltration of single cell nucleus cells, increasing the number of Schwann cells, increasing neurotrophic growth factors, and reducing dysesthesia [22]. In some studies, LLLT has been shown to increase the concentration of VEGF and NGF and, at the same time, reduce the expression of HIF-1α (hypoxia-induced factor 1 alpha), TNF-α, and IL -1β [23, 24].

## 2.5 Stem Cells and Photobiomodulation Therapy

Mesenchymal stem cells (MSCs), such as dental pulp stem cells (DPSCs), play a significant role in the future of regenerative medicine. Important features of MSCs include relative ease in cell culturing, limited immunogenicity, ability to suppress immune activity, and multilineage ability. Hence, some laboratory studies have pointed to the positive effect of LLLT on the rate of proliferation and differentiation of MSCs. LLLT affects the expression of cellular genes by stimulating the cell proliferation/inhibition of cell death, as well as producing extracellular matrix proteins [25]. PBM causes stem cell differentiation by stimulating cellular optical receptors. The absorption of visible light (380–700 nm) and NIR (700–1070 nm) by mitochondrial optical receptors activates the respiratory chain—specifically NADH dehydrogenase, cytochrome C reductase, oxidase, and ATP synthase [26, 27].

It is also understood that infrared radiation results in the transmission of biological messages by activating ion channels, which increases cell membrane permeability and changes the concentrations of $Na^+$, $K^+$, and $Ca^{2+}$ ions across the cell membrane [28]. Theocharidou et al. showed that LLLI first increased the expression of Runt-related transcription factor 2 (RUNX2) and core-binding factor subunit alpha-1 (CBF-alpha-1) transcription factors and secondly increased Osterix expression—both of which are key factors in the process of differentiation of MSCs into bone marrow [25, 29]. Also, Manzano-Moreno et al. suggested that PBM significantly increases the expression of early marker differentiation of osteoblasts such as ALP, Osterix, Runx2, and BMP-2 [30]. Other effects of PBM include the activation and augmentation of growth factor synthesis, such as FGF, VEGF, TGF-β1, and cell death. The findings of this study indicate improvement in biological function of stem cells involved in dental pulp regeneration following PBM therapy.

PBM therapy has also been studied on stem cells from human exfoliated deciduous teeth (SHED). PBM therapy on the SHED culture medium has an effect on the induction of osteoblast differentiation and increases the expression and activity of alkaline phosphatase and dentin sialophosphoprotein, along with increasing collagen synthesis. Furthermore, other findings from PBM therapy on deciduous teeth-derived stem cells have been shown to increase viability, proliferation, and production of inorganic tissue.

## 3 The Combination of Laser Therapy and Nanotechnology in Dentistry

The two new technologies of laser and nanotechnology have made a great impact on biomedical engineering. Simultaneous application of these two technologies has introduced many novel biomedical approaches to procedures, such as cancer treatment and diagnosis, drug delivery and release, antimicrobial therapies, tooth hypersensitivity treatments, and improvement in the adhesion of materials to dental structures.

The interaction of lasers with different chromophores and its photothermal properties, in combination with the new physical effect of nanoparticles as a result of the dominant quantum properties, rather than classical ones, may result in fascinating new therapeutic effects [31].

### 3.1 Laser and Nanotechnology in Oral Cancer Therapy

Despite the great progress achieved in diagnosis and treatment of cancers in recent years, oral cancer is still considered a common malignant disease with low survival rates [32]. Since conventional treatments—like radiotherapy and chemotherapy—have severe complications, researchers are searching for more effective alternative treatment strategies with fewer side effects. Lasers are a promising technology for diagnosis and treatment in various types of cancers, including oral cancers. One such use of lasers has been through laser ablation of head and neck tumors using image-guided technologies instead of conventional surgical procedures. The tumor is destroyed by inducing heat using a small laser fiber placed inside it. The destructed area is usually very small and concentrated only around the fiber; however, it might not be absolutely confined to the tumor tissue, with the possibility of unintentional heating and damage of nearby tissue.

Using the benefit of materials at the nanoscale, such as a larger surface area to volume ratio, new optical and magnetic characteristics, nanomaterials have been investigated to overcome many biological hurdles to cancer treatment. Nanotechnology-based detection and treatment of cancers have the prospective to replace extremely aggressive conventional cancer detection and treatment [32]. Nanobased medicine and the use of nanoparticles have been shown to be a much better strategy for cancer therapy with enhanced safety and efficacy. They can be preferentially targeted to the tumor and result in minimally invasive destruction of the tumor tissue upon laser irradiation [33].

The combination of these two fascinating technologies of laser and nanotechnology has led to newly developed and encouraging phototherapeutics, known as photothermal therapy (PTT). This procedure combines two key components: light source (especially lasers with a spectral range of red and near-infrared (NIR) 650–900 nm photonic window region with deep tissue penetration) and optical absorbing particles (which can be in the form of a nanoparticle) that transform the optical irradiation into heat [32]. The generated heat can cause cancer cell thermal ablation and permanent cell injury by loosening cell membranes and denaturing proteins while causing minimal toxicity to normal tissue.

Agents activated by NIR light are suitable for these treatments, since NIR radiation is considered a favorable light source with its minimum absorption in human body chromophores and deep tissue penetration [34].

Noble metal nanoparticles, with their strong surface electric fields, enhance electromagnetic radiation absorption and scattering; these properties can potentially be used in designing new optically active agents used in molecular imaging and photothermal cancer therapy [34].

Many different nanoscale photoabsorbers with precise control of size, shape, and surface functionalization are providing innovative paths to carry several diagnostic and/or therapeutic agents for improved result and fewer side effects. This has made controlled and directed damage of tumor tissues possible. Different designs of nanoparticles, such as nanorings, nanoshells, nanorods, nanopores, nanowires, and nanocomposites carrying anticancer drugs, have been created and studied. When used with a laser wavelength matching their peak absorption, these particles can each have unique properties and applications [31].

In order to specifically direct nanoparticles and nanocarriers to malignant cells, various methods are used. First, conjugation with antibodies, such as anti-HER2 and anti-EGFR, binds to overexpressed HER2 and EGFR on malignant cell cytoplasmic membranes and second, the use of macrophages as biocarriers for nanoparticles [35, 36]. Elimination of tumors surrounding vital tissues is not easy due to unclear tumor margins, and cutting healthy tissue may also have unacceptable cosmetic and medical outcomes. Hopefully, this new approach of targeted application of nanoparticles to cancer cells can provide great accuracy in such conditions [34].

Nanodiagnosis, nanoimaging, and nanotreatment strategies of oral cancer have been key research fronts with many highly cited papers in recent years, all showing promising results of successful elimination of cancerous tissue, along with better tumor contrast for imaging intentions and early diagnosis. Many studies—mainly in the form of in vitro and animal research—have been conducted in oral cancer therapy. Some of the interesting studies are presented here.

In 2007, Huang et al. studied laser photothermal therapy (PTT) using conjugation of anti-EGFR antibodies to aggregated spherical gold nanoparticles and short near-infrared (NIR) laser pulsed irradiation in which oral cancer cells were specifically targeted. They observed that a laser threshold power 20 times lower than normal PTT was needed for photothermal destruction of cells with nanoparticle treatment. Destroyed cell count was quadratically dependent on the laser power. They considered the aggregated nanospheres as the reason for enhanced photothermal cell killing [37].

In a study by Fekrazad et al. in 2011, anti-HER2 immuno-nanoshells were studied for oral squamous cell carcinoma treatment. HER2-positive KB cells and HER2-negative HeLaS3 were bound to gold-silica nanoshells conjugated with anti-HER2 (100 nm). Using an 810 nm laser, cells were irradiated at 4 W/cm$^2$ for 2 min. They observed significant destruction of cells in the KB tumor cell cultures, while HeLaS3 cells showed no evidence of cell damage or death.

In a more recent report by Fekrazad et al. in 2017, core-shell gold-coated iron oxide NPs (Au-IONPs) were developed as a multimodal nanoplatform to be employed as a magnetic resonance imaging (MRI) contrast agent and a nanoheater for photothermal cancer therapy. Photothermal and cytotoxic effects of Au-IONPs on a KB cell line, derived from human oral epidermal carcinoma, were studied with laser irradiation with a 808 nm laser wavelength and 6.3 W/cm$^2$ for 5 min. Approximate cell death was 70%, which strongly depended on incubation period and the u-IONP concentration. There was more sensitive detection of cancer lesions using MRI (result from magnetic nanoparticles present in the Au-IONP nanocomplex); furthermore, there was enhanced laser therapy efficacy because of the presence of Au-NPs in the Au-IONP nanocomplex and due to the surface plasmon resonance effect, which makes them suitable for photothermal therapy [31].

A recent 2018 in vivo study by Lang Rao et al. has successfully reported platelets as new carriers for gold nanorods (AuNRs) in photothermal therapy, using a gene-knockout mouse model. PLTs were loaded with nanorod electroporation. The AuNR-loaded PLTs (PLT-AuNRs) inherited both the long blood circulation and cancer targeting characteristics of PLTs and the photothermal aspect of AuNRs. After administration of AuNRs and laser irradiation of head and neck squamous cell carcinoma (HNSCC), growth was effectively inhibited. In addition, their results show that the PTT treatment increases PLT-AuNRs targeting the tumor and a special self-reinforcing effect of PLT-PTT resulting in enhancement of the PTT effects.

An important area of research is concerned with challenges still being faced in complete elimination of cancer cells in vivo and prevention of cancer cell migration; nanotechnology and laser research have also shown promising results in the field of metastasis prevention.

In an interesting study by Ali et al. in 2017, integrins were targeted using Arg-Gly-Asp (RGD) peptide-functionalized gold nanorods and 808 nm laser irradiation, which successfully inhibited human oral squamous cell carcinoma cell migration. AuNRs seem to be a more promising antimetastatic clinical treatment method compared to small molecule drugs that target only a single protein [38].

The presence of cancer stem cells (CSCs) within the bulk of cancer cells is an important cause of cancer relapse, metastasis, drug resistance, and angiogenesis. In a recent 2018 study by Stapathy, a hybrid-nanoparticle (QAuNP) was formulated using quinacrine and gold to evaluate their anti-angiogenic and antimetastatic properties on Oral Squamous Cell Carcinoma (OSCC)-cancer stem cells [39].

These recent advances in nanotechnology and results of studies in cancer therapy with the novel method of nanophotothermal therapy have raised hope for successful noninvasive earlier diagnosis and treatment of cancers, especially in hard-to-treat areas, such as the head and neck region. In order to turn these results into clinical use, further animal studies and even clinical trials are needed. Effective clinical applications are hindered by challenges, such as high cost of these treatments, readily available advanced technology, and even sometimes the need for versatile and direct light delivery systems in deeper tissues [40] .

## *3.2 Laser-Assisted Antimicrobial Photodynamic Therapy Using Nanoparticles*

Caries and periodontal and endodontic diseases are considered important public health issues. Studies have proven that these biofilm-dependent oral diseases may act as infectious foci that could affect other physiological systems in the body. Prevention and cure of these conditions are therefore of great importance. Antimicrobial agents, especially antibiotics, have been successfully used to inactivate biofilm-state pathogens for many years. However, the dynamic pattern of antimicrobial resistance has become a challenge of modern medicine worldwide, and effectiveness of antimicrobial drugs is gradually declining, while numbers of pathogens that are resistant to antibiotics are increasing worldwide. This calls for new treatment approaches that do not cause resistance. In the era of nanotechnology, antimicrobial nanomaterials seem to be a promising solution. Since the antimicrobial effect of NPs is through multiple biological pathways, they can be effective in broad species of microbes, and microbial resistance seems to be very unlikely [41].

As previously mentioned, lasers have also brought dental science to a new level with their wide range of applications to the field. One very important property of laser irradiation is its antimicrobial effects, either through direct effects of laser light at different wavelengths on microorganisms and bacteria or by indirect effects and absorption of the light by specific chromophores as seen in antibacterial photodynamic therapies (aPDT).

Photodynamic therapy is a nonthermal photochemical reaction, which requires three essential elements of light source: a dye, photosensitizer (PS), and oxygen. It was first proposed as an approach for cancer therapies. In this process, light is used to activate the nontoxic photosensitizers (PSs) localized in certain tissues. Singlet oxygen, free radicals, and reactive oxygen species (ROS) lead to the destruction and death of cells.

Antimicrobial photodynamic therapy (aPDT), or photodynamic inactivation (PDI), is a similar process applicable in bacterial, fungal, and viral infection treatment. In dentistry, new PDT-based treatments of caries, candidiasis, periodontal disease, and mucosal and endodontic infections have been a topic of research in recent years.

Lasers with different wavelengths can be used as a light source to activate matching photosensitizers (PS). PDT/PDI is a localized, selective, and safe method that does not disturb the flora at distant sites.

PDI treatment causes nonspecific killing of pathogens by ROS production; resistance is unlikely with this method.

Although safety and efficiency are among the advantages of PDT, some PS molecules have shortcomings that affect their efficacy in vitro and in clinical situations. Many PDT photosensitizers usually have poor water solubility and also tend to aggregate in physiological conditions and aqueous environments. Efforts have been directed to improve delivery systems to overcome such deficiencies. Nanoparticles in PDT as a new modality may be a promising method of addressing these shortcomings [42].

Various kinds of nanoparticles have been developed as PS delivery vehicles with the potential of enhancing the photochemical effectiveness of PSs and improving aPDT results. These nanoparticles may be used in PDT a few different ways: as an accompaniment to a PS, as PS themselves, as nanocapsules loaded with a PS, or as particles that a PS has attached and bound to its surface. Therefore, they are either covalently bound to the nanostructure or encapsulated in them (Fig. 7.3).

A great number of studies have been completed on laser aPDT in dentistry. Nanobased antimicrobial photodynamic treatment in dentistry is a new growing research field with applications in bacterial-based diseases, such as dental caries,

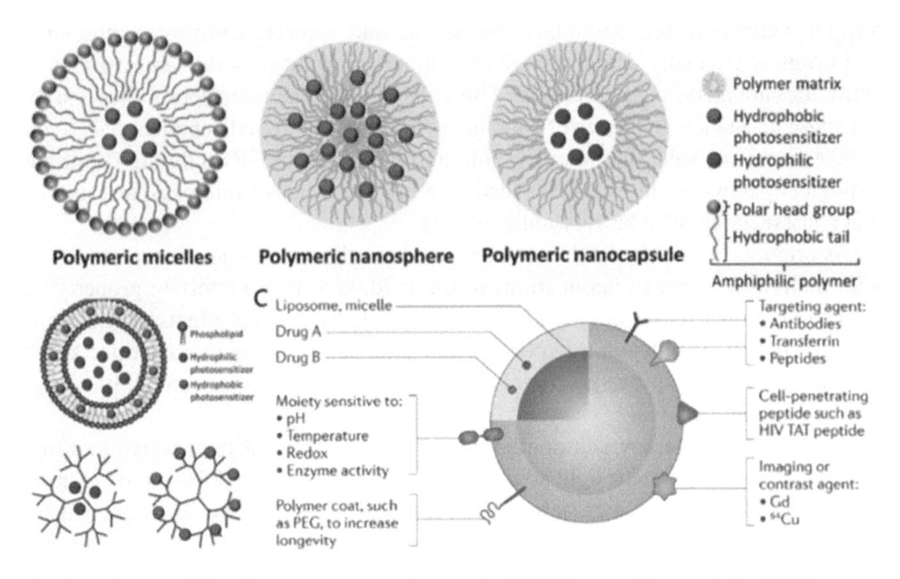


**Fig. 7.3** General PS loading approaches to be used in PDT. (Reuse with permission) [43]

periodontitis, peri-implantitis, and endodontic diseases, as well as in other fungi and viral-based oral infections. Here, we will review some of the recent studies in the field of combined nanotechnology and photodynamic treatments in dentistry.

## 3.3 *Nanophotodynamic Therapy and Dental Caries*

Dental caries is still a major health problem despite dental care improvements. It results from secretion of organic acids as a by-product of the metabolism of fermentable carbohydrates by cariogenic bacteria, such as Streptococcus mutans, Streptococcus sobrinus, and Lactobacillus species [44].

Some of the recent studies have focused on combining nanotechnology with laser photodynamic therapy to enhance the photosensitizing effects on these cariogenic bacteria. In 2016, Misba et al. studied the antibiofilm efficacy of toluidine blue O (TBO) conjugated with silver nanoparticles (AgNP) on Streptococcus mutans. A 630 nm laser light was applied for 70 s (9.1 J/cm$^2$). TBO-AgNP conjugates were able to inhibit biofilm formation, and a 4-log reduction in bacterial cell viability was observed. TBO-AgNP conjugates demonstrate greater phototoxic effects against S. mutans biofilm compared to TBO [45].

In 2017, Harris et al. evaluated the effect of a novel selenium nanoparticle-enhanced toluidine blue photodynamic therapy on S. mutans. A 630 nm diode laser was used for irradiation and activation of SeNP-TBO and TBO against S. mutans biofilm and cells. The results were confirmed by spectroscopic and microscopic techniques, along with biofilm reduction assay. SeNP-mediated S. mutans antibiofilm

PDT was shown to be an efficient and novel alternative to TBO alone. After 24 h of incubation, the SeNP-TBO conjugate group showed a 60% inhibition of S. mutans biofilm formation and 32% loss in viability, which was higher compared to TBO—with 20% and 22%, respectively [46].

In a recent report by Gholibeiglo et al. in 2018 [47], nanocarriers—including graphene oxide (GO), GO-carnosine (Car), and GO-Car/Hydroxyapatite (HAp)—were synthetized and loaded with indocyanine green (ICG). ICG is a photosensitizer with a main drawback of poor stability and concentration-dependent aggregation. aPDT causes a remarkable decline in S. mutans strain count; furthermore, GO-ICG, GO-Car-ICG, and GO-Car/Hap-ICG significantly suppress the S. mutans biofilm formation by 51.4%, 63.8%, and 56.8%, respectively. ICG loading, stability, and inhibitory effects against S. mutans could be enhanced dramatically using the novel multifunctionalized GO nanocarrier. Interestingly, in the PCR results, S. mutans gtfB gene expression reduction was greater with NCs + laser than NCs alone.

Other than positive reports of nanobased aPDT, there is great potential for application of this fascinating technology in operative dentistry. For instance, one of the many reasons for failure of dental restorations is secondary caries caused by bacteria invading the margins of the restoration. In recent years, advancements in nanotechnology and photodynamic-based antibacterial therapy research in the field of restorative dentistry have not only focused on elimination of cariogenic bacteria but also attempt to produce smarter restorative materials. There have been attempts to overcome secondary caries caused by bacteria invading the margins of the restoration and even promote regeneration of dental structures by loading them with photoactive antimicrobial nanoparticles. Long et al. reported a successful production of this kind of materials in their recent study [48].

Photodynamic therapy targeting cariogenic bacteria shows great promise. The results of in vitro investigations are hopeful; however, a lack of trustworthy clinical trial evidence has not permitted photodynamic therapy to be established as an effective technique to prevent, control, and treat caries. More clinical and laboratory studies are needed for optimization of treatment parameters and for better exploration of the anticariogenic potential of photodynamic therapy.

## *3.4 Nanophotodynamic Therapy in Periodontitis and Peri-implantitis*

Periodontal pathogens cause inflammation and degeneration of gingiva, supporting bone and the periodontal ligament. This can lead to periodontal pockets that provide an ideal environment for the growth and proliferation of colonizing microorganisms. These periodontal pockets contain as many as 400 species of bacteria that are organized in biofilms, which make their elimination even more difficult [49]. Photodynamic therapy has been a hot topic recently for nonsurgical periodontal treatments. Although many positive results have been reported in periodontal aPDT in vitro and in vivo studies, clinically there still seems to be variations in treatment techniques and results.

Plaque-induced peri-implantitis is a similar inflammatory condition that influences soft and hard tissues neighboring an osseointegrated dental implant, which may lead to its failure. A variety of experimental studies have been performed to evaluate the treatment of peri-implantitis using adjunctive PDT—results indicate considerable promise [50] .

However, as mentioned for other oral infections, scientists have been working on designing better photosensitizing agents and studying new nanobased photosensitizers to enhance photodynamic therapy efficacy in periodontal and peri-implant infections.

For instance, Nagahara et al. in 2013 studied ICG-loaded chitosan-coated nanospheres (ICG-Nano/c) as a photosensitizer for PDT on Porphyromonas gingivalis. A 0.5 W, 805 nm diode laser irradiation with 10% duty cycle for 3–100 ms, in repeated pulse (RPT) or continuous wave mode, was applied on cell cultures. The negative control was a nonirradiated group. After 7 days of culturing, bacterial CFU were counted in an anaerobic situation. ICG-Nano/c attached to P. gingivalis, and, with irradiation, a significant bactericidal effect was observed using these particles, especially with the RPT 100 ms irradiation, which also demonstrated the lowest increase in temperature.

In 2016, de Freitas et al. performed an in vitro and clinical study that used methylene blue-loaded polylactic-co-glycolic nanoparticles for aPDT in chronic periodontitis patients; results for this experiment were shown to be successful. In this study, dental plaque samples were treated with the aforementioned aPDT agent or simple methylene blue (25 μg/mL) and red 660 nm laser light 20 J/cm$^2$ in planktonic and biofilm phases. Clinical application of the MB-loaded nanoparticles as an aPDT agent and an adjunct to scaling and root planning was also compared with SRP alone in a split-mouth design. The results showed a 25% greater elimination of bacteria compared to MB. Clinically, both groups had similar results after 1 month; however, the aPDT group had better effects on gingival bleeding index compared to Scaling and Root Planning (SRP) alone after 3 months [51].

Although there are still only a limited number of reports on the combination of nano and laser in photodynamic therapy of periodontal and peri-implant infections, the results have been promising in this new field of nonsurgical periodontology. Nanobased aPDT studies in the field of biofilm-dependent and infectious oral diseases are mainly focused on improving current photosensitizers or developing new formulations for targeted delivery vehicles. Hopefully in the near future, these in vitro studies will lead to clinical studies and evidenced-based therapeutic guidelines for use in clinical practice [52].

# 4 Summary

Understanding the applications of low-intensity lasers and PBM, along with its accompaniment to nanotechnology, can be helpful for diagnosis, regeneration of damaged tissues, and treatment of malignancies. Rehabilitation and improvement of the function of tissues and organs is another advantage of laser technology in dentistry.

While many studies have investigated the role of low-intensity lasers in dentistry, the lack of applicable clinical protocols is still a major challenge of these studies. Echoing this sentiment, the World Association for Laser Therapy (WALT)—in the 12th International Congress, Nice, 2018—decided to launch several systematic review studies under the supervision of a group of international researchers to introduce the clinical protocols of PBM therapy for dentistry. Generally, clinicians' access to a practical protocol in low-intensity laser radiation can lead to widespread advancements in the diagnosis and treatment of many oral and maxillofacial diseases.

## References

1. Romanos, G. (2015). Current concepts in the use of lasers in periodontal and implant dentistry. *Journal of Indian Society of Periodontology, 19*(5), 490.
2. Karandish, M. (2014). The efficiency of laser application on the enamel surface: A systematic review. *Journal of Lasers in Medical Sciences, 5*(3), 108.
3. Walsh, L. (2003). The current status of laser applications in dentistry. *Australian Dental Journal, 48*(3), 146–155.
4. Anders, J. J., Lanzafame, R. J., & Arany, P. R. (2015). *Low-level light/laser therapy versus photobiomodulation therapy*. New Rochelle, NY: Mary Ann Liebert, Inc..
5. Chiari, S. (2016). Photobiomodulation and lasers. In *Tooth movement, 118–123*. Karger Publishers.
6. Fujita, S., et al. (2008). Low-energy laser stimulates tooth movement velocity via expression of RANK and RANKL. *Orthodontics & Craniofacial Research, 11*(3), 143–155.
7. Moslemi, N., et al. Effect of 660nm low power laser on pain and healing in palatal donor sites a randomized controlled clinical trial. *Journal of Dental Medicine, 27*(1), 71–77.
8. Hamblin, M. R., & Demidova, T. N. (2006). Mechanisms of low level light therapy. In *Mechanisms for low-light therapy*. International Society for Optics and Photonics, *6140*, 61001–61012.
9. Jere, S. W., Houreld, N. N., & Abrahamse, H. (2019). Role of the PI3K/AKT (mTOR and GSK3β) signalling pathway and photobiomodulation in diabetic wound healing. *Cytokine & Growth Factor Reviews*, 1–8.
10. Blair, J., Zheng, Y., & Dunstan, C. (2007). RANK ligand. *The International Journal of Biochemistry & Cell Biology, 39*(6), 1077–1081.
11. Lopes, C. B., et al. (2007). Infrared laser photobiomodulation (λ 830 nm) on bone tissue around dental implants: A Raman spectroscopy and scanning electronic microscopy study in rabbits. *Photomedicine and Laser Surgery, 25*(2), 96–101.
12. Uzêda-e-Silva, V. D., et al. (2016). Laser phototherapy improves early stage of cutaneous wound healing of rats under hyperlipidic diet. *Lasers in Medical Science, 31*(7), 1363–1370.

13. Arany, P. (2016). Craniofacial wound healing with photobiomodulation therapy: New insights and current challenges. *Journal of Dental Research, 95*(9), 977–984.
14. Ribeiro, M. A. G., et al. (2009). Immunohistochemical assessment of myofibroblasts and lymphoid cells during wound healing in rats subjected to laser photobiomodulation at 660 nm. *Photomedicine and Laser Surgery, 27*(1), 49–55.
15. Calil, J., et al. (2001). Clinical application of the VY posterior thigh fasciocutaneous flap. *Revista da Associação Médica Brasileira, 47*(4), 311–319.
16. Singer, A. J., & Clark, R. A. (1999). Cutaneous wound healing. *New England Journal of Medicine, 341*(10), 738–746.
17. Ruh, A. C., et al. (2018). Laser photobiomodulation in pressure ulcer healing of human diabetic patients: Gene expression analysis of inflammatory biochemical markers. *Lasers in Medical Science, 33*(1), 165–171.
18. de Andrade, A. L. M., Bossini, P. S., & Parizotto, N. A. (2016). Use of low level laser therapy to control neuropathic pain: A systematic review. *Journal of Photochemistry and Photobiology B: Biology, 164*, 36–42.
19. Forootan, S., et al. (2014). The comparison of treatment results of standard repair of traumatic injury of the distal third of the median nerve with the case of applying laser therapy after repair. *Iranian Journal of Surgery, 22*(1), 37–43.
20. Schwartz, F., et al. (2002). Effect of helium/neon laser irradiation on nerve growth factor synthesis and secretion in skeletal muscle cultures. *Journal of Photochemistry and Photobiology B: Biology, 66*(3), 195–200.
21. Freeman, R. S., et al. (2004). NGF deprivation-induced gene expression: after ten years, where do we stand? *Progress in Brain Research, 146*, 111–126.
22. Andreo, L., et al. (2017). Effects of photobiomodulation on experimental models of peripheral nerve injury. *Lasers in Medical Science, 32*(9), 2155–2165.
23. Hsieh, Y. L., et al. (2012). Low-level laser therapy alleviates neuropathic pain and promotes function recovery in rats with chronic constriction injury: Possible involvements in hypoxia-inducible factor 1α (HIF-1α). *Journal of Comparative Neurology, 520*(13), 2903–2916.
24. Chen, Y.-J., et al. (2014). Effect of low level laser therapy on chronic compression of the dorsal root ganglion. *PLoS One, 9*(3), e89894.
25. Theocharidou, A., et al. (2017). Odontogenic differentiation and biomineralization potential of dental pulp stem cells inside Mg-based bioceramic scaffolds under low-level laser treatment. *Lasers in Medical Science, 32*(1), 201–210.
26. Karu, T. I. (2008). Mitochondrial signaling in mammalian cells activated by red and near-IR radiation. *Photochemistry and Photobiology, 84*(5), 1091–1099.
27. Karu, T., & Kolyakov, S. (2005). Exact action spectra for cellular responses relevant to phototherapy. *Photomedicine and Laser Therapy, 23*(4), 355–361.
28. Smith, K. C. (1991). The photobiological basis of low level laser radiation therapy. *Laser Therapy, 3*(1), 19–24.
29. Sheykhhasan, M., & Ghiasi, M. (2017). Key transcription factors involved in the differentiation of mesenchymal stem cells. *Tehran University Medical Journal TUMS Publications, 75*(9), 621–631.
30. Manzano-Moreno, F. J., et al. (2015). The effect of low-level diode laser therapy on early differentiation of osteoblast via BMP-2/TGF-β1 and its receptors. *Journal of Cranio-Maxillo-Facial Surgery, 43*(9), 1926–1932.
31. Fekrazad, R., et al. (2016). The combination of laser therapy and metal nanoparticles in cancer treatment originated from epithelial tissues: A literature review. *Journal of Lasers in Medical Sciences, 7*(2), 62.
32. Virupakshappa, B. (2012). Applications of nanomedicine in oral cancer. *Oral Health and Dental Management, 11*(2), 62–68.
33. Melancon, M. P., et al. (2011). Targeted multifunctional gold-based nanoshells for magnetic resonance-guided laser ablation of head and neck cancer. *Biomaterials, 32*(30), 7600–7608.

34. Kennedy, L. C., et al. (2011). T cells enhance gold nanoparticle delivery to tumors in vivo. *Nanoscale Research Letters, 6*(1), 283.
35. Chanmee, T., et al. (2014). Tumor-associated macrophages as major players in the tumor microenvironment. *Cancers, 6*(3), 1670–1690.
36. Bazak, R., et al. (2015). Cancer active targeting by nanoparticles: A comprehensive review of literature. *Journal of Cancer Research and Clinical Oncology, 141*(5), 769–784.
37. Huang, X., et al. (2007). The potential use of the enhanced nonlinear properties of gold nanospheres in photothermal cancer therapy. *Lasers in Surgery and Medicine, 39*(9), 747–753.
38. Ali, M. R., et al. (2017). Targeting cancer cell integrins using gold nanorods in photothermal therapy inhibits migration through affecting cytoskeletal proteins. *Proceedings of the National Academy of Sciences*, 201703151.
39. Satapathy, S. R., et al. (2018). Metallic gold and bioactive quinacrine hybrid nanoparticles inhibit oral cancer stem cell and angiogenesis by deregulating inflammatory cytokines in p53 dependent manner. *Nanomedicine, 14*(3), 883–896.
40. Bansal, A., et al. (2018). In vivo wireless photonic photodynamic therapy. *Proceedings of the National Academy of Sciences*, 201717552.
41. Das, B., & Patra, S. (2017). Chapter 1-Antimicrobials: Meeting the challenges of antibiotic resistance through nanotechnology. In *Nanostructures for antimicrobial therapy*, Ficai, A., Grumezescu, A.M.,(Eds.) (pp. 1–22). Elsevier: Atlanta, GA, USA.
42. Fekrazad, R., Nejat, A., & Kalhori, K. A. (2017). Antimicrobial photodynamic therapy with nanoparticles versus conventional photosensitizer in oral diseases. In *Nanostructures for antimicrobial therapy* (pp. 237–259). Elsevier Inc.
43. Wang, Y., et al. (2019). Construction of nanomaterials with targeting phototherapy properties to inhibit resistant bacteria and biofilm infections. *Chemical Engineering Journal, 358*, 74–90.
44. Soukos, N. S., & Goodson, J. M. (2011). Photodynamic therapy in the control of oral biofilms. *Periodontology 2000, 55*(1), 143–166.
45. Misba, L., Kulshrestha, S., & Khan, A. U. (2016). Antibiofilm action of a toluidine blue O-silver nanoparticle conjugate on Streptococcus mutans: A mechanism of type I photodynamic therapy. *Biofouling, 32*(3), 313–328.
46. Haris, Z., & Khan, A. U. (2017). Selenium nanoparticle enhanced photodynamic therapy against biofilm forming streptococcus mutans. *International Journal of Life-Sciences Scientific Research, 3*(5), 1287–1294.
47. Gholibegloo, E., et al. (2018). Carnosine-graphene oxide conjugates decorated with hydroxyapatite as promising nanocarrier for ICG loading with enhanced antibacterial effects in photodynamic therapy against Streptococcus mutans. *Journal of Photochemistry and Photobiology B: Biology, 181*, 14–22.
48. Long, F., et al. (2015). Imaging of smart dental composites using mesoscopic fluorescence molecular tomography: An ex vivo feasibility study. *International Journal of Advanced Computer Science and Information Technology, 2*, 43–46.
49. Paster, B. J., & Dewhirst, F. E. (2009). Molecular microbial diagnosis. *Periodontology 2000, 51*(1), 38–44.
50. Fraga, R. S., et al. (2018). Is antimicrobial photodynamic therapy effective for microbial load reduction in peri-implantitis treatment? A systematic review and meta-analysis. *Photochemistry and Photobiology, 94*, 752.
51. de Freitas, L. M., et al. (2016). Polymeric nanoparticle-based photodynamic therapy for chronic periodontitis in vivo. *International Journal of Molecular Sciences, 17*(5), 769.
52. Paszko, E., et al. (2011). Nanodrug applications in photodynamic therapy. *Photodiagnosis and Photodynamic Therapy, 8*(1), 14–29.

# Chapter 8
# Applications of Hard and Soft Tissue Engineering in Dentistry

**Mohammadreza Tahriri, Regine Torres, Emelia Karkazis, Alexander Karkazis, Rizwan Bader, Daryoosh Vashaee, and Lobat Tayebi**

## 1 Introduction

It is vital that teeth and oral tissues are protected since they play a crucial role in human function. Strong masticatory stresses and physical changes can result in changes in oral tissues, such as dental caries and periodontitis [1]. As a therapeutic measure, the use of biomaterials has played a role in helping to repair damaged oral tissue. Concerns are arising from exposure to body fluids within the mouth leading to a degradation of the material. Moreover, potential cytotoxic and harmful products can be released through the use of products in the oral environment. Therefore, tissue engineering has replaced more conventional biomaterial innovations.

Tissue engineering has been widely implemented to develop functional alternates for the damaged tissues [2–12]. Tissue engineering application can be based on three components—the cell source, scaffold, and bioactive molecules [9, 11, 13–19]. Research has been conducted with a vast amount of scaffold materials, such as natural polymers [20–29], natural silk [30], synthetic polymers [9, 15, 20, 31–33], and ceramics [34], as an attempt to regenerate dental tissues. Tissue engineering has been developed to be effective with pulp-dentin complex regeneration [20], guided tissue regeneration [35], and tooth [36] and salivary glands [37].

The increasing amount of research regarding tissue engineering and regeneration has made it an emerging field. However, due to many complications and challenges, only a few products have been used for clinical applications. We hope that concepts regarding tissue engineering and their applications toward dentistry are made aware to the public, and challenges regarding these applications are faced.

M. Tahriri · R. Torres · E. Karkazis · A. Karkazis · R. Bader · L. Tayebi (✉)
Marquette University School of Dentistry, Milwaukee, WI, USA
e-mail: Lobat.tayebi@marquette.edu

D. Vashaee
Electrical and Computer Engineering Department, North Carolina State University, Raleigh, NC, USA



L. Tayebi (ed.), *Applications of Biomedical Engineering in Dentistry*,
https://doi.org/10.1007/978-3-030-21583-5_8

# 2 Tissue Engineering Strategies

Tissue engineering is poised to have a significant and exciting impact in the field of dentistry. As it relates to dentistry, bone, cartilage, dentin, dental pulp, salivary glands, skin, and oral mucosa can be bioengineered via three primary methods—conduction, induction, and cell transplantation [38].

The conductive method employs the use of a polymeric barrier membrane, which seals off the intended area of tissue regeneration solely to cells that enhance tissue growth, while preventing unnecessary, or potentially harmful, cells from entering the site of the regeneration [38]. Nyman et al. demonstrated such a method, as they were able to enhance the growth of periodontal supporting cells while preventing gingival epithelial cells and connective tissue cells from entering the area of regeneration [39]. One significant benefit of this method is its ability to form bone in a well-controlled and usual manner [38].

Another approach to tissue engineering, known as the inductive method, sends biological messages to cells near the site of damage, facilitating the formation of new bone [38]. Urist demonstrated that BMPs can form new bone at places that usually are unable [40]. This process is made possible through polymeric carriers transporting inductive factors, like bone morphogenic proteins (BMPs), to the desired site of regeneration [38]. Major polymers include collagen of animal origin and synthetic polymers of lactic acid and glycolic acid [38]. The speed and quantity at which inductive factors are released are dictated by the rate of carrier breakdown [41]. Discoveries in this area of research have led to the widespread production of BMPs, now enabling individuals with bone defects to regrow and heal such wounds successfully [38].

The last method is cell transplantation, which transplants cells cultivated in a laboratory into the desired target [38]. This method requires interaction and cooperation between a doctor, engineer, and a cell biologist [38]. First, an individual is biopsied by a doctor to acquire information regarding the cells present in the individual [38]. Then, the biopsy is sent to the laboratory, where a cell biologist appropriately reproduces the specific cells [1]. Next, an engineer will fabricate a biodegradable polymeric scaffold, which is ultimately integrated with the cells of interest [38]. Finally, the scaffold is transplanted into the individual by the doctor [38]. After successful cell transplantation, the scaffold eventually breaks down but also guides the successful formation of healthy tissue [38].

The schematic representation of the cell-matrix tissue engineering strategy has been given in Fig. 8.1.

# 3 Application of Tissue Engineering in Dentistry

## 3.1 *Tooth Regeneration*

Whole tooth regeneration poses a difficult, yet vastly improving, area of research. Multiple studies have been performed with varying success in this area of study.

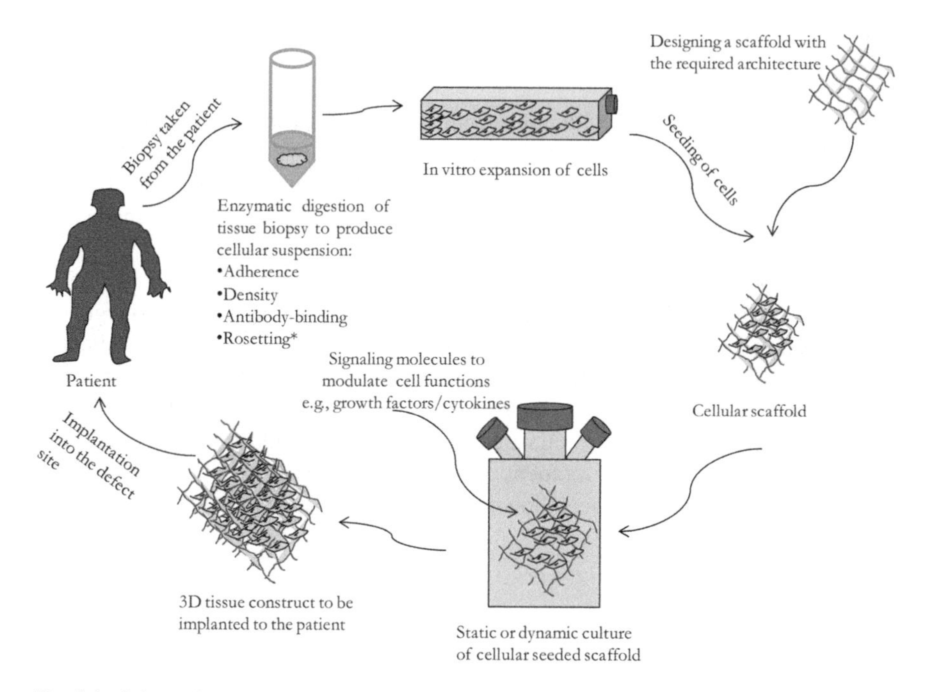


**Fig. 8.1** Schematic representation of cell-matrix tissue engineering strategy [42]

Using tooth buds from the third molars of pigs, Young et al. were the first to successfully regenerate tooth structure containing enamel and dentin [43]. Biodegradable scaffolds containing pig tooth bud cells were transplanted into rats, and 20–30 weeks later, defined tooth structure was present, although the size of the tooth was very small [43]. Likewise, Duailibi et al. were able to regenerate teeth using tooth buds from rats [44]. Tooth bud cells were isolated from the rats between 3 and 7 days postnatally and grown in vitro for 6 days with polyglycolic acid (PGA) and polylactic-co-glycolic acid (PLGA) scaffolds [44]. It was determined that tooth bud cells isolated from rats 4 days postnatally and seeded onto PGA and PLGA scaffolds resulted in the most mature tooth structure [44]. Xu et al. designed a novel silk scaffold, with specified pore sizes of 250 and 550 μm, to facilitate the growth of tooth bud cells from a 4-day postnatal rat [45]. It was determined that scaffolds with pore sizes of 550 μm best supported the development of osteodentin-like tissue and the intended tooth shape; however, no enamel was detected [45]. With a more unique approach, Nakao et al. placed epithelial and mesenchymal cells within collagen gel drops for 2 days, promoting growth before transplantation into mice; after 14 days, ameloblasts and odontoblasts were detected in the mice teeth [46].

Although many complex factors are required to achieve a structurally sound and morphologically acceptable tooth, research is currently progressing towards this desired outcome. Imagine a world where teeth can be regenerated with relative ease to replace missing teeth—it surely will be a revolutionary advancement.

## 3.2 Bone Tissue Regeneration

Bone damage is a serious health concern that may result from injuries, infections, and birth defects [38]. Conventional surgical methods—like autografts, allografts, and synthetic biomaterials—are not without their shortcomings; as a result, bone tissue regeneration has become an area of research interest to offset the inadequacies of conventional bone repair methods [38].

All three primary methods of tissue engineering may be employed for successful bone regeneration [38]. Conductive and inductive methods may be used to regenerate areas of minor bone damage [38]. When conductive measures cannot sufficiently repair bone, BMPs are then inductively bioengineered [38]. Lastly, cell transplantation uniquely enables researchers to create large bony structures, like the mandible, before surgery. Bone precursor cells are cultured onto scaffolds with careful consideration for the essential environment and factors needed for proper functioning. Gradually, the scaffold will break down, leaving bone shaped in the form of a mandible [38].

## 3.3 Cartilage Tissue Regeneration

Cartilaginous tissue has become an area of interest for researchers in developing cartilage transplantation methods, as this tissue has a limited ability to repair itself. Trauma and degenerative diseases, such as osteoarthritis, can lead to cartilage destruction, precisely at the temporomandibular joint (TMJ). Polymer scaffolds have been constructed to mimic the same mechanical properties as cartilage, leading to a novel discovery in cartilage reconstruction. At the forefront of this engineering project is the development of cartilaginous cell transplantation to counteract the limited regeneration capability of the tissue and its lack of inductive molecules. The newest technique in cartilage transplantation is to use cells without a carrier to repair small defects. Animal models have proven that new cartilaginous tissue relating to the maxillofacial region, such as the nasal septum and temporomandibular joint, can be scientifically engineered using biodegradable scaffolds to transplant these new cells [38].

The TMJ is a bilateral joint connecting the mandibular condyles and temporal bones of the skull, with a fibrocartilaginous disc between these two bones. This disc functions as the support of the joint and absorbs any stresses and trauma. Due to the complex structure of the TMJ, there are minimal treatment options available for the management of disorders relating to this joint. In 1991, Thomas et al. [47] produced the first in vitro cartilage tissue analog in an animal model by way of organ culture. The tissue produced had the same clinical appearance and physical properties of the TMJ disc; this experiment provided a method for in vivo autografting as an alternative way to treat TMJ disc problems. Three years later, Puelacher et al. [48] tested the effectiveness of the newly engineered tissue growth of the TMJ disc by placing dissociated chondrocytes on a synthetic biodegradable polymer in vitro and then transplanting this into mice, and the resultant engineered cartilage was visualized. At the conclusion of the study, all implants that were seeded with the chondrocytes displayed hyaline cartilage, while still allowing the scaffolds to maintain their original shape. This study proved the imminent possibility of scientifically engineered synthetic TMJ disc tissue.

The research conducted in the 1990s was followed by studies targeting TMJ tissues. Abukawa et al. [49] successfully reconstructed the mandibular condyle by using similar tissue-engineered bone constructs that were made by combining biodegradable polymers and porcine mesenchymal stem cells (pMSCs). Weng et al. [50] determined in their study that bone and cartilage composites can be successfully engineered to serve as substitutes to the mandibular condyle. The junction of bone and cartilage was proven to be similar to the common junction of these composite tissues in articulating joints.

Although these studies have shown many advances in engineering synthetic TMJ disc tissue, the presence of multiple tissues on the TMJ (bone, cartilage, fibrocartilage) presents a challenge. Researchers must be able to engineer the TMJ to withstand normal pressure and shock that the TMJ disc bears typically to have any reliable clinical application [1].

## *3.4 Enamel Regeneration*

Enamel is the outer surface of a tooth; it is avascular, acellular, and non-vital, making it a problematic tissue to attempt to regenerate. Enamel is subject to many forces to the tooth, such as chewing forces, temperature, pH, caries, bruxism, and chemical erosion. Ameloblasts, the enamel-forming cells, form a protective layer on the outer surface of the enamel before the eruption. However, at the eruption, ameloblasts are lost, therefore leaving behind a highly mineralized acellular enamel structure. Due to the difficulty in regenerating an acellular, avascular, and non-vital tissue, very little research has been published on tissue engineering of enamel. Therefore, the focus of enamel regeneration research is mainly concerned with the remineralization of demineralized or defective enamel [1].

In a study conducted by Fan et al. [51], amelogenin was used with a modified biomimetic deposition method to remineralize the surface of etched enamel, forming mineral layers containing hydroxyapatite crystals. Amelogenin was an essential modulator in the study, as it promoted bundle formation of fluoridated hydroxyapatite as the dose was increased. The biomimetic synthesis of amelogenin-fluoridated hydroxyapatite crystals is one of the initial steps necessary in developing biomaterials that would be applied in future applications for enamel regeneration in restorative dentistry. Although the research conducted in this study was novel in promoting remineralization of affected enamel in its earliest stage, producing enamel tissue itself is a significant challenge to researchers today. Many factors must be considered: the highly mineralized state of the enamel (96% mineralized); the arrangement, morphology, and size (2–3 mm) of the hydroxyapatite crystals; and the acellularity of enamel. Additionally, ameloblasts originate from epithelial cells and require the differentiation of odontoblasts before they can form the enamel. This epithelial-mesenchymal interaction is very complex and necessary for adequate enamel and dentin formation. Thus, although there has been some research conducted in the regeneration of the enamel, there are still many barriers present in achieving this new feat.

### 3.5 Dentin and Dental Pulp Regeneration

Animal and laboratory studies have successfully engineered dentin and dental pulp production. The biggest need for regeneration in this field of dentistry would be due to damage to the dentin and other structures in the dentin from tooth decay. Dental caries cause significant damage to the tooth structure, with the most insult to dentin. Caries is one of the most prevalent diseases in children and young adults; successful dentin regeneration through tissue engineering could be a potential future breakthrough solution to this epidemic [38].

There are many approaches to engineer lost dentin and pulp. Even if the odontoblasts (dentin-producing cells) have been lost due to the carious process, these odontoblastic cells still can be regenerated, unlike ameloblasts (enamel-producing cells). Specific bone morphogenetic proteins can be utilized, allowing the newly synthesized odontoblasts to form new dentin. A study conducted by M. Nakashima [52] proved this hypothesis correct. Reparative dentin was developed in the cavity of an amputated pulp and capped with a bone morphogenetic protein, allowing for a cell-mediated immune response, resorption of the BMP, and vascular invasion. Four weeks post-op, osteodentinoblasts were found in the matrix, and other parts of the pulp were filled with pulpal tissue. It was determined that the osteodentine found in this study may be involved in the differentiation of odontoblasts into dentin and dental pulp. This study was followed by a survey conducted by Lianjia Y et al. [53]; it was determined that the primary inductive factor in odontoblast differentiation has not been identified, but BMP, which induces the formation of cartilage and bone when implanted in muscle tissue, is found in dentin matrix, hence the reason why BMPs are used in this area of research. BMP exists in odontoblasts, ameloblasts, and dentin matrix and induces the formation of osteodentin, as found in the previous study. Thus, BMP plays a tremendous role and could be the primary inductive factor in odontoblast differentiation.

In addition to dentin, the dental pulp can be scientifically engineered by using fibroblasts and synthetic polymer matrices. The ability to successfully apply regenerated dentin and pulp is a future breakthrough to restorative dentistry, as it can potentially be the solution to dental caries, a disease common to many around the world.

## 3.6 *Periodontal Tissue Regeneration*

Periodontal disease is the result of accumulated bacterial biofilm and a subsequent inflammatory response that leads to the progressive destruction of the supporting tissues surrounding teeth and can eventually lead to tooth loss. Conventional therapy aims to decrease bacterial loads to a level tolerable by the body, thereby halting the disease process and allowing periodontal tissues to heal. However, traditional treatment is unlikely to result in the regeneration of lost periodontal structures. Tissue engineering techniques are alternative or adjunct treatments aimed at regenerating lost periodontal tissues. As with other tissue engineering approaches, periodontal tissue regeneration requires cells, growth factors, and scaffold or extracellular matrix. Effective treatment should result in the formation of cementum, ligament fibers, alveolar bone, and reattachment of the epithelial seal [1, 54].

A technique, termed guided tissue regeneration (GTR), involves the use of a physical barrier, either a resorbable (polylactic acid, polyglycolic acid, collagen) or non-resorbable (methylcellulose acetate, polytetrafluoroethylene) membrane that prevents the migration of the more rapidly forming epithelial and connective tissues, providing a space for the migration of cells onto the affected root surface and promoting the formation of bone. There is no clinically significant difference between the use of resorbable and non-resorbable membrane [55]. GTR is an established and widely used treatment for periodontal defects. Guided bone regeneration (GBR) is another technique used for the treatment of bone defects, such as dehiscence, apical fenestration, and socket defects [56].

Tissue engineering approaches may be improved by the use of bioactive molecules or growth factors, which may result in better cell migration and behavior [57]. A study by Nevins et al. [58] demonstrated the effect of purified recombinant human platelet-derived growth factor BB (rhPDGF-BB) on Class II furcations and interproximal intrabony defects. rhPDGF-BB incorporated into bone allograft resulted in histologically evident regeneration of the periodontal attachment apparatus, including new cementum and PDL, in four of the six interproximal defects and four of four furcation defects treated with PDGF. A subsequent randomized control trial demonstrated the safety and efficacy of rhPDGF-BB in the treatment of periodontal osseous defects, and the results showed a significant increase in the rate of CAL gain, reduced gingival recession at 3 months post-surgery, and improved bone fill at 6 months [56].

## 3.7 *Oral Mucosa Regeneration*

Soft tissue defects are commonly repaired using autologous grafts taken from a different part of the patient's own oral cavity. In these cases, rejection of the graft is not a risk, as the patient's own tissue is used, yet autologous grafting is not without limitations. Potential issues with autologous grafting include donor site morbidity, tissue shortage, and retention of donor tissue characteristics. An alternative approach to oral mucosal regeneration is the use of tissue-engineered products, produced by cultured keratinocytes on dermal matrices in vitro [59].

Oral mucosal equivalents have been developed for clinical applications and for use in in vitro studies of biocompatibility, mucosal irritation, disease, and other fundamental oral biology phenomena [60]. Such equivalents have been used in the surgical reconstruction of the lips, oral vestibule, and tongue and have been proposed for use in tissue engineering of other mucocutaneous structures [61].

### *3.8 Salivary Gland Regeneration*

Salivary glands may be damaged by diseases such as Sjogren's syndrome or radiotherapy, as they are particularly sensitive to radiation. The loss of salivary gland tissue or function has a significant impact on quality of life for those affected individuals, as saliva has a vital role in aiding food digestion and moistening and protecting the oral mucosa. Hyposalivation can cause dysgeusia, dysphagia, increased dental caries, and increased incidence of candidiasis, among many other sequelae [38]. Currently available therapies, which include saliva substitutes and sialagogues, are mostly supportive and are often insufficient. Tissue engineering of glands could improve treatment but is complicated by the intricate anatomy and histology of salivary glands [1]. Inductive gene therapy has been used to treat salivary gland deficiencies. The goals of this type of treatment include repair of hypofunctional gland tissue, production of secretory transgene products, and induction of a phenotypic change in existing ductal epithelial cells. This approach has demonstrated success in animal models [62]. In cases of extensive loss of salivary gland tissue, an alternative treatment is the transplantation of artificial salivary glands. This was demonstrated in a study by Baum et al. [63], in which synthetic salivary gland substitutes were developed from polymer tubes lined by epithelial cells. These devices could be grafted into buccal mucosa and would have the ability to deliver aqueous fluid into the oral cavity. These regenerative approaches have the potential to treat patients with insufficient saliva production due to salivary gland tissue dysfunction and/or destruction, thereby treating and preventing the sequelae of hyposalivation.

### *3.9 Temporomandibular Joint Regeneration*

The temporomandibular joint (TMJ) is a bilateral synovial joint composed of, in part, a shock-absorbing fibrocartilaginous disc located between the mandibular condyles and temporal bones of the skull. It is a complex structure consisting of many tissue types, including bone, cartilage, and ligament, which are bound posteriorly by blood vessels and nerves. There are only a few treatments available for the management of TMJ disorders, including pharmacotherapy, physiotherapy, and surgical intervention. Tissue engineering has a potential application in the treatment of TMJ dysfunction resulting from degeneration [1].

A study by Thomas et al. [47] from 1991 reported the in vitro development of TMJ cartilage using type I collagen meshes to culture chondrocyte-like cells. The study indicated that the "resultant tissue analog had the clinical appearance and characteristics of the temporomandibular joint disc" and concluded that such an analog could alternatively be used in vivo for disc repair. Not long after, another study by Puelacher et al. [48] engineered the fibrocartilaginous disc of the TMJ. TMJ disc replacements were made by seeding dissociated chondrocytes on synthetic, bioresorbable polylactic (PLA) and polyglycolic (PGA) acid fiber scaffolds. The constructs were incubated in vitro and then transplanted into test animals. The scaffolds maintained their shape, and all implants seeded with chondrocytes showed gross evidence of histologically organized hyaline cartilage. This study demonstrated the potential use of tissue-engineered cartilage grown on scaffolds in reconstructive surgery of the TMJ and also in craniomaxillofacial, plastic, and orthopedic surgery.

Engineering of other TMJ tissues followed the previously discussed studies. Abukawa et al. [49] proposed the fabrication of bone to eliminate donor site morbidity. Engineered constructs that closely resembled a modeled condyle were made using porcine mesenchymal stem cells and porous polymer scaffolds of biodegradable PLGA. A study by Bailey et al. [64] compared engineered condylar cartilage made from human umbilical cord matrix (HUCM) stem cells and TMJ condylar chondrocytes seeded onto PGA scaffolds. Samples were cultured either in a medium containing chondrogenic factors or in a control medium. The HUCM constructs showed increased levels of biosynthesis and higher cellularity, demonstrating that the HUCM stem cells outperformed the TMJ condylar cartilage cells.

Another study by Schek et al. [65] demonstrated the engineering of osteochondral implants using biphasic composite scaffolds to simultaneously generate bone and cartilage in discrete regions and a stable interface between cartilage and subchondral bone. Due to the presence of multiple tissues in addition to the complex anatomy of the TMJ, tissue engineering to treat TMJ dysfunction is challenging. Additionally, for engineered constructs to have a clinical application, they must be biologically and mechanically functional and can remodel according to functional loading stresses.

## 4 Tissue Engineering: Challenges and Opportunities in Dentistry

Tissue engineering introduces the exciting possibility of replacing lost or damaged tissue. This could be a reality for practitioners and patients in the near future, but there are undoubtedly many challenges before this approach can be regularly utilized clinically. There have been many significant contributions made to the literature, but still, relatively few tissue-engineered products have reached clinical trials, and applications are primarily limited to the skin, bone, cartilage, capillary, and periodontal tissue [66]. More research and interdisciplinary collaboration are still needed to shift clinical treatment from repair and reconstruction to regeneration. Research to date has illuminated the fundamental processes of tissue engineering, but many issues remain, as tissue engineering is a field that involves many disciplines of the health sciences and bioengineering. This requires the collaboration of many research groups and professionals, including but not limited to dentists, dental biomaterial experts, physicists, bioengineers, and biotechnologists [1].

Key challenges that the field of tissue engineering faces include the complexity and current lack of knowledge of oral tissues, tissue-specific problems, ethical concerns of stem cell research, the cost-effectiveness of treatments using tissue-engineered products, regulation of such products, and the need for training and funding.

It is crucial to understand the composition of the tissue and how it is produced in nature before one can successfully engineer the tissues. An article by Zafar et al. [1] discusses an example of the challenging complexity of enamel, which is the hardest substance in the body due to its highly mineralized structure and is secreted by ameloblasts. Scientists are unable to stimulate ameloblasts to secrete enamel tissue in vitro with structure and properties similar to that of natural enamel. Besides, the enamel is acellular, avascular, and cannot remodel. Many tissue-specific challenges complicate tissue engineering efforts.

The use of stem cells brings up ethical concerns. Stem cells have great potential to reveal the mechanisms of cell and tissue development and differentiation. However, religious and legal dilemmas arise due to debates about when the cells in question are considered a human being, consent to donate biological materials, oversight of research, local and international regulations, and more. Also, these concerns differ depending on geographical location, creating a limitation for research groups that develop partnerships and potentially involve the transport of biological materials across the globe [67].

Cost-effectiveness is inevitably a concern with any medical therapy on the market. One must consider the costs of research and development and the comparative value of currently available treatments. These factors are essential to labs, patients, and practitioners alike. As the development of tissue-engineered products continues, the cost-effectiveness of these products is something to consider.

Biomaterials and the regulation of such materials are additional challenges. A fundamental component of tissue engineering is the use of scaffolds. While it does not yet exist, an ideal scaffold would match the mechanical, physical, and biological properties of the natural tissue of interest, be able to support the tissues' cells throughout their lifespan, and be non-immunogenic and non-allergenic. Of course, infected or contaminated biomaterials cannot be used; however, maintaining a sterile environment during the process of tissue engineering, which can take months, is very challenging. Conventional heat or chemical sterilization may harm cells and tissues or affect the integrity of scaffold materials [66].

Last, as engineered tissue products become available, dental providers will need training and experience in the use of these products. This would require the introduction of these materials in the dental school curriculum and additional continuing education courses for current practitioners to increase the familiarity of such treatments among those in the profession. Additional specialty training in oral surgery and periodontology would need to be introduced, as the use of tissue-engineered products often involves surgical procedures. There is a need for interdisciplinary collaboration to further tissue engineering research efforts, as well as financial support via government funding agencies and private industry.

While there are still many barriers to the clinical use of tissue-engineered products, the possibilities grow with continued research and the contributions of many different groups around the globe. The paradigm shift from simple repair and reconstruction to regeneration is an exciting prospect for the future of dentistry.

## 5 Conclusions and Future Trends

Although tissue engineering is an emerging field in the career of dentistry, many challenges must be faced before many applications can be clinically practiced. We must be able to solve how we can apply this type of technology as a whole into the field. Some of the major issues to this problem have come down to the cost of having these applications available and how we are going to distribute and apply this technology in healthcare centers. There will also be a new rise of training programs to utilize this type of technology.

Moreover, ethical issues have arisen regarding tissue engineering. When applying this technology, the source of the cells, whether they are the patient's own or donated, would need to be considered. Furthermore, the type of people receiving these therapies is questioned. Many concerns regarding the implementation of this technology exist and will take time for the application of this technology to be used in an actual clinical setting. Much research regarding the field is being accomplished at dental schools and postgraduate programs to make many more advances in this field. Using the basic sciences and incorporating that knowledge into a clinical setting—such as in oral surgery, periodontics, and oral medicine—has been implemented with the use of translational research. For practitioners, continuing education programs in the field of tissue engineering will allow a better understanding in this area, facilitating awareness of newer and better treatments.

## References

1. Zafar, M. S., Khurshid, Z., & Almas, K. (2015). Oral tissue engineering progress and challenges. *Tissue Engineering and Regenerative Medicine, 12*(6), 387–397.
2. Langer, R., & Vacanti, J. P. (1993). Tissue engineering. *Science, 80*(260), 920–926.

3. Almela, T., Al-Sahaf, S., Brook, I. M., Khoshroo, K., Rasoulianboroujeni, M., Fahimipour, F., Tahriri, M., Dashtimoghadam, E., Bolt, R., Tayebi, L., & Moharamzadeh, K. (2018). 3D printed tissue engineered model for bone invasion of oral cancer. *Tissue & Cell, 52*, 71–77.
4. Del Monico, M., Tahriri, M., Fahmy, M. D., Ghassemi, H., Vashaee, D., & Tayebi, L. (2018). Manufacturing, cartilage and facial muscle tissue engineering and regeneration: A mini review. *Bio-Design and Manufacturing, 1*(2), 115–122.
5. Del Monico, M., Tahriri, M., Nicholson, Z., Khoshroo, K., & Tayebi, L. (2018). Facial muscle tissue engineering. *Biomaterials for Oral and Dental Tissue Engineering*, 353–365.
6. Eslami, H., Lisar, H. A., Kashi, T. S. J., Tahriri, M., Ansari, M., Rafiei, T., Bastami, F., Shahin-Shamsabadi, A., Abbas, F. M., & Tayebi, L. (2018). Poly (lactic-co-glycolic acid)(PLGA)/TiO2 nanotube bioactive composite as a novel scaffold for bone tissue engineering: In vitro and in vivo studies. *Biologicals, 53*, 51–62.
7. Jazayeri, H. E., Tahriri, M., Razavi, M., Khoshroo, K., Fahimipour, F., Dashtimoghadam, E., Almeida, L., & Tayebi, L. (2017). A current overview of materials and strategies for potential use in maxillofacial tissue regeneration. *Materials Science & Engineering. C, Materials for Biological Applications, 70*, 913–929.
8. Khoshroo, K., Kashi, T. S. J., Moztarzadeh, F., Tahriri, M., Jazayeri, H. E., & Tayebi, L. (2017). Development of 3D PCL microsphere/TiO2 nanotube composite scaffolds for bone tissue engineering. *Materials Science & Engineering. C, Materials for Biological Applications, 70*, 586–598.
9. Naghavi Alhosseini, S., Moztarzadeh, F., Kargozar, S., Dodel, M., & Tahriri, M. (2015). Development of polyvinyl alcohol fibrous biodegradable scaffolds for nerve tissue engineering applications: In vitro study. *International Journal of Polymeric Materials and Polymeric Biomaterials, 64*(9), 474–480.
10. Nojehdehian, H., Moztarzadeh, F., Baharvand, H., Nazarian, H., & Tahriri, M. (2009). Preparation and surface characterization of poly-L-lysine-coated PLGA microsphere scaffolds containing retinoic acid for nerve tissue engineering: In vitro study. *Colloids and Surfaces B: Biointerfaces, 73*(1), 23–29.
11. Touri, R., Moztarzadeh, F., Sadeghian, Z., Bizari, D., Tahriri, M., & Mozafari, M. (2013). The use of carbon nanotubes to reinforce 45S5 bioglass-based scaffolds for tissue engineering applications. *BioMed Research International, 2013*, 465086.
12. Yadegari, A., Fahimipour, F., Rasoulianboroujeni, M., Dashtimoghadarm, E., Omidi, M., Golzar, H., Tahriri, M., & Tayebi, L. (2018). Specific considerations in scaffold design for oral tissue engineering. *Biomaterials for Oral and Dental Tissue Engineering*, 157–183.
13. Galler, K. M., D'Souza, R. N., & Hartgerink, J. D. (2010). Biomaterials and their potential applications for dental tissue engineering. *Journal of Materials Chemistry, 20*(40), 8730–8746.
14. Shahin-Shamsabadi, A., Hashemi, A., & Tahriri, M. (2017). A viscoelastic study of poly (ε-Caprolactone) microsphere sintered bone tissue engineering scaffold. *Journal of Medical and Biological Engineering 38*(3), 359–369.
15. Fahimipour, F., Rasoulianboroujeni, M., Dashtimoghadam, E., Khoshroo, K., Tahriri, M., Bastami, F., Lobner, D., & Tayebi, L. (2017). 3D printed TCP-based scaffold incorporating VEGF-loaded PLGA microspheres for craniofacial tissue engineering. *Dental Materials, 33*(11), 1205–1216.
16. Jazayeri, H. E., Fahimipour, F., Tahriri, M., Almeida, L., & Tayebi, L. (2018). Oral nerve tissue repair and regeneration. *Biomaterials for Oral and Dental Tissue Engineering*, 319–336.
17. Khojasteh, A., Fahimipour, F., Eslaminejad, M. B., Jafarian, M., Jahangir, S., Bastami, F., Tahriri, M., Karkhaneh, A., & Tayebi, L. (2016). Development of PLGA-coated β-TCP scaffolds containing VEGF for bone tissue engineering. *Materials Science and Engineering: C, 69*, 780–788.
18. Khoshroo, K., Almela, T., Tahriri, M., Fahimipour, F., Metalwala, Z., Moharamzadeh, K., & Tayebi, L. (2016). 3D-printing of porous calcium phosphate cements for bone tissue engineering. *Dental Materials, 32*, e56–e57.

19. Raz, M., Moztarzadeh, F., Shokrgozar, M. A., & Tahriri, M. (2014). Synthesis of nano calcium phosphate via biomimetic method for bone tissue engineering scaffolds and investigation of its phase transformation in simulated body fluid. *Key Engineering Materials, Trans Tech Publications, 587*, 86–92.
20. Huang, G. T. (2009). Pulp and dentin tissue engineering and regeneration: Current progress. *Regenerative Medicine, 4*(5), 697–707.
21. Ayati Najafabadi, S., Keshvari, H., Ganji, Y., Tahriri, M., & Ashuri, M. (2012). Chitosan/heparin surface modified polyacrylic acid grafted polyurethane film by two step plasma treatment. *Surface Engineering, 28*(9), 710–714.
22. Davoudi, Z., Rabiee, M., Houshmand, B., Eslahi, N., Khoshroo, K., Rasoulianboroujeni, M., Tahriri, M., & Tayebi, L. (2018). Development of chitosan/gelatin/keratin composite containing hydrocortisone sodium succinate as a buccal mucoadhesive patch to treat desquamative gingivitis. *Drug Development and Industrial Pharmacy, 44*(1), 40–55.
23. Emami, S. H., Abad, A. M. A., Bonakdar, S., Tahriri, M. R., Samadikuchaksaraei, A., & Bahar, M. A. (2010). Preparation and evaluation of chitosan-gelatin composite scaffolds modified with chondroitin-6-sulphate. *International Journal of Materials Research, 101*(10), 1281–1285.
24. Heidari, F., Razavi, M., Bahrololoom, M. E., Tahriri, M., Rasoulianboroujeni, M., Koturi, H., & Tayebi, L. (2018). Preparation of natural chitosan from shrimp shell with different deacetylation degree. *Materials Research Innovations, 22*(3), 177–181.
25. Heidari, F., Razavi, M., Bahrololoom, M. E., Tahriri, M., & Tayebi, L. (2018). Investigation of the mechanical properties and degradability of a modified chitosan-based scaffold. *Materials Chemistry and Physics, 204*, 187–194.
26. Heidari, F., Razavi, M., Bahrololoom, M. E., Yazdimamaghani, M., Tahriri, M., Kotturi, H., & Tayebi, L. (2018). Evaluation of the mechanical properties, in vitro biodegradability and cytocompatibility of natural chitosan/hydroxyapatite/nano-$Fe_3O_4$ composite. *Ceramics International, 44*(1), 275–281.
27. Nejat, H., Rabiee, M., Varshochian, R., Tahriri, M., Jazayeri, H. E., Rajadas, J., Ye, H., Cui, Z., & Tayebi, L. (2017). Preparation and characterization of cardamom extract-loaded gelatin nanoparticles as effective targeted drug delivery system to treat glioblastoma. *Reactive and Functional Polymers, 120*, 46–56.
28. Raz, M., Moztarzadeh, F., Shokrgozar, M., Ashuri, M., & Tahriri, M. (2013). Preparation, characterization and evaluation of mechanical and biological characteristics of hybrid apatite/gelatin-chitosan nanocomposite bone scaffold via biomimetic method. *Journal of Advanced Materials in Engineering (Esteghlal), 32*(2), 25–42.
29. Raz, M., Moztarzadeh, F., Shokrgozar, M. A., Azami, M., & Tahriri, M. (2014). Development of biomimetic gelatin–chitosan/hydroxyapatite nanocomposite via double diffusion method for biomedical applications. *International Journal of Materials Research, 105*(5), 493–501.
30. Zafar, M. S., & Al-Samadani, K. H. (2014). Potential use of natural silk for bio-dental applications. *Journal of Taibah University Medical Sciences, 9*(3), 171–177.
31. Tahriri, M., Moztarzadeh, F., Hresko, K., Khoshroo, K., & Tayebi, L. (2016). Biodegradation properties of PLGA/nano-fluorhydroxyapatite composite microsphere-sintered scaffolds. *Dental Materials, 32*, e49–e50.
32. Tahriri, M., & Moztarzadeh, F. (2014). Preparation, characterization, and in vitro biological evaluation of PLGA/nano-fluorohydroxyapatite (FHA) microsphere-sintered scaffolds for biomedical applications. *Applied Biochemistry and Biotechnology, 172*(5), 2465–2479.
33. Zamani, Y., Rabiee, M., Shokrgozar, M. A., Bonakdar, S., & Tahriri, M. (2013). Response of human mesenchymal stem cells to patterned and randomly oriented poly (vinyl alcohol) nano-fibrous scaffolds surface-modified with Arg-Gly-Asp (RGD) ligand. *Applied Biochemistry and Biotechnology, 171*(6), 1513–1524.
34. Tonomura, A., Mizuno, D., Hisada, A., Kuno, N., Ando, Y., Sumita, Y., Honda, M. J., Satomura, K., Sakurai, H., & Ueda, M. (2010). Differential effect of scaffold shape on dentin regeneration. *Annals of Biomedical Engineering, 38*(4), 1664–1671.

35. Goyal, B., Tewari, S., Duhan, J., & Sehgal, P. (2011). Comparative evaluation of platelet-rich plasma and guided tissue regeneration membrane in the healing of apicomarginal defects: A clinical study. *Journal of Endodontics, 37*(6), 773–780.
36. Ohara, T., Itaya, T., Usami, K., Ando, Y., Sakurai, H., Honda, M. J., Ueda, M., & Kagami, H. (2010). Evaluation of scaffold materials for tooth tissue engineering. *Journal of Biomedical Materials Research Part A, 94*(3), 800–805.
37. Lim, J.-Y., Yi, T., Choi, J.-S., Jang, Y. H., Lee, S., Kim, H. J., Song, S. U., & Kim, Y.-M. (2013). Intraglandular transplantation of bone marrow-derived clonal mesenchymal stem cells for amelioration of post-irradiation salivary gland damage. *Oral Oncology, 49*(2), 136–143.
38. Kaigler, D., & Mooney, D. (2001). Tissue engineering's impact on dentistry. *Journal of Dental Education, 65*(5), 456–462.
39. Nyman, S., Lindhe, J., Karring, T., & Rylander, H. (1982). New attachment following surgical treatment of human periodontal disease. *Journal of Clinical Periodontology, 9*(4), 290–296.
40. Urist, M. R. (1965). Bone: Formation by autoinduction. *Science, 150*(3698), 893–899.
41. Sheridan, M., Shea, L., Peters, M., & Mooney, D. (2000). Bioabsorbable polymer scaffolds for tissue engineering capable of sustained growth factor delivery. *Journal of Controlled Release, 64*(1–3), 91–102.
42. Neel, E. A. A., Chrzanowski, W., Salih, V. M., Kim, H.-W., & Knowles, J. C. (2014). Tissue engineering in dentistry. *Journal of Dentistry, 42*(8), 915–928.
43. Young, C. S., Terada, S., Vacanti, J. P., Honda, M., Bartlett, J. D., & Yelick, P. C. (2002). Tissue engineering of complex tooth structures on biodegradable polymer scaffolds. *Journal of Dental Research, 81*(10), 695–700.
44. Duailibi, M. T., Duailibi, S. E., Young, C. S., Bartlett, J. D., Vacanti, J. P., & Yelick, P. C. (2004). Bioengineered teeth from cultured rat tooth bud cells. *Journal of Dental Research, 83*(7), 523–528.
45. Xu, W.-P., Zhang, W., Asrican, R., Kim, H.-J., Kaplan, D. L., & Yelick, P. C. (2008). Accurately shaped tooth bud cell–derived mineralized tissue formation on silk scaffolds. *Tissue Engineering Part A, 14*(4), 549–557.
46. Nakao, K., Morita, R., Saji, Y., Ishida, K., Tomita, Y., Ogawa, M., Saitoh, M., Tomooka, Y., & Tsuji, T. (2007). The development of a bioengineered organ germ method. *Nature Methods, 4*(3), 227.
47. Thomas, M., Grande, D., & Haug, R. H. (1991). Development of an in vitro temporomandibular joint cartilage analog. *Journal of Oral and Maxillofacial Surgery, 49*(8), 854–856.
48. Puelacher, W. C., Wisser, J., Vacanti, C. A., Ferraro, N. F., Jaramillo, D., & Vacanti, J. P. (1994). Temporomandibular joint disc replacement made by tissue-engineered growth of cartilage. *Journal of Oral and Maxillofacial Surgery, 52*(11), 1172–1177.
49. Abukawa, H., Terai, H., Hannouche, D., Vacanti, J. P., Kaban, L. B., & Troulis, M. J. (2003). Formation of a mandibular condyle in vitro by tissue engineering. *Journal of Oral and Maxillofacial Surgery, 61*(1), 94–100.
50. Weng, Y., Cao, Y., Arevalo, C., Vacanti, M. P., & Vacanti, C. A. (2001). Tissue-engineered composites of bone and cartilage for mandible condylar reconstruction. *Journal of Oral and Maxillofacial Surgery, 59*(2), 185–190.
51. Fan, Y., Sun, Z., & Moradian-Oldak, J. (2009). Controlled remineralization of enamel in the presence of amelogenin and fluoride. *Biomaterials, 30*(4), 478–483.
52. Nakashima, M. (1990). The induction of reparative dentine in the amputated dental pulp of the dog by bone morphogenetic protein. *Archives of Oral Biology, 35*(7), 493–497.
53. Lianjia, Y., Yuhao, G., & White, F. H. (1993). Bovine bone morphogenetic protein-induced dentinogenesis. *Clinical Orthopaedics and Related Research*, (295), 305–312.
54. Caton, J. G., & Greenstein, G. (1993). Factors related to periodontal regeneration. *Periodontology 2000, 1*, 9–15.
55. Villar, C. C., & Cochran, D. L. (2010). Regeneration of periodontal tissues: Guided tissue regeneration. *Dental Clinics, 54*(1), 73–92.

56. Nevins, M., Giannobile, W. V., McGuire, M. K., Kao, R. T., Mellonig, J. T., Hinrichs, J. E., McAllister, B. S., Murphy, K. S., McClain, P. K., & Nevins, M. L. (2005). Platelet-derived growth factor stimulates bone fill and rate of attachment level gain: Results of a large multicenter randomized controlled trial. *Journal of Periodontology, 76*(12), 2205–2215.
57. Alsberg, E., Hill, E., & Mooney, D. (2001). Craniofacial tissue engineering. *Critical Reviews in Oral Biology & Medicine, 12*(1), 64–75.
58. Nevins, M., Camelo, M., Nevins, M. L., Schenk, R. K., & Lynch, S. E. (2003). Periodontal regeneration in humans using recombinant human platelet-derived growth factor-BB (rhPDGF-BB) and allogenic bone. *Journal of Periodontology, 74*(9), 1282–1292.
59. Hotta, T., Yokoo, S., Terashi, H., & Komori, T. (2007). Clinical and histopathological analysis of healing process of intraoral reconstruction with ex vivo produced oral mucosa equivalent. *The Kobe Journal of Medical Sciences, 53*(1–2), 1–14.
60. Moharamzadeh, K., Brook, I., Van Noort, R., Scutt, A., & Thornhill, M. (2007). Tissue-engineered oral mucosa: A review of the scientific literature. *Journal of Dental Research, 86*(2), 115–124.
61. Sauerbier, S., Gutwald, R., Wiedmann-Al-Ahmad, M., Lauer, G., & Schmelzeisen, R. (2006). Clinical application of tissue-engineered transplants. Part I: Mucosa. *Clinical Oral Implants Research, 17*(6), 625–632.
62. Baum, B., & O'connell, B. (1999). In vivo gene transfer to salivary glands. *Critical Reviews in Oral Biology & Medicine, 10*(3), 276–283.
63. Baum, B. J., Wang, S., Cukierman, E., Delporte, C., Kagami, H., Marmary, Y., Fox, P. C., Mooney, D. J., & Yamada, K. M. (1999). Re-engineering the functions of a terminally differentiated epithelial cell in vivo. *Annals of the New York Academy of Sciences, 875*(1), 294–300.
64. Bailey, M. M., Wang, L., Bode, C. J., Mitchell, K. E., & Detamore, M. S. (2007). A comparison of human umbilical cord matrix stem cells and temporomandibular joint condylar chondrocytes for tissue engineering temporomandibular joint condylar cartilage. *Tissue Engineering, 13*(8), 2003–2010.
65. Schek, R., Taboas, J., Hollister, S. J., & Krebsbach, P. (2005). Tissue engineering osteochondral implants for temporomandibular joint repair. *Orthodontics & Craniofacial Research, 8*(4), 313–319.
66. Ikada, Y. (2006). Challenges in tissue engineering. *Journal of the Royal Society Interface, 3*(10), 589–601.
67. Lo, B., & Parham, L. (2009). Ethical issues in stem cell research. *Endocrine Reviews, 30*(3), 204–213.

# Chapter 9
# 3D Printing in Dentistry

**Samaneh Hosseini, Majid Halvaei, Amin Ebrahimi,
Mohammad Amin Shamekhi, and Mohamadreza Baghaban Eslaminejad**

## 1 Introduction

Tissue loss due to diseases, genetic disorders, and traumas is a major global health problem. Lack of tissue in the oral-maxillofacial region may result in problems with severe tooth loss that involves several soft and hard tissues [1]. The oral cavity is composed of the maxilla (upper jaw), mandible (lower jaw), and teeth that create a natural, complex three-dimensional (3D) structure. A critical challenge in regenerative dentistry is fabrication of functional 3D constructs for craniofacial reconstruction. There is an essential need to fabricate these complicated tissues in a controllable manner. Biomanufacturing methods used for regeneration of various dental structures are very limited and lead to tooth loss in most cases [2, 3]. High-level progressive periodontitis changes alveolar bone morphology, resulting in loss of tooth-supporting tissues with subsequent tooth extraction. Socket preservation or alveolar ridge preservation (ARP) and strengthening with bone grafting materials are available methods to preserve resting bone following a tooth extraction in clinic [4, 5]. Computer-aided design (CAD) and computer-aided manufacturing (CAM)

---

Majid Halvaei, Amin Ebrahimi and Mohammad Amin Shamekhi contributed equally with all other contributors.

---

S. Hosseini · A. Ebrahimi · M. Baghaban Eslaminejad (✉)
Department of Stem Cells and Developmental Biology, Cell Science Research Center, Royan Institute for Stem Cell Biology and Technology, ACECR, Tehran, Iran
e-mail: eslami@royaninstitute.org

M. Halvaei
Department of Cell Engineering, Cell Science Research Center, Royan Institute for Stem Cell Biology and Technology, ACECR, Tehran, Iran

M. A. Shamekhi
Department of Polymer Engineering, Islamic Azad University, Sarvestan Branch, Sarvestan, Iran



L. Tayebi (ed.), *Applications of Biomedical Engineering in Dentistry*,
https://doi.org/10.1007/978-3-030-21583-5_9

are promising technologies to create customized structures. CAD and CAM are of interest in medicine because of their ability to produce a range of medical devices, orthopedic implants, and artificial tissues and organs [6]. CAD and CAM make it possible to produce reliable restorations that have accurate dimensions and a more consistent quality, in addition to reduced manufacturing time. Among the various medical fields, dentistry has greatly exploited CAD/CAM technologies. CAD/CAM can be used for various applications in dentistry that include maxillofacial implants, dental models, dentures, crowns, and tooth tissue engineering [7]. For example, crown and bridge restoration and dentures are routinely fabricated by a wax technique, and metal casting can be replaced by more rapid, cost-effective 3D printing. Here, we describe 3D printing approaches currently used in dentistry. We mainly focus on the application of 3D printing in regenerative dentistry and dental tissue engineering. This chapter also explores the importance of biomolecules and vasculature in 3D-printed constructs.

## 2 3D Printing Methodology

Fabrication of 3D objects is one of the main challenges in industry and medicine. To date, different methods have been utilized to manufacture 3D objects. Along with the advances in computers, manually operated machines have been replaced by automated machines. CAD and CAM pave the way for minimizing operator error and help fabricate objects with higher repeatability. Briefly, in CAD/CAM, a 3D file is designed with different software (CATIA, SolidWorks, Maya, 3ds Max); 3D scanners provide this opportunity to create a primary 3D file. In addition to industrial 3D scanners, medical imaging systems such as magnetic resonance imaging (MRI) for soft tissues, and computed tomography [8] and cone beam computed tomography (CBCT) for hard tissues, provide volumetric data to create 3D files of implants, prostheses, tissues, and organs. These files can be used directly or modified by software to give a final 3D CAD file. The CAD/CAM methods are divided into two main manufacturing groups, subtractive and additive. Below, we describe their subgroups and provide a detailed description of their applications in medicine and dentistry.

### *2.1 Subtractive Manufacturing (SM)*

Subtractive manufacturing (SM) has a long history in dentistry. In the 1970s, Duret and Preston fabricated a fixed dental prosthesis by using a numerically controlled SM miller. In this method, a block of material undergoes a milling process to create a 3D structure. This process is very similar to carving a statue from a stone block. However, computer numerical controlled (CNC) machining is automated and performs the carving by a milling mechanism via a computer. Various materials have been used in dental milling, such as metals (Ti, Co-Cr) [9], ceramics ($ZrO_2$) [10, 11], and polymers (or composites) [12, 13]. Computer numerical controlled machining has been used to build personal anatomic implants, such as dental and craniofacial prostheses, as well as crown and bridge restorations [11]. EpiBone uses this method to create anatomically viable bone structures. They first decellularize the bone tissue, then create an anatomic 3D structure with the use of a CNC milling machine, and eventually recellularize the tissue with a perfusion system. The resultant product could be utilized as an anatomical, viable bone graft for craniofacial and orthopedic defects [14]. However, drawbacks related to the subtractive methods have hampered their extensive use in dental applications. The drawbacks include a high amount of wasted raw materials, macroscopic cracks due to machining, and limited precision fit. Fabrication of dental articles by CNC machining is a troublesome task due to the presence of overhangs and sharp corners.

## 2.2 *Additive Manufacturing (AM)*

Additive manufacturing (AM), which is often referred to as 3D printing, creates a 3D object with layer-by-layer addition of materials. Hull, the father of 3D printing, developed the first laser-based 3D printing method in the early 1980s [15]. Initial application of 3D printing in tissue engineering was reported in the mid-1990s [16–18], while a 3D bioprinting method was developed in the early 2000s [19]. 3D bioprinting is an exciting technology with tremendous potential to address critical issues in regenerative dentistry. Since the 3D bioprinting technique patterns cells and biomaterials, selection of a proper material for 3D bioprinting is more difficult than conventional 3D printing. Cells are one of the printing components, and biological considerations are needed to select a proper bioink [20]. Among various 3D printing methods, the most popular for medical and dental applications are described below.

### 2.2.1 Laser-Based Methods

In laser-based methods, a laser beam with different powers, intensities, and dimensions is applied to crosslink a resin, melt/sinter powder, or eject a microdroplet of material placed on a laser-absorbing layer.

*Stereolithography (SLA)* Stereolithography (SLA) is defined as the fabrication of a 3D model from a light-sensitive material. This technique is a 3D photolithography method in which a liquid-like photopolymer is exposed to a specific wavelength range of light to initiate the polymerization process. The photopolymer undergoes a change in its mechanical properties and gives rise to a solid material. A laser beam scans a predefined area of the surface of the photopolymer vat and crosslinks this point by laser radiation. A 3D structure is fabricated by layer-by-layer iteration of this procedure. The SLA technique has been applied in tissue engineering (TE) to fabricate a 3D structure with or without cells. Photosensitive biomaterials, such as poly(ethylene oxide) (PEO), polyethylene glycol diacrylate (PEGDA), and gelatin methacryloyl (GelMA), have been used in the SLA method to print a 3D scaffold [21, 22]. Although SLA is based on the photo-polymerization of photosensitive materials, ceramic materials like alumina combined with a photosensitive resin can be used. These ceramic materials are proper candidates for producing a dental crown framework [23, 24].

*Selective laser melting (SLM)* Selective laser melting (SLM) uses a laser beam to melt different materials, such as ceramics, polymers, and metal powders. Although SLM is akin to SLA, there are two main differences. First, the printing material in SLM is a powder instead of a photosensitive resin. Each layer is prepared by a roller prior to laser exposure. Second, the solidification mechanism is based on the melting of a powder in contrast to crosslinking of the photopolymer. Selective laser melting has been used to fabricate 3D metallic dental structures. Both Co-Cr and Ti are widely used to fabricate 3D dental structures and porous 3D implants by the SLM method [9, 25, 26].

*Selective laser sintering (SLS)* The selective laser sintering (SLS) method is similar to SLM, but differs in the fusion mechanism. In SLM, the powder particles reach their melting point and subsequently fuse together. In contrast, in the SLS technique, the powder particles do not melt; rather, they are heated with a laser beam to a critical temperature that enables the small particles of powder to fuse to each other at the molecular level. Various biomaterials can be utilized to manufacture 3D objects by SLS, such as polymers [poly(ε-caprolactone) (PCL) and polyamide] [27, 28], metals (steel and titanium, alloys) [29–31], and ceramic powders [calcium phosphate-based materials and hydroxyapatite (HA)] [32]. The composite of a polymer and a ceramic material would also provide an ideal biomaterial for hard tissue regeneration purposes [32–34].

*Laser-assisted bioprinting (LAB)* Laser-assisted bioprinting (LAB) is composed of a pulsed laser source, a ribbon coated with a printing material, and a receiving substrate. The ribbon is normally composed of a transparent supportive layer, a laser-absorbing interlayer, and the printing material. Although there is no laser-absorbing layer, the printing material is thermosensitive. For bioprinting applications, it is recommended to use an interlayer in order to protect the encapsulated cells in the printing material from directly sensing the laser's heat [35]. This technique is used to print biomaterials that have a high cell density and high precision pattering of the cell's microenvironment [36–39].

### 2.2.2 Flash Technology

Digital light processing (DLP) is one of the most widely used 3D printing methods. In this technology, the 3D printing material is a photosensitive material similar to SLA. In DLP, each layer is cured by projection of a picture from a projector onto the surface of the resin. The DLP technique has the capability to print 3D objects with the cells, in contrast to the SLS technique where cell printing is impossible due to its harsh conditions [40–44]. Biomaterials, such as PEGDA and GelMA, can be cured with visible light, which lack cytotoxicity and do not affect cell viability. In addition, DLP appears to be more convenient in terms of the precision and accuracy of dental models compared to the SLA technique [45].

### 2.2.3 Extrusion

Extrusion is extensively used in tissue engineering. The printing mechanism is layer-by-layer like other 3D printing techniques, yet nozzle-based. The most usable extrusion methods are fused deposition modeling (FDM) and dough deposition modeling (DMM).

*Fused deposition modeling (FDM)* A thermoplastic material, polylactic acid (PLA), is extruded from a heated nozzle and lies on the printing stage in the FDM method. After each layer is printed, the nozzle moves upward one step that is equal to the dimension of a printing layer. This process continues layer-by-layer until the formation of a 3D object is complete. Printing materials include PCL [46], PLA [47], or a mixture of a thermoplastic material with other materials (ceramics) [48, 49]. Osteoplug™ and Osteomesh™ are 3D-printed and patient-specific skull and craniofacial implants printed by the FDM method [50].

*Dough deposition modeling (DMM)* Among 3D bioprinting methods, DMM is broadly used for tissue engineering applications. In this technique, a vast range of materials, such as polymers, metals, and ceramics, can be used to print a 3D object. Materials with proper mechanical and rheological properties are placed into a reservoir. The printing material extrudes through a nozzle under hydrostatic pressure that is generated by movement of a plunger through a syringe [51–53], by pneumatic pressure exerted over the printing material [54–57], or by rotation of a screw inside the reservoir where the rotation exudes the material [58, 59]. Viscosity, gelation time, thixotropic behavior, and the shape and dimensions of the nozzle determine the printing quality [60]. It is possible to combine two different methods, such as FDM and DMM, to print a 3D structure that has the desired mechanical and biological parameters [52].

### 2.2.4 Jet Printing

Jet printing is one of the oldest methods used in tissue engineering. In the late 1980s, researchers used the jet printing method to print the word "fibronectin" on a non-cell-adhesive substrate. Then, by patterning fibronectin and culturing cells over this substrate, they observed that these cells only attached to the patterned areas [61]. In 1994, cells and biomaterials were patterned on a substrate with the use of an inkjet printer [62]. Inkjet printers use piezoelectric [63, 64] or thermal actuators [65, 66] to eject droplets from their nozzles. The simplest mode of a jet printing technique directly prints a material layer-by-layer. In some cases, the printing material is photo-curable and it is necessary to crosslink each layer by exposing the layers to light. A suitable biomaterial for jet printing is PEG-GelMA, a UV crosslink material [67]. Jet printing can be used to print a powder that needs a binder to bind the powder particles to each other. In this technique, as with SLS for patterning each layer, a layer of powder is initially prepared and then the binder solution is ejected from the nozzle [68]. Sajio et al. have used this technique to print maxillofacial 3D structures with calcium phosphate powder [69].

## 3 Biomaterials for 3D Printing in Dentistry

According to the 3D printing methodology, printing is normally accomplished via two approaches: an acellular structure that uses solid freeform fabrication (SLF), FDM, and stereolithography (SLA) or cell-containing constructs that use inkjet-based, extrusion-based, and laser-assisted bioprinting. The inks without cells are acellular inks, whereas the cell-containing inks are regarded as bioinks [70–72]. Biomaterials used for printing should mimic the natural environment of the host tissue in order to contribute to the function of those cells [73]. However, because of the various 3D printable materials used in biomaterial inks, precise matching of the materials to specific tissue types is a challenge. Understanding the structure-property relationship of the bioinks has led to construction of numerous specific tissues that have a variety of physical, mechanical, biochemical, and electrical properties [74].

Different types of materials, such as polymers, ceramics, and metals, are used for 3D printing in dentistry. Selection of these materials strictly depends upon where they are to be precisely applied. For example, Ti and calcium phosphate have been used to fabricate maxillary and mandibular implants, whereas partial and complete dentures have been created with metals such as cobalt and ceramics like zirconia and alumina [75, 76]. Numerous natural biomaterials (collagen, fibrin, silk, chitosan, hyaluronic acid, alginate, and agarose) and synthetic materials [PLA, poly(glycolic acid) (PGA), poly(lactic-co-glycolic acid) (PLGA), and PCL] have been used for tooth tissue engineering applications. Other synthetic materials include inorganic calcium phosphate materials, like HA or beta tricalcium phosphate (β-TCP), and composites of silicate and phosphate glasses [77]. Studies are underway to find the proper materials and bioinks for 3D printing.

The 3D-printed scaffolds used for tooth tissue engineering should fulfill general requirements of appropriate porosity, biodegradability, low immunogenic response, and angiogenesis capabilities. In load-bearing tissues, such as dental and maxillofacial tissues, it is necessary to have high mechanical properties of the 3D-printed scaffolds to withstand the applied loads and in vitro bioreactor maturation [78]. Thus, investigation of the fracture behavior of ceramic tissue scaffolds is of crucial importance [79]. Special architecture of the 3D-printed scaffolds, such as orientation, pore size, and porosity, in addition to the types of biomaterials, strictly determines both physical and mechanical properties of the final product [80]. Polymer coating is an efficient approach used to improve the mechanical properties of 3D-printed scaffolds. The results have indicated that PCL coating enhances compressive strength and biocompatibility of 3D-printed HA scaffolds in bone tissue engineering applications [81].

Extracellular matrix (ECM)-derived scaffolds have attracted considerable attention for regenerative purposes. A hydrogel bioink made of dentin has been used for 3D printing of cell-laden scaffolds in regenerative dentistry. Researchers developed a novel bioink composed of printable alginate (3% w/v) and dentin matrix where the higher percentage of dentin proteins considerably improved cell viability. Odontogenic differentiation of apical papilla (SCAP) stem cells considerably increased after addition of 100 μg/ml dentin soluble materials [82].

# 4 Incorporation of Cells and Biomolecules in 3D Printing

Limitations in 3D printing technology preclude incorporation of biomolecules and cells. For example, printing performed at high temperatures using organic solvents causes loss of biomolecule functionality and cell death. Advances in 3D printing technology and feasibility of low temperature 3D printing and development of a biocompatible structure that uses aqueous binder solutions and composite biomaterials provide proper circumstances with which to apply the biomolecules and cells.

The combination of signaling molecules with various materials in 3D printing that needs a cell-friendly requirement has changed the term of "3D printing" to "bioprinting." Over the last decade, considerable progress has been made to develop AM procedures that process distinct biomaterials into predesigned 3D constructs. Thus, the constructs are becoming increasingly complex with incorporation of biological components [83, 84]. This approach remarkably affects the performance of the 3D constructs by adjustments to the biological, mechanical, drug delivery, and degradation properties. Regeneration of craniomaxillofacial injuries that are comprised of hard and soft tissues shows the crucial need for bioprinters [85].

# 5 Growth Factor (GF) and Drug Delivery Using 3D Printing

One application for dental tissue engineering is the regeneration of soft and hard oral tissues by using cells, scaffolds, and soluble molecules. There are a number of interesting approaches that can reconstruct craniofacial defects, including periodontal, alveolar ridge, and large mandibular defects. Delivery of signaling and bioactive molecules, such as low-molecular-weight drugs, peptides, proteins, and oligonucleotides, is applied alone or in combination with engineered constructs in order to accelerate tissue regeneration. Numerous reports have confirmed the efficiency of signaling molecules in cell-scaffold constructs [86]. Among all types of biological components, growth factors (GFs) are widely used to regenerate damaged tissues. Growth factors regulate a variety of cellular functions, including survival, proliferation, migration, and differentiation, via specific binding to their receptors on target cells [87]. In turn, they initiate signaling pathways that mediate tissue and organ development. Human tooth development is dependent on epithelial-mesenchymal interactions mediated by multiple signaling pathways that include bone morphogenetic proteins (BMPs), FGFs, Shh, and Wnt pathways [88]. Bone morphogenetic proteins, more precisely BMP-7 and BMP-2, are widely used for bone regeneration in maxillofacial reconstruction due to their osteoinduction and osteogenesis potencies. Stromal cell-derived factor 1 (SDF-1) and platelet-derived GF (PDGF) are common GFs in dental applications (Table 9.1) [89, 90]. Although the mitogenic and chemotactic effects of GFs are apparent at extremely low concentrations, their sensitivity, low stability, and short half-life have prompted scientists to develop novel delivery methods to stringently control the release rate [91]. Numerous studies used GF in AM to create functional tissues. These sensitive polypeptides must be used under mild conditions in order to exert their effects on cellular functions. Among the different methods of AM, three methods of SLA, SLS, and direct metal laser sintering (DMLS) cannot be used to manufacture 3D constructs with biological components due to high temperature, hard conditions, and potential for free radical production [92, 93]. Attempts that have used GF in 3D-printed constructs in order to regenerate dental tissues are discussed below.

*Dental pulp regeneration* Dental pulp, the only vascularized dental tissue, is a part of the endodontium comprised of living connective tissue and odontoblasts. Pulpectomy is a conventional endodontic therapy or root canal therapy for irreversible pulpitis [94, 99]. Over recent years, efforts in regeneration of dental pulp have focused on cell transplantation, which encounters clinical and commercialization

**Table 9.1** Application of growth factors (GFs) in 3D printing for dental applications

| Growth factors | Printing method | Cells | Material | Target tissue | Animal | Ref. |
|---|---|---|---|---|---|---|
| BMP-7<br>SDF-1 | 3D layer-by-layer manufacturing | – | PCL/HA | Mandibular incisor regeneration | Rat | [94] |
| BMP-7 | 3D wax printing | HGFCs | PCL/PGA | Tooth-ligament regeneration | Nude mouse | [95] |
| BMP-7 | 3D wax printing | PDLCs | PCL fiber | Mandibular periodontal regeneration | Rat | [96] |
| Amelogenin<br>CTGF<br>BMP-2 | 3D layer-by-layer deposition | DPSCs, PDLSCs, or ABSCs | PCL/HA | Periodontium regeneration | Immune-deficient mice | [97] |
| BMP-7<br>SDF-1 | 3D layer-by-layer apposition | – | PCL/HA | Formation of alveolar bone, dentin-like tissue | Rat | [98] |

barriers [100]. Among various AM methods, 3D bioprinting possesses advantages of precise control of pore size, stiffness, anatomic dimensions, and interconnectivity [101]. The use of GF would promote the ultimate goal of regeneration. Kim et al. generated anatomically shaped tooth scaffolds by 3D printing of the PCL/HA composite. The scaffold microchannels were permeated with a blended cocktail of SDF-1 and BMP-7 in a collagen gel solution. Their findings showed significantly higher cell infiltration and angiogenesis in the group that contained SDF-1 and BMP-7. In addition, they suggested that SDF-1 and BMP-7 had the capability to recruit multiple cell lineages, as evidenced by histological analysis. The combination of SDF-1 and BMP-7 has led to regeneration of tooth-like arrangements and periodontal integration after 9 weeks. SDF-1 is chemotactic for bone marrow progenitor cells and endothelial cells (ECs), both of which are critical for angiogenesis [101].

*Periodontium regeneration* The periodontium tissue is composed of cementum, periodontal ligament (PDL), and alveolar bone. The PDL connects the alveolar bone root to the cementum, providing a tensile strength of less than 0.5 mm and support for mastication [102]. Although the development of multilayered scaffolds for bone-ligament regeneration with a 3D printer [96] does not appear to be a complicated process, the generation of a 3D submicron scaled construct with GF loaded to precisely control fibrous PDL formation with specific corners remains a major challenge [103]. Thus far, different approaches have been proposed to deal with this challenge. Park et al. developed multiscale computational manufacture of a PCL-PGA hybrid scaffold with a treated tooth dentin slice by using a 3D wax printing system. The hybrid scaffold was subsequently filled with adenovirus encoding murine BMP-7 (AdCMVBMP-7), transduced primary human gingival fibroblast (hGF) cells, and human PDL (hPDL) cells and then implanted subcutaneously into a surgically created pocket on the dorsa of immunodeficient mice. The hybrid scaffold with hPDL cells and osteogenic stimulation (BMP-7) enhanced regeneration of the multilayered periodontal complex and produced periodontium-like tissue 6 weeks after implantation [95].

Lee et al. reported that biophysical cues and spatial release of bioactive cues led to periodontium regeneration. They fabricated multiphasic PCL/HA (90:10 wt %) scaffolds with different pore sizes (phases A, B, and C) that resembled the periodontium tissue. Next, three recombinant human proteins (connective tissue GF, amelogenin, and BMP-2) encapsulated in PLGA microspheres were delivered and time-released in the A, B, and C phases. Spatiotemporal delivery of amelogenin led to mineralization of dentin/cementum, connective tissue GF (CTGF)-stimulated bone marrow stromal cells, and PDL regeneration. BMP-2, as an osteoinductive agent, induced alveolar bone regeneration [97]. Despite the promising advancements in dental regeneration, there is scant information about biological cues and biophysical parameters that would be considered crucial for the regeneration of the periodontium complex [96, 104].

*Tooth regeneration* A tooth is a complicated organ organized by a variety of soft (dental pulp) and hard (dentin, enamel, and cementum) tissues with different regenerative capacities [105]. Re-mineralization of teeth can restore the injuries to a particular level; however, it cannot repair large defects. Maintenance and repair of human tooth enamel is one of the primary dental concerns. In contrast to enamel, dentin grows throughout life and growth can be initiated in response to stimuli, such as tooth failure or attrition by the odontoblasts of dental pulp [106]. Different 3D printing methods and various biomaterials, like collagen, agarose, alginate, PLA, and fibrin, have been utilized with dental mesenchymal stem cells (MSCs) to regenerate different parts of the teeth – dental pulp, dentin, the crown, and root [102]. Yildirim et al. fabricated a tooth-shaped 3D scaffold that consisted of PCL (80%) and HA (20%) with an SDF-1/BMP-7 cocktail to induce tooth-like structures in rat mandibular central incisors. The harvested scaffold showed the development of various dental tissues that included fresh formed alveolar bone, PDL-like tissue, dentin-like tissue, and dental pulp-like tissue with blood vessels after 9 weeks. Binding of SDF-1 to CXCR4, a chemokine receptor for ECs and bone marrow stem/progenitor cells, led to angiogenesis. Additionally, BMP-7 triggered the phosphorylation of SMAD-1 and SMAD-5, which subsequently induced the transcription of numerous osteogenic/odontogenic genes that led to enhanced mineralization. Ultimately, the use of molecular cues instead of cell transplantation could represent a cost-effective cell homing approach in tooth regeneration [98].

## 6 Cells in 3D Printing

Tissue engineering approaches that use cell or gene deliveries have the capability to address existing challenges in regulating bone loss and enhance clinical alternatives for regeneration of intraoral bony tissues. Towards this goal, cells such as MSCs should be seeded in a precise and orderly manner onto the scaffolds. In classical tissue engineering approaches, cells are seeded onto polymeric scaffolds or natural porous biomaterials. The physical and mechanical properties of the scaffolds and their effects on cell viability and ECM secretion must be taken into consideration for scaffold-based approaches [107]. However, controlled positioning of cells is impossible in traditional tissue engineering approaches. 3D printing methods that provide a patient-specific anatomical bone defect scaffold with structural integrity have been used as a cell therapy and GF delivery platform to facilitate tissue restoration. However, to achieve the ultimate goal of healing, the cell viability rate must be preserved at the highest level. Cell viability greatly depends on the 3D printing methods. Laser-assisted bioprinting, particularly DLP-based bioprinting, exhibits a very high viability rate in comparison to other methods (Table 9.2) [108].

According to the various printing methods, proper hydrogels (bioink) must be selected to preserve cell viability during the printing procedure. Bioink supports proliferation and physicochemical control of cell differentiation. It has been reported that fibrin and collagen are suitable bioinks for bioprinting of ECs [112]. For dental pulp cells, the dentin matrix is an appropriate biological reservoir for specific bioinks. Dental ECM consists of insoluble non-collagenous components, such as proteoglycans, glycosaminoglycans, and chemokines, that support cell adhesion and

**Table 9.2** Comparison of the different bioprinting techniques [75, 109–111]

| Parameters | Extrusion | Inkjet | SLA | LAB | DLP |
|---|---|---|---|---|---|
| Cost | Moderate | Low | Low | High | Moderate |
| Resolution | 5 μm | 50 μm | 100 μm | >500 nm | 1 μm |
| Cell viability | 40–80% | >85% | >85% | >85% | 85–95% |
| Speed | Slow | Medium | Fast | Medium | Fast |
| Material choice | Medium range | Wide range | Limited | Limited | Limited |

proliferation and possess high odontogenic differentiation potential [113]. The cell viability rate, regardless of regeneration plan and type of tissue, stringently depends on nature of the bioink and printing method.

Appropriate cell sources are needed to obtain the desired structure that mimics human tissue anatomy. For example, bone and dentin are analogous in their matrix protein formation, but their organ anatomies completely differ. Batouli et al. have demonstrated that bone marrow MSCs (BMMSCs) and dental pulp stem cells (DPSCs) have the capability to differentiate into osteoblast/odontoblast cells, though the dentinogenesis capability of these cells is different. Only DPSCs could directly generate a reparative dentin-like structure on the surface of human dentin [114]. Appropriate cell sources that have the adequate cell density and culture conditions to obtain optimal craniofacial regeneration are challenges in tissue engineering and regenerative medicine. Cell spatial information in the desired tissue (cell location) is also crucial for functional tissue manufacturing. The utilized cell population for premeditated differentiation (homogeneous/heterogeneous) and features of this cell population (stem/adult/progeny) can determine the cell fate in a 3D-printed construct.

Various cell sources, particularly MSCs, have been used to direct bone/dental tissue regeneration in 3D-printed constructs. Mesenchymal stem cells are considered to be an appropriate type of stem cell due to their ability to differentiate into both osteoblasts/odontoblasts and ECs that support hematopoiesis [115]. Additionally, they can be isolated from dental tissues (dental pulp, PDL, dental follicles, and dental apical papilla) and are the most promising sources of MSCs for regenerative dentistry [116]. Although most MSCs have common features, some are more specific for regeneration of dental defects. Table 9.3 lists the various types of MSCs used in 3D-printed constructs for dental tissue regeneration [97].

## 6.1 *Dental Pulp Stem Cells (DPSCs)*

Dental pulp stem cells are mesenchymal stem-like cell populations derived from adult third molars. They are clonogenic cells and highly proliferative and have the capability to give rise into odontoblast-like cells and form dentin–/pulp-like complexes [121, 122]. In 2009, data from a successful clinical trial of alveolar bone regeneration that used DPSCs suggested that a DPSC/collagen sponge bio-complex could completely restore human mandible bone defects [123]. Several

**Table 9.3** Mesenchymal stem cells (MSCs) used in dental tissue regeneration with 3D printing

| Cell type | Type of scaffold | Printing method | Results | Ref. |
|---|---|---|---|---|
| DPSCs & SCAPs | 3D-printed HA construct | Stereolithography | Vascularized pulp-like tissue and mineralized tissue formation occurred after 12 wks | [117] |
| SCAPs | Alginate-dentin hydrogel | Extrusion | Remarkable increase in ALP and RUNX2 at both protein and gene levels | [82] |
| SHED | 3D-printed tricalcium phosphate paste | Inkjet | Scaffold material itself promotes osteogenic differentiation of the cells, resulted in increased osteocalcin expression level | [118, 119] |
| Shed | PLA scaffold | Fused deposition modeling (FDM) | Higher expression level of osteocalcin and osteonectin was observed on PLA scaffold | [92] |
| PDLSCs | PCL scaffold embedded with PLGA microspheres | Extrusion | Enhancement of CEMP1 mRNA expression and newly formed cementum-like layer. Activation of canonical Wnt signaling pathway in PDLSCs | [120] |

materials with diverse manufacturing methods have been used to estimate the regenerative potential of DPSCs. Hilkens et al. used 3D-printed HA scaffolds that contained either DPSCs or stem cells from the apical papilla (SCAPs) and their combination to evaluate the angiogenic capacity in an ectopic transplantation model of dental pulp regeneration. There were no significant differences among all cell-seeded 3D-printed scaffolds and the negative control in terms of amount of newly formed blood vessels 12 weeks after implantation into immunocompromised mice compared to in vitro studies. These results were attributed to the scaffold properties that could affect the cellular behaviors. Moreover, an adequate stem cell density within the best time frame would provide ideal environment for regeneration [117].

## 6.2 Stem Cells from Human Exfoliated Deciduous Teeth (SHED)

Human exfoliated deciduous teeth contain an MSC population that has the ability to generate adherent cell clusters and induce bone and dentin formation in vivo. Stem cells derived from human exfoliated deciduous teeth (SHED) represent a more immature subpopulation that expand and proliferate more quickly in comparison with DPSCs or BMMSCs. These SHED are collected from the dental pulp of exfoliated deciduous teeth [124, 125]. In contrast to DPSCs, SHED lack the capability to regenerate a complete dentin pulp-like tissue in vivo [126]. It has been reported that cultivation of SHED on an osteoconductive 3D-printed ceramic scaffold with a gradient distribution of porosity and phase composition resulted in enhanced cell adhesion and proliferation [118, 119]. In a recent work, Islam et al. proposed that the combination of a human SHED-PLA 3D-printed scaffold could be a convenient osteogenic filling material for regenerative dentistry [92].

### 6.3 Periodontal Ligament Stem Cells (PDLSCs)

The multiple properties of PDL stem cells (PDLSCs) include expression of cementum-associated markers and the ability to make mineralized nodules. They are considered potential cell sources for periodontitis regeneration. These cells play a key role in formation of new bone, cementum, and functional PDL in unhealthy periodontium [127, 128]. A study of subcutaneous cell transplantation has shown that PDLSCs created periodontal tissue-like tissue, including a PDL-like structure, while BMSCs and DPSCs formed bone-like tissue and dentin/pulp complex-like tissue, respectively [129]. Choe et al. attempted to fabricate a PCL scaffold embedded with PLGA microspheres loaded with BMP-7/BMP-2/CTGF to evaluate the cementum layer formation potential of PDLSCs on extracted human dentin. After 6 weeks, gene expression analysis of *CEMP1*, *ColI*, and *BSP*, as well as tissue formation analysis, verified the cementum formation capability and showed the different responses of PDLSCs to various GFs [120].

### 6.4 Stem Cells from the Apical Papilla (SCAP)

Stem cells from the apical papilla are widely applied in regenerative dentistry due to their remarkable characteristics. These cells have a high proliferation rate and STRO-1 expression, as well as mineralization and regeneration capabilities. In addition, SCAPs exhibit a higher expression of survivin and telomerase, two proteins that play a key role in cell proliferation [130]. Bakopoulou et al. have reported a significantly higher mineralization rate of SCAPs compared to DPSCs after osteogenic induction. In 2017, Athirasala et al. developed a novel alginate-dentin (1:1 ratio) bioink and bioprinted SCAPs with the hybrid gel. The encapsulated SCAPs in alginate-dentin had a survival rate of 90% at 5 days after bioprinting. Differentiation of SCAPs encapsulated in the developed bioink resulted in increased ALP and RUNX2 activities. They observed that addition of soluble dentin matrix molecules at 1, 10, and 100 μg/mL concentrations led to a remarkable increase in ALP and RUNX2 expressions at both the protein and gene levels. These increases were dose-dependent and confirmed that dentin ECM content (especially PGs and GAGs) could precisely control the spatial presentation of signaling factors, as well as cell interactions for engineering of the pulp-dentin complex [82]. Therefore, in addition to the importance of the cell type, other biological and non-biological components played a regulatory role in local regeneration.

# 7 3D Printing Approaches for Vasculature in Tissue-Engineered Constructs

Angiogenesis is a critical parameter in tissue engineering that affects both design and manufacturing. The vascular network provides transport and exchange of nutrients, biomolecules, wastes, and gases in a scaffold or tissue-engineered construct. Diffusion is considered to be a dominant mechanism for transportation of materials in small engineered tissues. Although this mechanism is for transporting materials, it is not an efficient method for human scale tissues. The formation of a vascular network is a fundamental phase during tooth development. Dental pulp is a highly vascularized tissue where blood capillaries traverse centrally through the pulp and extend towards the tooth crown. Rapid vascularization of the engineered dental pulp is required for pulp regeneration in root canal therapy. Thus far, numerous studies have utilized angiogenic GFs in a variety of delivery approaches; however, they could not fulfill the desired angiogenesis in 3D constructs. Advances in manufacturing techniques and development of rapid prototyping methods have enabled researchers to create very complex 3D structures with distinct internal porosities. The 3D bioprinting methods provide the possibility of printing 3D structures with vascular networks for tissue engineering applications. The most important 3D printing techniques used to create vascular networks in an engineered scaffold are described below. These techniques are especially useful for printing hydrogels where the diffusion of nutrition is decreased toward the center of scaffold.

## *7.1 Hollow Fiber Printing*

This method is principally based on 3D patterning of hollow fibers instead of solid fibers. The hollow fibers enable perfusion of culture medium throughout a 3D-engineered tissue, which enables the cells to survive inside the 3D structure for extended periods of time. A coaxial nozzle and proper materials are prerequisites to extrude hollow fibers from the printer head. The outer needle injects the printing material and the inner needle injects the crosslinker fluid. Ionic crosslink materials like alginate are appropriate. Since hollow fibers have low mechanical properties, it is essential to perform post-processing tasks. Once a single component ink, such as alginate, is used as a printing material, the final structure can be immersed into a $CaCl_2$ bath to complete the crosslinking process [131–134]. The combination of other materials, such as thermos-responsive materials with suitable printing properties (e.g., gelatin), can improve the printing quality of the hollow fibers in an ionic crosslink material [135].

In another method, two different crosslinking mechanisms are applied to improve the final mechanical properties of the 3D structure. In this approach, the printing material is composed of an ionic crosslink material (alginate) and a covalently crosslinked material (GelMA). The former acts as a pre-crosslink mechanism to form hollow fibers, whereas the latter renders the final mechanical strength of the structure [136]. In order to increase the efficiency of ionic crosslinking, we can use a multilayer needle that has three coaxial needles. In this nozzle, the middle needle injects the hydrogel, and both the inner and outer needles inject the ionic cross-linker. Since the inner and outer surface of the fibers are in contact with the cross-linker, the strength of the final fiber is higher relative to the method that has only inner crosslinking [136, 137].

## 7.2 *Sacrificial Method*

In the sacrificial method, one of the printing components is removed from the final structure. The sacrificial material acts as a supportive material that prevents the 3D structure from collapsing when the main material is printing. Once the cross-linking procedure is completed and the printed structure reaches a suitable mechanical strength, the supportive material is removed from the 3D structure. If cells are printed without hydrogel, cell-cell contact (fusion of printed aggregates) occurs before removal of the supporting material [138]. It is very important that the main structure be intact prior to removal of the supporting material. Thus far, various sacrificial materials have been introduced for tissue engineering applications. Physically reversible hydrogels, like thermos-responsive materials, appear to be suitable sacrificial materials and include Pluronic F127, which is mostly used in bioprinting. Pluronic F127 is a liquid at 4 °C, but forms a gel at 37 °C. We can print Pluronic F127 at 37 °C and remove it at 4 °C because of its physically reversible gelation mechanism [52, 56]. In addition, this technique can be employed to create micro-channels in microchip fabrication for microfluidic applications [139].

Carbohydrate glass is another sacrificial material that dissolves in culture medium after several minutes. After printing, the carbohydrate glass can be removed from the main structure by immersion in aqueous media where it forms a hollow vascular network [140]. Bertassoni et al. have mechanically removed a hydrogel-like agarose and used the hollow space as a channel for culture medium transportation under in vitro conditions [141, 142]. In a recent, important work, they used this technique to vascularize dental pulp tissue constructs. After the preparation of the root canal with endodontic files, a microchannel was created by a sacrificial agarose fiber via a 3D printing-inspired method. A cell-laden hydrogel was then located in the microchannel and photo-polymerized. After the polymerization of the hydrogel, the sacrificial fiber was removed to leave a hollow microchannel. Endothelial cells were seeded into the created microchannel to construct a pre-vascularized complete dental pulp tissue [82].

## 7.3 *Cell Spheroid-Based 3D Bioprinting*

The assembly of a cell spheroid into 3D tissues was introduced to overcome the challenges associated with scaffold-based constructs in tissue engineering. Cyfuse Biomedical developed a cell spheroid-based 3D bioprinting method, known as the Kenzan method. Cell spheroids are manipulated with a robotic system and placed into microneedle arrays. This method is independent of the hydrogels as bioink or supportive materials. Once cell spheroids fuse to each other, the entire structure detaches from the microneedle array. This technique has the ability to directly generate cellular tube-like structures [143, 144]. The potential of a cell spheroid for angiogenesis and dental pulp regeneration has been investigated. Dissanayaka et al. used DPSCs and human umbilical vein endothelial cells (HUVECs) to create 3D scaffold-free microtissue spheroids that mimicked the microenvironment of dental pulp cells. They used agarose 3D petri dishes to fabricate the spheroids that could be replaced by 3D bioprinting.

## 7.4 *Sprouting*

Creation of microvascular networks is one of the main issues in 3D printing techniques. These structures with some lithographic methods are achievable, though they cannot be used for bioprinting a scaffold. In this technique, a macro-vascular network is first printed and its cells are allowed to sprout toward each other and create a complex microvascular network. It is important to use angiogenesis factors to promote ECs to create this microvascular structure [145, 146].

## 7.5 *Direct Printing of Vessel-like Structures*

3D printing techniques provide the possibility for direct printing of a vessel-like structure. In this method, one of the previously mentioned methods may be utilized in combination to form this structure [147]. The addition of a roller to an extrusion base 3D printer makes it possible to print hollow structures with multi-level fluidic microchannels. This technique helps to directly create a vessel-like structure for feeding cells inside a 3D structure [148].

Of note, different 3D printing methods are utilized to overcome the challenges related to vascularization. These methods facilitate the transportation of nutrition, oxygen, and wastes within a 3D object. Although these methods are useful, they only create pre-vascular networks and cannot mimic the microvascular network of native tissue. Thus, the necessity of using biochemical cues cannot be eliminated and the use of angiogenesis factors is inevitable. The combination of different methods will give better outcomes.

# 8 Advances in 3D Printing for Dental Tissue Engineering

CAD/CAM and 3D printing have been applied in different fields of dentistry. Numerous attempts have been made with 3D printing to fabricate dental models, maxillofacial implants, and dental devices, such as crown and bridge restorations, and dentures [149, 150]. Other dental applications of CAD/CAM include prosthodontics, in addition to oral surgery applications such as endodontics, orthodontics, and dental bioengineering research (Fig. 9.1) [151].

3D printing has been used to fabricate proper scaffolds for dental tissue engineering. Tissue engineering is a multidisciplinary field of research that combines the principles of biology, materials science, and medicine. Advances in tissue engineering have sparked scientists' hopes for organ and tissue repair, and it offers a regenerative strategy for dental tissues. Typically, several types of tissues, such as cartilage, bone, muscle, tendons, cranial sutures, temporomandibular joints (TMJ), salivary glands, periodontium, and teeth, are involved in oral cavity and craniomaxillofacial injuries. The complexity of the tissues necessitates application of advanced scaffolds and medications, as well as strategies for regeneration of tissues and interfaces. Dental tissue regeneration is ideally focused on two purposes: regeneration of an entire tooth and regeneration of individual components such as dentin, enamel, cementum, pulp, alveolar bone, and PDLs [152, 153]. Tissue-engineered teeth should fulfill requirements of suitable physical and mechanical properties in order to withstand different deformational loadings and appropriate contacts with

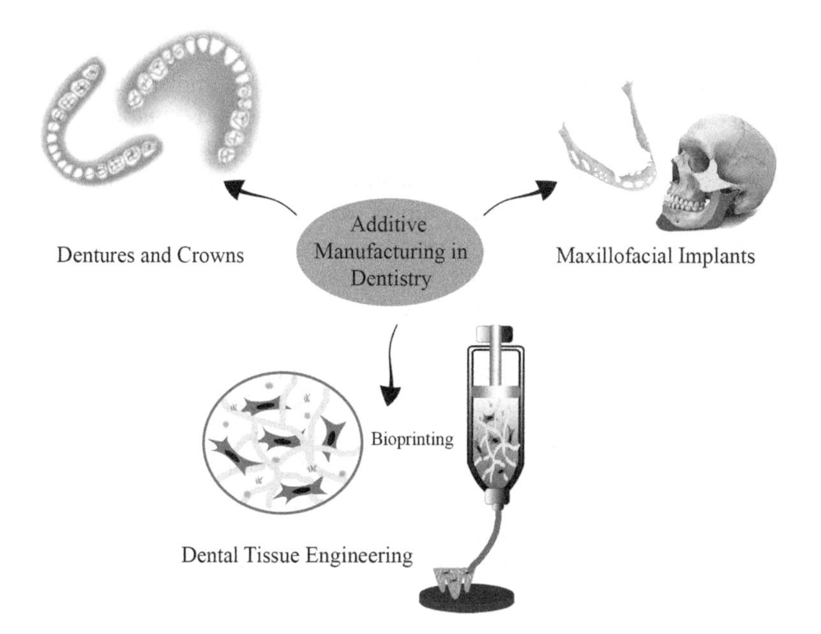


**Fig. 9.1** Various applications of additive manufacturing in dentistry

adjacent teeth. 3D printing plays an important role in design and mimicking the natural structures of the injured tissues. 3D-printed scaffolds have attracted considerable attention due to patient-specific designs, high structural complications, and comparatively rapid, fully automated construction that is cost-effective. Fabrication of dental articles with diverse requirements is also available by AM. Dentin-like scaffolds have been constructed by the combination of 3D printing and biomineralization [154]. The novel concept of four-dimensional (4D) printing of scaffolds for tissue engineering may soon be applied for tooth regeneration. Four-dimensional printing denotes 3D printing of shape memory materials. The printed object slowly converts into a shape after completion of printing and the fourth dimension is related to time [155].

There are a number of studies, particularly for additive manufacturing of periodontium and tooth tissue engineering. With the combination of 3D-printed periodontium scaffolds and native dentin pieces, complex tissues can be regenerated [156]. Pilpchuck et al. have succeeded in achieving an aligned collagenous tissue formation by using a 3D-printed scaffold combined with a micropatterned region in the preclinical setting [110].

3D-printed implants have been used in oral and maxillofacial sections. Patient-specific bones were prepared by CT. The results indicated incorporation of cells and GF would enhance the bone formation capability of the implanted scaffolds, due to induction of osteogenic activity [157]. Micro-CT was used in an attempt to fabricate a 3D-printed PCL patient-specific scaffold to treat a large periodontal osseous defect. The results showed complete restoration of the defective site 12 months after surgery [158]. Regarding the difficulties with traditional bone grafting materials, the 3D-printed implants are being considered as successful alternatives [159]. A long-term follow-up study in a clinical setting has revealed that 3D-printed titanium dental implants had an overall survival rate of 94.5% and an implant-crown success of 94.3% [75]. Restoration of the TMJ and involved bones was completely investigated by using 3D-printed scaffolds and techniques. Bioprinting has been used for engineering craniofacial tissues and investigations of diverse tissues such as bone, periodontal complex, cartilage, and pulp of the craniofacial region [160, 161]. Numerous studies evaluated different aspects of bioprinting such as image processing, bio-modelling, bioink, the bioprinting process, and bioreactors.

However, drawbacks related to these techniques include limited measuring circumstances due to existence of adjacent teeth, gingiva, and saliva, all of which cause difficulties in precise determination of the support margin [162]. This phenomenon may cause an internal gap in the final product that is the space between the prepared teeth and the prosthesis. Recent developments in CBCT and optical scan technology, in particular, have revolutionized and are profoundly changing many aspects of restorative and implant dentistry. X-ray micro-CT is a noninvasive imaging method for evaluation of internal structures of the products. It has been used for efficient assessment of this gap [163, 164]. Micro-CT is usually combined with AM for fabrication of endoprosthetics, surgical guides, anatomical models, and tissue engineering scaffolds. The patient micro-CT is used to design

AM processes [165]. In a research, micro-CT and 3D printing have been used for preparation of dual architecture scaffolds with adjustment of fiber orientation for PDL tissue engineering [166]. In another attempt, AM has also been used to fabricate surgical templates in complicated endodontic surgery. In a case report, a 3D-printed surgical template was used to perform endodontic microsurgery on a 57-year-old woman with symptomatic apical periodontitis. The customized surgical template was fabricated after CBCT imaging of the lesion site. Despite the time-consuming process of 3D printing, the surgical templates reduced the length of surgical process [167].

Investigations in the field of 3D printing are rapidly advancing to overcome current obstacles. Recently, traditional 3D printing has been replaced by organ printing along with advances in bioprinting, micro-well-mediated tissue formation, cell sheet engineering, and self-assembled hydrogels that utilize cell aggregates as a building block to construct the complete organ [168]. Organ printing is assisted by CAD/CAM with self-assembly of tissue spheroids. Organ printing is not a one-step method, as bioreactors and other technologies are also needed. Computer-assisted design and bio-imaging techniques must be developed in order to construct a detailed blueprint that reflects the complexity of an organ. Next, bioink and biopaper technologies are used to fabricate the bio-printer. Finally, maturation and monitoring are conducted in the bioreactors [169].

## 9 Summary

Customized implants and devices are a necessity in the dental industry. 3D printing can be considered as the only technology that provides this opportunity and thus can impact the dental industry in the near future. For example, fabrication of patient-specific crowns, removable prosthetic metal frameworks, and implants could possibly be created from digital data by dentists in their laboratories. In addition to customizations, advanced 3D printers would provide ease of manufacturing of any type of complicated geometry with versatile materials compared to conventional methods. 3D printings create highly detailed complex surface objects with minimal waste and cost-saving materials. Nevertheless, it is not accurate to assume that 3D printing does not have drawbacks. This technology currently costs a tremendous amount in terms of materials, equipment, and maintenance. High-resolution printing methods are needed for fabrication of small objects with marginal fit. 3D printing is indeed in its infancy, and further experiments are required to address and optimize the printing parameters to support accuracy of the 3D-printed structures. Finally, additional research in the clinical and preclinical settings is necessary to provide adequate evidence for successful 3D printing outcomes in humans.

## References


1. Harris, C. M., & Laughlin, R. (2013). Reconstruction of hard and soft tissue maxillofacial defects. *Atlas of the Oral and Maxillofacial Surgery Clinics of North America, 21*(1), 127–138.
2. Obregon, F., et al. (2015). Three-dimensional bioprinting for regenerative dentistry and craniofacial tissue engineering. *Journal of Dental Research, 94*(9 Suppl), 143S–152S.
3. Hacking, S. A., & Khademhosseini, A. (2009). Applications of microscale technologies for regenerative dentistry. *Journal of Dental Research, 88*(5), 409–421.
4. Pilipchuk, S. P., et al. (2015). Tissue engineering for bone regeneration and osseointegration in the oral cavity. *Dental Materials, 31*(4), 317–338.
5. Peck, M. T., Marnewick, J., & Stephen, L. (2011). Alveolar ridge preservation using leukocyte and platelet-rich fibrin: A report of a case. *Case Reports in Dentistry, 2011*, 345048.
6. Frame, M., & Leach, W. (2014). DIY 3D printing of custom orthopaedic implants: A proof of concept study. *Surgical Technology International, 24*, 314–317.
7. Susic, I., Travar, M., & Susic, M. (2017). The application of CAD/CAM technology in dentistry. *IOP Conference Series: Materials Science and Engineering, 200*(1), 012020.
8. Rubio-Palau, J., et al. (2016). Three-dimensional planning in craniomaxillofacial surgery. *Ann Maxillofac Surg, 6*(2), 281–286.
9. Al Jabbari, Y., et al. (2014). Metallurgical and interfacial characterization of PFM Co–Cr dental alloys fabricated via casting, milling or selective laser melting. *Dental Materials, 30*(4), e79–e88.
10. Reich, S., et al. (2005). Clinical fit of all-ceramic three-unit fixed partial dentures, generated with three different CAD/CAM systems. *European Journal of Oral Sciences, 113*(2), 174–179.
11. Anadioti, E., et al. (2014). 3D and 2D marginal fit of pressed and CAD/CAM lithium disilicate crowns made from digital and conventional impressions. *Journal of Prosthodontics, 23*(8), 610–617.
12. Gandolfi, M., et al. (2015). Calcium silicate/calcium phosphate biphasic cements for vital pulp therapy: Chemical-physical properties and human pulp cells response. *Clinical Oral Investigations, 19*(8), 2075–2089.
13. Gandolfi, M. G., et al. (2018). Polylactic acid-based porous scaffolds doped with calcium silicate and dicalcium phosphate dihydrate designed for biomedical application. *Materials Science and Engineering: C, 82*, 163–181.
14. Grayson, W. L., et al. (2010). Engineering anatomically shaped human bone grafts. *Proceedings of the National Academy of Sciences, 107*(8), 3299–3304.
15. Kietzmann, J., Pitt, L., & Berthon, P. (2015). Disruptions, decisions, and destinations: Enter the age of 3-D printing and additive manufacturing. *Business Horizons, 58*(2), 209–215.
16. Giordano, R. A., et al. (1997). Mechanical properties of dense polylactic acid structures fabricated by three dimensional printing. *Journal of Biomaterials Science, Polymer Edition, 8*(1), 63–75.
17. Kim, S. S., et al. (1998). Survival and function of hepatocytes on a novel three-dimensional synthetic biodegradable polymer scaffold with an intrinsic network of channels. *Annals of Surgery, 228*(1), 8.
18. Zein, I., et al. (2002). Fused deposition modeling of novel scaffold architectures for tissue engineering applications. *Biomaterials, 23*(4), 1169–1185.
19. Mironov, V., et al. (2003). Organ printing: Computer-aided jet-based 3D tissue engineering. *Trends in Biotechnology, 21*(4), 157–161.
20. Atala, A., & Yoo, J. J. (2015). *Essentials of 3D biofabrication and translation*. Boston: Academic Press.
21. Arcaute, K., Mann, B. K., & Wicker, R. B. (2006). Stereolithography of three-dimensional bioactive poly (ethylene glycol) constructs with encapsulated cells. *Annals of Biomedical Engineering, 34*(9), 1429–1441.

22. Dhariwala, B., Hunt, E., & Boland, T. (2004). Rapid prototyping of tissue-engineering constructs, using photopolymerizable hydrogels and stereolithography. *Tissue Engineering, 10*(9–10), 1316–1322.
23. Dehurtevent, M., et al. (2017). Stereolithography: A new method for processing dental ceramics by additive computer-aided manufacturing. *Dental Materials, 33*(5), 477–485.
24. Song, X., et al. (2015). Ceramic fabrication using Mask-Image-Projection-based Stereolithography integrated with tape-casting. *Journal of Manufacturing Processes, 20*, 456–464.
25. Fukuda, A., et al. (2011). Osteoinduction of porous Ti implants with a channel structure fabricated by selective laser melting. *Acta Biomaterialia, 7*(5), 2327–2336.
26. Matena, J., et al. (2015). SLM produced porous titanium implant improvements for enhanced vascularization and osteoblast seeding. *International Journal of Molecular Sciences, 16*(4), 7478–7492.
27. Du, Y., et al. (2017). Selective laser sintering scaffold with hierarchical architecture and gradient composition for osteochondral repair in rabbits. *Biomaterials, 137*, 37–48.
28. Mueller, A., et al. (2011). Missing facial parts computed by a morphable model and transferred directly to a polyamide laser-sintered prosthesis: An innovation study. *British Journal of Oral and Maxillofacial Surgery, 49*(8), e67–e71.
29. Badiru, A. B., Valencia, V. V., & Liu, D. (2017). *Additive manufacturing handbook: Product development for the defense industry*. Boca Raton, FL: CRC Press.
30. Xie, F., et al. (2013). Influence of pore characteristics on microstructure, mechanical properties and corrosion resistance of selective laser sintered porous Ti–Mo alloys for biomedical applications. *Electrochimica Acta, 105*, 121–129.
31. Harun, W., et al. (2017). A review of powder additive manufacturing processes for metallic biomaterials. *Powder Technology, 327*, 128–151.
32. Duan, B., et al. (2010). Three-dimensional nanocomposite scaffolds fabricated via selective laser sintering for bone tissue engineering. *Acta Biomaterialia, 6*(12), 4495–4505.
33. Wiria, F., et al. (2007). Poly-ε-caprolactone/hydroxyapatite for tissue engineering scaffold fabrication via selective laser sintering. *Acta Biomaterialia, 3*(1), 1–12.
34. Velu, R., & Singamneni, S. (2014). Selective laser sintering of polymer biocomposites based on polymethyl methacrylate. *Journal of Materials Research, 29*(17), 1883–1892.
35. Guillemot, F., et al. (2010). Laser-assisted cell printing: Principle, physical parameters versus cell fate and perspectives in tissue engineering. *Nanomedicine, 5*(3), 507–515.
36. Guillemot, F., et al. (2010). High-throughput laser printing of cells and biomaterials for tissue engineering. *Acta Biomaterialia, 6*(7), 2494–2500.
37. Guillotin, B., et al. (2010). Laser assisted bioprinting of engineered tissue with high cell density and microscale organization. *Biomaterials, 31*(28), 7250–7256.
38. Barron, J., et al. (2004). Biological laser printing: A novel technique for creating heterogeneous 3-dimensional cell patterns. *Biomedical Microdevices, 6*(2), 139–147.
39. Keriquel, V., et al. (2017). In situ printing of mesenchymal stromal cells, by laser-assisted bioprinting, for in vivo bone regeneration applications. *Scientific Reports, 7*(1), 1778.
40. Lin, H., et al. (2013). Application of visible light-based projection stereolithography for live cell-scaffold fabrication with designed architecture. *Biomaterials, 34*(2), 331–339.
41. Wang, Z., et al. (2015). A simple and high-resolution stereolithography-based 3D bioprinting system using visible light crosslinkable bioinks. *Biofabrication, 7*(4), 045009.
42. Seo, H., et al. (2017). Preparation of PEG materials for constructing complex structures by stereolithographic 3D printing. *RSC Advances, 7*(46), 28684–28688.
43. Sun, A. X., et al. (2015). Projection stereolithographic fabrication of human adipose stem cell-incorporated biodegradable scaffolds for cartilage tissue engineering. *Frontiers in Bioengineering and Biotechnology, 3*, 115.
44. Neiman, J. A. S., et al. (2015). Photopatterning of hydrogel scaffolds coupled to filter materials using stereolithography for perfused 3D culture of hepatocytes. *Biotechnology and Bioengineering, 112*(4), 777–787.

45. Kim, S. Y., et al. (2018). Precision and trueness of dental models manufactured with different 3-dimensional printing techniques. *American Journal of Orthodontics and Dentofacial Orthopedics, 153*(1), 144–153.
46. Muller, D., et al. (2011). Vascular guidance: Microstructural scaffold patterning for inductive neovascularization. *Stem Cells International, 2011*, 1.
47. Kao, C.-T., et al. (2015). Poly (dopamine) coating of 3D printed poly (lactic acid) scaffolds for bone tissue engineering. *Materials Science and Engineering: C, 56*, 165–173.
48. Lam, C. X., et al. (2009). Evaluation of polycaprolactone scaffold degradation for 6 months in vitro and in vivo. *Journal of Biomedical Materials Research Part A, 90*(3), 906–919.
49. Schantz, J.-T., et al. (2005). Osteogenic differentiation of mesenchymal progenitor cells in computer designed fibrin-polymer-ceramic scaffolds manufactured by fused deposition modeling. *Journal of Materials Science: Materials in Medicine, 16*(9), 807–819.
50. Teoh, S. H., et al. (2011). *Three-dimensional bioresorbable scaffolds for tissue engineering applications*. US Patent: US8071007B1. Assignee: Osteopore International Pte Ltd.
51. Srivas, P. K., et al. (2017). Osseointegration assessment of extrusion printed Ti6Al4V scaffold towards accelerated skeletal defect healing via tissue in-growth. *Bioprinting, 6*, 8–17.
52. Kang, H.-W., et al. (2016). A 3D bioprinting system to produce human-scale tissue constructs with structural integrity. *Nature Biotechnology, 34*(3), 312–319.
53. Bae, E.-B., et al. (2018). Efficacy of rhBMP-2 loaded PCL/β-TCP/bdECM scaffold fabricated by 3D printing technology on bone regeneration. *BioMed Research International, 2018*, 1.
54. Seyednejad, H., et al. (2012). In vivo biocompatibility and biodegradation of 3D-printed porous scaffolds based on a hydroxyl-functionalized poly (ε-caprolactone). *Biomaterials, 33*(17), 4309–4318.
55. Serra, T., Planell, J. A., & Navarro, M. (2013). High-resolution PLA-based composite scaffolds via 3-D printing technology. *Acta Biomaterialia, 9*(3), 5521–5530.
56. Kolesky, D. B., et al. (2014). 3D bioprinting of vascularized, heterogeneous cell-laden tissue constructs. *Advanced Materials, 26*(19), 3124–3130.
57. Shim, J.-H., et al. (2014). Efficacy of rhBMP-2 loaded PCL/PLGA/β-TCP guided bone regeneration membrane fabricated by 3D printing technology for reconstruction of calvaria defects in rabbit. *Biomedical Materials, 9*(6), 065006.
58. Visser, J., et al. (2013). Biofabrication of multi-material anatomically shaped tissue constructs. *Biofabrication, 5*(3), 035007.
59. Liu, F., et al. (2018). Structural evolution of PCL during melt extrusion 3D printing. *Macromolecular Materials and Engineering, 303*(2).
60. Donderwinkel, I., van Hest, J. C., & Cameron, N. R. (2017). Bio-inks for 3D bioprinting: Recent advances and future prospects. *Polymer Chemistry, 8*(31), 4451–4471.
61. Klebe, R. J. (1988). Cytoscribing: A method for micropositioning cells and the construction of two-and three-dimensional synthetic tissues. *Experimental Cell Research, 179*(2), 362–373.
62. Klebe, R. J., et al. (1994). Cytoscription: Computer controlled micropositioning of cell adhesion proteins and cells. *Methods in Cell Science, 16*(3), 189–192.
63. Ferris, C. J., et al. (2013). Bio-ink for on-demand printing of living cells. *Biomaterials Science, 1*(2), 224–230.
64. Saunders, R. E., Gough, J. E., & Derby, B. (2008). Delivery of human fibroblast cells by piezoelectric drop-on-demand inkjet printing. *Biomaterials, 29*(2), 193–203.
65. Zheng, Q., et al. (2011). Application of inkjet printing technique for biological material delivery and antimicrobial assays. *Analytical Biochemistry, 410*(2), 171–176.
66. Cui, X., et al. (2010). Cell damage evaluation of thermal inkjet printed Chinese hamster ovary cells. *Biotechnology and Bioengineering, 106*(6), 963–969.
67. Gao, G., et al. (2015). Improved properties of bone and cartilage tissue from 3D inkjet-bioprinted human mesenchymal stem cells by simultaneous deposition and photocrosslinking in PEG-GelMA. *Biotechnology Letters, 37*(11), 2349–2355.

68. Khalyfa, A., et al. (2007). Development of a new calcium phosphate powder-binder system for the 3D printing of patient specific implants. *Journal of Materials Science: Materials in Medicine, 18*(5), 909–916.
69. Saijo, H., et al. (2009). Maxillofacial reconstruction using custom-made artificial bones fabricated by inkjet printing technology. *Journal of Artificial Organs, 12*(3), 200–205.
70. Chia, H. N., & Wu, B. M. (2015). Recent advances in 3D printing of biomaterials. *Journal of Biological Engineering, 9*, 4.
71. Guvendiren, M., et al. (2016). Designing biomaterials for 3D printing. *ACS Biomaterials Science & Engineering, 2*(10), 1679–1693.
72. Ji, S., & Guvendiren, M. (2017). Recent advances in bioink design for 3D bioprinting of tissues and organs. *Frontiers in Bioengineering and Biotechnology, 5*, 23.
73. Sears, N. A., et al. (2016). A review of three-dimensional printing in tissue engineering. *Tissue Engineering. Part B, Reviews, 22*(4), 298–310.
74. Mondschein, R. J., et al. (2017). Polymer structure-property requirements for stereolithographic 3D printing of soft tissue engineering scaffolds. *Biomaterials, 140*, 170–188.
75. Murphy, S. V., & Atala, A. (2014). 3D bioprinting of tissues and organs. *Nature Biotechnology, 32*, 773.
76. Maleksaeedi, S., et al. (2014). Property enhancement of 3D-printed alumina ceramics using vacuum infiltration. *Journal of Materials Processing Technology, 214*(7), 1301–1306.
77. Sharma, S., et al. (2014). Biomaterials in tooth tissue engineering: A review. *Journal of Clinical and Diagnostic Research, 8*(1), 309–315.
78. Geong, C. G., & Atala, A. (2015). 3D printing and biofabrication for load baring tissue engineering. In L. E. Bertassoni & P. G. Coelho (Eds.), *Engineering mineralized and load bearing tissues*. Cham: Springer.
79. Entezari, A., et al. (2016). Fracture behaviors of ceramic tissue scaffolds for load bearing applications. *Scientific Reports, 6*, 28816.
80. Roohani-Esfahani, S. I., Newman, P., & Zreiqat, H. (2016). Design and fabrication of 3D printed scaffolds with a mechanical strength comparable to cortical bone to repair large bone defects. *Scientific Reports, 6*, 19468.
81. Kim, B. S., et al. (2017). Improvement of mechanical strength and osteogenic potential of calcium sulfate-based hydroxyapatite 3-dimensional printed scaffolds by epsilon-polycarbonate coating. *Journal of Biomaterials Science. Polymer Edition, 28*(13), 1256–1270.
82. Athirasala, A., et al. (2018). A dentin-derived hydrogel bioink for 3D bioprinting of cell laden scaffolds for regenerative dentistry. *Biofabrication, 10*(2), 024101.
83. Ahlfeld, T., et al. (2017). Design and fabrication of complex scaffolds for bone defect healing: Combined 3D plotting of a calcium phosphate cement and a growth factor-loaded hydrogel. *Annals of Biomedical Engineering, 45*(1), 224–236.
84. Roseti, L., et al. (2017). Scaffolds for bone tissue engineering: State of the art and new perspectives. *Materials Science & Engineering. C, Materials for Biological Applications, 78*, 1246–1262.
85. Gadre, K. S., et al. (2013). Incidence and pattern of cranio-maxillofacial injuries: A 22 year retrospective analysis of cases operated at major trauma hospitals/centres in Pune, India. *Journal of Oral and Maxillofacial Surgery, 12*(4), 372–378.
86. Ikada, Y. (2006). Challenges in tissue engineering. *Journal of the Royal Society Interface, 3*(10), 589–601.
87. Akter, F. (2016). Principles of tissue engineering, Chapter 2. In *Tissue engineering made easy* (pp. 3–16). London, United Kingdm: Academic Press.
88. Huang, X. F., & Chai, Y. (2012). Molecular regulatory mechanism of tooth root development. *International Journal of Oral Science, 4*(4), 177–181.
89. Mao, J. J., Giannobile, W. V., Helms, J. A., Hollister, S. J., Krebsbach, P. H., Longaker, M. T., & Shi, S. (2006). Craniofacial tissue engineering by stem cells. *Journal of Dental Research, 85*(11), 966–979.

90. Raj Rai, R. R., Khandeparker, R. V. S., Chidrawar, S. K., Khan, A. A., & Ganpat, M. S. (2015). Tissue engineering: Step ahead in maxillofacial reconstruction. *Journal of International Oral Health, 7*(9), 138–142.
91. Mina, M. (2015). Growth factors: Biochemical signals for tissue engineering, Chapter 7. In *Stem cell biology and tissue engineering in dental sciences*. Amsterdam, Netherlands: Elsevier/Academic Press.
92. Islam, A., et al. (2017). In vitro cultivation, characterization and osteogenic differentiation of stem cells from human exfoliated deciduous teeth on 3D printed polylactic acid scaffolds. *Iranian Red Crescent Medical Journal, 19*(8).
93. Saijo, H., et al. (2009). Maxillofacial reconstruction using custom-made artificial bones fabricated by inkjet printing technology. *Journal of Artificial Organs, 12*(3), 200–205.
94. Kim, J. Y., et al. (2010). Regeneration of dental-pulp-like tissue by chemotaxis-induced cell homing. *Tissue Engineering. Part A, 16*(10), 3023–3031.
95. Park, C. H., et al. (2010). Biomimetic hybrid scaffolds for engineering human tooth-ligament interfaces. *Biomaterials, 31*(23), 5945–5952.
96. Park, C. H., et al. (2012). Tissue engineering bone-ligament complexes using fiber-guiding scaffolds. *Biomaterials, 33*(1), 137–145.
97. Lee, C. H., et al. (2014). Three-dimensional printed multiphase scaffolds for regeneration of periodontium complex. *Tissue Engineering. Part A, 20*(7–8), 1342–1351.
98. Yildirim, S., et al. (2011). Tooth regeneration: A revolution in stomatology and evolution in regenerative medicine. *International Journal of Oral Science, 3*(3), 107–116.
99. Roshene, R. (2015). Regeneration of dental pulp- A review. *Journal of Pharmaceutical Sciences and Research, 7*(10), 858–860.
100. Sloan, A. J., & Smith, A. J. (2007). Stem cells and the dental pulp: Potential roles in dentine regeneration and repair. *Oral Diseases, 13*(2), 151–157.
101. Kim, K., et al. (2010). Anatomically shaped tooth and periodontal regeneration by cell homing. *Journal of Dental Research, 89*(8), 842–847.
102. Gaviria, L., Pearson, J. J., Montelongo, S. A., Guda, T., & Ong, J. L. (2017). Three-dimensional printing for craniomaxillofacial regeneration. *Journal of the Korean Association of Oral and Maxillofacial Surgeons, 43*, 288–298.
103. Park, C. H., et al. (2014). Spatiotemporally controlled microchannels of periodontal mimic scaffolds. *Journal of Dental Research, 93*(12), 1304–1312.
104. Dangaria, S. J., et al. (2011). Apatite microtopographies instruct signaling tapestries for progenitor-driven new attachment of teeth. *Tissue Engineering. Part A, 17*(3–4), 279–290.
105. Guo, W., et al. (2009). The use of dentin matrix scaffold and dental follicle cells for dentin regeneration. *Biomaterials, 30*(35), 6708–6723.
106. Nanci, A. (2012). *Ten cate's oral histology* (8th ed.). Quebec: Mosby.
107. Monteiro, N., & Yelick, P. C. (2017). Advances and perspectives in tooth tissue engineering. *Journal of Tissue Engineering and Regenerative Medicine, 11*(9), 2443–2461.
108. Zhu, W., et al. (2016). 3D printing of functional biomaterials for tissue engineering. *Current Opinion in Biotechnology, 40*, 103–112.
109. Zhang, X., & Zhang, Y. (2015). Tissue engineering applications of three-dimensional bioprinting. *Cell Biochemistry and Biophysics, 72*(3), 777–782.
110. Mandrycky, C., et al. (2016). 3D bioprinting for engineering complex tissues. *Biotechnology Advances, 34*(4), 422–434.
111. Bajaj, P., et al. (2014). 3D biofabrication strategies for tissue engineering and regenerative medicine. *Annual Review of Biomedical Engineering, 16*, 247–276.
112. Benning, L., et al. (2018). Assessment of hydrogels for bioprinting of endothelial cells. *Journal of Biomedical Materials Research. Part A, 106*(4), 935–947.
113. Salehi, S., et al. (2016). Dentin matrix components extracted with phosphoric acid enhance cell proliferation and mineralization. *Dental Materials, 32*(3), 334–342.
114. Batouli, S., Miura, M., Brahim, J., Tsutsui, T. W., Fisher, L. W., Gronthos, S., Robey, P. G., & Shi, S. (2003). Comparison of stem-cell-mediated osteogenesis and dentinogenesis. *Journal of Dental Research, 82*(12), 976–981.

115. Hosseini, S., et al. (2018). Regenerative medicine applications of mesenchymal stem cells. *Advances in Experimental Medicine and Biology, 1089*, 115–141.
116. Khorsand, A., et al. (2013). Autologous dental pulp stem cells in regeneration of defect created in canine periodontal tissue. *The Journal of Oral Implantology, 39*(4), 433–443.
117. Hilkens, P., et al. (2017). The angiogenic potential of DPSCs and SCAPs in an in vivo model of dental pulp regeneration. *Stem Cells International, 2017*, 2582080.
118. Barinov, S. M., et al. (2015). 3D printing of ceramic scaffolds for engineering of bone tissue. *Inorganic Materials: Applied Research, 6*(4), 316–322.
119. Vakhrushev, I., Vdovin, A., Fedotov, A. Y., Mironov, A. V., Komlev, V. S., & Yarygin, K. N. (2014). Bone tissue engineering utilizing mesenchymal stem cells from deciduous teeth and 3D printed ceramic scaffolds. *Journal of Tissue Engineering and Regenerative Medicine, 8*, 207–518.
120. Cho, H., et al. (2016). Periodontal ligament stem/progenitor cells with protein-releasing scaffolds for cementum formation and integration on dentin surface. *Connective Tissue Research, 57*(6), 488–495.
121. Arthur, A., Shi, S., & Gronthos, S. (2015). Dental Pulp Stem Cells, Chapter 21. In *Stem cell biology and tissue engineering in dental sciences*. Amsterdam, Netherlands: Elsevier/Academic Press.
122. Eslaminejad, M. B., Bordbar, S., & Nazarian, H. (2013). Odontogenic differentiation of dental pulp-derived stem cells on tricalcium phosphate scaffolds. *Journal of Dental Sciences, 8*(3), 306–313.
123. Chen, F.-M., & Shi, S. (2014). Periodontal tissue engineering, Chapter 72. In *Principles of tissue engineering (4th ed.)*. Amsterdam, Netherlands: Elsevier/Academic Press.
124. Leyendecker Junior, A., et al. (2018). The use of human dental pulp stem cells for in vivo bone tissue engineering: A systematic review. *Journal of Tissue Engineering, 9*, 2041731417752766.
125. Eslaminejad, M. B., et al. (2010). In vitro growth and characterization of stem cells from human dental pulp of deciduous versus permanent teeth. *Journal of Dentistry (Tehran), 7*(4), 185–195.
126. Miura, M., et al. (2003). SHED: Stem cells from human exfoliated deciduous teeth. *Proceedings of the National Academy of Sciences of the United States of America, 100*(10), 5807–5812.
127. Wada, N., et al. (2015). Immunomodulatory properties of PDLSC and relevance to periodontal regeneration. *Current Oral Health Reports, 2*(4), 245–251.
128. Ma, Y., et al. (2015). Bioprinting 3D cell-laden hydrogel microarray for screening human periodontal ligament stem cell response to extracellular matrix. *Biofabrication, 7*(4), 044105.
129. Seo, B.-M., et al. (2004). Investigation of multipotent postnatal stem cells from human periodontal ligament. *The Lancet, 364*(9429), 149–155.
130. Bakopoulou, A., et al. (2011). Comparative analysis of in vitro osteo/odontogenic differentiation potential of human dental pulp stem cells (DPSCs) and stem cells from the apical papilla (SCAP). *Archives of Oral Biology, 56*(7), 709–721.
131. Gao, Q., et al. (2015). Coaxial nozzle-assisted 3D bioprinting with built-in microchannels for nutrients delivery. *Biomaterials, 61*, 203–215.
132. Gao, G., et al. (2017). Tissue engineered bio-blood-vessels constructed using a tissue-specific bioink and 3D coaxial cell printing technique: A novel therapy for ischemic disease. *Advanced Functional Materials, 27*(33).
133. Liu, W., et al. (2018). Coaxial extrusion bioprinting of 3D microfibrous constructs with cell-favorable gelatin methacryloyl microenvironments. *Biofabrication, 10*(2), 024102.
134. Luo, Y., Lode, A., & Gelinsky, M. (2013). Direct plotting of three-dimensional hollow fiber scaffolds based on concentrated alginate pastes for tissue engineering. *Advanced Healthcare Materials, 2*(6), 777–783.
135. Dai, X., et al. (2017). Coaxial 3D bioprinting of self-assembled multicellular heterogeneous tumor fibers. *Scientific Reports, 7*(1), 1457.

136. Jia, W., et al. (2016). Direct 3D bioprinting of perfusable vascular constructs using a blend bioink. *Biomaterials, 106*, 58–68.
137. Lee, K. H., et al. (2009). Synthesis of cell-laden alginate hollow fibers using microfluidic chips and microvascularized tissue-engineering applications. *Small, 5*(11), 1264–1268.
138. Norotte, C., et al. (2009). Scaffold-free vascular tissue engineering using bioprinting. *Biomaterials, 30*(30), 5910–5917.
139. Hur, D., et al. (2018). 3D micropatterned all-flexible microfluidic platform for microwave-assisted flow organic synthesis. *ChemPlusChem, 83*(1), 42–46.
140. Miller, J. S., et al. (2012). Rapid casting of patterned vascular networks for perfusable engineered three-dimensional tissues. *Nature Materials, 11*(9), 768.
141. Bertassoni, L. E., et al. (2014). Direct-write bioprinting of cell-laden methacrylated gelatin hydrogels. *Biofabrication, 6*(2), 024105.
142. Bertassoni, L. E., et al. (2014). Hydrogel bioprinted microchannel networks for vascularization of tissue engineering constructs. *Lab on a Chip, 14*(13), 2202–2211.
143. Moldovan, N. I., Hibino, N., & Nakayama, K. (2017). Principles of the Kenzan method for robotic cell spheroid-based three-dimensional bioprinting. *Tissue Engineering Part B: Reviews, 23*, 237.
144. Kizawa, H., et al. (2017). Scaffold-free 3D bio-printed human liver tissue stably maintains metabolic functions useful for drug discovery. *Biochemistry and Biophysics Reports, 10*, 186–191.
145. Lee, V. K., et al. (2014). Creating perfused functional vascular channels using 3D bio-printing technology. *Biomaterials, 35*(28), 8092–8102.
146. Lee, V. K., et al. (2014). Generation of multi-scale vascular network system within 3D hydrogel using 3D bio-printing technology. *Cellular and Molecular Bioengineering, 7*(3), 460–472.
147. Tabriz, A. G., et al. (2015). Three-dimensional bioprinting of complex cell laden alginate hydrogel structures. *Biofabrication, 7*(4), 045012.
148. Gao, Q., et al. (2017). 3D bioprinting of vessel-like structures with multilevel fluidic channels. *ACS Biomaterials Science & Engineering, 3*(3), 399–408.
149. das Neves, F. D., et al. (2014). Micrometric precision of prosthetic dental crowns obtained by optical scanning and computer-aided designing/computer-aided manufacturing system. *Journal of Biomedical Optics, 19*(8), 088003.
150. McLaughlin, J. B., Ramos, V., Jr., & Dickinson, D. P. (2019). Comparison of fit of dentures fabricated by traditional techniques versus CAD/CAM technology. *Journal of Prosthodontics, 28*(4), 428–435.
151. Shah, P., & Chong, B. S. (2018). 3D imaging, 3D printing and 3D virtual planning in endodontics. *Clinical Oral Investigations, 22*(2), 641–654.
152. Hosseini, S., Jahangir, S., & Eslaminejad, M. B. (2017). Tooth tissue engineering, Chapter 27. In *Biomaterials for oral and dental tissue engineering* (pp. 467–501). Kidlington, United Kingdom: Elsevier/Woodhead Publishing.
153. Bakhtiar, H., et al. (2017). Histologic tissue response to furcation perforation repair using mineral trioxide aggregate or dental pulp stem cells loaded onto treated dentin matrix or tricalcium phosphate. *Clinical Oral Investigations, 21*(5), 1579–1588.
154. Wu, Y., et al. (2016). Fabrication of dentin-like scaffolds through combined 3D printing and bio-mineralisation. *Cogent Engineering, 3*(1), 1222777.
155. Hendrikson, W. J., et al. (2017). Towards 4D printed scaffolds for tissue engineering: Exploiting 3D shape memory polymers to deliver time-controlled stimulus on cultured cells. *Biofabrication, 9*(3), 031001.
156. Gaviria, L., et al. (2017). Three-dimensional printing for craniomaxillofacial regeneration. *Journal of the Korean Association of Oral and Maxillofacial Surgeons, 43*(5), 288–298.
157. Hikita, A., et al. (2017). Bone regenerative medicine in Oral and maxillofacial region using a three-dimensional printer<sup/>. *Tissue Engineering. Part A, 23*(11–12), 515–521.

158. Rasperini, G., et al. (2015). 3D-printed bioresorbable scaffold for periodontal repair. *Journal of Dental Research, 94*(9 Suppl), 153S–157S.
159. Asa'ad, F., et al. (2016). 3D-printed scaffolds and biomaterials: Review of alveolar bone augmentation and periodontal regeneration applications. *International Journal of Dentistry, 2016*, 1239842.
160. Yu, H. Y., Ma, D. D., & Wu, B. L. (2017). Gelatin/alginate hydrogel scaffolds prepared by 3D bioprinting promotes cell adhesion and proliferation of human dental pulp cells in vitro. *Nan Fang Yi Ke Da Xue Xue Bao, 37*(5), 668–672.
161. Zhai, X., et al. (2018). 3D-bioprinted osteoblast-laden nanocomposite hydrogel constructs with induced microenvironments promote cell viability, differentiation, and osteogenesis both in vitro and in vivo. *Advanced Science (Weinheim), 5*(3), 1700550.
162. Carneiro, T. A. P. N., et al. (2018). Micro-CT analysis of in-office computer-aided designed/computer-aided manufactured dental restorations. *Computer Methods in Biomechanics and Biomedical Engineering, 6*(1), 68–73.
163. Tapie, L., et al. (2016). Adaptation measurement of CAD/CAM dental crowns with X-ray micro-CT: Metrological chain standardization and 3D gap size distribution. *Advances in Materials Science and Engineering, 2016*, 13.
164. Rungruanganunt, P., Kelly, J. R., & Adams, D. J. (2010). Two imaging techniques for 3D quantification of pre-cementation space for CAD/CAM crowns. *Journal of Dentistry, 38*(12), 995–1000.
165. Thompson, A., et al. (2017). X-ray computed tomography and additive manufacturing in medicine: A review. *International Journal of Metrology and Quality Engineering, 8*, 17.
166. Park, C. H., et al. (2014). Image-based, fiber guiding scaffolds: A platform for regenerating tissue interfaces. *Tissue Engineering. Part C, Methods, 20*(7), 533–542.
167. Ahn, S. Y., et al. (2018). Computer-aided design/computer-aided manufacturing-guided endodontic surgery: Guided osteotomy and apex localization in a mandibular molar with a thick buccal bone plate. *Journal of Endodontia, 44*(4), 665–670.
168. Achilli, T. M., Meyer, J., & Morgan, J. R. (2012). Advances in the formation, use and understanding of multi-cellular spheroids. *Expert Opinion on Biological Therapy, 12*(10), 1347–1360.
169. Rezende, R. A., et al. (2013). An organ biofabrication line: Enabling technology for organ printing. Part I: From biocad to biofabricators of spheroids. *Biomedical Engineering, 47*(3), 116–120.

# Chapter 10
# Clinical Functions of Regenerative Dentistry and Tissue Engineering in Treatment of Oral and Maxillofacial Soft Tissues

**Mohammad Reza Jamalpour, Farshid Vahdatinia, Jessica Vargas, and Lobat Tayebi**

## 1 Introduction

Over the last 20 years, soft tissue regeneration in the craniomaxillofacial region has attracted attention due to developments in allotransplantation techniques. The most common method employed for the restoration of different tissues (such as skin, muscle, the oral mucosa, and neurovascular bundles) includes the utilization of local, regional, and distal flaps to fill and cover the area of the defect. However, there are several limitations associated with this technique including the lack of function, poor esthetics in the recipient site and donor site morbidity, immune responses, tissue interactions, and difficulties with capillary formation. Combining allotransplantation and tissue-engineered construct techniques has recently made significant improvements in multilayer soft tissue restoration [1–4], which will be discussed in this chapter. More specifically, this chapter will discuss tissue engineering approaches in wound dressing as well as regeneration of the oral mucosa, skeletal muscle, osteochondral and nervous tissues of oral and maxillofacial region.

M. R. Jamalpour
Dental Implants Research Center, Dental School, Hamadan University of Medical Sciences, Hamadan, Iran

F. Vahdatinia
Dental Implants Research Center, Hamadan University of Medical Sciences, Hamadan, Iran

J. Vargas · L. Tayebi (✉)
Marquette University School of Dentistry, Milwaukee, WI, USA
e-mail: lobat.tayebi@marquette.edu



L. Tayebi (ed.), *Applications of Biomedical Engineering in Dentistry*,
https://doi.org/10.1007/978-3-030-21583-5_10

## 2 Regeneration of the Oral Mucosa

The mucous membrane is comprised of stratified squamous epithelium that lines the inner surfaces of the digestive, urinary, and respiratory systems. The inner surface of the oral cavity is lined with a mucous membrane of ectodermal origin, comprised of both keratinized and non-keratinized tissues.

The oral mucosa extends to the vermillion border of the lips anteriorly and posteriorly to the pharyngeal mucosa. There are differences, both physically and histologically, within respective areas of the oral mucosa. The dorsal surface of the tongue is comprised of epithelial papillae, whereas the ventral surface of the tongue, floor of mouth, lips, cheeks, and vestibules are composed of non-keratinized epithelium. Keratinized epithelium can be found in both the gingiva and hard palate [5].

The usage of autologous cells has replaced split-thickness skin grafts (STSG) due to recent improvements in mucosal layer restoration. STSG can be used for restoration of soft tissue defects throughout the body, including the oral cavity. The unique anatomy of skin and its composition of uneven keratinization, however, are not in accordance with the natural function of the oral mucosa [1, 6].

In order to regenerate the oral mucosa, the scaffolds used must be permeable to fibroblasts without inducing shrinkage and also biodegradable in a controlled manner. The following are some examples of said scaffold: artificial extracellular matrix (ECM), protein-based scaffolds, synthetic materials, and hybrid scaffolds of both natural and synthetic matrices [7].

One of the most common strategies of classifying tissue-engineered oral mucosa (TEOM) substitutes is according to the type and number of reconstructed layers: mono-layered structures, such as epithelial sheets or dermal substitutes (made of allogeneic and acellular dermis or artificial matrices), and bilayered products, which combine epithelial sheets or dermal substitutes as a full-thickness graft (Fig. 10.1, Table 10.1) [8].

Ex Vivo-Produced Oral Mucosa Equivalent (EVPOME) is a type of dermal scaffold, like AlloDerm, that keratinized autogenous epithelial cells can be cultured in it. This dermal scaffold can be used for the restoration of oral cavity defects that occur from trauma, tumors, and periodontal diseases. The utilization of autologous cells with the scaffolds can prevent immunosuppression or rejection [1, 2, 9].

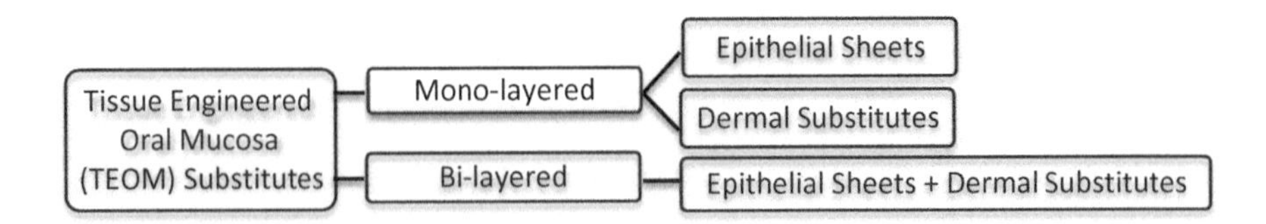


**Fig. 10.1** Tissue-engineered oral mucosa (TEOM) substitutes diagram. The concept is from reference [8]

**Table 10.1** Applications and important points of tissue-engineered oral mucosa (TEOM) substitutes. The concept is from reference [8]

| Tissue-engineered oral mucosa (TEOM) substitutes | Applications | Important considerations |
|---|---|---|
| Epithelial sheets (cultured epidermal autografts) | Regeneration of large intraoral mucosa defects and full-thickness wounds | Time-consuming cell growth<br>Variable rates of engraftment<br>Difficult handling due to the thin, fragile cell layers<br>Severe wound contraction<br>Blister formation when exposed to minor shearing forces<br>Limited capacity to reconstruct epithelial structures |
| Dermal substitutes | Full-thickness wounds | Prevention of wound contraction and scarring<br>Providing physical support and a functional tissue with mechanical stability<br>Lack of epithelial-mesenchymal interactions |
| Epithelial sheets + dermal substitutes | Regeneration of intraoral mucosa defects and full-thickness wounds | The most common approach for producing a TEOM<br>Low immunogenicity in comparison to allogeneic fibroblasts and keratinocytes |

EVPOME has been successfully employed in the restoration of keratinized gingiva and also in creating a musculocutaneous flap to restore the opening function of the oral cavity in animal models (Fig. 10.2) [2, 10].

Other biodegradable scaffolds, such as polylactide meshes, tendon collagen-glycosaminoglycan constructs, and collagen membranes, are used in restoration of autologous oral mucosa. Vicryl mesh is a type of absorbable construct that is applied in the area of mucosal regeneration, and due to its mesh-like structure, its potential for fibroblast migration and growth is not as successful when compared with collagen-based scaffolds [11].

## 3 Wound Dressing

A wound can be described as a type of anatomical-functional disruption within a tissue. Various factors will determine the extent and characteristics of a skin wound. These factors include genetic disorders, severe trauma (resulting from cold temperatures, radiation, electricity, etc.), chronic diseases (such as diabetes and cardiovascular disease), and surgical procedures [12, 13].

Skin injuries are categorized into three types, based on the amount of layers involved: superficial, partial thickness, and full thickness. In superficial skin

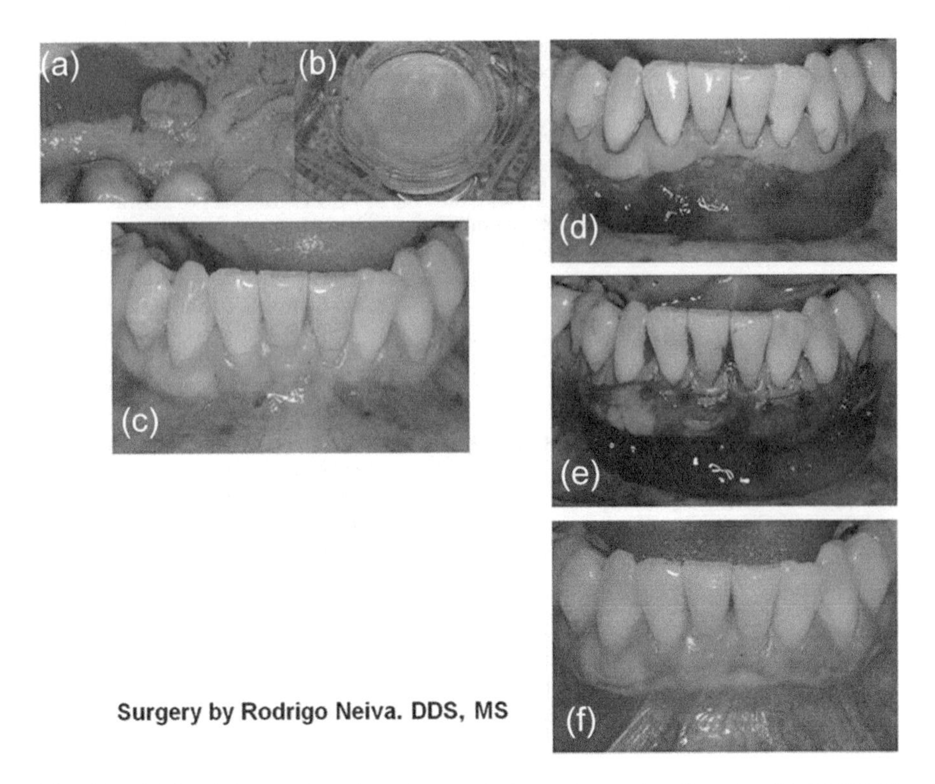


**Fig. 10.2** (**a**) Punch biopsy from the palate to obtain autologous keratinocytes. (**b**) EVPOME construct. (**c**) Preoperative view. (**d**) Recipient site of EVPOME graft. (**e**) EVPOME secured in position with multiple sutures, (**f**) 6-month postoperative follow-up with a significant gain of keratinized gingiva [8]. (Surgery by Rodrigo Neiva. DDS, MS)

wounds, only the epidermal layers are damaged. Partial-thickness wounds pertain to those that have a greater depth of injury, which involves blood vessels, hair follicles, and sweat glands. The full-thickness type of skin injury is the most profound wound type that penetrates not only the epidermal and dermal layers but also the subcutaneous region [14].

Another method of classification of wounds is based on the healing time. Acute wounds completely heal in 12 weeks with minimal scar tissue formation. Chronic wounds have a prolonged healing time and may present as recurring. Arrested wounds are those that exist in an inflammatory condition. They possess an extensive amount of cytotoxic enzymes, oxygen-free radicals, inflammatory mediators, and matrix metalloproteases released by polymorphonuclear leukocytes [15–17].

Wound healing process and the manipulation of different methods to condense healing time have been studied extensively throughout history. Skin injury healing is dependent on the functions of various cells, such as fibroblasts, leukocytes, monocytes, macrophages, endothelial cells, and epidermal cells. Other factors, such as cytokines and growth factors, also affect healing. The wound healing process occurs in four stages: hemostasis, inflammation, proliferation, and remodeling.

In the hemostasis stage, platelet aggregation and clot formation occur. During the inflammatory stage, macrophages and neutrophils stimulate an immune attack in the site of the wound. Then, granulation tissue formation, matrix deposition, angiogenesis, and reepithelialization occur during the proliferation stage. The remodeling stage includes collagen deposition and formation, increased tensile strength, and wound contraction.

Skin wounds need dressings in order to prevent infection and to maintain proper functioning of the tissue. An ideal wound dressing is biocompatible, protects against trauma, prevents bacterial infections, absorbs secretions properly, applies sufficient pressure to prevent edema, and minimizes the amount of necrotic tissue. In addition, sufficient water vapor transmission rate (WVTR) is another important characteristic of an adequate wound dressing, which helps to improve healing and avoid adherence of the wound to the dressing during dressing change [18–21].

Natural, synthetic, and combined origin wound dressings are produced in the form of films, sponges, hydrogels, and hydrocolloids. Due to their high biocompatibility, biodegradability, and similarity to extracellular matrix (ECM), natural compounds prevent immunological responses; thus they are a much more superior candidate for wound dressing compared to synthetic composites [17, 22].

Cellulose, chitosan, chitin, pullulan, starch, and β-glucan are examples of homopolysaccharide natural polymers that are used in wound dressings. The combination of biopolymers with metals, antibiotics, proteins, and other substances of bioactive origin can promote the wound healing process. Among various biopolymers, bacterial cellulose and chitosan have been investigated the most.

Bacterial cellulose is low cost and possesses high water absorption capacity, high tensile strength, flexibility, and great biocompatibility. These characteristics make it a suitable polymer to be used in wound dressing. Disadvantages of bacterial cellulose include lack of antibacterial activity and not being able to improve wound healing. Chitosan does possess antibacterial activity in addition to positive effects on fibroblast proliferation, collagen deposition, and hyaluronic acid synthesis. Due to the benefits of chitosan that make up for the disadvantages of bacterial cellulose, it has been combined with bacterial cellulose and applied in wound dressings [17, 23, 24].

As mentioned previously, synthetic polymers are another type of polymers used in wound dressings that are classified into two groups: passive and active. Similar to gauze and tulle, passive synthetic polymer dressings are non-occlusive. They are used only to cover the wound and help with the regeneration of the covered area. Active synthetic polymer dressings, such as foams, hydrogels, or hydrocolloids, are occlusive or semiocclusive; they provide protection against bacterial infection (Fig. 10.3) [25, 26].

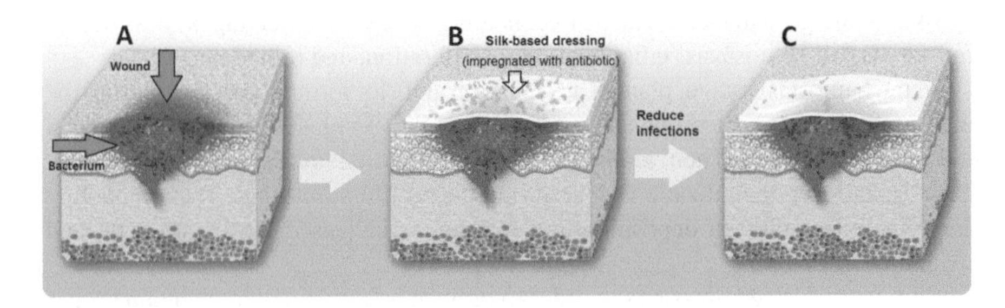


**Fig. 10.3** Interactive synthetic polymer dressings with antibacterial agents (a silk wound dressing) [27]

## 4 Skeletal Muscle Regeneration

Muscles have different important functions, such as locomotion, prehension, mastication, ocular movement, and metabolism regulation. Skeletal muscles consist of approximately 40% of the human body. They are exposed to various injuries, such as mechanical trauma, heat stress, neurological damage, myotoxic agents, ischemia, and other pathogenic conditions.

Mechanical trauma is the most common type of muscular injury. Due to the disruption in the integrity of the myofiber plasma membrane and basal lamina, it causes the entry of extracellular calcium into skeletal muscle cells. This leads to muscle protein disruption and necrosis [28–31].

In addition to traumatic injury, surgical and aesthetic treatments are also made essential due to conditions such as myopathies, radical and extensive tumor resections, and muscle denervation. Thus, 4.5 million surgical reconstructive procedures, due to traumatic injury, car accidents, cancer, ablation, and cosmetics, are performed annually [32, 33].

The natural regeneration process in muscular tissue occurs through swelling and hematoma formation resulting from inflammation and muscle degeneration activation. Following early muscle degeneration, muscle regeneration begins immediately by muscle stem cells.

The injured myofibers have healing potential, thus the contraction and metabolism functions of natural cells can be restored again. The muscle-resident progenitors and innate and adaptive immune cells play important roles in skeletal muscle regeneration.

Muscle stem cells (satellite cells or SCs), which are located in membrane-enclosed niches, between the sarcolemma (plasma membrane) and the basal lamina surrounding muscular fibers, are the main cells in muscle tissue regeneration [31, 34–37].

The cells involved in skeletal muscle cell restoration are regarded as non-satellite stem cells and include mesenchymal stem/stromal cells (MSCs), PW1+/PAX7− interstitial cells (PICs), fibro/adipogenic progenitors/mesenchymal stem cells (FAPs/MSCs), muscle side population (SP) cells, and muscle resident pericytes.

Following skeletal muscle injuries, activated SCs release chemotactic and pro-inflammatory cytokine factors. This leads to aggregation of monocytes and macrophages in the damaged area. Subsequently, activated SCs proliferate and migrate to the wound site and cause myoblasts production [37–40]. The adaptive method of skeletal muscle regeneration is performed using tissue engineering techniques, both in vivo and in vitro. In vitro, the skeletal muscle structure is prepared under the experimental conditions and then transplanted in the desired region. In vivo, the scaffolds are placed in the defect area and the injured tissue will be treated and regenerated in its place [41, 42]. The first in vitro skeletal muscle tissue culture was performed 100 years ago by Lewis and was created from a chicken embryo leg. Research in this area has continued in order to build large-scale muscle tissues with functional properties. In the early 1990s, Strohman et al. grew the first three-dimensional (3D) muscle construct of myoblasts on a membrane in vitro.

Recently, in the study by Lam et al., it has been reported that aligned myotubes formed by the realignment of myoblasts on a micropatternal polydimethylsiloxane (PDMS) layer can transfer PDMS into a fibrin gel. This led to the formation of a 3D freestanding construct that provides higher muscle fiber content and greater capacity for force production.

Nowadays, technological advancements have made the production of synthetics possible. Patterning techniques, as well as skeletal muscle tissue engineering (SMTE), have improved considerably. As a result, the following methods are the main techniques of in vitro muscle cell culturing [43]:

- Cell alignment by topography
- Cell alignment by surface patterning
- Cell alignment by mechanical stimulation
- Cell alignment by magnetic or electrical fields

In vivo, scaffolds consisting of synthetic polymers, such as polyglycolic acid (PGA) and poly-ε-caprolactone (PCL), are utilized, along with materials like decellularized ECM. Additionally, natural polymers are utilized, like alginate, collagen, and fibrin [44–49].

# 5 Nerve Regeneration

Peripheral nerve injury treatment is a challenging therapy. Injuries of the oral and maxillofacial region are the most common requiring this kind of treatment. Contusion and compression injuries are common peripheral nerve injuries in the oral and maxillofacial region that frequently occur due to maxillofacial trauma, orthognathic surgery, dentoalveolar surgery, surgical removal of the impacted lower third molars, implant placement, and injection of local anesthesia [50].

After serious peripheral nerve injury and axon disruption, the terminal part of a damaged nerve enters a destruction process, termed Wallerian degeneration. In Wallerian degeneration, the destruction of the damaged terminal part of the nerve creates adequate conditions necessary for axon and nerve regeneration [51–54]. At the same time, Schwann cells that are located in the terminal part of injured nerves differentiate into their non-myelinated phenotype and proliferate. Then, through the mechanisms of phagocytosis and macrophage aggregation in the damaged region, they clean the cellular debris and myelin resulting from Wallerian degeneration.

Subsequently, the Schwann cells align along their basement membrane in a tubular form, called bands of Büngner. Then, the regenerating axons are guided through this tubular canal into their target organ [55, 56].

In most cases, there is a need for surgical intervention to create and conduct proper contact between the two separated neural parts by autologous nerve transplant or an engineered scaffold [57].

The most common method utilized in damaged nerve regeneration, when there is a gap between the separated parts in the nerve, is creating a contact between the injured parts with an autologous donor nerve. However, with this technique, the donor nerve is somewhat injured and a secondary scar is created at the surgery site.

In the past, autologous biological tubular structures, such as arteries, veins, inside-out vein conduits, skeletal muscle, and decalcified bone channels, were applied in the reconstruction of the injured terminal part of a nerve. Although cadaveric nerve allografts and xenografts are being used frequently, the results of autografts are much more preferable [58–60].

## 5.1 Tissue Engineering and Peripheral Nerve Regeneration

In recent years, the use of artificial nerve conduits based on tissue engineering techniques has received considerable attention in regard to the reconstruction of the peripheral nerve system (PNS) and central nerve system (CNS). Compared with autografts, artificial nerve conduits have several advantages, including the avoidance of a secondary surgery and scarring. In comparison to allografts and xenografts, composition and structure modifications are able to take place with artificial nerve conduits. In addition, they allow for a decreased rate of graft rejection (Fig. 10.4) [61, 62].

Nerve guides are tubular biomaterials that support the injured nerves and promote the regeneration along the lumen via regenerating nerve factors. The most common polymers utilized in nerve guides include polyglycolic acid (PGA), polylactide-co-glycolide, polylactide-co-caprolactone (PLCL), poly(2-hydroxyethyl methacrylate) or (PHEMA), and polyurethane (Fig. 10.5).

Another new method employed in the repair and regeneration in nervous system diseases (e.g., Parkinson's, Alzheimer's) is creating a 3D cell culture that simulates the function and growth of PNS cells. The main characteristics of 3D cell culture models are monitoring and evaluating possibilities of cell activity and accurate observation of the results under the controlled experimental condition.

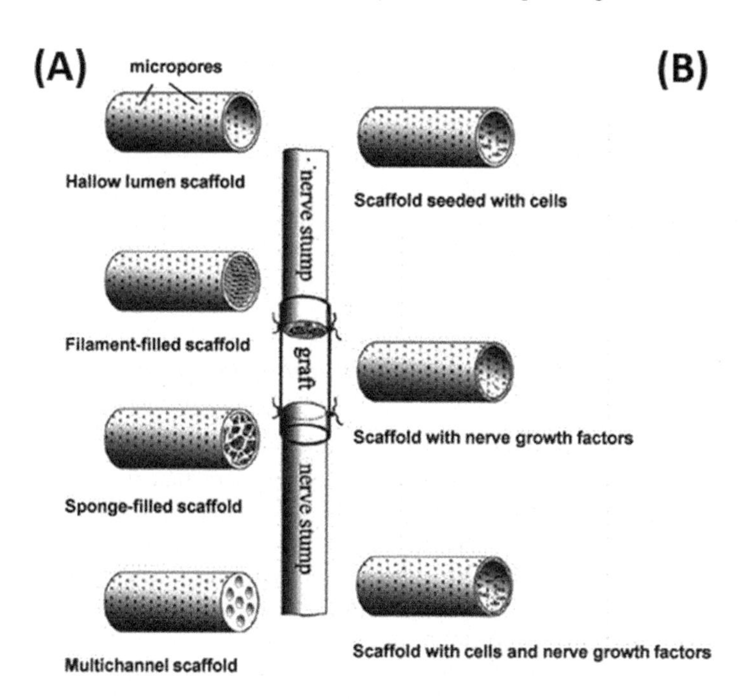


**Fig. 10.4** Schematic configurations of nerve scaffolds (**a**) and various compositions of tissue-engineered nerve grafts (**b**) [63]

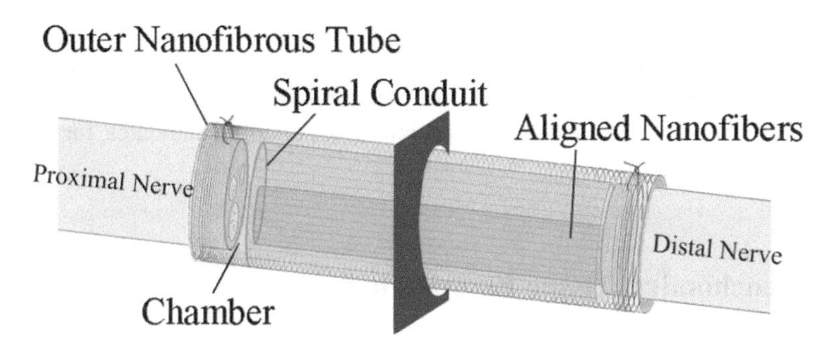


**Fig. 10.5** Tissue-engineered spiral nerve guidance conduit schematic [64]

A proper 3D cell culture should provide the opportunity to regenerate the native ECM and promote cell migration, proliferation, and differentiation. Regeneration of the native ECM depends on four major elements. These elements include collagen and related molecules as structural parts (e.g., types I, II, III, IV, and V), non-collagenous glycoproteins (e.g., laminin, fibronectin, entactin, and vitronectin.), glycosaminoglycans (e.g., hyaluronic acid, dermatan, chondroitin, keratan, heparan), and proteoglycans (e.g., chondroitin sulfate, heparin sulfate) [65, 66]. The other essential element in 3D cell culture is a polymeric scaffold that provides mechanical support to maintain the cell connection and growth in a three-dimensional space.

The polymers applied in the scaffold structures can be classified into two major categories: natural and synthetic. Collagen, hyaluronic acid (HA), silk, etc. are examples of natural polymers. Polyethylene glycol (PEG), poly-lactic-co-glycolic acid (PLGA), and poly-e-caprolactone (PCL) are the samples of synthetic polymers used in scaffold structures [57, 67].

### 5.2 *Role of Stem Cells in Regeneration of Peripheral Nerves*

Application of stem cells is a new method used in the regeneration and treatment of neural tissue injuries. Stem cells have the ability to differentiate into Schwann cells and affect the peripheral nerve regeneration by promoting myelinogenesis in healing axons through secretion of neurotrophic factor (e.g., nerve growth factor (NGF), brain-derived growth factor (BDNF), glial cell-derived neurotrophic factor (GDNF), NT-3 and NT-4/5), extracellular matrix formation, and moderation of the immune response. The mechanisms, however, are not known yet.

These cells, in the form of stem cells or Schwann-like differentiated cells in a cell-conditioned medium, possess the potential to be transplanted into patients. The stem cells can be transferred by synthetic or local injections. Also, it is possible to culture them on biological scaffolds (such as conduits or neural grafts without cells) and, subsequently, transplant them into the injured area [57, 68, 69].

In order to be applied in clinical experiments, the ideal stem cells should be easily extracted, expanded, and proliferated in a cell culture properly, survive in the host body, and show no tumorigenicity. Regarding these features, the adipose, cutaneous, hair follicle, and placental stem cells are suitable candidates for clinical applications [70, 71].

## 6 Osteochondral Tissue Engineering

Osteochondral defect healing is a challenging issue in clinical medicine due to the low efficiency of cartilaginous tissue to regenerate and heal. Osteochondral defects or damages can occur in any joint and affect the cartilaginous structure, the underlying subchondral bone, or the interstitial tissues. Osteoarthritis, in addition to articular cartilage and subchondral bone tissue degeneration and loss, is a notable cause of cartilage and osteochondral defects. There are some drawbacks to methods utilizing autografts and allografts to treat osteochondral defects. Nowadays, techniques based on tissue engineering and biodegradable scaffolds, with or without cells and growth factors, are alternative methods.

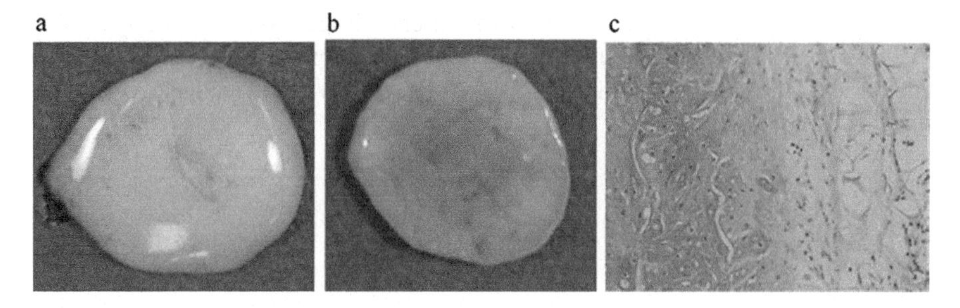


**Fig. 10.6** Gross appearance of cartilage layer (**a**) and subchondral bone layer (**b**) of osteochondral implant and safranin O/fast green staining of the implant (**c**) [76]

The major challenge in osteochondral tissue engineering is designing a structure with both satisfying physicochemical and biological properties to regenerate and replace the bone and cartilaginous tissues simultaneously. The advanced tissue-engineered grafts, such as monophasic, biphasic, triphasic, and gradient configurations, have received attention in regard to the repair and regeneration of complex structures like osteochondral tissue. The designed grafts should simulate the cartilage and bone layer formation with an interdigitating transitional zone (i.e., bone-cartilage interface) (Fig. 10.6) [72–75].

In tissue and organ regeneration, porous scaffolds play a major role in maintaining a temporary support for growth and controlled function of seeded cells. Therefore, various biodegradable polymers and calcium phosphate can be applied with bioactive factors to control stem cell differentiation. In addition, the 3D structure of porous scaffolds is an important factor in both cell adhesion and spatial distribution [76].

Different materials and compounds are utilized to maintain interactions and formation of ECM during osteochondral regeneration. Therefore, bilayered scaffold designs with restorative capacity for both cartilage and subchondral bone are regarded as the most common technique in comparison to scaffolds composed of only cartilage or bone [77, 78].

The composition and biomaterials utilized in osteochondral regeneration should be able to simulate the extracellular matrix (ECM) and the complex function of the cells. In other words, because of the essential role of biomaterials in natural cell proliferation and growth, critical consideration must be taken when choosing their physical and chemical properties.

From a chemical perspective, natural polymers (e.g., collagen, gelatin, and chitosan) provide sufficient biocompatibility and interaction with cell receptors, as well as minimize the risk of producing metabolized degradation products. However, synthetic materials have higher feasibility to control their composition and greater stability and reproducibility [79–81]. Some physical properties of structures used in osteochondral tissue engineering include the ability to tolerate stress in the site and the ability to support cell integration maintenance. The microstructure of the scaffold is important in the success of both chondrogenesis and osteogenesis. A porosity less than 300 μm improves cell growth and promotes the formation of capillaries. The interconnectivity (>100 μm) of scaffolds makes adequate cell colonization possible [82–86].

## 7 Conclusion

In light of the findings of the aforementioned studies on tissue engineering capabilities and 3D printing technology for the reconstruction of soft tissue in the oral and maxillofacial region, it can be concluded that the use of natural structures with autogenic cells is more efficient. However, the role of synthetic polymers in improving mechanical properties and controlling the biodegradability of scaffolds can also be helpful. Given the strength and manufacturing control of synthetic materials, and the biocompatibility and low immunogenicity of natural materials, combined synthetic and natural polymer scaffolds seem to possess the best properties. In spite of the myriad of studies conducted in this area during the recent years, further animal and human studies are required in order to optimize clinical features and achieve reliable therapeutic outcomes.

## References

1. Shah, G., & Costello, B. J. (2017). Soft tissue regeneration incorporating 3-dimensional biomimetic scaffolds. *Oral and Maxillofacial Surgery Clinics of North America, 29*(1), 9–18.
2. Kim, R. Y., Fasi, A. C., & Feinberg, S. E. (2014). Soft tissue engineering in craniomaxillofacial surgery. *Ann Maxillofac Surg, 4*(1), 4–8.
3. Costello, B. J., et al. (2010). Regenerative medicine for craniomaxillofacial surgery. *Oral and Maxillofacial Surgery Clinics of North America, 22*(1), 33–42.
4. Susarla, S. M., Swanson, E., & Gordon, C. R. (2011). Craniomaxillofacial reconstruction using allotransplantation and tissue engineering: Challenges, opportunities, and potential synergy. *Annals of Plastic Surgery, 67*(6), 655–661.
5. Evans, E. W. (2017). Treating scars on the oral mucosa. *Facial Plastic Surgery Clinics of North America, 25*(1), 89–97.
6. Izumi, K., Song, J., & Feinberg, S. E. (2004). Development of a tissue-engineered human oral mucosa: From the bench to the bed side. *Cells, Tissues, Organs, 176*(1–3), 134–152.
7. Scheller, E., Krebsbach, P., & Kohn, D. (2009). Tissue engineering: State of the art in oral rehabilitation. *Journal of Oral Rehabilitation, 36*(5), 368–389.
8. Izumi, K., Kato, H., & Feinberg, S. E. (2015). Tissue engineered oral mucosa. In *Stem cell biology and tissue engineering in dental sciences* (pp. 721–731). Elsevier.
9. Kato, H., et al. (2015). Fabrication of large size ex vivo-produced oral mucosal equivalents for clinical application. *Tissue Engineering. Part C, Methods, 21*(9), 872–880.
10. Izumi, K., Neiva, R. F., & Feinberg, S. E. (2013). Intraoral grafting of tissue-engineered human oral mucosa. *The International Journal of Oral & Maxillofacial Implants, 28*(5), e295–e303.
11. Kriegebaum, U., et al. (2012). Tissue engineering of human oral mucosa on different scaffolds: In vitro experiments as a basis for clinical applications. *Oral Surgery, Oral Medicine, Oral Pathology, Oral Radiology, 114*(5 Suppl), S190–S198.

12. Velnar, T., Bailey, T., & Smrkolj, V. (2009). The wound healing process: An overview of the cellular and molecular mechanisms. *Journal of International Medical Research, 37*(5), 1528–1542.
13. Girard, D., et al. (2017). Biotechnological management of skin burn injuries: Challenges and perspectives in wound healing and sensory recovery. *Tissue Engineering Part B: Reviews, 23*(1), 59–82.
14. Boateng, J., & Catanzano, O. (2015). Advanced therapeutic dressings for effective wound healing—A review. *Journal of Pharmaceutical Sciences, 104*(11), 3653–3680.
15. Parani, M., et al. (2016). Engineered nanomaterials for infection control and healing acute and chronic wounds. *ACS Applied Materials & Interfaces, 8*(16), 10049–10069.
16. Wong, S. Y., Manikam, R., & Muniandy, S. (2015). Prevalence and antibiotic susceptibility of bacteria from acute and chronic wounds in Malaysian subjects. *The Journal of Infection in Developing Countries, 9*(09), 936–944.
17. Naseri-Nosar, M., & Ziora, Z. M. (2018). Wound dressings from naturally-occurring polymers: A review on homopolysaccharide-based composites. *Carbohydrate Polymers, 189*, 379.
18. Merei, J. M. (2004). Pediatric clean surgical wounds: Is dressing necessary? *Journal of Pediatric Surgery, 39*(12), 1871–1873.
19. Mirzania, H. and S. Abbasifard, The effect of dressing in surgical wound complications. 2006.
20. Archana, D., Dutta, J., & Dutta, P. (2013). Evaluation of chitosan nano dressing for wound healing: Characterization, in vitro and in vivo studies. *International Journal of Biological Macromolecules, 57*, 193–203.
21. Farzamfar, S., et al. (2017). Taurine-loaded poly (ε-caprolactone)/gelatin electrospun mat as a potential wound dressing material: In vitro and in vivo evaluation. *Journal of Bioactive and Compatible Polymers*, 0883911517737103.
22. Mano, J., et al. (2007). Natural origin biodegradable systems in tissue engineering and regenerative medicine: Present status and some moving trends. *Journal of the Royal Society Interface, 4*(17), 999–1030.
23. Sulaeva, I., et al. (2015). Bacterial cellulose as a material for wound treatment: Properties and modifications. A review. *Biotechnology Advances, 33*(8), 1547–1571.
24. Paul, W., & Sharma, C. P. (2004). Chitosan and alginate wound dressings: A short review. *Biomaterials and Artificial Organs, 18*(1), 18–23.
25. Dhivya, S., Padma, V. V., & Santhini, E. (2015). Wound dressings–a review. *Biomedicine, 5*(4), 22.
26. Mir, M., et al. (2018). Synthetic polymeric biomaterials for wound healing: A review. *Progress in Biomaterials, 7*, 1–21.
27. Farokhi, M., et al. (2018). Overview of silk fibroin use in wound dressings. *Trends in Biotechnology, 36*, 907.
28. Schmalbruch, H., & Lewis, D. (2000). Dynamics of nuclei of muscle fibers and connective tissue cells in normal and denervated rat muscles. *Muscle & Nerve: Official Journal of the American Association of Electrodiagnostic Medicine, 23*(4), 617–626.
29. Huard, J., Li, Y., & Fu, F. H. (2002). Muscle injuries and repair: Current trends in research. *JBJS, 84*(5), 822–832.
30. Järvinen, T. A., et al. (2000). Muscle strain injuries. *Current Opinion in Rheumatology, 12*(2), 155–161.
31. Yang, W., & Hu, P. (2018). Skeletal muscle regeneration is modulated by inflammation. *Journal of Orthopaedic Translation, 13*, 25.
32. Klumpp, D., et al. (2010). Engineering skeletal muscle tissue–new perspectives in vitro and in vivo. *Journal of Cellular and Molecular Medicine, 14*(11), 2622–2629.
33. Grasman, J. M., et al. (2015). Biomimetic scaffolds for regeneration of volumetric muscle loss in skeletal muscle injuries. *Acta Biomaterialia, 25*, 2–15.
34. Mauro, A. (1961). Satellite cell of skeletal muscle fibers. *The Journal of Biophysical and Biochemical Cytology, 9*(2), 493.

35. Chang, N. C., & Rudnicki, M. A. (2014). Satellite cells: the architects of skeletal muscle. *Current Topics in Developmental Biology 107*, 161–181.
36. Madaro, L., & Bouché, M. (2014). From innate to adaptive immune response in muscular dystrophies and skeletal muscle regeneration: The role of lymphocytes. *BioMed Research International, 2014*, **1**.
37. Judson, R. N., Zhang, R. H., & Rossi, F. (2013). Tissue-resident mesenchymal stem/progenitor cells in skeletal muscle: Collaborators or saboteurs? *The FEBS Journal, 280*(17), 4100–4108.
38. Joe, A. W., et al. (2010). Muscle injury activates resident fibro/adipogenic progenitors that facilitate myogenesis. *Nature Cell Biology, 12*(2), 153.
39. Uezumi, A., et al. (2011). Fibrosis and adipogenesis originate from a common mesenchymal progenitor in skeletal muscle. *Journal of Cell Science, 124*(21), 3654–3664.
40. Klimczak, A., Kozlowska, U., & Kurpisz, M. (2018). Muscle stem/progenitor cells and mesenchymal stem cells of bone marrow origin for skeletal muscle regeneration in muscular dystrophies. *Archivum Immunologiae et Therapiae Experimentalis 66*(5), 341–354.
41. Stern-Straeter, J., et al. (2007). Advances in skeletal muscle tissue engineering. *In Vivo, 21*(3), 435–444.
42. Koning, M., et al. (2009). Current opportunities and challenges in skeletal muscle tissue engineering. *Journal of Tissue Engineering and Regenerative Medicine, 3*(6), 407–415.
43. Ostrovidov, S., et al. (2014). Skeletal muscle tissue engineering: Methods to form skeletal myotubes and their applications. *Tissue Engineering Part B: Reviews, 20*(5), 403–436.
44. Saxena, A. K., et al. (1999). Skeletal muscle tissue engineering using isolated myoblasts on synthetic biodegradable polymers: Preliminary studies. *Tissue Engineering, 5*(6), 525–531.
45. Sicari, B. M., et al. (2014). An acellular biologic scaffold promotes skeletal muscle formation in mice and humans with volumetric muscle loss. *Science Translational Medicine, 6*(234), 234ra58–234ra58.
46. Page, R. L., et al. (2011). Restoration of skeletal muscle defects with adult human cells delivered on fibrin microthreads. *Tissue Engineering Part A, 17*(21–22), 2629–2640.
47. Borselli, C., et al. (2010). Functional muscle regeneration with combined delivery of angiogenesis and myogenesis factors. *Proceedings of the National Academy of Sciences, 107*(8), 3287–3292.
48. San Choi, J., et al. (2008). The influence of electrospun aligned poly (ε-caprolactone)/collagen nanofiber meshes on the formation of self-aligned skeletal muscle myotubes. *Biomaterials, 29*(19), 2899–2906.
49. Kroehne, V., et al. (2008). Use of a novel collagen matrix with oriented pore structure for muscle cell differentiation in cell culture and in grafts. *Journal of Cellular and Molecular Medicine, 12*(5a), 1640–1648.
50. Bayram, B., et al. (2018). Effects of platelet-rich fibrin membrane on sciatic nerve regeneration. *Journal of Craniofacial Surgery, 29*(3), e239–e243.
51. Noble, J., et al. (1998). Analysis of upper and lower extremity peripheral nerve injuries in a population of patients with multiple injuries. *Journal of Trauma and Acute Care Surgery, 45*(1), 116–122.
52. Dubový, P. (2011). Wallerian degeneration and peripheral nerve conditions for both axonal regeneration and neuropathic pain induction. *Annals of Anatomy-Anatomischer Anzeiger, 193*(4), 267–275.
53. Gaudet, A. D., Popovich, P. G., & Ramer, M. S. (2011). Wallerian degeneration: Gaining perspective on inflammatory events after peripheral nerve injury. *Journal of Neuroinflammation, 8*(1), 110.
54. Ghayour, M. B., Abdolmaleki, A., & Fereidoni, M. (2015). *Use of stem cells in the regeneration of peripheral nerve injuries: An overview* (Vol. 3, p. 84).
55. Hall, S. (2001). Nerve repair: a neurobiologist's view. *Journal of hand surgery, 26*(2), 129–136.
56. Ide, C. (1996). Peripheral nerve regeneration. *Neuroscience Research, 25*(2), 101–121.
57. Ayala-Caminero, R., et al. (2017). Polymeric scaffolds for three-dimensional culture of nerve cells: A model of peripheral nerve regeneration. *MRS Communications, 7*(3), 391–415.

58. Siemionow, M., & Sonmez, E. (2007). Nerve allograft transplantation: A review. *Journal of Reconstructive Microsurgery, 23*(08), 511–520.
59. Chung, J.-R., et al. (2017). Effects of nerve cells and adhesion molecules on nerve conduit for peripheral nerve regeneration. *Journal of dental anesthesia and pain medicine, 17*(3), 191–198.
60. Pfister, B. J., et al. (2011). Biomedical engineering strategies for peripheral nerve repair: Surgical applications, state of the art, and future challenges. *Critical Reviews™ in Biomedical Engineering, 39*(2), 81.
61. Colen, K. L., Choi, M., & Chiu, D. T. (2009). Nerve grafts and conduits. *Plastic and Reconstructive Surgery, 124*(6S), e386–e394.
62. Hadlock, T., et al. (1998). A tissue-engineered conduit for peripheral nerve repair. *Archives of Otolaryngology–Head & Neck Surgery, 124*(10), 1081–1086.
63. Gu X., Ding F., Yang Y., Liu J., So K. F., & Xu X. M. (2015). Tissue engineering in peripheral nerve regeneration. In So K. F., & Xu X. M. (Eds). *Neural Regeneration* (pp. 73–99), Oxford: Academic Press.
64. Chang, W., et al. (2018). Tissue-engineered spiral nerve guidance conduit for peripheral nerve regeneration. *Acta Biomaterialia, 73*, 302.
65. Rutka, J. T., et al. (1988). The extracellular matrix of the central and peripheral nervous systems: Structure and function. *Journal of Neurosurgery, 69*(2), 155–170.
66. Carbonetto, S. (1984). The extracellular matrix of the nervous system. *Trends in Neurosciences, 7*(10), 382–387.
67. Painter, P. C., & Coleman, M. M. (2008). *Essentials of polymer science and engineering*. DEStech Publications, Lancaster.
68. Gu, X., Ding, F., & Williams, D. F. (2014). Neural tissue engineering options for peripheral nerve regeneration. *Biomaterials, 35*(24), 6143–6156.
69. di Summa, P. G., et al. (2010). Adipose-derived stem cells enhance peripheral nerve regeneration. *Journal of Plastic, Reconstructive & Aesthetic Surgery, 63*(9), 1544–1552.
70. Azizi, S. A., et al. (1998). Engraftment and migration of human bone marrow stromal cells implanted in the brains of albino rats—Similarities to astrocyte grafts. *Proceedings of the National Academy of Sciences, 95*(7), 3908–3913.
71. Tavassoli, A., et al. (2010). In vitro experimental study of interactions between blastema tissue and three-dimensional matrix derived from bovine cancellous bone and articular cartilage. *Journal of cell and tissue, 1*(1), 53–62.
72. Spencer, V., et al. (2018). Osteochondral tissue engineering: Translational research and turning research into products. *Advances in Experimental Medicine and Biology, 1058*, 373–390.
73. Giannini, S., et al. (2013). One-step repair in talar osteochondral lesions: 4-year clinical results and t2-mapping capability in outcome prediction. *The American Journal of Sports Medicine, 41*(3), 511–518.
74. Ribeiro, V. P., et al. (2018). Silk fibroin-based hydrogels and scaffolds for osteochondral repair and regeneration. *Advances in Experimental Medicine and Biology, 1058*, 305–325.
75. Nukavarapu, S. P., & Dorcemus, D. L. (2013). Osteochondral tissue engineering: Current strategies and challenges. *Biotechnology Advances, 31*(5), 706–721.
76. Chen, G., & Kawazoe, N. (2018). *Porous scaffolds for regeneration of cartilage, bone and Osteochondral tissue.*. Advances in experimental medicine and biology (Vol. 1058, pp. 171–191).
77. Dormer, N. H., Berkland, C. J., & Detamore, M. S. (2010). Emerging techniques in stratified designs and continuous gradients for tissue engineering of interfaces. *Annals of Biomedical Engineering, 38*(6), 2121–2141.
78. Swieszkowski, W., et al. (2007). Repair and regeneration of osteochondral defects in the articular joints. *Biomolecular Engineering, 24*(5), 489–495.
79. Canadas, R. F., Pina S., Marques A. P., et al (2016). Cartilage and bone regeneration—how close are we to bedside? In: *Transl. Regen. Med. to Clin*, (pp. 89–106). Elsevier, Amsterdam.

80. Lutolf, M., & Hubbell, J. (2005). Synthetic biomaterials as instructive extracellular microenvironments for morphogenesis in tissue engineering. *Nature Biotechnology, 23*(1), 47.
81. Nair, L. S., & Laurencin, C. T. (2005). Polymers as biomaterials for tissue engineering and controlled drug delivery. In *Tissue engineering I* (pp. 47–90). Springer, Berlin, Heidelberg.
82. Benders, K. E., et al. (2013). Extracellular matrix scaffolds for cartilage and bone regeneration. *Trends in Biotechnology, 31*(3), 169–176.
83. Oliveira, J. T., & Reis, R. (2011). Polysaccharide-based materials for cartilage tissue engineering applications. *Journal of Tissue Engineering and Regenerative Medicine, 5*(6), 421–436.
84. Ge, Z., Jin, Z., & Cao, T. (2008). Manufacture of degradable polymeric scaffolds for bone regeneration. *Biomedical Materials, 3*(2), 022001.
85. Karageorgiou, V., & Kaplan, D. (2005). Porosity of 3D biomaterial scaffolds and osteogenesis. *Biomaterials, 26*(27), 5474–5491.
86. Habibovic, P., et al. (2005). 3D microenvironment as essential element for osteoinduction by biomaterials. *Biomaterials, 26*(17), 3565–3575.

# Chapter 11
# Challenges in the Rehabilitation Handling of Large and Localized Oral and Maxillofacial Defects

**Arash Khojasteh and Sepanta Hosseinpour**

## 1 Introduction

Bone defects in the oral and maxillofacial region are caused mainly by trauma, various pathology and their surgical treatment, and congenital situations that have functional, esthetic, and psychological effects on patients. These defects remain a major health problem that commonly challenges oral and maxillofacial surgeons, scientists, and healthcare systems. Clinician scientists have been studying and applying various materials and methods to retrieve function and esthetic appearance. In this regard, the size of bony defects and possible radiotherapy in that specific region are the main restricting factors in order to achieve a successful bone reconstruction [1, 2]. The current chapter provides information regarding challenges in reconstruction of large and localized bone defects in oral and craniofacial sites.

A. Khojasteh (✉)
Department of Tissue Engineering and Applied Cell Sciences, School of Advanced Technologies in Medicine, Shahid Beheshti University of Medical Sciences, Tehran, Iran

Department of Oral and Maxillofacial Surgery, Dental School, Shahid Beheshti University of Medical Sciences, Tehran, Iran
e-mail: arashkhojasteh@sbmu.ac.ir

S. Hosseinpour
Department of Tissue Engineering and Applied Cell Sciences, School of Advanced Technologies in Medicine, Shahid Beheshti University of Medical Sciences, Tehran, Iran

School of Dentistry, The University of Queensland, Brisbane, Australia



L. Tayebi (ed.), *Applications of Biomedical Engineering in Dentistry*,
https://doi.org/10.1007/978-3-030-21583-5_11

# 2 Bone Defects' Classifications in Oral and Maxillofacial Region

## 2.1 Large Bone Defects

The success of bone regenerating process is closely correlated with the defect size, its location in oral and maxillofacial region, and patient's health status and age [3]. Studies in animal models lead to the determination of a "critical-sized" defect (CSD) as a bony defect that cannot totally heal without additional intervention, like bone regenerative approaches, within the lifetime of the animal model or the time period of the scientific survey [3]. The diameter or size of a CSD depends on the species and is altered by anatomical site [4, 5]. For instance, in mice, the size of a CSD in the cranium is 4 mm [6], in rabbits is 15 mm [7], in rats is 8 mm [8], and in sheep is 20 mm [9] in diameter. However, due to thousands of considerations in human studies, the exact CSD for various anatomical regions is still unknown [10]. Hren and Milijavec reported that spontaneous >90% bone healing occurred even in 30–50-mm-diameter mandibular defects after 12 months. The "6 cm rule" for defining a large bone defect has been accepted by many authors—for reconstructing bone defects larger than 6 cm, the best approach is to apply vascularized bone grafts (VBG). Although this rule may be helpful for classifying some oral and maxillofacial bone defects, determining the critical size for classifying bone defect is closely related to its anatomic location. For instance, cranial bony defects commonly categorized into small-sized (less than 25 $cm^2$), the medium-sized (25–200 $cm^2$), and the large-sized (greater than 200 $cm^2$) [11].

Another important aspect for classification of bone defects in oral and maxillofacial region is the effect on the adjacent anatomical structures. For example, maxillary defects have been classified by Brown and Shaw [12] into five different classes (Fig. 11.1). Class I shows the least defect area and class IV shows the largest affected area based on vertical dimension. If the defect includes orbital region in addition to

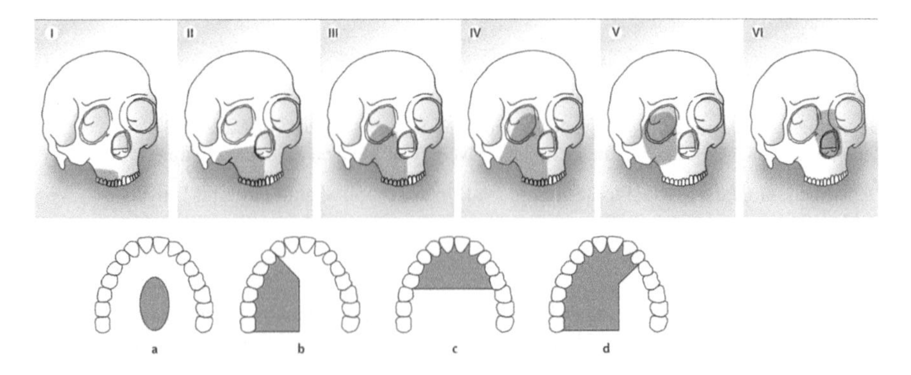


**Fig. 11.1** Various categories of maxillectomy and midface bony defects. Pink areas show the defect parts. (Reuse with permission) [12]

maxillary bone, it will be considered as class V. Class VI defects consist of only nasomaxillary region without involvement of alveolar or palatal bones (Fig. 11.1).

Moreover, Brown et al. proposed one of the most comprehensive and appropriate classification systems [13]. They have reviewed existing evidence regarding mandibular defects classification and proposed a diagrammatic categorization which is depicted in Fig. 11.2.

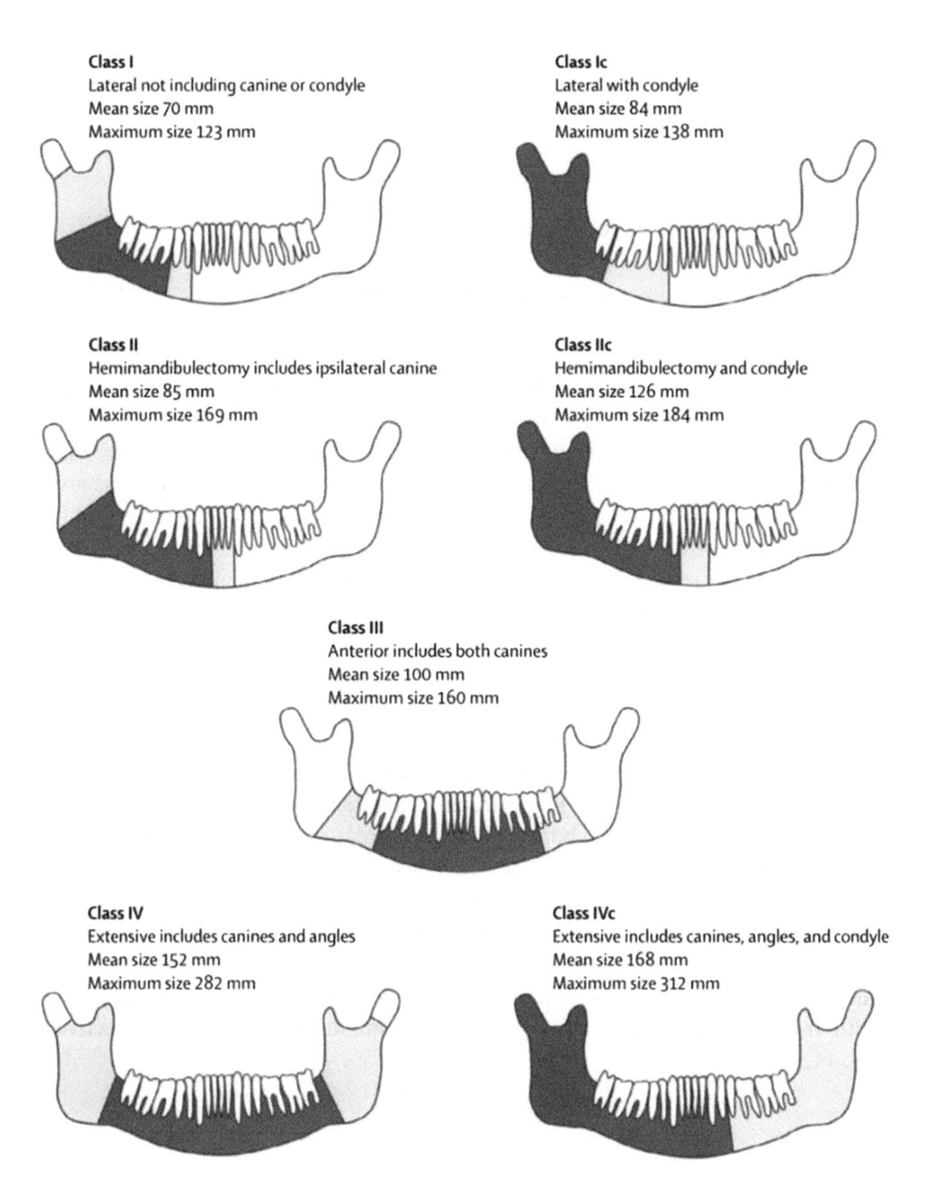


**Fig. 11.2** Mandibular bone defects categorization based on the mean (dark shading) and total (light shading) defect size. (Reuse with permission) [13]

A mandibular continuity defect is a 2 cm or greater portion of bone loss in the mandible [14–16], which commonly occurs due to an acquired etiology, such as various pathologies or traumas [17–19]. Reconstruction of these defects is also a great challenge for oral and maxillofacial surgeons due to biomechanical forces present in this region and anatomical form of the bone [20–22]. In the following sections, comprehensive therapeutic charts will address each of these challenges.

## 2.2 *Localized Bone Defects in Oral and Maxillofacial Region*

### 2.2.1 Alveolar Bone Defects

#### Horizontal and Vertical Alveolar Defects

Nowadays, different classifications exist to describe alveolar ridge defects [23–25]. In this regard, there are various approaches. For instance, Seibert et al. categorized the alveolar bone defects according to the dimension that the resorption had occurred. Class I shows horizontal defects with the prevalence of 33%, followed by class II vertical defects (3%) and the most common frequent type, class III that is a mixed horizontal and vertical defect (56%) [24]. In addition, some other classifications were recommended by other researchers based on the morphology of the alveolar bone defects. CCARD approved and applied a three-part codes pattern at the 8th European Consensus of the European Association of Dental Implantologists (*BDIZ EDI*) to depict the effect of the alveolar ridge as comprehensively as possible with a view to existing therapeutic approaches.

#### Khojasteh's Classification for Alveolar Ridge

In a 2013 literature review, Khojasteh et al. accentuate the clinical impact of defect site properties for vertical ridge reconstruction and demonstrated that data about the condition of the initial vertical bone defect is not precisely incorporated in the existing evidence [26]. Thus, Khojasteh et al. proposed the first quantitative categorization of alveolar bone defects by anticipating demand for reconstructing the deficiencies. In the Khojasteh et al. classification, alveolar bony defects were divided into three groups based on the surrounding bony walls (A, two walls; B, one wall; and C, without wall) which can consists of classes I–III according to their width from greater than 5 mm, 3–5 mm, to smaller than 3 mm, respectively (Fig. 11.3) [26].

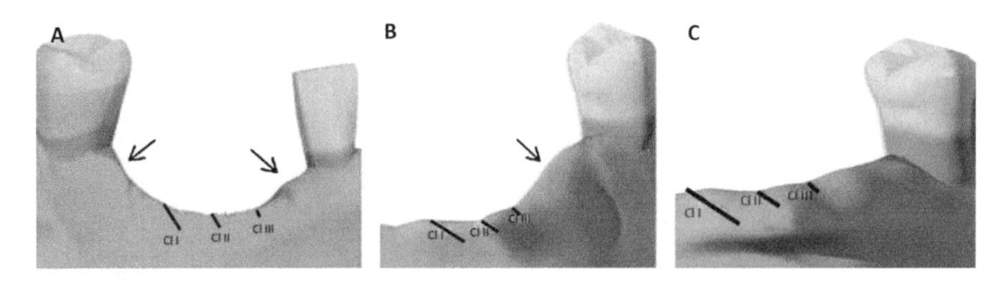


**Fig. 11.3** ABC classification of alveolar bone defects. (**a**) panel depicts the defect surrounded by two walls indicated by black arrows. (**b**) panel shows a defect which only has one wall (black arrow), and panel (**c**) indicates a defect without any wall. Classes I–III were shown in the figure which refer to >5 mm (Cl I), 3–5 mm (Cl II), and <3 mm (Cl III). (Reuse with permission) [27]

Fenestration and Dehiscence

Fenestrations—derived from Latin word for "window"—is defined as secluded areas of denuded tooth root with the root surface only covered by periosteum and soft tissue, while the marginal bone over the area remains intact. Sometimes the buccal/labial covering bone is very thin and this denudation extends to the marginal bone. When the marginal bone is affected, the defect is called a dehiscence rather than fenestration [28]. Davies et al. [29] proposed that dehiscence is the absence of at least 4 mm of root covering bone that continues from the apical aspect to the marginal level of bone, whereas a fenestration is an isolated bone defect that resulted in an exposure of root surface. These defects can occur both in maxilla and mandible, and many studies have reported a wide range of prevalence among various populations, from 0.23% to 69.57% for fenestration and geographic distribution 0.99–53.62% for dehiscence [30, 31].

### 2.2.2 Clefts

The American Cleft Palate–Craniofacial Association (ACPA) Reclassification Committee [32] proposed the most practical classification of clefts for surgeons.

In 1981, the ACPA Ad Hoc Committee on Nomenclature and Classification of Craniofacial Anomalies introduced a reclassification of craniofacial anomalies. The 1981 Committee determined that the Kernahan and Stark Classification of 1958 [33] and the ACPA Classification of 1962 [34] were better systems based on the literature, ease of use, and clarity of categorizing. The Kernahan "striped-Y" diagram (Fig. 11.4) [35] was presented to simplify record keeping with a visual diagram. Their striped Y which has been provided in Fig. 11.4 was also modified by Elsahy and Millard to be more appropriate in clinical practice [36, 37].

It is estimated that 3/4 of all CL/P patients have alveolar bone defects [38]. It is the alveolar cleft that will be discussed in this chapter. In fact, alveolar cleft creates a critical disruption of dentition and causes a collapsed alveolar segment. The major

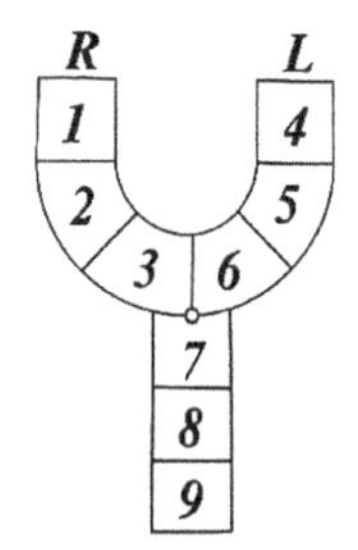


**Fig. 11.4** Kernahan's striped-Y design for cleft categories. (Reuse with permission) [35]

goal of bone reconstruction in clefts is to provide a normal facial and dental function. Failing to rehabilitate and unite the maxillary bone leads to a poor function and significantly comprises the restoring process [39].

## 3 Treatment Approaches and Challenges

Application of autologous bone grafting is the current gold standard in both orthopedic and cranio-maxillofacial bone repair [40]. Autogenous bone grafts are often easily available in surrounding tissues of the bone defect site. In addition, they can also be obtained from distant anatomical sites, such as iliac crest or rib. Extra collected bone can even be stored for a long period of time by means of cryopreservation. The major risk related to autogenous bone grafts is postoperative infection leading to failure of the reconstruction, which requires further intervention later. Failure in the long-term outcome can also be observed as massive resorption of the regenerated bone [41]. Moreover, the main risks at the donor site consist of nerve injury, discomfort and pain, and postoperative wound infections. There are many risk factors that are related to the patient—such as poor nutrition, compromised immune system, weakened microcirculation after chemo-/radiotherapy, and smoking—that can influence the regenerative treatment outcome [42]. Since the local sources for autologous grafts are restricted and other long-distance donor sites, like pelvic bones and limbs, cause serious and prolonged morbidity and discomfort, new methods for bone tissue engineering are being developed. Reconstruction of large bone defects are always a challenge and must meet high functional and esthetic requisites. Albeit autologous bone is preferred, bone substitutes—such as titanium, acrylic, polylactic acid [43], and hydroxyapatite (HA)—are available and have been used in many clinical investigations [44, 45]. Alloplastic alternatives are often used for specific indications. Patient-oriented regenerative approaches are becoming more common as custom-made applications fused with imaging technologies are gaining popularity [46]. By its nature, reconstruction in the oral and maxillofacial region is a highly individualized process, according to the location and type of bony defect. In addition, it is important to notice that success rate in treating small- or medium-sized defects by using conventional autogenous bone grafting method is up to 98% [47], but in the case of larger defects, autogenous custom-manufactured smart scaffolds and stem cells could provide new beneficial alternatives.

## *3.1 Reconstruction of Large Bone Defects and Suggested Treatment Algorithm*

### 3.1.1 Midface Region

Managing midface bone defects is among the most intricate and controversial regions for reconstruction. There are a wide range of treatment options from prosthetic obturators to pedicled-, free-, or non-vascularized bone grafts [48]. Nowadays, the application of pedicled flaps has decreased due to its restricted volume and reach. In addition, for large defects, obturators—especially in edentulous patients—may be impractical or difficult to retain [49]. Prosthetic obturators are also inappropriate in orbital content, orbital floor, or soft tissue resected cases. On the other hand, various flaps and bone graft techniques have been described, but the best evidence-based treatment method is still being debated [50–53]. One of the basic challenges is that the defects are usually highly variable in shape and size due to their etiology, which is mainly oncologic resection or trauma. Moreover, these defects usually do not only involve the bony structures but also influence adjacent soft tissues. Thus, successful outcomes of reconstruction encompass a wide range of regenerative knowledge, craniofacial plating techniques, and comprehensive understanding of prosthetic rehabilitation. In Fig. 11.5, a suggested protocol for treatment of midface bone defects has been provided. This protocol is based on the

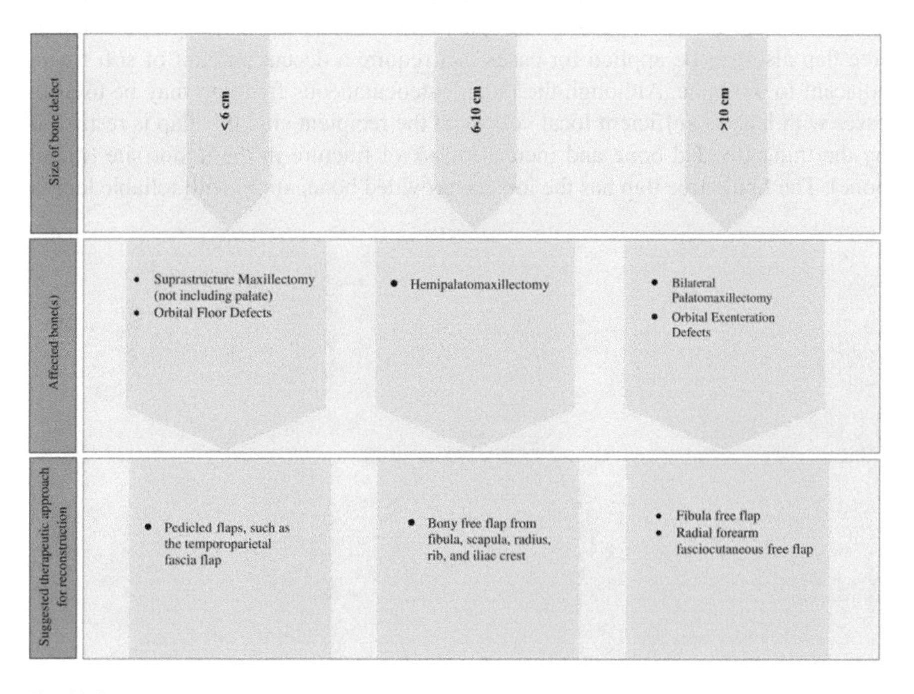


**Fig. 11.5** Reconstruction algorithm of midfacial bone defects according to the size of the defects (except alveolar and cleft bone defects)

defect size and includes bony structures [53–55]. In this protocol, there are several considerations, the first of which is the condition of palatal bone, which is one of the main determinants of selecting the best suited plan for reconstruction [49]. The status of the orbital floor is also important; grafts, bony flaps, and implants are required in order to preserve eye's function. For instance, if an extended maxillectomy reaches to the orbital floor, a free flap is necessary to separate orbit, nasal cavity/sinuses, or even intracranial spaces.

### 3.1.2 Mandibular Defects

Although many advancements have been introduced in past decades—consisting of vascularized bone grafts, various reconstruction plates, osseointegrated dental implants, and computer-aided surgical planning—goals of reconstructing mandibular defects are not sufficiently addressed in one treatment modality, such as restoring mastication and preserving temporomandibular joint function. A suggested algorithm for reconstructing large mandibular defects has been provided in Fig. 11.6. The size and type of defect play a pivotal role in the treatment planning [49, 53, 56–59].

For selecting among various types of flaps for mandibular bone reconstruction, it is important to consider length of pedicle, adjacent soft tissue and skin, flap length, the capacity to accept dental implants, and donor site morbidity. The free fibula or iliac crest flaps are most reliably accepted flaps for this region [60]. The scapular free flap also can be applied for cases that require a decent amount of soft tissue adjacent to the bone. Although the radial osteocutaneous free flap may be used in cases with lack of sufficient local vessels in the recipient site, this flap is restricted by the thin provided bone and increased risk of fracture in the donor site (radial bone). The fibula free flap has the longest provided bone, along with reliable length

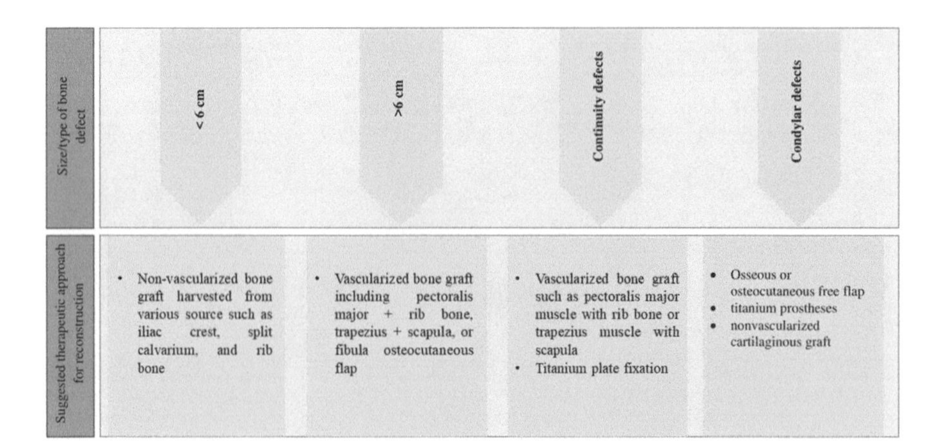


**Fig. 11.6** Reconstruction algorithm of large mandibular bone defects based on the size/type of the defects (except alveolar defects)

and caliber of pedicle. This flap is a good choice in defects more than 6 cm requiring vascularized bone graft. However, for this selection, clinician should consider donor site availability and morbidity, risk for complications, and patient positioning. The specific location of the defect on mandibular bone also influences reconstructive decisions. For instance, bone defects in the anterior part of mandible involve parasymphysis and symphysis regions. Moreover, posterior defects can involve condyle and temporomandibular joint which make the placement of titanium fixation plate more complicated. Nowadays, the gold standard method to rehabilitate continuity bone defects is vascularized grafts, due to its capability of maintaining blood supply to the graft and also the defect region. Vascularized bone grafting represents faster regeneration, lower infection risk, and greater resistance to radiation [61, 62]. However, vascularized bone grafting is an intricate method that requires high practical skill and specific technology and materials. Moreover, its disadvantages are longer surgery time, intensified blood loss, and increased cost [61, 62]. Thus, non-vascularized bone grafts attempt to address these issues that consist of harvesting bone tissue from donor (the ilium, mandibular ramus, rib, etc.) [63–65]. Non-vascularized bone grafts application was successful in 84.7% for bone defects in craniofacial reconstructions. In addition, in a cohort investigation, 95% of vascularized bone grafts were successful which was higher than non-vascularized bone grafts application with 72% promising results. One of the explanations of this failure of the non-vascularized grafts is the length of the recipient site (defect site), which shows the fact that large defects require alternative treatment approaches compared to small bony defects. In this regard, only 17% of bone grafts were failed in the smaller than 6 cm defects, whereas 75% of them were unsuccessful in greater than 12 cm defects. In addition, Pogrel et al. demonstrated a higher rate of failure in defects which are greater than 9 cm. They suggested the application of alternative tissue engineering approaches in these cases to ameliorate the results. Foster et al. compared vascularized bone versus non-vascularized bone grafts, reporting a total success rate of 88% for vascularized bone grafts and 68% for non-vascularized bone defects, of which there was 75% success rate for bone defects <6 cm, 44% for >6 cm, 46% for 6–10 cm, and 40% for 10–14 cm [63–65].

### 3.1.3 Cranial Defects

Reconstruction of cranial defects is crucial in order to conserve underlying important anatomical structures—the brain and meninges. The cranium in adults does not have the capability to spontaneously regenerate, as it does in infancy. Hence, there is a need for more rapid and consistent reconstruction of the adult skull with autografts and bone substitutes. In 2013, Ugur et al. suggested a specific algorithm for clinicians to choose the best evidence-based therapeutic modality [11]. In this algorithm, they categorized the best treatment according to the size of bone defect. For small (<25 $cm^2$) or moderate defects (25–200 $cm^2$), split calvarial grafts, bone substitutes such as HA cement, and allogenic bone grafts have been recommended.

Reconstruction of large cranial bone defects are always a challenge, and the outcomes have to meet high esthetic and functional requirements. In this regard, though autografts are preferred, biomaterials such as titanium, polylactic acid (PLA), acrylic, and hydroxyapatite (HA) are accessible and have been applied by clinicians [66, 67]. In some cases, there is no possibility to use cranial harvested bone grafts for reconstructive purposes due to the size of the defect. The autogenous bone graft can be obtained as a non-vascularized graft from long-distance anatomical regions, such as iliac crest, scapula, or ribs. Although using scapular angle flaps showed good esthetic results and low morbidity in donor site for bone reconstruction in head and neck region, iliac crest and fibular grafts remain more popular [68].

In cranial defects, the demand for the direct loadbearing capability of the scaffold is minimal. Ideally, in order to preserve cranial esthetic contours, the scaffold resorption should be synchronized in all parts of the regenerated site. This functional capacity consists of the potential to mimic the natural bone microstructure of the surrounding bone tissue in detail and to establish an appropriate mechanical biocompatibility [69]. Moreover, this structure should consist of a gradually biodegradable composite scaffold that has osteoinductive, osteoconductive, and anti-inflammatory properties, inducing revascularization to enable regeneration throughout the defect area. Many existing scaffolds are being tested in combination with different stem cell types in CSD models of calvarial bone defects. A good example of the application of bone tissue engineering triangle is the study of Taub et al., in which skeletal muscle-derived stem cells were evaluated in a rat calvarial full-thickness CSD in combination with polyglycolic acid (PGA) mesh, resulting in better new bone formation in the PLA in combination with stem cells group, compared to the PLA scaffold and empty defect groups [70]. In addition, vascularized new bone was formed in rats by subcutaneously wrapping around vascular bundles with stem cell loaded ß-TCP scaffolds [71]. This novel approach for preparing vascularized scaffolds may enhance reconstruction of large bone defects, especially in a cranium that has insufficient vascularization.

### 3.1.4 Tissue Engineering as an Alternative Therapeutic Approach

Conventional treatment modalities for regenerating of oral and maxillofacial bone defects commonly need to apply autograft or alloplastic materials. Both, however, have detriments that limit their clinical applications [72, 73]. The concept of isolating stem cells followed by expansion and their implantation to patients for bone regeneration has been proposed to address drawbacks of the aforementioned methods. A completely new field of technology—tissue engineering—has emerged to address the aforementioned issues [74]. In order to achieve an ideal result in bone regeneration, tissue engineering needs to utilize the optimal combination of a selected stem cell population, which is differentiated and cultured in a laboratorial environment. This is then seeded onto a biocompatible scaffold, a supporting template that serves as a structure to anchor both seeded and endogenous stem cells to conserve differentiating cells [75] in an in vivo setting. Biomaterial is kind of material that is intended to face biological systems in order to evaluate, treat, and regenerate cells, tissues, or organs in body. This concept to apply organic or synthetic materials is not a novel paradigm, as they have been broadly applied even in old cultures for various medical applications. Later, in clinical approaches, biomaterials such as silk or animal gut have been replaced with either biodegradable or biologically stable scaffolds [76], which consists of custom-printed three-dimensional constructions for oral and maxillofacial bone reconstructions [77, 78].

In 2004, Warnke et al. reported a novel approach of bone-engineered reconstruction of subtotal mandibulectomy defect (>7 cm) that was successfully applied in a 56-year-old man. In this study, they used natural bovine bone mineral (NBBM) scaffold loaded with bone morphogenic protein-7 (BMP-7) and bone marrow aspirate and preserved in a custom-made computer-assisted titanium cage. This specific cage was used to maintain the required shape of arch for reconstructing mandibular anatomical form. The cage first implanted into the latissimus dorsi muscle for 7 weeks and was then transplanted to the defect size as a custom-made free bone-muscle flap [79]. The authors later updated some information regarding their previous study for further application of their method [80]. They mentioned that titanium cage was not the best option for fabricating a customized engineered bone tissue due to its lack of biodegradability; however, it can sufficiently preserve the desired shape. On the other hand, other factors can influence the results, such as the appropriate dosage of growth factor, patient age, and general health status.

Another successful application of bone tissue engineering in reconstructing massive oral and maxillofacial bone defects was reported by Mesimaki et al. [80]. They had implanted a custom-made shaped titanium cage containing adipose-derived stem cells (ASCs) and BMP-2 loaded on beta-tricalcium phosphate (TCP) into left rectus abdominis muscle for 8 months. Then, a vascularized flap was removed from the muscle and transplanted to the defect site in order to reconstruct a large hemimaxillectomy bone defect. Their study represented a successful reconstruction of a large craniofacial bone defect via ASCs and customized engineered bone.

In 2013, Sandor et al. reported a clinical ASCs tissue-engineered construct for treating large anterior mandibular defect. In contrast to the previous study, they had completely produced the engineered tissue in the laboratory and transplanted it to the patient's body in one step. In this study, they rehabilitated a 10 cm anterior mandibular defect in length via application of beta-TCP granules loaded with ASCs and BMP-2. After 21 days of in situ expansion and differentiation of ASCs on the scaffold, they transplanted the construct to the defect site, which was protected via a specific titanium mesh and plate [81]. Although this method of patient-specific hardware and engineered bone revealed successful clinical result, treatment of patients who received radiotherapy or have complicated defects still require vascularized tissue grafts.

## 3.2 *Algorithm-Based Selection of Treatment Options Based on the Defect Site and Type*

### 3.2.1 Alveolar Bone Defects

Several techniques have been proposed to enhance the result of augmentative approaches of alveolar regeneration; however, the type of bone deficiency and recipient-site properties can influence the outcome of these interventions [82]. Morphologic oriented categorization for homogenizing the study designs on various types of bone defects have been carried out for extraction socket defects [83], peri-implant defects [84], posterior maxillary defects (including sinus pneumatization) [85], and vertical alveolar bone defects [86]. Tinti et al. presented a classification of alveolar bone defects associated with immediate or delayed placement of dental implant, which was only according to the amount of deficiency. Nevertheless, complicated bone defects with combined deficiencies could not be assessed with Tinti classification [87].

The anatomic location of the alveolar bone defect might affect the outcome of bone healing. Anterior and posterior parts of the maxilla and mandible represent dissimilar bone qualities [88]; thus, it might be reasonable to elect a donor site similar to the recipient site, if feasible. It is necessary to measure the baseline bone defect size and the amount of augmentation instantly after bone graft surgery due to the size, area, and contour of the bone healing and resorption, depending on the shape and size of the atrophic alveolar bone (baseline condition of the bone) [89]. In addition, width of the bone base in the defect site facilitates space supplied for bone augmentation in guided bone regeneration (GBR). It has been shown that in small alveolar bone defects, the demand for bone augmentation and thus the expected gain are slightly less compared to larger bone defects [90]. The healing and augmentation of large alveolar bone defects is more challenging and complicated and is mainly performed by incorporation of block bone grafts [82]. In Fig. 11.7, a reconstruction algorithm is shown for alveolar bone defects in maxilla.

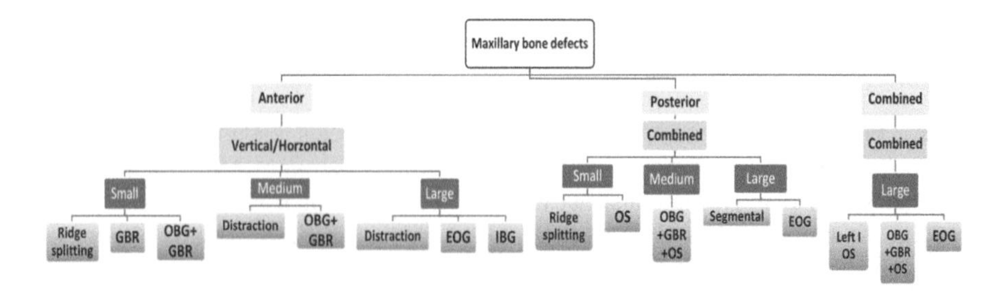


**Fig. 11.7** Reconstruction algorithm of alveolar bone defects in maxilla. Yellow boxes show the location of defects. Green boxes indicate the type of defects and blue ones indicate size of defects. Suggested therapeutic approaches represented by red boxes on the bottom. **Abbreviations: GBR* guided bone regeneration, *IBG* inlay bone graft, *left* LeFort osteotomy, *OBG* onlay bone graft, *OS* osteotomy

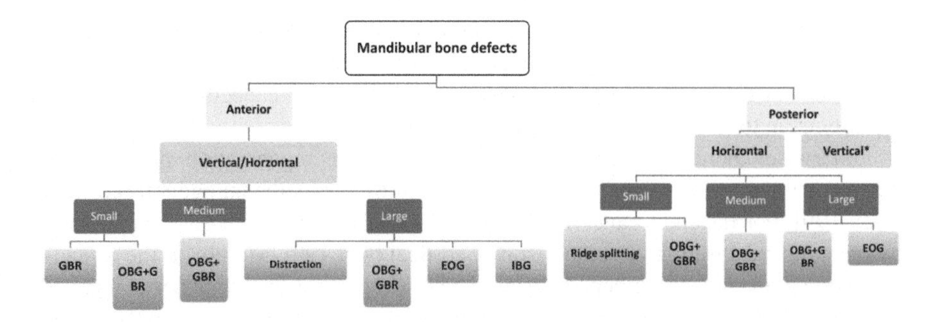


**Fig. 11.8** Reconstruction algorithm of alveolar bone defects in mandible. The vertical alveolar bone defects in the posterior mandible have been explained in the next figure. Yellow boxes show the location of defects. Green boxes indicate the type of defects and blue ones indicate size of defects. Suggested therapeutic approaches represented by red boxes on the bottom. *∗Abbreviations: GBR* guided bone regeneration, *IBG* inlay bone graft, *OBG* onlay bone graft

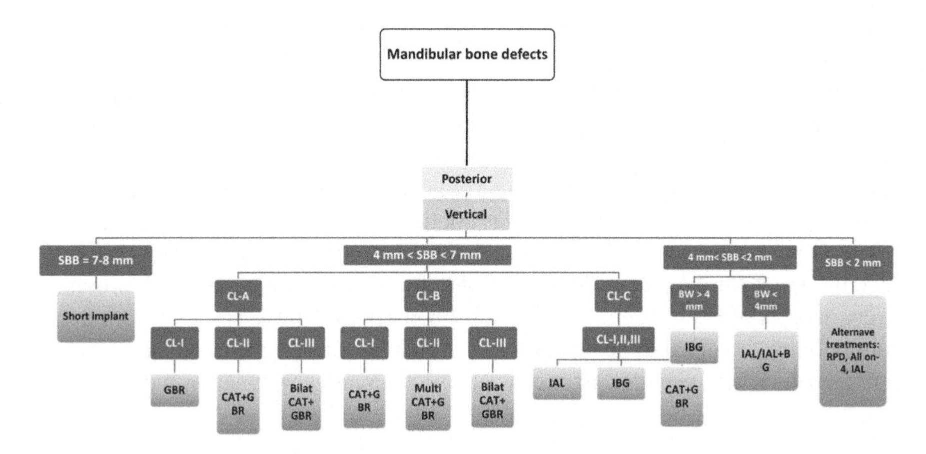


**Fig. 11.9** Reconstruction algorithm of vertical alveolar bone defects in posterior mandible region. Yellow boxes show the location of defects. Green boxes indicate the type of defects and blue ones indicate the size of defects. Suggested therapeutic approaches are represented by red boxes on the bottom. *∗Abbreviations: Bilat* bilateral, *CAT* cortical autogenous tenting, *GBR* guided bone regeneration, *IAL* inferior alveolar nerve lateralization, *IBG* inlay bone graft, *RPD* removable partial denture

This categorization is based on the location of the bone defects (anterior, posterior, and the combination of both locations) and the size of defects (small, medium, and large).

In addition, Figs. 11.8 and 11.9 provide information regarding recommended algorithm for reconstructing mandibular alveolar defects. These algorithms have been organized based on the previous evidence [91–98].

Although cancellous block autografts can be reshaped to comply with the shape and size of new generated bone, cortical bone graft features are difficult to modify due to their inherent shape [89]. Moreover, cortical block grafts are not capable of preserving long-term three-dimensional cohesion, as they have a resorption rate of up to 60% at the time of implant placement; whereas, the cancellous block bone represents up to 10% of bone resorption [89].

Otherwise, there are significant differences in the regeneration process and mechanical properties of the autogenous cancellous versus the autogenous cortical grafts [99]. For instance, cancellous bone revascularizes better and is strengthened by creeping substitution in comparison to cortical bone [99]. Moreover, the cancellous bone grafts are strengthened during the bone regeneration, while cortical grafts are debilitated [99]. Bone augmentation by block bone grafts is frequently correlated to bone resorption [100]. To prevent bone resorption during the regenerative process, membranes are helpful; nevertheless, bone resorption still occurs slightly [100, 101].

Tissue engineering approaches—including cell-based therapies that have been rapidly growing as an alternative therapy [102]—attempt to compensate for the conventional methods' drawbacks and present patients with "personalized autologous bone grafts" [103]. Bone marrow mesenchymal stem cells (BMMSCs) are evidently the most widely studied and utilized adult stem cells [103]. BMMSCs with a proper carrier were also investigated in several articles. Moreover, iliac bone is the most common source for BMMSCs, and the harvesting process was frequently well tolerated by patients. The other pivotal element of bone regeneration is the scaffold that acts as a carrier for stem cells and bioactive molecules to the defect site. Demineralized bovine bone mineral was applied as a carrier for BMMSCs and represented proper biocompatibility, osteoconduction, and mechanical properties. In fact, until now, finding the "perfect scaffold" for bone regeneration which provides every aspects of bone regeneration is still on progress. Nowadays, there is a trend for applying "composite" scaffolds with various bioactive molecules such as various growth factors, peptides, or nucleic acids to increase new bone formation [104].

### Alveolar Fenestration and Dehiscence

Fenestration and dehiscence alveolar bone defects commonly have been managed by membranes or periodontal flap surgeries, bone grafts [105, 106]. It has been shown that the membrane treatment is superior to the bone fill [107]. There are also several studies that demonstrate membrane barrier application for dehiscence on the dental implants [108, 109]. A 1-year study was completed on 55 Branemark implants with alveolar bone dehiscence in 45 patients [110]. In this study, all patients were treated with expanded polytetrafluoroethylene membrane, and findings showed an average 82% of bone fill after a year of follow-up. The survival rate of implant was 84.7% cumulatively during the follow-up period. Another study demonstrated successful application of titanium-reinforced membrane in severe dehiscence (mean 8.2 mm) at implant sites [111]. After 7–8 months, a complete bone coverage was observed around the implants. There was not any clinical comparison between membrane application and bone grafts. However, it has been represented that the use of various bone substitutes—such as demineralized freeze dried bone allograft [105], hydroxyapatite [112], and composite graft [113] by GBR technique—can significantly improve bone healing in these cases. GBR with freeze dried bone allograft showed a 96.8% complete bone fill in dehiscence defect adjacent to 110 implants even after 29% of membrane exposure [109].

### 3.2.2 Clefts

Alveolar cleft reconstruction was first treated with autologous tissue by von Eiselsberg [114], and then Lexer [115] introduced a non-vascular bone graft. Drachter et al. revealed that tibial bone graft can be used for alveolar bone regeneration [116]. Until the 1970s, clinicians commonly used primary bone grafting [117–119] at the infant stage. However, long-term follow-up studies showed that retrusion of midface and anterior cross-bite mostly occur after primary bone grafting [120, 121]. Reconstructing alveolar clefts by secondary bone grafting (SBG) is the most beneficial treatment plan [117]. The main aim of SBG is to omit oronasal communication and impede inflammation [122]. In fact, this technique stabilizes maxillary bone segment and symmetry and esthetic of face. Figure 11.10 represented an algorithm for reconstructing alveolar bone cleft. At first step and orthodontic treatment, bone grafting is needed for reinforcing bone support, nasal cartilage, and dental implant placement [123–125].

Unilateral and bilateral CL/P patients require a broad orthodontic and surgical management. In order to retain the orthodontic treatment's appropriate outcomes, lifetime retention is suggested as an essential protocol [126, 127]. Bone graft stability is closely related to the cleft width, existence of unilateral or bilateral defect, and cleft/nasal cavity ratio [128]. For instance, wide bone gap, insufficient wound closure, wound infection, and lack of attached gingiva can lead to failure [129]. After SBG, as seen in Fig. 11.10, it is recommended to place dental implants after 6 months. Placed implants in this region varied in length (10–15 mm) and diameter (3.25–4 mm). Survival rate of dental implants in unilateral cases showed promising outcomes (more than 94%) [129–131].

At first, Bergland et al. [132] introduced Bergland scale (1986) to measure amount of bone graft, after that scientists presented various evaluation guides, such as the Enemark score, the Long rating scale, the Kindelan scale, and the Chelsea scale [133–136]. Nowadays, most techniques for assessing the results of an alveolar bone regeneration use periapical radiographs and cone-beam computed tomography. Feichtinger et al. [136] assessed the volumetric alterations of 24 cases during a 3-year follow-up period. The implanted autogenous bone was absorbed by 49.5% after the first year and 52% after 3 years. Another study [137] assessed the volume of implanted bone in 15 cases after 3 months and 1-year post-surgery. The mean grafted bone volume was $1.1 \pm 0.3\ cm^3$ immediately after surgery, $1.2 \pm 0.6\ cm^3$ and $1.1 \pm 0.5\ cm^3$ at 3 months and 1 year after surgery, respectively. However, the volume revealed a considerable degree of variability, ranging from 0.3 to 2.0 $cm^3$. In 2005, Trindade et al. [138] assessed 65 alveolar bone grafts for a 1-year follow-up.

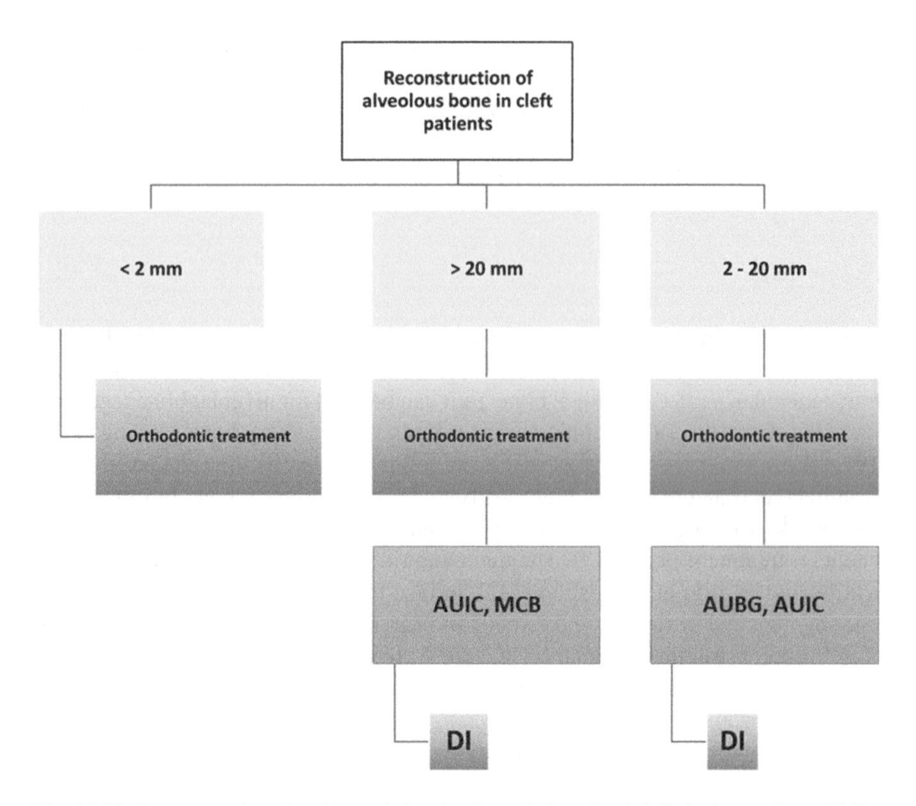


**Fig. 11.10** Reconstruction algorithm of alveolus bone defects in cleft lip/palate patients. Yellow boxes show the location of defects. Suggested therapeutic approaches represented by red boxes on the bottom. ∗*Abbreviations: AUBG* autogenous bone grafts, *AUIC* autogenous iliac crest, *DI* dental implant, *MCB* microvascular corticocancellous bone

They classified 68–71% of their cases as Bergland type I and 15% as type II. In the remaining cases, the grafted bone absorption could not be measured, since the volume continued to alter due to the eruption of the permanent teeth and the orthodontic treatment [138].

In another study conducted on 100 cases for 5 years [139], long-term changes in the implanted bone were evaluated. At the end of the follow-up, they reported that 84.6% of the bilateral clefts patients and 88.9% of the unilateral clefts patients were scored as Bergland type I. Enemark et al. [133] assessed 95 cases of bilateral and unilateral alveolar clefts for 4 years. 76 patients showed no difference in the amount of the bone, and the rest 14 cases, the bone volume only reduced to 75% of the volume of normal alveolar bone. Thus, it is logical to expect a slight change in the amount of implanted graft bone over time. In this regard, despite autologous bone is the ideal choice with a slight resorption over a long period of time, in recent years, bone tissue engineering helped surgeons to restrict this amount. Growth factor-rich materials, such as platelet-rich plasma (PRP) and platelet-rich fibrin (PRF) [140], and application of other additives, such as recombinant human bone morphogenic protein (rhBMP), have been used. rhBMP has also been used in combination with various scaffolds, such as TCP, HA, etc. [141, 142]. In 2012, Behnia et al. showed the enhancing impact of biphasic scaffold in combination with platelet-derived growth factor (PDGF) for alveolar bone regeneration in cleft patients [143]. However, this study did not have any control group due to ethical issues which may influence their conclusion.

## 4 Conclusion and Future Direction

Despite regenerative methods are not usually entailed in the healing process of small bone defects in oral and maxillofacial region, large bone defects need different interventions to treat. Although fabrication of various organic and synthetic scaffolds offers various choices, the treatment results is yet questionable in comparison to autogenous bone grafts based on newly formed bone quality and healing time. The postoperative complications, such as greater price, have been reported in bone regenerative treatments that scientists try to address by new innovative bone tissue engineering techniques. It is necessary to investigate therapeutic impact and mechanism of these techniques in order to precisely understand them, especially in human clinical trials.

## References

1. Singaram, M., & Udhayakumar, R. K. (2016). Prevalence, pattern, etiology, and management of maxillofacial trauma in a developing country: A retrospective study. *Journal of the Korean Association of Oral and Maxillofacial Surgeons, 42*(4), 174–181.
2. Oh, J.-h. (2018). Recent advances in the reconstruction of cranio-maxillofacial defects using computer-aided design/computer-aided manufacturing. *Maxillofacial Plastic and Reconstructive Surgery, 40*(1), 2.
3. Schmitz, J. P., & Hollinger, J. O. (1986). The critical size defect as an experimental model for craniomandibulofacial nonunions. *Clinical Orthopaedics and Related Research, 205*, 299–308.
4. Hollinger, J. O., & Kleinschmidt, J. C. (1990). The critical size defect as an experimental model to test bone repair materials. *The Journal of Craniofacial Surgery, 1*(1), 60–68.
5. Hosseinpour, S., & Bastami, F. (2017). Critical-sized bone defects in mandible of canine model. *Tissue Engineering Part A, 23*(9–10), 470–470.
6. Carvalho, P. P., et al. (2014). Undifferentiated human adipose-derived stromal/stem cells loaded onto wet-spun starch–polycaprolactone scaffolds enhance bone regeneration: Nude mice calvarial defect in vivo study. *Journal of Biomedical Materials Research Part A, 102*(9), 3102–3111.
7. Lam, C. X., et al. (2009). Evaluation of polycaprolactone scaffold degradation for 6 months in vitro and in vivo. *Journal of Biomedical Materials Research Part A, 90*(3), 906–919.
8. Li, L., et al. (2015). Controlled dual delivery of BMP-2 and dexamethasone by nanoparticle-embedded electrospun nanofibers for the efficient repair of critical-sized rat calvarial defect. *Biomaterials, 37*, 218–229.

9. Haberstroh, K., et al. (2010). Bone repair by cell-seeded 3D-bioplotted composite scaffolds made of collagen treated tricalciumphosphate or tricalciumphosphate-chitosan-collagen hydrogel or PLGA in ovine critical-sized calvarial defects. *Journal of Biomedical Materials Research Part B: Applied Biomaterials, 93*(2), 520–530.
10. Hren, N. I., & Miljavec, M. (2008). Spontaneous bone healing of the large bone defects in the mandible. *International Journal of Oral and Maxillofacial Surgery, 37*(12), 1111–1116.
11. Uygur, S., et al. (2013). Management of cranial bone defects: A reconstructive algorithm according to defect size. *Journal of Craniofacial Surgery, 24*(5), 1606–1609.
12. Brown, J. S., & Shaw, R. J. (2010). Reconstruction of the maxilla and midface: Introducing a new classification. *The Lancet Oncology, 11*(10), 1001–1008.
13. Brown, J. S., et al. (2016). A new classification for mandibular defects after oncological resection. *The Lancet Oncology, 17*(1), e23–e30.
14. Adamo, A. K., & Szal, R. L. (1979). Timing, results, and complications of mandibular reconstructive surgery: Report of 32 cases. *Journal of Oral Surgery, 37*(10), 755–763.
15. Tidstrom, K. D., & Keller, E. E. (1990). Reconstruction of mandibular discontinuity with autogenous iliac bone graft: Report of 34 consecutive patients. *Journal of Oral and Maxillofacial Surgery, 48*(4), 336–346. discussion 347.
16. August, M., et al. (2000). Factors influencing the long-term outcome of mandibular reconstruction. *Journal of Oral and Maxillofacial Surgery, 58*(7), 731–737; discussion 738.
17. Pogrel, M. A., et al. (1997). A comparison of vascularized and nonvascularized bone grafts for reconstruction of mandibular continuity defects. *Journal of Oral and Maxillofacial Surgery, 55*(11), 1200–1206.
18. Chiapasco, M., et al. (2008). Long-term results of mandibular reconstruction with autogenous bone grafts and oral implants after tumor resection. *Clinical Oral Implants Research, 19*(10), 1074–1080.
19. Obiechina, A. E., et al. (2003). Mandibular segmental reconstruction with iliac crest. *West African Journal of Medicine, 22*(1), 46–49.
20. Hayden, R. E., Mullin, D. P., & Patel, A. K. (2012). Reconstruction of the segmental mandibular defect: Current state of the art. *Current Opinion in Otolaryngology & Head and Neck Surgery, 20*(4), 231–236.
21. Sajid, M. A., et al. (2011). Reconstruction of mandibular defects with autogenous bone grafts: A review of 30 cases. *Journal of Ayub Medical College, Abbottabad, 23*(3), 82–85.
22. Ardary, W. C. (1993). Reconstruction of mandibular discontinuity defects using autogenous grafting and a mandibular reconstruction plate: A prospective evaluation of nine consecutive cases. *Journal of Oral and Maxillofacial Surgery, 51*(2), 125–130; discussion 131-2.
23. Cawood, J., & Howell, R. (1988). A classification of the edentulous jaws. *International Journal of Oral and Maxillofacial Surgery, 17*(4), 232–236.
24. Seibert, J. (1983). Reconstruction of deformed, partially edentulous ridges, using full thickness onlay grafts, Part I. Technique and wound healing. *The Compendium of Continuing Education in Dentistry, 4*(5), 437–453.
25. Tinti, C., Parma-Benfenati, S., & Polizzi, G. (1996). Vertical ridge augmentation: What is the limit? *International Journal of Periodontics & Restorative Dentistry, 16*(3).
26. Khojasteh, A., Morad, G., & Behnia, H. (2013). Clinical importance of recipient site characteristics for vertical ridge augmentation: A systematic review of literature and proposal of a classification. *Journal of Oral Implantology, 39*(3), 386–398.
27. Khojasteh, A., Nazeman, P., & Tolstunov, L. (2016). Tuberosity-alveolar block as a donor site for localised augmentation of the maxilla: A retrospective clinical study. *British Journal of Oral and Maxillofacial Surgery, 54*(8), 950–955.
28. Singh, S., Panwar, M., & Arora, V. (2013). Management of mucosal fenestration by multidisciplinary approach: A rare case report. *Medical Journal, Armed Forces India, 69*(1), 86.
29. Davies, R., et al. (1974). Alveolar defects in human skulls. *Journal of Clinical Periodontology, 1*(2), 107–111.

30. Nimigean, V. R., et al. (2009). Alveolar bone dehiscences and fenestrations: An anatomical study and review. *Romanian Journal of Morphology and Embryology, 50*(3), 391–397.
31. Rupprecht, R. D., et al. (2001). Prevalence of dehiscences and fenestrations in modern American skulls. *Journal of Periodontology, 72*(6), 722–729.
32. Whitaker, L. A., Pashayan, H., & Reichman, J. (1981). A proposed new classification of craniofacial anomalies. *The Cleft Palate Journal, 18*(3), 161–176.
33. Kernahan, D. A., & Stark, R. B. (1958). A new classification for cleft lip and cleft palate. *Plastic and Reconstructive Surgery, 22*(5), 435–441.
34. Harkins, C. S., et al. (1962). A classification of clfft lip and cleft palatf. *Plastic and Reconstructive Surgery, 29*(1), 31–39.
35. Kernahan, D. A. (1971). The striped Y—A symbolic classification for cleft lip and palate. *Plastic and Reconstructive Surgery, 47*(5), 469–470.
36. Elsahy, N. (1973). The modified striped Y--a systematic classification for cleft lip and palate. *The Cleft Palate Journal, 10*, 247–250.
37. Millard, D. (1976). The naming and classifying of clefts. In *Cleft craft: The evolution of its surgery* (pp. 41–55). Boston: Little, Brown.
38. Waite, P. D., & Waite, D. E. (1996). Bone grafting for the alveolar cleft defect. In *Seminars in orthodontics, 2*(3), (pp. 192–196). Philadelphia, USA, WB Saunders. Elsevier.
39. Boyne, P. J. (1972). Secondary bone grafting of residual alveolar and palatal clefts. *Journal of Oral Surgery, 30*, 87–92.
40. Piitulainen, J. M., et al. (2015). Outcomes of cranioplasty with synthetic materials and autologous bone grafts. *World Neurosurgery, 83*(5), 708–714.
41. Iaccarino, C., et al. (2015). Preliminary results of a prospective study on methods of cranial reconstruction. *Journal of Oral and Maxillofacial Surgery, 73*(12), 2375–2378.
42. Reddy, S., et al. (2014). Clinical outcomes in cranioplasty: Risk factors and choice of reconstructive material. *Plastic and Reconstructive Surgery, 133*(4), 864–873.
43. Bhumiratana, S., et al. (2011). Nucleation and growth of mineralized bone matrix on silk-hydroxyapatite composite scaffolds. *Biomaterials, 32*(11), 2812–2820.
44. Rotaru, H., et al. (2006). Silicone rubber mould cast polyethylmethacrylate-hydroxyapatite plate used for repairing a large skull defect. *Journal of Cranio-Maxillofacial Surgery, 34*(4), 242–246.
45. Vignes, J.-R., et al. (2007). Cranioplasty for repair of a large bone defect in a growing skull fracture in children. *Journal of Cranio-Maxillofacial Surgery, 35*(3), 185–188.
46. Goldstein, J. A., Paliga, J. T., & Bartlett, S. P. (2013). Cranioplasty: Indications and advances. *Current Opinion in Otolaryngology & Head and Neck Surgery, 21*(4), 400–409.
47. Bernal-Sprekelsen, M., et al. (2014). Management of anterior skull base defect depending on its size and location. *BioMed Research International, 2014*, 1.
48. Archibald, S., Jackson, S., & Thoma, A. (2005). Paranasal sinus and midfacial reconstruction. *Clinics in Plastic Surgery, 32*(3), 309–325.
49. Okay, D. J., et al. (2001). Prosthodontic guidelines for surgical reconstruction of the maxilla: A classification system of defects. *The Journal of Prosthetic Dentistry, 86*(4), 352–363.
50. Chang, Y.-M., et al. (2004). Maxillary reconstruction with a fibula osteoseptocutaneous free flap and simultaneous insertion of osseointegrated dental implants. *Plastic and Reconstructive Surgery, 113*(4), 1140–1145.
51. Yazar, S., et al. (2006). Osteomyocutaneous peroneal artery perforator flap for reconstruction of composite maxillary defects. *Head & Neck, 28*(4), 297–304.
52. Heredero, S., et al. (2016). Osteomyocutaneous peroneal artery perforator flap for reconstruction of the skull base. *British Journal of Oral and Maxillofacial Surgery, 54*(1), 99–101.
53. Hanasono, M. M. (2014). Reconstructive surgery for head and neck cancer patients. *Advances in Medicine, 2014*, 1.
54. Wehage, I. C., & Fansa, H. (2011). Complex reconstructions in head and neck cancer surgery: Decision making. *Head & Neck Oncology, 3*(1), 14.

55. George, R. K., & Krishnamurthy, A. (2013). Microsurgical free flaps: Controversies in maxillofacial reconstruction. *Annals of Maxillofacial Surgery, 3*(1), 72.
56. Wei, F.-C., et al. (2003). Complications after reconstruction by plate and soft-tissue free flap in composite mandibular defects and secondary salvage reconstruction with osteocutaneous flap. *Plastic and Reconstructive Surgery, 112*(1), 37–42.
57. Allsopp, B. J., Hunter-Smith, D. J., & Rozen, W. M. (2016). Vascularized versus nonvascularized bone grafts: what is the evidence? *Clinical Orthopaedics and Related Research®, 474*(5), 1319–1327.
58. Akinbami, B. O. (2016). Reconstruction of continuity defects of the mandible with non-vascularized bone grafts. Systematic literature review. *Craniomaxillofacial Trauma & Reconstruction, 9*(3), 195.
59. Osborn, T. M., Helal, D., & Mehra, P. (2018). Iliac crest bone grafting for mandibular reconstruction: 10-year experience outcomes. *Journal of Oral Biology and Craniofacial Research, 8*(1), 25–29.
60. Disa, J. J., et al. (1999). Evaluation of bone height in osseous free flap mandible reconstruction: An indirect measure of bone mass. *Plastic and Reconstructive Surgery, 103*(5), 1371–1377.
61. Pogrel, M., et al. (1997). A comparison of vascularized and nonvascularized bone grafts for reconstruction of mandibular continuity defects. *Journal of Oral and Maxillofacial Surgery, 55*(11), 1200–1206.
62. Foster, R. D., et al. (1999). Vascularized bone flaps versus nonvascularized bone grafts for mandibular reconstruction: An outcome analysis of primary bony union and endosseous implant success. *Head & Neck, 21*(1), 66–71.
63. Gadre, P. K., et al. (2011). Nonvascularized bone grafting for mandibular reconstruction: Myth or reality? *Journal of Craniofacial Surgery, 22*(5), 1727–1735.
64. Ndukwe, K. C., et al. (2014). Reconstruction of mandibular defects using nonvascularized autogenous bone graft in nigerians. *Nigerian Journal of Surgery, 20*(2), 87–91.
65. Adenike, O. A., et al. (2014). Perioperative findings and complications of non-vascularised iliac crest graft harvest: The experience of a Nigerian tertiary hospital. *Nigerian Medical Journal, 55*(3), 224.
66. Motamedian, S. R., et al. (2015). Smart scaffolds in bone tissue engineering: A systematic review of literature. *World Journal of Stem Cells, 7*(3), 657.
67. Hosseinpour, S., et al. (2017). Application of selected scaffolds for bone tissue engineering: A systematic review. *Oral and Maxillofacial Surgery, 21*(2), 109–129.
68. Ferrari, S., Ferri, A., & Bianchi, B. (2015). Scapular tip free flap in head and neck reconstruction. *Current Opinion in Otolaryngology & Head and Neck Surgery, 23*(2), 115–120.
69. Mazza, E., & Ehret, A. E. (2015). Mechanical biocompatibility of highly deformable biomedical materials. *Journal of the Mechanical Behavior of Biomedical Materials, 48*, 100–124.
70. Taub, P. J., et al. (2009). Bioengineering of calvaria with adult stem cells. *Plastic and Reconstructive Surgery, 123*(4), 1178–1185.
71. Nakano, K., et al. (2016). Promotion of osteogenesis and angiogenesis in vascularized tissue-engineered bone using osteogenic matrix cell sheets. *Plastic and Reconstructive Surgery, 137*(5), 1476–1484.
72. Nkenke, E., et al. (2002). Morbidity of harvesting of retromolar bone grafts: A prospective study. *Clinical Oral Implants Research, 13*(5), 514–521.
73. Nkenke, E., et al. (2001). Morbidity of harvesting of chin grafts: A prospective study. *Clinical Oral Implants Research, 12*(5), 495–502.
74. Berthiaume, F., Maguire, T. J., & Yarmush, M. L. (2011). Tissue engineering and regenerative medicine: History, progress, and challenges. *Annual Review of Chemical and Biomolecular Engineering, 2*, 403–430.
75. Wolff, J., et al. (2013). GMP-level adipose stem cells combined with computer-aided manufacturing to reconstruct mandibular ameloblastoma resection defects: Experience with three cases. *Annals of Maxillofacial Surgery, 3*(2), 114.

76. Best, S., et al. (2008). Bioceramics: Past, present and for the future. *Journal of the European Ceramic Society, 28*(7), 1319–1327.
77. Kang, H.-W., et al. (2016). A 3D bioprinting system to produce human-scale tissue constructs with structural integrity. *Nature Biotechnology, 34*(3), 312.
78. Kohan, E., et al. (2015). Customized bilaminar resorbable mesh with BMP-2 promotes cranial bone defect healing. *Annals of Plastic Surgery, 74*(5), 603–608.
79. Warnke, P., et al. (2004). Growth and transplantation of a custom vascularised bone graft in a man. *The Lancet, 364*(9436), 766–770.
80. Warnke, P. H., et al. (2006). Man as living bioreactor: Fate of an exogenously prepared customized tissue-engineered mandible. *Biomaterials, 27*(17), 3163–3167.
81. Sándor, G. K., et al. (2013). Adipose stem cell tissue–engineered construct used to treat large anterior mandibular defect: A case report and review of the clinical application of good manufacturing practice–level adipose stem cells for bone regeneration. *Journal of Oral and Maxillofacial Surgery, 71*(5), 938–950.
82. Khojasteh, A., Morad, G., & Behnia, H. (2013). Clinical importance of recipient site characteristics for vertical ridge augmentation: A systematic review of literature and proposal of a classification. *The Journal of Oral Implantology, 39*(3), 386–398.
83. Caplanis, N., Lozada, J. L., & Kan, J. Y. (2005). Extraction defect assessment, classification, and management. *Journal of the California Dental Association, 33*(11), 853–863.
84. Vanden Bogaerde, L. (2004). A proposal for the classification of bony defects adjacent to dental implants. *The International Journal of Periodontics & Restorative Dentistry, 24*(3), 264–271.
85. Wang, H. L., & Katranji, A. (2008). ABC sinus augmentation classification. *The International Journal of Periodontics & Restorative Dentistry, 28*(4), 383–389.
86. Khojasteh, A., et al. (2013). Vertical bone augmentation with simultaneous implant placement using particulate mineralized bone and mesenchymal stem cells: A preliminary study in rabbit. *The Journal of Oral Implantology, 39*(1), 3–13.
87. Tinti, C., Parma-Benfenati, S., & Polizzi, G. (1996). Vertical ridge augmentation: What is the limit? *The International Journal of Periodontics & Restorative Dentistry, 16*(3), 220–229.
88. Hassani, A., Khojasteh, A., & Shamsabad, A. N. (2005). The anterior palate as a donor site in maxillofacial bone grafting: A quantitative anatomic study. *Journal of Oral and Maxillofacial Surgery, 63*(8), 1196–1200.
89. Aghaloo, T. L., & Moy, P. K. (2007). Which hard tissue augmentation techniques are the most successful in furnishing bony support for implant placement? *The International Journal of Oral & Maxillofacial Implants, 22 Suppl*, 49–70.
90. Beitlitum, I., Artzi, Z., & Nemcovsky, C. E. (2010). Clinical evaluation of particulate allogeneic with and without autogenous bone grafts and resorbable collagen membranes for bone augmentation of atrophic alveolar ridges. *Clinical Oral Implants Research, 21*(11), 1242–1250.
91. Khojasteh, A., et al. (2017). The influence of initial alveolar ridge defect morphology on the outcome of implants in augmented atrophic posterior mandible: An exploratory retrospective study. *Clinical Oral Implants Research, 28*(10), e208–e217.
92. Morad, G., & Khojasteh, A. (2013). Cortical tenting technique versus onlay layered technique for vertical augmentation of atrophic posterior mandibles: A split-mouth pilot study. *Implant Dentistry, 22*(6), 566–571.
93. Khojasteh, A., et al. (2016). Cortical bone augmentation versus nerve lateralization for treatment of atrophic posterior mandible: A retrospective study and review of literature. *Clinical Implant Dentistry and Related Research, 18*(2), 342–359.
94. Behnia, H., et al. (2015). Accuracy and reliability of cone beam computed tomographic measurements of the bone labial and palatal to the maxillary anterior teeth. *International Journal of Oral & Maxillofacial Implants, 30*(6).
95. Khodayari, A., et al. (2011). Spontaneous regeneration of the mandible after hemimandibulectomy: Report of a case. *Journal of Dentistry (Tehran, Iran), 8*(3), 152.

96. Behnia, H., et al. (2013). Multidisciplinary reconstruction of a palatomaxillary defect with nonvascularized fibula bone graft and distraction osteogenesis. *Journal of Craniofacial Surgery, 24*(2), e186–e190.
97. Behnia, H., et al. (2008). Treatment of arteriovenous malformations: Assessment of 2 techniques—Transmandibular curettage versus resection and immediate replantation. *Journal of Oral and Maxillofacial Surgery, 66*(12), 2557–2565.
98. Khojasteh, A., & Sadeghi, N. (2016). Application of buccal fat pad-derived stem cells in combination with autogenous iliac bone graft in the treatment of maxillomandibular atrophy: A preliminary human study. *International Journal of Oral and Maxillofacial Surgery, 45*(7), 864–871.
99. Donos, N., Mardas, N., & Chadha, V. (2008). Clinical outcomes of implants following lateral bone augmentation: Systematic assessment of available options (barrier membranes, bone grafts, split osteotomy). *Journal of Clinical Periodontology, 35*(8 Suppl), 173–202.
100. Nissan, J., et al. (2011). Implant-supported restoration of congenitally missing teeth using cancellous bone block-allografts. *Oral Surgery, Oral Medicine, Oral Pathology, Oral Radiology, and Endodontics, 111*(3), 286–291.
101. Penarrocha-Diago, M., et al. (2013). Localized lateral alveolar ridge augmentation with block bone grafts: Simultaneous versus delayed implant placement: A clinical and radiographic retrospective study. *The International Journal of Oral & Maxillofacial Implants, 28*(3), 846–853.
102. Soltan, M., Smiler, D. G., & Gailani, F. (2005). A new "platinum" standard for bone grafting: Autogenous stem cells. *Implant Dentistry, 14*(4), 322–327.
103. Bhumiratana, S., & Vunjak-Novakovic, G. (2012). Concise review: Personalized human bone grafts for reconstructing head and face. *Stem Cells Translational Medicine, 1*(1), 64–69.
104. Bose, S., Roy, M., & Bandyopadhyay, A. (2012). Recent advances in bone tissue engineering scaffolds. *Trends in Biotechnology, 30*(10), 546–554.
105. Bhatsange, A., et al. (2017). Management of fenestration using bone allograft in conjunction with platelet-rich fibrin. *Journal of Indian Society of Periodontology, 21*(4), 337.
106. Ricucci, D., et al. (2018). Management and Histobacteriological findings of mucosal fenestration: A report of 2 cases. *Journal of Endodontia, 44*, 1583.
107. Mulyar, M. K. Y. (2015). Bone fenestration: A case report of management of a lower anterior buccal bone fenestration. *International Dental Journal of Students Research, 3*.
108. Jensen, O. T., et al. (1995). Vertical guided bone-graft augmentation in a new canine mandibular model. *International Journal of Oral & Maxillofacial Implants*, 10(3).
109. Klokkevold, P., Han, T., & Camargo, P. (1999). Aesthetic management of extractions for implant site development: Delayed versus staged implant placement. *Practical Periodontics and Aesthetic Dentistry, 11*(5), 603–610. quiz 612.
110. Dahlin, C., et al. (1995). Treatment of fenestration and dehiscence bone defects around oral implants using the guided tissue regeneration technique: A prospective multicenter study. *International Journal of Oral & Maxillofacial Implants*, 10(3).
111. Newman, M. G., et al. (2011). *Carranza's clinical periodontology*. Philadelphia: Elsevier Health Sciences.
112. Bains, V. K., et al. (2015). Management of dehiscence and fenestration alveolar defects around incisors using platelet-rich fibrin: Report of two cases. *Journal of Interdisciplinary Dentistry, 5*(2), 92.
113. Rosen, P. S., & Reynolds, M. A. (2001). Guided bone regeneration for dehiscence and fenestration defects on implants using an absorbable polymer barrier. *Journal of Periodontology, 72*(2), 250–256.
114. Von Eiselsberg, F. (1901). Zur technik der uranoplastik. *Arch Klin Chir, 64*(64), 509–529.
115. Lexer, E. (1908). Die verwendung der freien knochenplastic nebst versuchen uber gelenkversteifung & gelenk-transplantation. *Arth Klin Chir, 86*, 939.
116. Drachter, R. (1914). Die Gaumenspalte und deren operative Behandlung. *Deutsche Zeitschrift für Chirurgie, 131*(1–2), 1–89.

117. Kang, N. H. (2017). Current methods for the treatment of alveolar cleft. *Archives of Plastic Surgery, 44*(3), 188.
118. Schmid, E. (1960). Die Osteoplastik bei Lippen-Kiefer-Gaumenspalten. *Langenbecks Archiv für klinische Chirurgie, 295*(1), 868–876.
119. Skoog, T. (1967). The use of periosteum and Surgicel® for bone restoration in congenital clefts of the maxilla: A clinical report and experimental investigation. *Scandinavian Journal of Plastic and Reconstructive Surgery, 1*(2), 113–130.
120. Coots, B. K. (2012). Alveolar bone grafting: Past, present, and new horizons. In *Seminars in plastic surgery, 26*(4), (pp. 178–183). Stuttgart, Germany, Thieme Medical Publishers.
121. Borba, A. M., et al. (2014). Predictors of complication for alveolar cleft bone graft. *British Journal of Oral and Maxillofacial Surgery, 52*(2), 174–178.
122. Bajaj, A. K., Wongworawat, A. A., & Punjabi, A. (2003). Management of alveolar clefts. *Journal of Craniofacial Surgery, 14*(6), 840–846.
123. Koh, K. S., et al. (2013). Treatment algorithm for bilateral alveolar cleft based on the position of the premaxilla and the width of the alveolar gap. *Journal of Plastic, Reconstructive & Aesthetic Surgery, 66*(9), 1212–1218.
124. Tanimoto, K., et al. (2013). Longitudinal changes in the height and location of bone bridge from autogenous iliac bone graft in patients with cleft lip and palate. *Open Journal of Stomatology, 3*(01), 58.
125. Wahaj, A., Hafeez, K., & Zafar, M. S. (2016). Role of bone graft materials for cleft lip and palate patients: A systematic review. *The Saudi Journal for Dental Research, 7*(1), 57–63.
126. Scott, J. K., Webb, R. M., & Flood, T. R. (2007). Premaxillary osteotomy and guided tissue regeneration in secondary bone grafting in children with bilateral cleft lip and palate. *The Cleft Palate-Craniofacial Journal, 44*(5), 469–475.
127. Murthy, A. S., & Lehman, J. A., Jr. (2006). Secondary alveolar bone grafting: An outcome analysis. *Canadian Journal of Plastic Surgery, 14*(3), 172–174.
128. Santiago, P. E., & Grayson, B. H. (2009). Role of the craniofacial orthodontist on the craniofacial and cleft lip and palate team. In *Seminars in orthodontics, 15*(4), (pp. 225–243). Philadelphia, USA, WB Saunders. Elsevier.
129. Duskova, M., et al. (2007). Bone reconstruction of the maxillary alveolus for subsequent insertion of a dental implant in patients with cleft lip and palate. *Journal of Craniofacial Surgery, 18*(3), 630–638.
130. Giudice, G., et al. (2007). The role of functional orthodontic stress on implants in residual alveolar cleft. *Plastic and Reconstructive Surgery, 119*(7), 2206–2217.
131. de Barros Ferreira Jr, S., et al. (2010). Survival of dental implants in the cleft area—A retrospective study. *The Cleft Palate-Craniofacial Journal, 47*(6), 586–590.
132. Bergland, O., Semb, G., & Abyholm, F. E. (1986). Elimination of the residual alveolar cleft by secondary bone grafting and subsequent orthodontic treatment. *The Cleft Palate Journal, 23*(3), 175–205.
133. Enemark, H., Sindet-Pedersen, S., & Bundgaard, M. (1987). Long-term results after secondary bone grafting of alveolar clefts. *Journal of Oral and Maxillofacial Surgery, 45*(11), 913–918.
134. Long, R. E., Jr., Spangler, B. E., & Yow, M. (1995). Cleft width and secondary alveolar bone graft success. *The Cleft Palate-Craniofacial Journal, 32*(5), 420–427.
135. Kindelan, J. D., Nashed, R. R., & Bromige, M. R. (1997). Radiographic assessment of secondary autogenous alveolar bone grafting in cleft lip and palate patients. *The Cleft Palate-Craniofacial Journal, 34*(3), 195–198.
136. Feichtinger, M., Mossböck, R., & Kärcher, H. (2007). Assessment of bone resorption after secondary alveolar bone grafting using three-dimensional computed tomography: A three-year study. *The Cleft Palate-Craniofacial Journal, 44*(2), 142–148.
137. Honma, K., et al. (1999). Computed tomographic evaluation of bone formation after secondary bone grafting of alveolar clefts. *Journal of Oral and Maxillofacial Surgery, 57*(10), 1209–1213.

138. Trindade, I. K., et al. (2005). Long-term radiographic assessment of secondary alveolar bone grafting outcomes in patients with alveolar clefts. *Oral Surgery, Oral Medicine, Oral Pathology, Oral Radiology and Endodontics, 100*(3), 271–277.
139. Tan, A. E., et al. (1996). Secondary alveolar bone grafting—Five-year periodontal and radiographic evaluation in 100 consecutive cases. *The Cleft Palate-Craniofacial Journal, 33*(6), 513–518.
140. Khojasteh, A., et al. (2016). The effect of a platelet-rich fibrin conduit on neurosensory recovery following inferior alveolar nerve lateralization: A preliminary clinical study. *International Journal of Oral and Maxillofacial Surgery, 45*(10), 1303–1308.
141. Khojasteh, A., et al. (2019). Buccal fat pad-derived stem cells with anorganic bovine bone mineral scaffold for augmentation of atrophic posterior mandible: An exploratory prospective clinical study. *Clinical Implant Dentistry and Related Research, 21*, 292.
142. Khojasteh, A., et al. (2018). Antibody-mediated osseous regeneration for bone tissue engineering in canine segmental defects. *BioMed Research International, 2018*, 1.
143. Behnia, H., et al. (2012). Repair of alveolar cleft defect with mesenchymal stem cells and platelet derived growth factors: A preliminary report. *Journal of Cranio-Maxillo-Facial Surgery, 40*(1), 2–7.

# Chapter 12
# Recent Advances in Nanodentistry

**Zhila Izadi, Hossein Derakhshankhah, Loghman Alaei, Emelia Karkazis, Samira Jafari, and Lobat Tayebi**

## 1 Introduction

To have general health and well-being, oral health is of great importance. A lot of genius drug delivery systems were developed for local treatment to prevent various diseases in the oral cavity. However, there are a few optimized systems and many therapeutic challenges that remain unsolved, including weak drug effectiveness and maintenance at targeted centers [1, 2].

Oral drug delivery is the most favored and helpful way of drug administration due to high patient compliance, cost-effectiveness, lowest amount of sterility limitations, adaptability in the designing of dosage form, and facility of generation [3]. In any case, the challenges confronted in oral drug delivery include low bioavailability of drug; this limitation is identified by three important factors—dissolution, permeability, and solubility [4–6].

The oral cavity (mouth) is discussed as the first section of the digestive tract, which includes various anatomical sectors: teeth, gingiva (gum) and their escort tissues, hard and soft palate, tongue, lips, and a mucosal membrane which lines the interior surface of the cheek [7]. The most known oral disorders among the world are dental caries, periodontal diseases, oral malignancies, and oral infections. In these cases, local therapy proposes numerous advantages over systemic drug administration, such as directly targeting the affected area while minimizing systemic side effects [8].

Z. Izadi · H. Derakhshankhah · L. Alaei · S. Jafari (✉)
Pharmaceutical Sciences Research Center, Health Institute, Kermanshah University of Medical Sciences, Kermanshah, Iran
e-mail: samira.jafari@kums.ac.ir

E. Karkazis · L. Tayebi (✉)
Marquette University School of Dentistry, Milwaukee, WI, USA
e-mail: lobat.tayebi@marquette.edu



L. Tayebi (ed.), *Applications of Biomedical Engineering in Dentistry*,
https://doi.org/10.1007/978-3-030-21583-5_12

One of the most routine factors influencing human lifestyle is inevitable caries formation and other tooth-related diseases, as they often lead to loss of teeth. A large ratio of research has been devoted to introduce control and preventive approaches [9]. It seems that a current challenge in the endodontic therapy field may be the elimination of the microbial infection, specifically the multispecies infections induced by aerobic and anaerobic bacteria [10–12]. It appears to be a suitable approach to treat and control dental infections by antibiotics or other active agents (such as nanoparticles to load in specific drug vehicle systems), even if the used delivery systems are less established when compared with other tissues. Based on the importance of biomedical delivery compartments, this study aims to provide a clear review on the amendments in drug delivery systems for dental applications [13, 14].

One can use the oral cavity as a limited drug delivery route in such cases like periodontitis and dental caries or for oral mucosal drug delivery—such as alveolar osteitis, analgesia, transmucosal systemic effect, or delivery of new biotechnological products like proteins and peptides. The present chapter provides an overview of dental physiology, prevalent dental diseases, and some nano-/bio dental materials and drug delivery systems corresponding to the oral cavity [15].

Different diseases affecting the orodental region, along with conventional as well as new and emerging drug delivery and technologies that improve local drug therapy, are presented in this chapter. Various types of drug delivery, along with their important clinical views, will be discussed. This chapter will offer the reader with a general and inspiring landscape on recent and promising aspects of innovation in oral drug delivery.

Nanotechnology is a field that studies the matter at the levels of molecule and atom, which has evolved the territory of dentistry as "nanodentistry" [16, 17].

Nanodentistry, as a term and a field, was coined in the twentieth century. Parallel to advancement of nanomedicine, dentistry commenced evolving in the field of nanotechnology, too. It seems that the nanotechnology field will influence the fields of diagnosis, surgery, and restorative dentistry. These promising new tools—like nanorobotics, nanodiagnosis, nanomaterials, nanosurgery, and nanodrugs—will highly impact clinical dentistry in the future [16–19].

The field of nanotechnology provides the diagnosis and treatment of oral cancer. Nanotechnology identifies the biomarkers of tumor cells and thus discovers them earlier, increasing the sensitivity of the test [20]. Many nanomaterials exist that can be utilized for restoration and/or prevention of decayed, carious, missing, or fractured teeth. Current progress in nanomaterials has introduced nanocomposites, nanoimpression, and nanoceramic in the area of clinical dentistry [17, 19, 21].

Although many ideas have been proposed for nanodentistry, most of them are not applicable because of various difficulties like designing challenges, medical challenges, social challenges, and so on. It is difficult to place and assemble the molecular scale part in a precise manner [21]. Manipulating the functions of some nanorobots simultaneously is also challenging. Nanomaterials can also be pyrogenic, so it is also an obstacle to produce biocapable nanomaterials. Social concerns, such as ethics and public acceptance, can be obstacles as well [16, 18].

Nanodentistry is an interdisciplinary research area that discusses the new nanomaterials and device applications in all the areas of human functionality [22]. Taking into account the advances in nanotechnology, nanomaterials and nanorobots show great attraction [23]. Though there is long-term research activity for this promising field, the clinical results have a strong tendency to highly promote the diagnosis and treatment approach planning for improving esthetics in the dental field. However, more research and trials are needed for the application of nanotechnology in oral tract and dental care. Nanodentistry will maintain comprehensive oral health by linking nanomaterials and biotechnology, including tissue engineering and dental nanorobotics. Although it is at an early stage, it has made a sufficient clinical and commercial effect [24].

## 2 Nanodentistry

Nanotechnology is an interesting branch in which all disciplines of natural sciences meet at nanoscale; for instance, physical forces merge with biologic sciences, engineering, organic/inorganic chemistry, materials science, and computational means, which are all highly linked. This inherent interdisciplinary nature devotes wide potency for multidisciplinary functions [5, 14, 20].

Recent developments in dental field research have made treatment routes fast, precise, safe, and less painful in recent years. Newborn techniques—such as nanotechnology, dental implants, cosmetic surgery, laser application, and digital dentistry—have had remarkable influence on dental treatment and restoration time [25, 26]. In the medicine research area, nanotechnology has been integrated to diagnose, prevent, and treat diseases. The following sections of the chapter address the recent developments in this integrative field that bridges nanotechnology and dentistry, nano-/biomaterials in oral health research, and some usages of nano-/biomaterials in this field [22, 27]. Oral medicine is an evolving field of dentistry, in which its multidisciplinary approaches have led to advancement of other areas in prevention, diagnostics, and therapeutics [28, 29].

Nanotechnology concerns the study of materials at molecular and atomic scale, which has evolved the field of dentistry, namely nanodentistry. This newly born scope is established on four approaches (biomimetics, functional, top-down, and bottom-up) and can be defined as a promising discipline that provides nanotechnology based on next-generation devices and tools for use in oral health care [16, 17, 19].

### *2.1 The Bottom-Up Approach*

The bottom-up approach includes producing nanostructures and devices by arranging atom by atom. This approach involves self-assembly, using chemical or physical forces functioning at nanoscale to assemble smaller blocks to form larger structures.

Some instances of bottom-up path include synthesis of chemical materials, self-assembly, and molecular production. In other words, this approach is similar to building—taking many blocks and lining them together to fabricate the ultimate structure. Another tangible example from nature is that of body cells, which utilize enzymes to generate DNA by various components and assemble them to produce the final superstructure. Bottom-up approach fields in nanodentistry confine polymerization, precipitation, and micellar compartments [30, 31].

## 2.2 *The Top-Down Approach*

The top-down approach (that in some cases is recognized as the term decompose and also used as a synonym to stepwise design) refers to the breaking down of a collection to understand its components in a reverse engineering mode. In this approach, an original view of the system is figured out and characterized, but not in detail. Then, each subsystem component is studied in greater detail, sometimes in many additional sublevels, until the full specification is reached to elementary blocks. In this approach, synthesis of the particles is occurring in a routine manner and then made smaller by grinding or milling. Among all, the most successful industry that uses the top-down approach is the electronics industry [31]. Some applications of top-down and bottom-up approaches are summarized in Table 12.1.

## 2.3 *In the Functional Approach*

In the functional approach, the final goal is to create favored functionality components, regardless of the routine process. These desired properties might be electronic in the case of molecular scale electronics or materials with mechanical properties, like synthesized molecular motors.

**Table 12.1** Some applications based on top-down and bottom-up approaches [18, 30, 32–34]

| Top-down approach | Bottom-up approach |
|---|---|
| Nanomaterials for anesthesia | Nanocomposites |
| Major particles for tooth repair | Nanolight treatment glasses as ionomer restorative |
| Particles for repositioning tooth | Impression materials |
| Hypersensitive cure | Nanocomposite denture teeth |
| Dental sturdiness and apparent features | Nanosolution |
| Dental robots | Nanoencapsulation |
| Cancer diagnostic tools | Applying the laser plasma for periodontia |
| Therapeutic aid in oral disorders | Prosthetic implant |
| | Nanoneedles |
| | Materials for bone replacement |

### *2.4 The Biomimetic Approach*

The biomimetic approach is also called bionics. This name comes from the properties, which mimic the biological systems to form nanoscale devices. This approach refers to the inspiration and application of concepts from nature for generating new compositions, tools, and systems. The technology is still at its beginning stages and has not yet reached commercialization [35].

## 3 Nano-/Bio Dental Materials

Medical application of nano-/biomaterials in dentistry has been the focus of research laboratories worldwide [36]. Nowadays, nanotechnology is conducting dental materials industry to important growth areas. It seems that the prevalence of nanotechnology in dentistry answers the mysteries or challenges concerning routine materials, because they have the potential to mimic surface and interface properties of biological tissues [16, 18, 19]. Similar to nanomedicine, nanotechnology used in dentistry is expected to possible nearly perfect oral health by using nanomaterials and biotechnologies, such as tissue engineering and different technologies [37].

Nanotechnology, as a drastic field, has the power to control the individual particles in the nanometer scale. Some of these results are to a large extent relevant and remain impactful to human life. Although over the last few decades the fields of regenerative medicine and tissue engineering have gained a lot, still a large amount of research is required to innovate new materials in order to overcome the defects of existing biomaterials [5, 14, 20].

Orthodontic nanomaterials have come into practice widely, due to the industrialization process of nanotechnology and the patients having the opportunity to come into contact with them. These materials have resulted in remarkable improvements in medical treatments and have driven the creation of multiple routine dental materials. Some principal applications of nanomaterials in the field of dentistry are discussed in this section, and a summary of these functions is illustrated in Table 12.2.

## 4 Nano-/Biomaterials as Dental Drug Carriers

Drug carrier considerations include approaches, formulations, techniques, and systems for transporting pharmaceutical compounds in the human body as needed to safely reach therapeutic effect. This concept has been merged with dosage form and method of administration. The term "target drug delivery system" was coined by Ehrlich, who proposed the term "magic bullet" in 1906. The main difficulty in target drug delivery carriers was based on three important factors: finding the target of the disease, identifying the drug that will sufficiently cure the disease, and selecting

Table 12.2 Summary of some common nanomaterials in dentistry field and their characteristics

| Major applications | Nanomaterial type | Particle size | Significant characteristics | References |
|---|---|---|---|---|
| Composite resins | Nano-ZnO | 125 nm | Better antibacterial and mechanical properties | [25] |
| | Nanosilica | 7 nm<br>70 nm | Better mechanical properties | [38, 39] |
| | Nano-Ca3$(PO_4)_2$ and $CaF_2$ | 112 nm<br>53 nm | Better stress-bearing capabilities and the inhibition of caries | [40] |
| | Nano-$TiO_2$ | <20 nm | Improved microhardness and flexural strength | [41] |
| Dental adhesives | Nano-HAp | 20–70 nm | Better bonding strength to dentin | [42] |
| | Nanosilver and calcium phosphate | <10 nm<br>112 nm | Improved antibacterial properties | [43] |
| | Nanosilica | 7 nm | High mechanical strength and good thermostability | [44, 45] |
| Root canal fillings | Nano-HAp | – | Better osteogenesis and improved bacteriostatic and antibacterial effects | [46, 47] |
| Bone repair materials | Nano-HAp | 100 nm<br>20 nm<br>3 nm | Guiding the regeneration of periodontal and bone tissue | [48–50] |
| Bioceramics | Nano-$ZrO_2$/HAp composite | 70–90 nm/<br>500–1000 nm | Guiding bone reconstruction | [51] |
| | Nano-$ZrO_2$/$Al_2O_3$ | – | Better resistance to crack propagation | [52] |
| | Nanosilver | 10 nm | Increased fracture toughness and Vickers hardness | [53] |
| Silicone elastomer material | Nano-Ti-, Zn-, Ceoxide | 30–40 nm<br>20 nm<br>50 nm | Improved mechanical properties | [54] |
| Denture base materials | Nanosilver | 10–20 nm | Better antifungal properties and biocompatibility | [55] |
| Coating materials for dental implants | Nanoporous alumina | 20–200 nm | Good cell adhesion and no adverse effect on cell activity | [56] |
| | Nano-zirconia/calcium phosphate | 360 nm/151 nm | High bioactivity potential and good mechanical stability | [57] |
| | Nano-ZnO | 10–100 nm | Better antimicrobial and biocompatible properties | [58] |
| | Nano-HAp | – | Achieving rapid osseointegration | [59] |

(continued)

**Table 12.2** (continued)

| Major applications | Nanomaterial type | Particle size | Significant characteristics | References |
|---|---|---|---|---|
| Drug delivery | Nanosilica | 150 nm | Sustained and controlled release of anticancer drugs (as drug carriers) | [60] |
| | Polymeric NPs (vitamin e TPGS) | 300–1000 nm | Controlled release of anticancer drugs (as drug carriers) | [27] |
| Tumor imaging | Superparamagnetic iron oxide NPs | 82 ± 4.4 nm | Good superparamagnetic and optical properties | [61] |

suitable target mediums transport the drug in a stable shape while preventing other interactions and harm to the healthy tissues.

The delivery of targeted particles has the potential to transport high-density drug molecules while expressing ligands on the surface of the particle at the same time. Nanomedicine is the field of development and use of nanotechnology in the area of medicine to block, detect, and treat diseases at the cellular and molecular level. Nanoproducts delivered through target drug delivery carriers use the pathophysiological and anatomical variances within the defected tissue to differentiate it from healthy tissues to get site-specific targeted drug delivery. Thus, the goal of this section is to show a brief landscape of the targeted drug delivery system using nanoparticles and nanovectors for different treatment purposes in dentistry.

## 4.1 *Various Delivery Vehicles*

Nanoparticles are used as potent carriers along with targeting ligands for the target drug. These materials have multiple advantages over larger systems because of their submicron size. The principal characteristics of these systems are that they should be biodegradable, biocompatible, toxic-free, and physicochemically durable. Drug release should be even, scheduled, predictable, and without any side effect to the main drug [62, 63]. The main advantages of nanoparticle drug delivery carriers are their small size, which makes them a suitable candidate to be extravasated through blood vessels and tissues, especially in tumors. Targeted drugs can be designed to avoid first-pass metabolism. Moreover, they may also show properties like optical and electrical characteristics. These features make it possible to chase and localize the drug intracellularly. However, it has its disadvantages, such as toxicity, requiring skill to administer, and limited drug durability. A variety of submicron colloidal nanosystems of size <1 μm are included. They may have various structures and compositions like inorganic, liposome, or polymer-based colloidal systems, which have acted as effective drug carriers for several decades [63, 64].

### 4.1.1 Liposomes

Liposomes are structures composed of two components—amphiphilic phospholipids and cholesterol in bilayers that confine an aqueous interior. Liposomes as a reservoir for target drug delivery were first introduced by Gregoriadis [65]. These bodies have provided promising results in improving therapeutic benefits, diminishing side effects, and increasing patient relief, as they mimic the biologic membrane. They can also be designed as bio-adhesives that are retained by the enamel, increasing the exposure time and residence in the oral cavity [28, 29]. They break down into smaller structures that can surround hydrophilic drugs in the aqueous interior or hydrophobic drugs in the bilayer. There are two methods for encapsulation, namely, by the pH gradient and ammonium sulfate method. Adding polyethylene glycol (PEG) to the lipid surface enhances its surface properties via functioning as an obstacle to avoid interaction with the plasma proteins, thereby retarding detection by the reticuloendothelial system (RES). This results in an increased circulation time of the liposomes. Phosphatidylcholine-based liposomes are used to target bacterial biofilms, whereas succinylated concanvalin A (conA) liposomes are targeted for delivery of triclosan to the biofilm of *Staphylococcus epidermidis* and *Proteus vulgaris*. However, application of liposomes in target drug delivery displays the following disadvantages: low control over drug release, poor encapsulation yield, and poor stability during encapsulation [66].

### 4.1.2 Solid Biodegradable Nanoparticles

Solid biodegradable nanoparticles are another kind of carriers that are widely seen because they have different polymer compositions and morphologies than liposomes, which can sufficiently control release features over a long period of time. These families of materials include aliphatic polyesters, specifically hydrophobic polylactic acid, hydrophilic polyglycolic acid, and their copolymers, such as polylactide-co-glycolide. These materials have been utilized for various clinical applications for over three decades and are regarded as safe to use in human body [64].

### 4.1.3 Micelles

Micelles are another group of polymers, which are composed of lipids and have spherical structure, but lack a lipid bilayer or an inner hole. Their typical size is about 10–80 nm, and they can transport various drugs with better longevity, low circulation time, and stability. They have better penetration and flexibility to enter the target sites because of their size, which allows them to enhance the drug effect on the target site. These drug delivery elements target cancer cells and are presumed to have magnetic resource imaging (MRI) contrast characteristics [67].

#### 4.1.4 Dendrimers

Dendrimers are molecules that possess three-dimensional, multi-branched structures. They are well-defined, unimolecular, monodisperse materials ranging from 1 to 10 nm in size. These structures, due to their branching pattern, offer a larger surface area for drug binding. Dendrimers are the best way to deliver both water-soluble and insoluble drugs [65, 68]. Multifunctional types of them are synthetically formulated in conjugation with fluorescein isothiocyanate used for imaging and folic acid for targeting cancer cells, which overexpress folate receptors and paclitaxel as a chemotherapeutic drug [69].

#### 4.1.5 Polymers

Polymeric nanoparticles can deliver low-molecular-weight drugs, macromolecular proteins, and genes. Unlike liposomes, these nanoparticles show less toxicity, high durability, higher loading capacity for water-soluble drugs with sustained release of drugs, and many physicochemical properties [65, 70]. Due to their slow clearance by RES, their use as biodegradable nanoparticles is rapidly increased; the dosage of the drugs has been decreased due to enhanced plasma half-life. Polyketals are biocompatible, hydrophobic polymers and have been synthesized recently for use as biodegradable ketal linkages. This linkages aid in creating nanoparticles to encapsulate and enrich hydrophobic drugs or proteins [71]. PEG is a hydrophilic polymer used to form a stealth layer to minimize the nonspecific enrichment of the drug. This advantage leads to more stability of the nanoparticles and targeting of the site [70, 72].

#### 4.1.6 Carbon Nanotubes

Carbon nanotubes are single or multiple sheets produced from graphene and rolled into a cylinder. They can pass into living cells without causing any cell death or defect to their size or shape. Although these nanoparticles show high potential in nanodrug delivery, their safety remains obscure because of needle-like fiber shape and toxicity [26, 65].

#### 4.1.7 Gold Nanoparticles

Gold nanoparticles can be synthesized in a range of sizes. They are biocompatible, easy functionable, highly dispersed, and able to conjugate with other molecules. Their high surface area/volume index, inert entity, and small size allow their use extensively as delivery systems [73]. Studies have addressed that monodisperse spheres can be synthesized using reducing agents, like citrate, by acting on some given gold salts, such as tetrachloraurate [74].

### 4.1.8 Nanodiamonds

Nanodiamonds are allotropes of carbon with a size of about 2–8 nm. These type of nanoparticles possess functional groups, which can attach a wide spectrum of compounds, such as chemotherapy agents and other drugs [75]. They possess unique physical characteristics like small size, less corrosion, high mechanically stable, and biocompatibility and function as biomarkers and biosensors [76]. Recently, these materials have been widely used to collect proteins and deliver drugs to the target areas. For example, when they are bound to doxorubicin and encapsulated into polymeric microfilms, they can be used to sustain release of drugs [65, 75] [76]. They can be formulated into dental materials and used as a filling or veneer, and their hardness makes them a good candidate for implant and cutting tools formation. When dry, nanodiamonds provide favorable appearance, such as natural enamel, and it is believed to treat gum illness when utilized as toothpaste [30].

### 4.1.9 Nanogel

Nanogel is a novel biocompatible polymer with a core-shell formulation. Nanogel nanoparticles are of submicron range size and have a gel-like appearance that contains colloidal aggregates, which come from hydrophilic polymers. Nanogels have both nanoparticle and hydrogel advantages and show a high potential to deliver genes and proteins [32].

## 5 Nano-/Biomaterials as Dental Filling Agents

In dental applications, fillers are the additives in solid form with various polymer composition and structure. These additives are comprised frequently of inorganic materials and partly organic material [31]. In recent decades, with advent nanotechnology incorporated into the medical field—particularly dentistry, considerable endeavors have been demonstrated for design of innovative promising dental restorative structures, for instance, nanofillers [33]. Nanofillers are nanosized reinforcement particles blended with resins of various properties, rather than traditional fillers that necessitate a shift from a top-down to a bottom-up construction methodology, which are usually blended with resins to create nano-filled resin composites [34].

Considering the excellent features of nanomaterials, these structures are currently considered as novel fillers to improve the mechanical and esthetic properties of polymer composites in dentistry. Nanofillers that possess greater aspect ratio—the ratio of largest to smallest dimension—depict an appropriate reinforcement for nanocomposites fabrication. To date, diverse materials with organic and inorganic nature are utilized for the preparation of nanofillers; silica, titanium dioxide, calcium carbonate, and polyhedral oligomeric silsesquioxane are examples of inorganic materials [35]. Coir nanofiller, carbon black, and cellulosic nanofiller can also be utilized as inorganic fillers [77].

Generally, nanofillers are able to improve/adjust the variable properties of the materials into which they are incorporated, like fire-retardant, optical or electrical, mechanical, as well as thermal properties, occasionally in synergy with conventional fillers. From the prevalent nanofillers in nanocomposites, nanoclays, nanooxides, and carbon nanotubes are some examples [78, 79].

## 6 Nano-/Biomaterials as Dental Adhesive Agents

Dental adhesives are systems that consist of monomers with hydrophilic and hydrophobic groups, creating the resin dental substrate interaction. Hydrophilic groups provide an appropriate wettability to dental hard tissues, whereas the presence of hydrophobic groups in adhesive systems leads to interaction and copolymerization with the restorative materials [80]. Curing initiators, inhibitors or stabilizers, solvents, and inorganic fillers are major chemical components of dental adhesives. Overall, considering the anatomy of the tooth is a pivotal issue in design of dental adhesives; particularly, composition and structure of enamel and dentin are requisite parameters for examination of their influence on adhesive bonds [81]. Indeed, enamel is composed of hydroxyapatite (HAp), as a hard solid crystalline structure, together with water and organic materials. In comparison with enamel, dentin has low intermolecular forces and low energy surfaces. This humid layer, which lies immediately underneath the enamel, is a component similar to enamel [82].

Resin composites, as esthetic components in dentistry, are being progressively employed as dental restorations owing to significant improvements in their properties and performance. Nevertheless, composites possess a tendency for accumulation of biofilm in vivo, which could lead to production of acids and subsequently cause dental caries. The principal reason for restoration fracture is recurrent caries and, therefore, for 50–70% of all operative work, it should be conducted for replacement of the failed restorations. To circumvent this drawback, several research groups designed antibacterial resins based on nanostructures. In recent research, to treat dental caries, antibacterial resins and silver (Ag) filler particles were used as an appropriate approach for management of caries [83]. It is well documented that nanoparticles of Ag are effective for antibacterial applications [84]. Another study introduced a new alternate method for inhibiting the caries, in which researchers applied center-filled calcium phosphate (CaP) composite particles that can release Ca and P ions and remineralize tooth lesions. Recently, calcium phosphate nanoparticles were fabricated using a spray-drying method. Some new nanocomposites were designed, which contain amorphous CaP. These nanoparticles can release calcium and phosphate ions in the same way as traditional calcium phosphate composites. Moreover, they possess higher mechanical properties for loading tooth restorations [85].

## 7 Nano-/Biomaterials as Dental Implants

When teeth are lost, endoosseus oral implants are—from the clinical point of view—"the last stand" of bite reconstruction. The idea of using Ti implants in dentistry began in the early 1980s and was based on Brennemark's definition of osseointegration, which explained the direct contact of a living bone with functionally loaded oral implants [86]. From that moment, implant dentistry has evolved, and the conceptions of treatment protocols have changed. One thing that remained the same was the struggle to improve implant–bone interconnection quality. Along with views on surface modifications, the classic approach to implant surface treatment—"the rougher-the better"—was rejected in the early 2000s. This was based on clinical observations that showed that a micro-rough surface, despite better stability in the beginning, may initiate subsequent bone osteolysis and favor biofilm formation and infection development, which is commonly known as "periimplantitis" [87, 88].

Along with the evolution of nanodentistry, the views on implant surface modification followed the general rule of mimicking nature. It was proposed that the implant surface may imitate the bone-like structure and properties at the nanoscale level, as bone is nothing more like a biological nanocomposite. Dental implants usually consist of three independently manufactured parts: intraosseous screw, transmucosal abutment, and prosthetic crown [89].

Among all dental sciences, oral implantology represents the fastest developing area and applies to all implant components, as well as surgical instruments. An approach to oral implants, with regard to their intraosseous portion, is focused on osseointegration improvement. The process of implant connection with bone consists of two phases: primary interlock corresponds to the mechanical anchorage and mostly macro design of implants, such as the screw shape of threads geometry. The second anchorage relies on bone remodeling at the implant interface and the creation of biological bonding. This process is related to surface micro-nano topography, chemical composition, wettability, and roughness which, taken together, has an impact on the biochemistry and dynamics of bone formation de novo [90, 91].

Clinically, a decrease in implant stability can be observed between the primary mechanical and secondary biological anchorage as a natural consequence of biological remodeling of bone tissue following surgical injury (osteotomy preparation, implant insertion, inflammatory response). Good modification of the surface from macro to nanoscale may promote the process of implant healing [92]. There are a lot of ways for modifying the surface in order to roughen it, based on direct surface tailoring (e.g., etching, sandblasting) and/or making functions (bio-glass coatings or polymers, peptides, etc.), or combinations of these techniques to commercially available implants to achieve roughness at the micro level. However, this technique could decrease surface hardness and, moreover, cause a loss of superficial material layer that damages screw threads, possibly negatively affecting proper implant anchorage to bone. Other techniques that provide modifications at the microscale could result in coating delamination, surface contamination with hydrocarbons (re-hydrophobization of the surface), and many others, which are elucidated in the detail in the recent work of Durracio et al. [93, 94].

As long as surface properties have a key role in long-term stability of bone tissues, dental implants are increasingly used as nanotechnology tools for surface modifications. To reach this purpose, it is necessary for implants to have direct contact with bone. This direct contact makes good biomechanical anchoring, rather than encapsulation via fibrous tissues [91]. The surface roughness of bone is approximately near 100 nm, and this nanoscale data is important to the surface of implants, as the proliferation of osteoblast is induced via production of nanosized particles on the surface of implants [95, 96]. Roughening the implant surface at the nanoscale level is important for the optimum cellular reaction that takes place in the tissue and stimulates merging of the implant into the bone [97, 98].

Using nanotechnology methods, some titanium implants were fabricated, then their surface was coated with calcium and inserted into rabbit tibias. Finally, their impact on osteogenesis was measured. As a result, the responsiveness of the bone around the implant was increased due to the insertion of the nanostructured calcium coat [99]. In vitro research on these materials illustrates that the most effective factor on osteogenic cells is the topography of the implant, and this nanosized surface enhances the surface area and the adhesion of osteoblastic cells. This enhanced surface provides an increased surface area that facilitates the reaction with biologic environment [99–101]. Recent nanostructured implant coatings are as follows:

1. *Nanostructured Diamond*: This coating type presents very high hardness, improved toughness over common microcrystalline diamond, low friction, and good adhesion to titanium alloys [102].
2. *Nanostructured Coatings of HA*: This type of coating material is applied to amend the favored mechanical characteristics and to enrich surface reactivity and has shown increment of osteoblast adhesion, proliferation, and mineralization [56, 90, 103].
3. *Metalloceramic-Based Nanostructured Coatings*: These coatings cover a vast range from nanocrystalline metallic bond at the interface to hard ceramic bond on the surface.

Nanostructured ceramics, carbon fibers, polymers, metals, and composites enhance osteoblast adhesion and calcium/phosphate mineral deposition.

Some researchers have shown that nanophase ZnO and $TiO_2$ may lower *Staphylococcus epidermidis* adhesion and intensify the osteoblast functions that are vital to elevate the effectiveness of orthopedic implants [91, 104, 105].

# 8 Nanodiagnosis in Dentistry

Nanodiagnosis technology uses nanodevices and nanosystems to detect disease in early stages at the cellular and molecular level. The development of nanoscale diagnostic methods on human fluids or tissue samples could increase efficiency of these methods. Nanodiagnosis devices will be able to detect and identify the early presence of diseases, such as tumor cells and toxic molecules, and quantify them inside the body. In cancer diagnosis, the advantages of this technology include being a less invasive and less uncomfortable method for identifying and measuring disease indicators, which will be applied in diagnosis as well as in monitoring recurrence or metastasis and types and behaviors of malignancies [106]. Here, some of the techniques used in nanodiagnosis are described briefly (Fig. 12.1).

Nanopores: Nanopores are a pore of tiny and nanometer size that allows DNA sequencing to pass more efficiently. Researchers can use this technology to decode coded information, including errors in a code known as cancer [107].

**Nanotubes:** hese are carbon rods that can help detect and pinpoint the presence of altered genes and their exact location. From this category, the quantum dots may help to identify DNA changes associated with cancer and designed quantum dots that match with altered genes in sequences of DNA responsible for disease [35]. The quantum dots are excited with light, then they emit their characteristic bar codes and visible cancer-associated DNA sequences [108].

**Nanoscale Cantilevers:** These flexible beams can be designed to bind to cancer-related molecules. They bind to altered DNA sequences or proteins in certain types of cancer and can provide rapid and sensitive detection of cancer-related molecules [109].

**Nanoelectromechanical Systems (NEMS):** NEMS-based biosensors based on nanotechnology that show a specific sensitivity to detect single-molecule levels are under development. These systems convert biochemical signals into electrical signals, monitoring the health status, disease progression, and result of treatment by noninvasive means [16, 110].

**Laboratory-on-a-Chip (LOC):** These are devices that integrate several laboratories on a single chip. This technology deals with a very low volume—less than

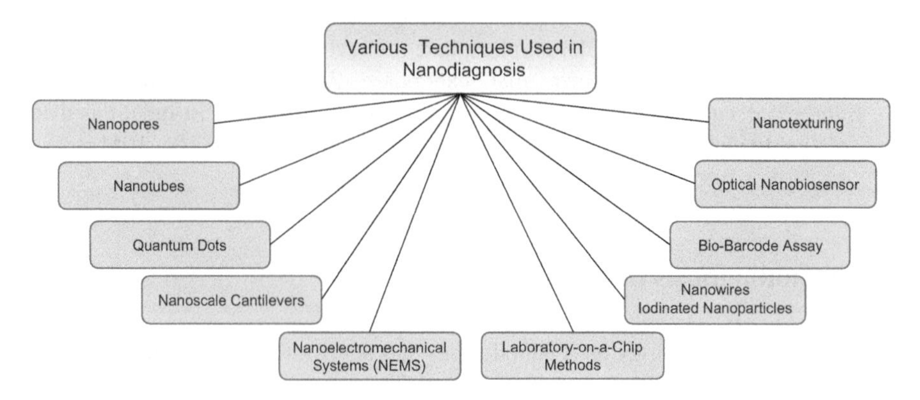


**Fig. 12.1** Some of the techniques used in nanodiagnosis

picoliters—of fluid. The basis of these assays is the use of chemical sensitivities that are embedded in silicon sheets in fluids and are capable of optical detection. The special advantage of LOC devices is performing complex tests with small sample size, short-time analysis, and reduction in reactive costs [111, 112].

**Oral Fluid Nanosensor Test (OFNASET):** This technology is a combination of self-assembled monolayers (SAM), microfluidics, and enzymatic amplification to identify salivary biomarkers for oral cancer. The high specificity and sensitivity of *OFNASET* technology was demonstrated in the detection of salivary proteomic and mRNA biomarkers in oral cancer.

**Optical Nanobiosensor:** An important feature of nanobiosensor is a unique fiberoptics-based tool that provides the analysis of intracellular components with the least invasion. For example, cytochrome C, an important protein involved in the production of cellular energy and in apoptosis, can be analyzed through optical nanobiosensor [113].

**Nanotexturing:** Physicochemical-modified surfaces under nanoscale allow the analysis of low-molecular-weight proteins from body fluids and other biologic samples. This will result in separation based on size, selective adsorption of proteins, and lead enhancement of specific regions of the proteins [110].

**Bio-Barcode Assay (BCA):** This technique was developed by a magnetic probe for specific detection of a target molecule using a monoclonal antibody or complementary oligonucleotide. Target-specific gold nanoparticles can be used to capture the target, distinguishing it and amplifying the signal and, thus, be detected using the scanometric method [110].

## 9 Clinical Applications of Nano-/Bio Dental Materials

Nanodentistry has been recognized as a very promising field, through which oral health care could be pulled to an unprecedented height via the utilization of various components of nanotechnology, nanomaterials, tissue engineering, and dental nanorobots. Applications of nanotechnology in dentistry are as follows.

### *9.1 Local Anesthesia*

In virtue of nanodentistry, a colloidal suspension composed of a myriad of active analgesic micron-sized dental robots is infused into the patient's gingiva. Next, these wandering nanorobots gain access to the pulp through the gingival sulcus, lamina propria, and dentinal tubules. Afterward, the dentist may control the analgesic dental robots to suppress all sensitivity in the tooth requiring treatment. When treatment of a specific tooth is completed, all sensations can be promptly recovered because nanorobots deny the control of nerve signals, having received the orders from the dentist, and leave from same path applied for entry [114].

### *9.2 Hypersensitivity Cure*

Any change in the hydrodynamic pressure transmitted to the pulp is most liable to bring about dentin hypersensitivity. This hypothesis is due to the fact that dentinal tubules and tubules with diameter twice as big as non-sensitive teeth are eight times more numerous on the surface than non-sensitive teeth. In the foreseeable future, this complaint of patients will be curbed by dental nanorobots, which can selectively occlude tubules by native biological materials [114].

### *9.3 Diagnosis of Oral Cancer*

- *Cantilever Array Sensors*: Based on ultrasensitive mass detection technology: picogram, bacterium; femtogram, virus; and attogram, DNA.
- *Nanoelectromechanical Systems (NEMS)*: Nanotechnology-based NEMS biosensors showing excellent sensitivity and specificity for analyte detection down to single-molecule levels are being developed. They can transform (bio)chemical to electrical signals.
- *Multiplexing Modality*: Sensing good numbers of diverse biomolecules at a time [114].
- *Oral Fluid NanoSensor Test (OFNASET)*: OFNASET technology is applied for multiplex detection of salivary biomarkers for early oral cancer diagnosis. It has been confirmed that the combination of two salivary proteomic biomarkers (thioredoxin and IL-8) and four salivary mRNA biomarkers (SAT, ODZ, IL-8, and IL-1b) can diagnose oral cancer with noticeable selectivity and sensitivity [18].
- *Optical Nanobiosensor*: Low invasive analysis of intracellular components, such as cytochrome c, a momentous protein in the process of producing cellular energy and the protein engaged in apoptosis, has become possible by the utilization of nanobiosensor, a sole fiber optics-based tool [110].

### *9.4 Treatment of Oral Cancer*

- *Nanomaterials for Brachytherapy*: BrachySilTM (Sivida, Australia) delivers 32P, clinical trial. Drug delivery across the blood-brain barrier. More effective therapy of brain tumors, Alzheimer's and Parkinson's are in development.

- *Nanovectors for Gene Therapy*: Non-viral gene delivery systems.
- *Photodynamic Therapy*: Hydrophobic porphyrins are molecules that inherently attract the photodynamic therapy (PDT) of solid tumors or ocular vascularization disorders [115].

## *9.5 Dental Durability, Appearance, and Dentifrobots*

The appearance and strength of the tooth may be intensified by substituting upper enamel layers with pure sapphire and diamond. This approach makes them more break safe as nanostructured materials. This could include entrenched carbon nanotube toothpaste or mouthwash that can be applied to deliver nanorobotic dentifrice. This would possess an inbuilt programmer to avoid the occlusal region. Their function would be similar to common dentifrices, yet the approach would be thoroughly diverse, as they would be infinitesimal [1–10 micron] mechanical devices, creeping at a speed of 1–10 microns/sec, performing by metabolizing trapped organic matter into safe and scentless vapors, and debriding calculus incessantly. Regarding the safety, if swallowed accidentally, they would be inactivated. Dentifrobots are programmed to recognize and demolish pathogenic bacteria dwelling in the plaque and the oral cavity while sparing around 500 species of safe oral microflora. Hence, by killing bacteria, dentifrobots would provide a blockade against halitosis on the grounds that bacterial putrefaction is the central metabolic process engaged in oral malodor [116]. With the assistance of this type of daily dental care available from an early age, common tooth decay and gingival disease will be eradicated.

## *9.6 Orthodontic Treatment*

Orthodontic nanorobots could directly impact the periodontal tissues, providing the chance for quick and painless tooth straightening, revolving, and vertical repositioning within minutes to hours. This is in contrast with the commonly used molar uprighting methods, which require weeks or even months to be completed [114].

## *9.7 Tooth Repair*

Nanodental methods for major tooth repair may thrive via several steps of technological progress: at first, taking modest steps of genetic engineering, tissue engineering, and regeneration and then making a great leap of development of whole new teeth in vitro and their installation [117].

## 9.8 Dentition Renaturalization

Esthetic dentistry would go into a fully novel era with the addition of dentition renaturalization procedures to the common dental practice armamentarium. Demand would observe an abrupt outburst for full coronal renaturalization procedures, in which all of the fillings, crowns, and other twentieth-century treatment methods will be substituted with the affected teeth remanufactured to become exactly similar to original teeth [118].

## 9.9 Nanocomposites

Corporation of nanoproducts has successfully produced non-agglomerated discrete NPs, which are homogeneously dispersed in resins or coatings to form nanocomposites. The nanofiller applied encompasses an aluminosilicate powder possessing a mean size for the particles about 80 nm and a 1:4 M proportion of alumina to silica and an index of refraction near 1.508. Merits have higher hardness, higher flexural strength, higher modulus of elasticity and translucency, 50% abatement in filling shrinkage, and adequate handling features [119].

***Trade Name:*** Filtek O Supreme Universal Restorative Pure Nano O

## 9.10 Nanosolution

Nanosolutions generate special and distributable NPs, which are able to be utilized in bonding agents. This guarantees both the homogeneousness and adhesive sticking well mixed [119].

***Trade Name:*** Adper O Single Bond Plus Adhesive Single Bond

## 9.11 Impression Materials

Nanomaterials that are used as fillers are incorporated in vinylpolysiloxanes, shaping a special expansion of siloxane impression materials. The material has more stream, improved hydrophilic virtues, and intensified detail accuracy [114].

***Business Name:*** Nanotech Elite H-D

## *9.12 Nanoencapsulation*

Latest evolution in the field of targeted release systems is attributed to SWRI [South West Research Institute], which has developed nanocapsules—such as novel vaccines, antibiotics, and drug delivery—with curtailed side effects. Among these series of evolutions, the most recent has come from Osaka University (Japan), which has improved targeted delivery of genes and drugs to the human liver in 2003. In this research, designed Hepatitis B virus encapsulated particles used to produce NPs showing a peptide momentous for liver-selective entry by the virus in humans. In the future, specialized NPs may be designed to reach oral texture corresponding to the cells originated from the periodontium [119].

## *9.13 Other Products of SWRI*

(a) Medical supplements for fast healing:
    - Biodegradable nanofibers will act as delivery platform for hemostasis.
    - Function of silk nanofibers in wound dressings is still under investigation.
    - Nanocrystalline silver particles with antimicrobial virtues on wound dressings [ActicoatTM, UK].

(b) Protective clothing and filtration masks using antipathogenic nanoemulsions and NPs.
(c) Bone targeting nanocarriers: Calcium phosphate-based biomaterial has been developed. It is a readily flowable, moldable paste that adapts to and interdigitates with host bone, providing support for the growth of cartilage and bone cells [114, 119].

## *9.14 Nanoneedles*

Suture needles including nanosized stainless-steel crystals have been developed.

***Trade Name:*** Sandvik Bioline, RK 91TM needles [AB Sandvik, Sweden]

Nanotweezers are under development. These materials possess the potential to make cell surgery possible in a foreseeable future [114, 119].

## *9.15 Materials Applied for Bone Replacement*

Hydroxyapatite NPs are utilized to heal bone defects are [8, 15]: VITOSSO (Orthovita, Inc., USA) HA + TCP; NanOSSTM (Angstrom Medica, USA) HA; Ostim® (Osartis GmbH, Germany) HA.

## 10 Possible Hazards Resulting from NPs

Nanobiotechnology could strikingly ameliorate public health, but there are concerns that technical improvements could breed unexpected adverse effects. Human beings have been exposed to NPs during their developing phases; nevertheless, this exposure has increased in the past century due to the industrial revolution. Nanotechnology is also being utilized in medical sciences with the effort to develop a more personalized medicine. Epidemiological investigations have revealed that the urban population—with airborne particulate matter along with NPs—created combustion sources, such as motor vehicle and industrial emissions. These emissions play a vital role in respiratory and cardiovascular morbidity and mortality. Likewise, NPs may also be involved in the toxicological profile of NPs in biological systems. These smaller particles possess larger surface area per unit mass, and this feature makes NPs very reactive in the cellular media. The respiratory system, blood, central nervous system, gastrointestinal tract, and skin have been demonstrated to be affected by NPs [120, 121].

## 11 Summary

Nanotechnology has made bright progress in science, especially in the field of dentistry with an extrapolation of current resources, and offers a clear vision with the possibility of great advances under resources available. Although this technology is still very young, many applications of it will be introduced. In this chapter, we discussed a few applications that have already been developed and used to help patients. More research related to dental health care should focus on drug delivery systems and toxicity by the emergence of more biocompatible materials. There is a need for extensive research on this technology in various fields, including public and dental care, biomedicine, food, and agriculture. In the future, many diseases that do not have a cure today may be cured by nanotechnology. We also discussed some concerns in this area, however, with proper care these problems can be avoided. Still, the arrival of nanotechnology in the dentistry field has grown increasingly during recent years, but it is noteworthy that biosafety assessment of nanostructures should be considered prior to apply them in dental applications in order to avoid many pathological conditions.

## References


1. Harris, D., & Robinson, J. R. (1992). Drug delivery via the mucous membranes of the oral cavity. *Journal of Pharmaceutical Sciences, 81*(1), 1–10.
2. World Health Organization. (2013). *Oral health surveys: Basic methods*. World Health Organization. School of Dentistry, University of São Paulo, Brazil

3. Ensign, L. M., Cone, R., & Hanes, J. (2012). Oral drug delivery with polymeric nanoparticles: The gastrointestinal mucus barriers. *Advanced Drug Delivery Reviews, 64*(6), 557–570.
4. Langer, R. (1998). Drug delivery and targeting. *Nature-London, 392*, 5–10.
5. Langer, R., & Peppas, N. A. (2003). Advances in biomaterials, drug delivery, and bionanotechnology. *AICHE Journal, 49*(12), 2990–3006.
6. Goldberg, M., & Gomez-Orellana, I. (2003). Challenges for the oral delivery of macromolecules. *Nature Reviews Drug Discovery, 2*(4), 289.
7. Scott, J. H., & Symons, N. B. B. (1982). *Introduction to dental anatomy* (Vol. 6). Edinburgh: Churchill Livingstone.
8. Petersen, P. E., et al. (2005). The global burden of oral diseases and risks to oral health. *Bulletin of the World Health Organization, 83*, 661–669.
9. Magalhães, A. C., et al. (2009). Insights into preventive measures for dental erosion. *Journal of Applied Oral Science, 17*(2), 75–86.
10. Friedman, S. (2002). Prognosis of initial endodontic therapy. *Endodontic Topics, 2*(1), 59–88.
11. Gomes, B. P., et al. (2004). Microbiological examination of infected dental root canals. *Oral Microbiology and Immunology, 19*(2), 71–76.
12. Pavarina, A. C., et al. (2003). An infection control protocol: Effectiveness of immersion solutions to reduce the microbial growth on dental prostheses. *Journal of Oral Rehabilitation, 30*(5), 532–536.
13. Ficai, D., et al. (2017). Drug delivery systems for dental applications. *Current Organic Chemistry, 21*(1), 64–73.
14. Nikalje, A. P. (2015). Nanotechnology and its applications in medicine. *Medicinal Chemistry, 5*(2), 081–089.
15. WHO. (2012). *World Health Organization: Oral health fact sheet N° 318*. WHO Media Centre. Malmö University, Sweden
16. Freitas, R. A., Jr. (2000). Nanodentistry. *The Journal of the American Dental Association, 131*(11), 1559–1565.
17. Kumar, P. S., et al. (2011). Nanodentistry: A paradigm shift-from fiction to reality. *The Journal of Indian Prosthodontic Society, 11*(1), 1–6.
18. Chandki, R., et al. (2012). 'Nanodentistry': Exploring the beauty of miniature. *Journal of Clinical and Experimental Dentistry, 4*(2), e119.
19. Ingle, E., & Gopal, K. S. (2011). Nanodentistry: A hype or hope. *Dentist, 3*, 7.
20. Hatziantoniou, S., & Demetzos, C. (2006). An introduction to nanotechnology in health care. *Pharmakeftiki, 19*(IV), 86–88.
21. Mitsiadis, T. A., Woloszyk, A., & Jiménez-Rojo, L. (2012). Nanodentistry: Combining nanostructured materials and stem cells for dental tissue regeneration. *Nanomedicine, 7*(11), 1743–1753.
22. Viswanathan, P., Muralidaran, Y., & Ragavan, G. (2017). Challenges in oral drug delivery: A nano-based strategy to overcome. In *Nanostructures for oral medicine* (pp. 173–201). Amsterdam: Elsevier.
23. Cavalcanti, A., et al. (2007). Nanorobot architecture for medical target identification. *Nanotechnology, 19*(1), 015103.
24. Sankar, V., et al. (2011). Local drug delivery for oral mucosal diseases: Challenges and opportunities. *Oral Diseases, 17*, 73–84.
25. Kasraei, S., et al. (2014). Antibacterial properties of composite resins incorporating silver and zinc oxide nanoparticles on Streptococcus mutans and Lactobacillus. *Restorative Dentistry & Endodontics, 39*(2), 109–114.
26. Khan, A., et al. (2014). Gold nanoparticles: Synthesis and applications in drug delivery. *Tropical Journal of Pharmaceutical Research, 13*(7), 1169–1177.
27. Mu, L., & Feng, S. (2003). A novel controlled release formulation for the anticancer drug paclitaxel (Taxol®): PLGA nanoparticles containing vitamin E TPGS. *Journal of Controlled Release, 86*(1), 33–48.
28. Munot, N. M., & Gujar, K. N. (2013). Orodental delivery systems: An overview. *International Journal of Pharmacy and Pharmaceutical Sciences, 5*(3), 74–83.

29. He, Z., & Alexandridis, P. (2017). Ionic liquid and nanoparticle hybrid systems: Emerging applications. *Advances in Colloid and Interface Science, 244*, 54–70.
30. Sung, J. (2009). *Diamond nanotechnology: Synthesis and applications*. Singapure: Pan Stanford.
31. Nakatuka, T., et al. (2003). *Dental fillers*. Google Patents. US6620861B1, United States
32. Raemdonck, K., Demeester, J., & De Smedt, S. (2009). Advanced nanogel engineering for drug delivery. *Soft Matter, 5*(4), 707–715.
33. Maleki, A., et al. (2018). Effect of nano-fillers on mechanical properties of dental PMMA based composites. *Journal of Advanced Chemical and Pharmaceutical Materials (JACPM), 1*(3), 73–76.
34. Sadat-Shojai, M., et al. (2010). Hydroxyapatite nanorods as novel fillers for improving the properties of dental adhesives: Synthesis and application. *Dental Materials, 26*(5), 471–482.
35. Klapdohr, S., & Moszner, N. (2005). New inorganic components for dental filling composites. *Monatshefte für Chemie/Chemical Monthly, 136*(1), 21–45.
36. Hannig, M., & Hannig, C. (2010). Nanomaterials in preventive dentistry. *Nature Nanotechnology, 5*(8), 565.
37. Bogunia-Kubik, K., & Sugisaka, M. (2002). From molecular biology to nanotechnology and nanomedicine. *Biosystems, 65*(2–3), 123–138.
38. Wang, Y., et al. (2013). Susceptibility of young and adult rats to the oral toxicity of titanium dioxide nanoparticles. *Small, 9*(9–10), 1742–1752.
39. Baloš, S., et al. (2013). Improving mechanical properties of flowable dental composite resin by adding silica nanoparticles. *Vojnosanitetski Pregled, 70*(5), 477–483.
40. Xu, H., et al. (2010). Strong nanocomposites with Ca, PO4, and F release for caries inhibition. *Journal of Dental Research, 89*(1), 19–28.
41. Xia, Y., et al. (2008). Nanoparticle-reinforced resin-based dental composites. *Journal of Dentistry, 36*(6), 450–455.
42. Wagner, A., et al. (2013). Biomimetically-and hydrothermally-grown HAp nanoparticles as reinforcing fillers for dental adhesives. *Journal of Adhesive Dentistry, 15*(5), 413–422.
43. Melo, M. A. S., et al. (2013). Novel dental adhesives containing nanoparticles of silver and amorphous calcium phosphate. *Dental Materials, 29*(2), 199–210.
44. Wang, W., et al. (2014). Structure–property relationships in hybrid dental nanocomposite resins containing monofunctional and multifunctional polyhedral oligomeric silsesquioxanes. *International Journal of Nanomedicine, 9*, 841.
45. Habekost, L. V., et al. (2012). Nanoparticle loading level and properties of experimental hybrid resin luting agents. *Journal of Prosthodontics, 21*(7), 540–545.
46. Jallot, E., et al. (2005). STEM and EDXS characterisation of physico-chemical reactions at the periphery of sol–gel derived Zn-substituted hydroxyapatites during interactions with biological fluids. *Colloids and Surfaces B: Biointerfaces, 42*(3–4), 205–210.
47. Krisanapiboon, A., Buranapanitkit, B., & Oungbho, K. (2006). Biocompatability of hydroxyapatite composite as a local drug delivery system. *Journal of Orthopaedic Surgery, 14*(3), 315–318.
48. Huber, F.-X., et al. (2006). First histological observations on the incorporation of a novel nanocrystalline hydroxyapatite paste OSTIM® in human cancellous bone. *BMC Musculoskeletal Disorders, 7*(1), 50.
49. Qi, X., et al. (2013). Development and characterization of an injectable cement of nanocalcium-deficienthydroxyapatite/multi (amino acid) copolymer/calcium sulfate hemihydrate for bone repair. *International Journal of Nanomedicine, 8*, 4441.
50. Yang, C., et al. (2013). Periodontal regeneration with nano-hyroxyapatite-coated silk scaffolds in dogs. *Journal of Periodontal & Implant Science, 43*(6), 315–322.
51. An, S.-H., et al. (2012). Porous zirconia/hydroxyapatite scaffolds for bone reconstruction. *Dental Materials, 28*(12), 1221–1231.
52. De Aza, A., et al. (2002). Crack growth resistance of alumina, zirconia and zirconia toughened alumina ceramics for joint prostheses. *Biomaterials, 23*(3), 937–945.

53. Uno, M., et al. (2013). Effects of adding silver nanoparticles on the toughening of dental porcelain. *The Journal of Prosthetic Dentistry, 109*(4), 241–247.
54. Han, Y., et al. (2008). Effect of nano-oxide concentration on the mechanical properties of a maxillofacial silicone elastomer. *The Journal of Prosthetic Dentistry, 100*(6), 465–473.
55. Acosta-Torres, L. S., et al. (2012). Cytocompatible antifungal acrylic resin containing silver nanoparticles for dentures. *International Journal of Nanomedicine, 7*, 4777.
56. Karlsson, M., et al. (2003). Initial in vitro interaction of osteoblasts with nano-porous alumina. *Biomaterials, 24*(18), 3039–3046.
57. Pardun, K., et al. (2015). Characterization of wet powder-sprayed zirconia/calcium phosphate coating for dental implants. *Clinical Implant Dentistry and Related Research, 17*(1), 186–198.
58. Memarzadeh, K., et al. (2015). Nanoparticulate zinc oxide as a coating material for orthopedic and dental implants. *Journal of Biomedical Materials Research Part A, 103*(3), 981–989.
59. Uezono, M., et al. (2013). Hydroxyapatite/collagen nanocomposite-coated titanium rod for achieving rapid osseointegration onto bone surface. *Journal of Biomedical Materials Research Part B: Applied Biomaterials, 101*(6), 1031–1038.
60. Lebold, T., et al. (2009). Nanostructured silica materials as drug-delivery systems for doxorubicin: Single molecule and cellular studies. *Nano Letters, 9*(8), 2877–2883.
61. Melancon, M. P., et al. (2011). Targeted multifunctional gold-based nanoshells for magnetic resonance-guided laser ablation of head and neck cancer. *Biomaterials, 32*(30), 7600–7608.
62. Patil, J. (2016). Encapsulation technology: Opportunity to develop novel drug delivery systems. *Journal of Pharmacovigilance, 4*, e156.
63. Maysinger, D. (2007). Nanoparticles and cells: Good companions and doomed partnerships. *Organic & Biomolecular Chemistry, 5*(15), 2335–2342.
64. Fahmy, T. M., et al. (2005). Targeted for drug delivery. *Materials Today, 8*(8), 18–26.
65. Reddy, R. S., & Dathar, S. (2015). Nano drug delivery in oral cancer therapy: An emerging avenue to unveil. *Journal of Medicine, Radiology, Pathology and Surgery, 1*, 17–22.
66. Krishna, K., Reddy, C., & Srikanth, S. (2013). A review on microsphere for novel drug delivery system. *International Journal of Research in Pharmacy and Chemistry, 3*(4), 763–767.
67. Nasongkla, N., et al. (2006). Multifunctional polymeric micelles as cancer-targeted, MRI-ultrasensitive drug delivery systems. *Nano Letters, 6*(11), 2427–2430.
68. Hu, C.-M. J., Aryal, S., & Zhang, L. (2010). Nanoparticle-assisted combination therapies for effective cancer treatment. *Therapeutic Delivery, 1*(2), 323–334.
69. Majoros, I. J., et al. (2006). PAMAM dendrimer-based multifunctional conjugate for cancer therapy: Synthesis, characterization, and functionality. *Biomacromolecules, 7*(2), 572–579.
70. Jain, N., et al. (2010). Nanotechnology: A safe and effective drug delivery system. *Asian Journal of Pharmaceutical and Clinical Research, 3*(3), 159–165.
71. Tang, M., et al. (2010). Recent progress in nanotechnology for cancer therapy. *Chinese Journal of Cancer, 29*(9), 775–780.
72. Barakat, N. S., BinTaleb, D., & Al Salehi, A. (2012). Target nanoparticles: An appealing drug delivery platform. *Journal of Nanomedicine & Nanotechnology, 3*(3), 1–9.
73. Bae, Y. H., & Park, K. (2011). Targeted drug delivery to tumors: Myths, reality and possibility. *Journal of Controlled Release, 153*(3), 198.
74. Chen, P. C., Mwakwari, S. C., & Oyelere, A. K. (2008). Gold nanoparticles: From nanomedicine to nanosensing. *Nanotechnology, Science and Applications, 1*, 45.
75. El-Say, K. M. (2011). Nanodiamond as a drug delivery system: Applications and prospective. *Journal of Applied Pharmaceutical Science, 1*(06), 29–39.
76. Tang, L., et al. (1995). Biocompatibility of chemical-vapour-deposited diamond. *Biomaterials, 16*(6), 483–488.
77. Saba, N., Tahir, P., & Jawaid, M. (2014). A review on potentiality of nano filler/natural fiber filled polymer hybrid composites. *Polymers, 6*(8), 2247–2273.
78. Atai, M., et al. (2009). PMMA-grafted nanoclay as novel filler for dental adhesives. *Dental Materials, 25*(3), 339–347.

79. Khurshid, Z., et al. (2015). Advances in nanotechnology for restorative dentistry. *Materials, 8*(2), 717–731.
80. Ruyter, I. (1992). The chemistry of adhesive agents. *Operative Dentistry, Suppl 5*, 32–43.
81. Breschi, L., et al. (2008). Dental adhesion review: Aging and stability of the bonded interface. *Dental Materials, 24*(1), 90–101.
82. Moszner, N., Salz, U., & Zimmermann, J. (2005). Chemical aspects of self-etching enamel–dentin adhesives: A systematic review. *Dental Materials, 21*(10), 895–910.
83. Cheng, Y. J., et al. (2011). In situ formation of silver nanoparticles in photocrosslinking polymers. *Journal of Biomedical Materials Research Part B: Applied Biomaterials, 97*(1), 124–131.
84. Melo, M. A. S., et al. (2013). Novel dental adhesive containing antibacterial agents and calcium phosphate nanoparticles. *Journal of Biomedical Materials Research Part B: Applied Biomaterials, 101*(4), 620–629.
85. Skrtic, D., et al. (2000). Physicochemical evaluation of bioactive polymeric composites based on hybrid amorphous calcium phosphates. *Journal of Biomedical Materials Research, 53*(4), 381–391.
86. Parr, G. R., Gardner, L. K., & Toth, R. W. (1985). Titanium: The mystery metal of implant dentistry. Dental materials aspects. *Journal of Prosthetic Dentistry, 54*(3), 410–414.
87. Avila, G., et al. (2009). Implant surface treatment using biomimetic agents. *Implant Dentistry, 18*(1), 17–26.
88. Mombelli, A., & Lang, N. (1992). Antimicrobial treatment of peri-implant infections. *Clinical Oral Implants Research, 3*(4), 162–168.
89. Anusavice, K. J., Shen, C., & Rawls, H. R. (2013). *Phillips' science of dental materials*. London: Elsevier Health Sciences.
90. Willmann, G. (1999). Coating of implants with hydroxyapatite–material connections between bone and metal. *Advanced Engineering Materials, 1*(2), 95–105.
91. Catledge, S. A., et al. (2002). Nanostructured ceramics for biomedical implants. *Journal of Nanoscience and Nanotechnology, 2*(3–4), 293–312.
92. Davies, J. E. (2003). Understanding peri-implant endosseous healing. *Journal of Dental Education, 67*(8), 932–949.
93. Duraccio, D., Mussano, F., & Faga, M. G. (2015). Biomaterials for dental implants: Current and future trends. *Journal of Materials Science, 50*(14), 4779–4812.
94. Pachauri, P., Bathala, L. R., & Sangur, R. (2014). Techniques for dental implant nanosurface modifications. *The Journal of Advanced Prosthodontics, 6*(6), 498–504.
95. Gümüşderelioğlu, M., et al. (2007). *Doku mühendisliğinde nanoteknoloji.* Bilim ve Teknik Dergisi Yeni Ufuklara Eki.
96. Tetè, S., et al. (2008). A macro-and nanostructure evaluation of a novel dental implant. *Implant Dentistry, 17*(3), 309–320.
97. Braceras, I., et al. (2009). In vivo low-density bone apposition on different implant surface materials. *International Journal of Oral and Maxillofacial Surgery, 38*(3), 274–278.
98. Ellingsen, J. E., Thomsen, P., & Lyngstadaas, S. P. (2006). Advances in dental implant materials and tissue regeneration. *Periodontology 2000, 41*(1), 136–156.
99. Suh, J. Y., et al. (2007). Effects of a novel calcium titanate coating on the osseointegration of blasted endosseous implants in rabbit tibiae. *Clinical Oral Implants Research, 18*(3), 362–369.
100. Meirelles, L., et al. (2008). The effect of chemical and nanotopographical modifications on the early stages of osseointegration. *International Journal of Oral & Maxillofacial Implants, 23*(4), 641–647.
101. Chiang, C.-Y., et al. (2009). Formation of TiO2nano-networkon titanium surface increases the human cell growth. *Dental Materials, 25*(8), 1022–1029.
102. Paul, W., & Sharma, C. P. (2006). Nanoceramic matrices: Biomedical applications. *American Journal of Biochemistry and Biotechnology, 2*(2), 41–48.

103. Zhang, L., & Webster, T. J. (2009). Nanotechnology and nanomaterials: Promisesfor improved tissue regeneration. *Nano Today, 4*(1), 66–80.
104. Colon, G., Ward, B. C., & Webster, T. J. (2006). Increased osteoblast and decreased Staphylococcus epidermidis functions on nanophase ZnO and TiO2. *Journal of Biomedical Materials Research Part A, 78*(3), 595–604.
105. Webster, T. J., & Ejiofor, J. U. (2004). Increased osteoblast adhesion on nanophase metals: Ti, Ti6Al4V, and CoCrMo. *Biomaterials, 25*(19), 4731–4739.
106. Pauwels, E. K., et al. (2008). Nanoparticles in cancer. *Current Radiopharmaceuticals, 1*(1), 30–36.
107. Sivaramakrishnan, S., & Neelakantan, P. (2014). Nanotechnology in dentistry-what does the future hold in store? *Dentistry, 4*(2), 1.
108. Salerno, M., & Diaspro, A. (2015). Dentistry on the bridge to nanoscience and nanotechnology. *Frontiers in Materials, 2*, 19.
109. Nguyen, S., et al. (2010). The influence of liposomal formulation factors on the interactions between liposomes and hydroxyapatite. *Colloids and Surfaces B: Biointerfaces, 76*(1), 354–361.
110. Li, Y., et al. (2005). The oral fluid MEMS/NEMS chip (OFMNC): Diagnostic & translational applications. *Advances in Dental Research, 18*(1), 3–5.
111. Christodoulides, N., et al. (2007). Lab-on-a-chip methods for point-of-care measurements of salivary biomarkers of periodontitis. *Annals of the New York Academy of Sciences, 1098*(1), 411–428.
112. Meagher, R. J., et al. (2008). An integrated microfluidic platform for sensitive and rapid detection of biological toxins. *Lab on a Chip, 8*(12), 2046–2053.
113. Song, J. M., et al. (2004). Detection of cytochrome C in a single cell using an optical nanobiosensor. *Analytical Chemistry, 76*(9), 2591–2594.
114. Kumar, S. R., & Vijayalakshmi, R. (2006). Nanotechnology in dentistry. *Indian Journal of Dental Research, 17*(2), 62–65.
115. Gau, V., & Wong, D. (2007). Oral fluid nanosensor test (OFNASET) with advanced electrochemical-based molecular analysis platform. *Annals of the New York Academy of Sciences, 1098*(1), 401–410.
116. Somerman, M., et al. (1999). Evolution of periodontal regeneration: From the roots' point of view. *Journal of Periodontal Research, 34*(7), 420–442.
117. Shellhart, W. C., & Oesterle, L. J. (1999). Uprighting molars without extrusion. *Journal of the American Dental Association (1939), 130*(3), 381–385.
118. Scott, N. (2007). Nanoscience in veterinary medicine. *Veterinary Research Communications, 31*(1), 139–144.
119. Jhaveri, H., & Balaji, P. (2005). Nanotechnology: The future of dentistry. *Journal of Indian Prosthodontic Society, 5*(1), 15–17.
120. Labhasetwar, V., & Leslie-Pelecky, D. L. (2007). *Biomedical applications of nanotechnology*. Hoboken: John Wiley & Sons.
121. Gaur, A., Midha, A., & Bhatia, A. L. (2014). Significance of nanotechnology in medical sciences. *Asian Journal of Pharmaceutics (AJP), 2*(2).

# Chapter 13
# Application of Stem Cell Encapsulated Hydrogel in Dentistry

**Abdolreza Ardeshirylajimi, Ali Golchin, Jessica Vargas, and Lobat Tayebi**

## 1 Introduction

As we know, regenerative medicine has become a game-changing area of advanced medicine that has created a promising viewpoint. Cell and tissue-based therapy is one of the important keys to regenerative medicine protocols. It has created a high expectancy in the treatment topics of medical specialties [1]. Dentistry and maxillofacial surgery have been able to employ this new therapy by the method of orofacial reconstruction. This has been accomplished by using cell-tissue products, which in turn has created a more unique tissue engineering method. One of the important branches of orofacial tissue engineering is the employment of degradable porous three-dimensional (3D) materials, such as hydrogels, which have been integrated with cells and bioactive factors to improve regeneration criteria. These criteria include the reconstruction of dental bone, stem cell-based regenerative endodontics, and tissue engineering of other oral tissues (Fig. 13.1). During the past years, hydrogels have explored as a hopeful platform for promoting delivery systems of cells and biological factors for tissue engineering applications in medicine—especially in the dental field, due to their excellent properties. The properties include control of degradation and release capabilities, minimally invasive utilization techniques, ability to match 3D defects, proper encapsulating of cells, increase

A. Ardeshirylajimi
Department of Tissue Engineering and Applied Cell Sciences, School of Advanced Technologies in Medicine, Shahid Beheshti University of Medical Sciences, Tehran, Iran

A. Golchin
Department of Tissue Engineering and Applied Cell Sciences, Student Research Committee, School of Advanced Technologies in Medicine, Shahid Beheshti University of Medical Sciences, Tehran, Iran

J. Vargas · L. Tayebi (✉)
Marquette University School of Dentistry, Milwaukee, WI, USA
e-mail: lobat.tayebi@marquette.edu



L. Tayebi (ed.), *Applications of Biomedical Engineering in Dentistry*,
https://doi.org/10.1007/978-3-030-21583-5_13

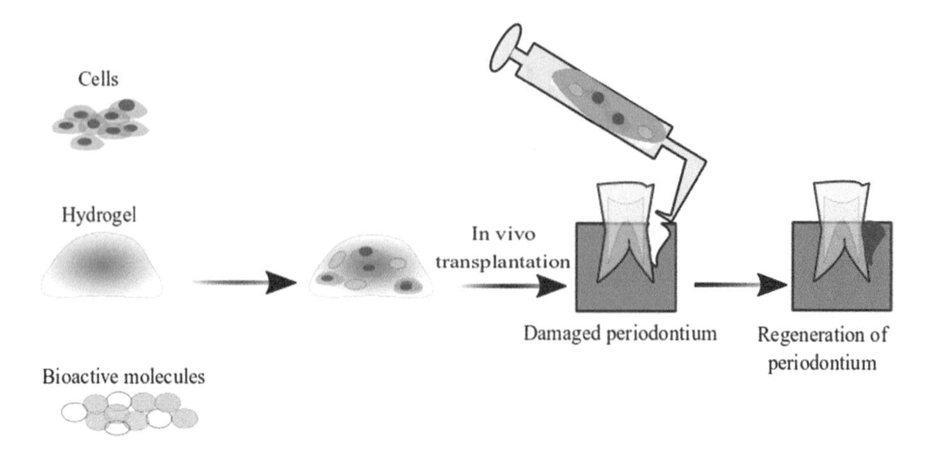


**Fig. 13.1** Application summary of hydrogels in periodontal tissue engineering

of cell viability, and adjustable tissue-like features [2]. Hydrogels can be used in different approaches in dentistry, such as enamel reconstruction [3], root canal treatment [4], artificial bone graft in the orofacial area [5], and/or other dental tissues engineering. Hydrogel physicochemical properties with changeable capabilities prepare a suitable condition for manipulation. For instance, gelation rates and stiffness of the hydrogels can be tuned by varying the HRP and $H_2O_2$, respectively. These properties can alter the stem cell fate from the aspect of differentiation [2, 6]. In the following sections, hydrogel properties and applications will be introduced, along with their applications in dental medicine and orofacial tissue engineering.

## 2 Hydrogel

Hydrogels were established and introduced by Wichterle and Lim in 1954 [7]. A hydrogel is a macromolecular gel constructed from a group of polymeric materials with the ability to hold large amounts of water in its network, which allows it to become a 3D structure. This permits for a wide amount of potential applications in regenerative medicine, especially as a cellular delivery system. Unique properties of hydrogels are dependent on several factors and most importantly its initial derived source. Hydrogels can be derived from natural sources (examples include alginate, hyaluronic acid, fibrin, collagen) and synthetic sources (examples include Poly 2-hydroxyethyl methacrylate (pHEMA), Polyethylene glycol (PEG)). Each of these derived hydrogel sources can present various properties for different therapeutic targets [8]. In addition, hydrogels that are saturated with water can also provide a safe and bio-tolerable matrix for cellular encapsulation [9]. Due to their network and crosslinking structure, hydrogels can also be used for sustained release of biomolecular content and provide prolonged periods of controlled release of biological factors [10, 11]. Hydrogels can be prepared in liquid form and then injected at the site of tissue defects in order to form into the shape of the irregular defect. After taking the shape of the defects, they can then solidify by various stimuli, which in turn are named in situ hybridization hydrogels [12]. These hydrogels are also able to regulate pH and extinguish free radicals within tissue lesions, thereby decreasing the oxidative stress and increasing survival and engraftment of the cells in the site of injury [13]. It should be considered that the porous framework of the hydrogels can provide an appropriate microenvironment condition for the cells' adhesion, migration, and proliferation and also stem cells' fate determination [12]. As per the mentioned reasons, hydrogels can be good conductors for delivery of cells and signaling molecules in a single structure that can play the role of the ECM itself [13]. However, the outline of hydrogels for regenerative medicine applications demands the simple synthesis, safety, efficacy, and capability to respond to multi-stimuli.

Hydrogel technologies were taken into consideration for regenerative medicine application, including tissue engineering of the bone [14], tooth [15], myocardium [16, 17], wound dressing [18], cell-based therapy as cell delivery systems [13], and cell signaling molecule delivery systems [19], from 1954 until now.

## 3 Biodegradable Hydrogels

In tissue engineering, biodegradability is a crucial parameter for biomaterials, which will be used at the defect site, and therefore, biodegradable hydrogels have been exploited in regenerative medicine applications. Generally, hydrogels are affected by three degradation mechanisms including solubilization, chemical hydrolysis, and enzyme-induced degradation. However, there are other mechanisms, such as ion-exchange, which lead to soluble or bio-absorbable moieties that some hydrogels utilize [20]. Environmental factors—such as enzymes, pH, metal ions, and mechanical stress—are the main features in the biological niche that may affect the biodegradation process of hydrogels [21]. Among biomaterials, natural ones have perfect biodegradability. Alongside their biocompatibility and ECM similarity, natural biomaterials have been strongly considered for maxillofacial and dental regenerative medicine. However, synthetic biomaterials are reproducible and controllable and can escape immune responses (see Table 13.1).

## 4 Hydrogels in Dental Tissue Engineering

There are several targets for hydrogels in dental tissue engineering. These include the creation of an entirely functional bioengineered tooth and tissue engineering of soft tissues (skin, mucosa, salivary glands), bone, and temporomandibular joints. Hydrogels, as a scaffold, play an important role in dental and periodontal tissue engineering. To fully reconstruct damaged orofacial tissues, it is important to synthesize scaffolds with proper biocompatibility and biodegradability that present an

**Table 13.1** Injectable biodegradable hydrogels for various tissue-engineering applications

| Hydrogels | Polymers | Gelation mechanism |
|---|---|---|
| Natural hydrogels | Collagen/gelatin | Thermal, chemical crosslinking |
| | Chitosan | Thermal, chemical, Schiff-base reaction, and free radical crosslinking |
| | Hyaluronic acid | Thermal, chemical, Schiff-base reaction, Michael-type addition, and free radical crosslinking |
| | Chondroitin sulfate | Free radical crosslinking |
| | Alginate | Ionic and free radical crosslinking |
| | Fibrin | Thermal crosslinking |
| Synthetic hydrogels | Methoxy polyethylene glycol | Thermal crosslinking |
| | PVA | Chemical and free radical crosslinking |
| | PPF/OPF | Free radical crosslinking |
| | PNIPAAm | Thermal crosslinking |
| | PEG | Thermal crosslinking |

desired delivery system for cell and growth factor while imitating the native specifications of the target tissues [12]. Another main goal in dentistry is developing of the innovative bactericidal, bioactive, and ion-releasing hydrogels that can accelerate periodontium defects repairing [22]. So far, different scaffolds alone and in combination with various stem cells and biological factors have been studied at the both in vitro and in vivo levels (Table 13.2). However, many of these studies are performed on periodontal tissue regeneration but rarely have been employed in clinical studies. Therefore, challenges remain for developing a suitable construct that can provide a suitable microenvironment for proper proliferation and differentiation of the stem cells to new tissue formation.

Due to their natural and inherent features, hydrogels can be used to provide a good cell delivery system combined with different growth factors and antibiotics for sustained release [24]. Some signs of progress have been observed in the chemistry of the hydrogels to improve cells function and fate controlling and adjusting cells and tissue responses versus various stresses such as oxidation and inflammation where transplanted [29]. Hydrogels as a delivery system have been used for dentine-pulp regeneration. For example, materials such as customized self-assembled peptide hydrogels [4] and PEGylated fibrin hydrogels [23] have been employed for encapsulating of stem cells for dental tissue engineering. Studies show that injectable hydrogels represent a suitable strategic approach for engineering the dentin-pulp complex, due to their size and confinement within the pulp and root canals [30].

## 5 Cell Delivery/Cell Encapsulation by Hydrogels

In regard to regenerative medicine, encapsulation protects the transplanted cells against the host immune system and can promote delivery of the cells/cellular products to the main therapeutic target [31]. Most of the recent studies have

**Table 13.2** Some examples of the hydrogel used in orofacial area reconstruction

| Materials | Study aim | Cell sources | Model of study | Results | Ref |
|---|---|---|---|---|---|
| Fibrin and PEG gel | Evaluate the suitability of PEGylated fibrin as a scaffold for dental stem cells | DPSCs | Mice | Enhancement of cell proliferation, osteogenic differentiation (after osteogenic induction) with increasing in dentin-specific markers expression, production of a collagenous matrix, and mineral deposition | [23] |
| Porcine-bladder derived ECM· Ag-doped BG (sol-gel) | Fabrication of the scaffold for pulp-dentin tissue engineering plus bactericidal effect | DPSCs | Mice | Ag-BG/ECM outstandingly increased cells proliferation and stemness markers, prevent apoptosis, enhances differentiation in in vitro, and mineralization with dentin formation in in vivo levels | [24] |
| Amelogenin-chitosan hydrogel | Enamel regrowth with a dense interface | RC (*E. coli*–BC21) | In vitro | Amelogenin-chitosan hydrogel showed suitable properties for the prevention, restoration, and treatment of defective enamel | [3] |
| $ZrO_2$ surface chemically coated with hyaluronic acid hydrogel loading GDF-5 | Providing a suitable osseointegration condition for dental implants in dentistry | Human osteosarcoma cells (MG-63) | In vitro | Cell proliferation and differentiation and showed good properties to deliver osteogenic differentiation factors | [5] |
| MDP hydrogel | Incorporating of stem cells and bioactive factors for dental tissue engineering | DPSCs | Mice | Formation of a neo-vascularized dental pulp-like soft tissue | [4] |
| HyStem-C (PEG-based injectable hydrogel blended with ECM derived proteins) | Enhancement of DPSC viability and expansion | hDPSCs | In vitro | Increased hDPSCs viability by hydrogels and improved cell proliferation and spreading—especially composite with ECM proteins | [25] |

(continued)

**Table 13.2** (continued)

| Materials | Study aim | Cell sources | Model of study | Results | Ref |
|---|---|---|---|---|---|
| Puramatrix™ | Assessment of the Puramatrix™ biocompatibility by stem cell viability and odontoblastic differentiation assessments | hDPSCs | In vitro – human tooth slice model | Stem cells seeded in Puramatrix™ hydrogel presented morphological features of healthy cells and expressed DMP-1 and DSPP (as odontoblastic markers) | [26] |
| Corn starch-based hydrogel loaded with hydroxyapatite or calcium carbonate | Fabrication of a scaffold for bone reconstruction after maxillofacial surgery | HO | In vitro | Starch-based hydrogels loaded with two different bioactive particles promoted osteoblast cells viability | [27] |
| PEGMEM and DEM | Development of an artificial antibacterial bone substitute | OC | In vitro | Beneficial effect on the osteoblast cells density on hydrogels and Zn bactericidal features | [28] |

*BG* bioactive glass, *DEM* [2(dimethylamine) ethyl methacrylate], *DPSCs* dental pulp stem cells, *ECM* extracellular matrix, *hDPSCs* human DPSCs, *HO* human osteoblasts, *MDPs* multidomain peptides, *OC* osteoblast cell, *PEG* polyethylene glycol, *PEGMEM* [poly (ethylene glycol) methyl ether methacrylate], *RC* recombinant cells

investigated injectable composite hydrogels at the nanoscale level to develop the stem cell delivery systems by addressing the often conflicting mechanical requirements and stages of the transplantation process. Cells encapsulating in the hydrogel can be easily accessible due to its similarities to the natural ECM. A desired injectable-hydrogel should be synthesized carefully to obtain the appropriate physicochemical and biological characteristics [32]. For instance, microbeads fabricated by oxidized-alginate are a newly introduced injectable scaffold that can well encapsulate periodontal ligament-derived stem cells (PDLSCs) and gingiva-derived MSCs (GMSCs). Hydrogels can be formed using sufficient concentrations of necessary molecules to maintain stable physical properties. Cell encapsulation in three dimensions prevents cellular morphology and cell cycle changes. Stem cells can also differentiate while growing under normal growth media and in the presence of small-molecule functional groups that can induce differentiation [33]. As mentioned before, the application of hydrogels as a cell delivery system has been attracting a considerable amount of attention in bone and maxillofacial regenerative medicine.

## 6 Role of Hydrogels in Bone Regeneration

Bony defects are one of the most commonly faced issues in dentistry, which influence dental treatment in the oral and maxillofacial area. Current therapies are not adequate, and autografting bony defects have several limitations, which include donor-site problems and several uncertain harmful effects. Consequently, bone tissue engineering has attracted considerable attention from researchers and clinicians as a promising strategy for repairing bony defects without the limitations and shortcomings of using autograft, allograft, and xenograft sources [34].

Hydrogels are considered a suitable candidate for cell delivery and creation of calcification nuclei. Osteoblasts are the main cellular component of bone tissue and play the role of secreting and mineralizing ECM in bone. Mineralized ECM contains dense collagen type I, collagen type IV, fibronectin, heparan sulfate, and other proteins found in bone. The encapsulation system of different biopolymeric hydrogels has been investigated as a suitable approach for bone tissue engineering (see Table 13.1). Cells encapsulated in hydrogels support bone ECM and bony tissue structure formation. The hydrogel and its incorporated growth factors provide a number of functional cues that affect the differentiated cells and/or stem cell proliferation, migration, metabolism, and secretion.

The investigation of a method to integrate the qualities of various biomaterials and synthesizing methods for fabrication of the suitable injectable and in situ hybridization hydrogels will play a significant role in the clinical uses of hydrogels in dentistry and bone tissue engineering.

## 7 Mineralization of Injectable Hydrogels and In Situ Hybridization

Hydrogels and their contents need to be in liquid form for injection, and after transplantation in the site of defects, need to undergo gelation. Gelation and then subsequent mineralization of the injectable hydrogels is an important issue in their employment in maxillofacial and dental regenerative medicine. With improvement of their mechanical properties, they can also enhance differentiation of different progenitor cells into the osteoblastic-like cells.

Presence of calcium phosphate (CaP) can improve osteoinductivity of the bone-substituting implants, similar to what occurs in the natural osteogenesis process; as a result, a chemical interaction with adjacent bony tissue is created after in vivo transplantation. After hydrogels mineralize, CaP bioceramics have inherent dependence for biological-active peptides, which stimulate healing procedure of the adjacent bony tissue [35]. Several different strategies can be considered for the mineralization of the hydrogels. These strategies for the injected hydrogels in the area of bone defects can be included via direct and indirect routes. Direct routes include incorporation of an inorganic phase, biomimetic of the physiological mineralization process, and/or structure functionalization with negatively charged groups [36]. Indirect routes include differentiated osteogenic lineage and/or the mixture of osteoinductive growth factors and stem cells that are encapsulated straightly into hydrogels before implantation/injection and subsequently mineralizes the carrier hydrogel in transplanted site [37].

Incorporation of inorganic phases is one of the more interesting routes to create a nucleation site for the promotion of hydroxyapatite (HA) precipitation. Calcium phosphates and bioglasses are two of the most routinely used inorganic phases to promote nucleation and proliferation of calcium phosphate crystals [36]. In the enzymatic mineralization route, the purpose is a natural enzyme use to create homogenous gel mineralization to improve its mechanical properties and provide more suitable properties for bone substitutes or regeneration applications. This is an alternative method for incorporating of CaP particles. Alkaline phosphatase is an important enzyme with a major role in natural bone remodeling. This enzyme's crucial role in mineralization of carbonated-apatite, self-assembling peptide-based hydrogels, covalently linking to collagen that derived from dentine for mineralization induction, and mineralization of various hydrogels was confirmed previously [38]. Hydrogels can also be hybridized using biomimetic techniques that take their creativity from the biomineralization process through in vivo local nanocrystalline apatites formation. This method can be performed by soaking in solutions containing Ca2þ and PO43 or their vesicles loaded in hydrogel [36, 39]. When there are no nucleation sites to provide sites of calcification, the third way of direct calcification includes chemical modification of hydrogel polymers. In this regard, studies have shown sequences of anionic carboxylate, hydroxyl, and phosphate groups along the backbone of hydrogel-forming polymers that provides the resulting in situ hybridization hydrogels in a swollen state with apatite-nucleating properties [40].

Therefore, injectable hydrogels, which can be delivered in a minimally invasive manner, can also form and hybridize in situ, which are then called in situ hybridization injectable hydrogels. In situ hybridization injectable hydrogels have found a crucial role in bony defects reconstruction (Table 13.3) which show its potential application in maxillofacial and dental regenerative medicine. In situ hybridization can be induced after transplantation or injection using artificial manipulation or in response to environmental stimuli such as temperature, pH, and other physiological conditions. Among them, injectable thermosensitive hydrogels with a lower sol-gel transition temperature range than physiological temperature have been a good candidate for bone and maxillofacial regenerative medicine targets. Another method that has promising potential for in situ hybridization of hydrogels in bone and maxillofacial tissue engineering is improvement of in situ crosslinkability of hydrogels. However, new investigations by novel and combination methods are in progress.

**Table 13.3** Some examples of in situ hybridization hydrogel studies for reconstruction in bone tissue

| Composite | Type of action | Result | Ref |
|---|---|---|---|
| PIPAAm/TGM/polyamidoamine crosslinker | Mineralization potential and biocompatibility measurement of injectable, dual-gelling hydrogels in rats | The appropriate mineralization potential of injectable/dual-gelling hydrogels | [41] |
| Copolymerization of acrylonitrile, 1-vinylimidazoleand polyethylene glycoldiacrylate | In situ precipitation mineralization for eliciting bone regeneration | Highly mineralized hydrogel and promoted bone reconstruction | [42] |
| PIPAAm-co-PEG dimethacrylate, with the addition of tri-methacryloxypro pyltrimethoxysilane (MPS) | Injectable in situ shape-forming hydrogel (apatite crystals) | Provide attachment sites for calcium and initiate mineral dissolution from the simulated biological environments | [43] |
| Calcium-crosslinkable polysaccharide gellan gum (GG) | Comparison of three bioglasses to prepare suitable injectable self-gelling composites for bone regeneration based on gellan gum hydrogel | Promotion GG mineralize—ability depending on bioglass type, antibacterial properties, and MSC differentiation | [44] |
| Hydroxyapatite nanoparticles (HANPs) contain MSC | Encapsulate MSCs within stable hydrogel composites when elevated to physiologic temperature | Form in situ while facilitating cell delivery and mineralization | [45] |
| HRGD6 elastin-like recombinamers hydrogel | Preparation of self-mineralizing hydrogels crosslinked with citric acid | Tailored hydrogels were able to rapidly self-mineralize in biomimetic conditions | [46] |
| Mixture of Graphene oxide (GO) and Co-responsive supramolecular hydrogel | In situ hybridization of CoOX nanoparticles on Co-responsive hydrogel | CoOX active sites anchored on the Graphene matrixplay a central role in the upgrading of the catalytic performance of Graphene aerogels | [47] |
| Zinc-doped chitosan/beta-glycerophosphate hydrogel | Synthesize and characterization of thermosensitive hydrogel for bone regeneration | Osteogenic differentiation promoted by hydrogel with bactericidal activity | [48] |
| Zinc-doped chitosan/nanohydroxyapatite/β--glycerophosphate-based hydrogel | Synthesize and characterization of thermosensitive hydrogel for bone tissue repair | Accelerated osteogenic differentiation in vitro and bone regeneration in rats | [49] |
| PEG-PCL-PEG copolymer/collagen/n-HA hydrogel | A novel three-component biomimetic hydrogel composite | Good biocompatibility and better performance in guided bone regeneration than the self-healing process | [50] |

*PIPAAm* poly(*N*-isopropylacrylamide), *TGM* thermo-gelling macromere, *PEG* poly(ethyleneglycol)

# 8 Conclusion

Hydrogel-based scaffolds are promising biomaterial for dental tissue engineering, especially when stem cells are encapsulated on it as a suitable cell delivery system. Hydrogels have applicable properties because of their minimally invasive nature and high capability to match with different irregular defects. In addition, stem cell encapsulation by hydrogels provides facilitated cell implantation via support of cell proliferation, high viability protection against the external physical environment, modulating of cell differentiation, and applicability to precede considered dentistry tissue engineering projects. Natural biomaterials including collagen/gelatin, chitosan, hyaluronic acid, chondroitin sulfate, alginate, and fibrin are the most commonly used biomaterials for the preparation of hydrogels for stem cell encapsulation. This is due to their ideal biocompatibility, biodegradability, low cytotoxicity, and the possibility to mimic natural ECM for dental biomedical engineering. However, synthetic biomaterials—such as PVA, PPF/OPF, PNIPAAm, and PEG—can be combined with natural polymers during different chemical and physical methods to improve some of the natural polymeric hydrogel features, like stability and mechanical properties. However, advanced fabrication methods require extra development to improve the mechanical properties, physiological stability, as well as decrease the cytotoxicity and adverse effects of the hydrogels in biological condition.

In summary, stem cells can be simply incorporated into the hydrogel matrix, and the interior condition of their matrix is suitable for differentiation and functions of the stem cells or the uptake of differentiated cells. Despite notable studies in the development of multifunctional hydrogel systems in dentistry, the regenerative tissue field, and stem cell encapsulation, most of the accessible instruments in dental biomedical engineering have limited and variable sequels. An ideal biological tissue regeneration method has not yet been accessible, and the studies continue in this field.

# References


1. Frese, L., Dijkman, P. E., & Hoerstrup, S. P. (2016). Adipose tissue-derived stem cells in regenerative medicine. *Transfusion Medicine and Hemotherapy, 43*(4), 268–274.
2. Toh, W. (2014). Injectable hydrogels in dentistry: Advances and promises. *Austin Journal of Dentistry, 1*(1), 1001.
3. Ruan, Q., & Moradian-Oldak, J. (2014). Development of amelogenin-chitosan hydrogel for in vitro enamel regrowth with a dense interface. *Journal of Visualized Experiments: JoVE*, (89).
4. Galler, K. M., et al. (2011). A customized self-assembling peptide hydrogel for dental pulp tissue engineering. *Tissue Engineering Part A, 18*(1–2), 176–184.
5. Bae, M. S., et al. (2013). ZrO2 surface chemically coated with hyaluronic acid hydrogel loading GDF-5 for osteogenesis in dentistry. *Carbohydrate Polymers, 92*(1), 167–175.
6. Toh, W. S., et al. (2012). Modulation of mesenchymal stem cell chondrogenesis in a tunable hyaluronic acid hydrogel microenvironment. *Biomaterials, 33*(15), 3835–3845.

7. Wichterle, O., & Lim, D. (1960). Hydrophilic gels for biological use. *Nature, 185*(4706), 117.
8. Vasani, D., et al. (2011). Recent advances in the therapy of castration-resistant prostate cancer: The price of progress. *Maturitas, 70*(2), 194–196.
9. Ungerleider, J. L., & Christman, K. L. (2014). Concise review: Injectable biomaterials for the treatment of myocardial infarction and peripheral artery disease: Translational challenges and progress. *Stem Cells Translational Medicine, 3*(9), 1090–1099.
10. Ruvinov, E., Leor, J., & Cohen, S. (2010). The effects of controlled HGF delivery from an affinity-binding alginate biomaterial on angiogenesis and blood perfusion in a hindlimb ischemia model. *Biomaterials, 31*(16), 4573–4582.
11. Zhao, Y., et al. (2011). Preparation of gelatin microspheres encapsulated with bFGF for therapeutic angiogenesis in a canine ischemic hind limb. *Journal of Biomaterials Science, Polymer Edition, 22*(4–6), 665–682.
12. Liu, M., et al. (2017). Injectable hydrogels for cartilage and bone tissue engineering. *Bone Research, 5*, 17014.
13. Golchin, A., Hosseinzadeh, S., & Roshangar, L. (2018). The role of nanomaterials in cell delivery systems. *Medical Molecular Morphology*, 1–12.
14. Korbelář, P., Vacik, J., & Dylevský, I. (1988). Experimental implantation of hydrogel into the bone. *Journal of Biomedical Materials Research, 22*(9), 751–762.
15. Pellico, M. A. (1998). Stabilized anhydrous tooth whitening gel. Google Patents.
16. Li, R.-K., & Weisel, R. D. (2014). *Cardiac regeneration and repair: Biomaterials and tissue engineering*. Oxford: Elsevier.
17. Hasan, A., et al. (2015). Injectable hydrogels for cardiac tissue repair after myocardial infarction. *Advanced Science, 2*(11), 1500122.
18. Farrar, D. (2011). *Advanced wound repair therapies*. New York: Elsevier.
19. Li, J., & Mooney, D. J. (2016). Designing hydrogels for controlled drug delivery. *Nature Reviews Materials, 1*(12), 16071.
20. Kamath, K. R., & Park, K. (1993). Biodegradable hydrogels in drug delivery. *Advanced Drug Delivery Reviews, 11*(1–2), 59–84.
21. Williams, D. F., & Zhong, S. P. (1994). Biodeterioration/biodegradation of polymeric medical devices in situ. *International Biodeterioration & Biodegradation, 34*(2), 95–130.
22. Sauro, S., et al. (2013). Novel light-curable materials containing experimental bioactive micro-fillers remineralise mineral-depleted bonded-dentine interfaces. *Journal of Biomaterials Science, Polymer Edition, 24*(8), 940–956.
23. Galler, K. M., et al. (2011). Bioengineering of dental stem cells in a PEGylated fibrin gel. *Regenerative Medicine, 6*(2), 191–200.
24. Wang, Y. Y., et al. (2015). Biological and bactericidal properties of Ag-doped bioactive glass in a natural extracellular matrix hydrogel with potential application in dentistry. *European Cells & Materials, 29*, 342–355.
25. Jones, T. D., et al. (2016). An optimized injectable hydrogel scaffold supports human dental pulp stem cell viability and spreading. *Advances in Medicine, 2016*, 7363579.
26. Cavalcanti, B. N., Zeitlin, B. D., & Nör, J. E. (2013). A hydrogel scaffold that maintains viability and supports differentiation of dental pulp stem cells. *Dental Materials, 29*(1), 97–102.
27. Flores-Arriaga, J. C., et al. (2014). Cell viability of starch-based hydrogels for maxillofacial bone regeneration. *Dental Materials, 30*, e108–e109.
28. Tommasi, G., Perni, S., & Prokopovich, P. (2016). An injectable hydrogel as bone graft material with added antimicrobial properties. *Tissue Engineering Part A, 22*(11–12), 862–872.
29. Toh, W. S., & Loh, X. J. (2014). Advances in hydrogel delivery systems for tissue regeneration. *Materials Science and Engineering: C, 45*, 690–697.
30. Neel, E. A. A., et al. (2014). Tissue engineering in dentistry. *Journal of Dentistry, 42*(8), 915–928.
31. Wan, A. C. A., & Ying, J. Y. (2010). Nanomaterials for in situ cell delivery and tissue regeneration. *Advanced Drug Delivery Reviews, 62*(7–8), 731–740.

32. Moshaverinia, A., et al. (2013). Encapsulated dental-derived mesenchymal stem cells in an injectable and biodegradable scaffold for applications in bone tissue engineering. *Journal of Biomedical Materials Research Part A, 101*(11), 3285–3294.
33. Benoit, D. S. W., et al. (2008). Small functional groups for controlled differentiation of hydrogel-encapsulated human mesenchymal stem cells. *Nature Materials, 7*(10), 816.
34. Khojasteh, A., et al. (2016). Development of PLGA-coated β-TCP scaffolds containing VEGF for bone tissue engineering. *Materials Science and Engineering: C, 69*, 780–788.
35. Bongio, M., et al. (2011). Biomimetic modification of synthetic hydrogels by incorporation of adhesive peptides and calcium phosphate nanoparticles: in vitro evaluation of cell behavior. *European Cells & Materials, 22*, 359–376.
36. Gkioni, K., et al. (2010). Mineralization of hydrogels for bone regeneration. *Tissue Engineering Part B: Reviews, 16*(6), 577–585.
37. Hunt, N. C., & Grover, L. M. (2010). Cell encapsulation using biopolymer gels for regenerative medicine. *Biotechnology Letters, 32*(6), 733–742.
38. Douglas, T. E. L., et al. (2012). Enzymatic mineralization of hydrogels for bone tissue engineering by incorporation of alkaline phosphatase. *Macromolecular Bioscience, 12*(8), 1077–1089.
39. Kimura, K., et al. (2018). Formation process of hydroxyapatite granules in agarose hydrogel by electrophoresis. *Crystal Growth & Design, 18*(4), 1961–1966.
40. Lu, Y., et al. (2017). Multifunctional copper-containing Carboxymethyl chitosan/alginate scaffolds for eradicating clinical bacterial infection and promoting bone formation. *ACS Applied Materials & Interfaces, 10*(1), 127–138.
41. Vo, T. N., et al. (2015). In vitro and in vivo evaluation of self-mineralization and biocompatibility of injectable, dual-gelling hydrogels for bone tissue engineering. *Journal of Controlled Release, 205*, 25–34.
42. Xu, B., et al. (2017). A mineralized high strength and tough hydrogel for skull bone regeneration. *Advanced Functional Materials, 27*(4), 1604327.
43. Ho, E., Lowman, A., & Marcolongo, M. (2007). In situ apatite forming injectable hydrogel. *Journal of Biomedical Materials Research Part A: An Official Journal of The Society for Biomaterials, The Japanese Society for Biomaterials, and The Australian Society for Biomaterials and the Korean Society for Biomaterials, 83*(1), 249–256.
44. Douglas, T. E. L., et al. (2014). Injectable self-gelling composites for bone tissue engineering based on gellan gum hydrogel enriched with different bioglasses. *Biomedical Materials, 9*(4), 045014.
45. Watson, B. M., et al. (2015). Biodegradable, in situ-forming cell-laden hydrogel composites of hydroxyapatite nanoparticles for bone regeneration. *Industrial & Engineering Chemistry Research, 54*(42), 10206–10211.
46. Sánchez-Ferrero, A., et al. (2015). Development of tailored and self-mineralizing citric acid-crosslinked hydrogels for in situ bone regeneration. *Biomaterials, 68*, 42–53.
47. He, T., et al. (2017). In situ fabrication of defective CoN x single clusters on reduced graphene oxide sheets with excellent electrocatalytic activity for oxygen reduction. *ACS Applied Materials & Interfaces, 9*(27), 22490–22501.
48. Niranjan, R., et al. (2013). A novel injectable temperature-sensitive zinc doped chitosan/β--glycerophosphate hydrogel for bone tissue engineering. *International Journal of Biological Macromolecules, 54*, 24–29.
49. Dhivya, S., et al. (2015). Nanohydroxyapatite-reinforced chitosan composite hydrogel for bone tissue repair in vitro and in vivo. *Journal of Nanobiotechnology, 13*(1), 40.
50. Fu, S., et al. (2012). Injectable and thermo-sensitive PEG-PCL-PEG copolymer/collagen/n-HA hydrogel composite for guided bone regeneration. *Biomaterials, 33*(19), 4801–4809.

# Chapter 14
# Tissue Engineering in Periodontal Regeneration

**Aysel Iranparvar, Amin Nozariasbmarz, Sara DeGrave, and Lobat Tayebi**

## 1 Introduction

Millions of people around the world suffer from tooth loss caused by irreversible periodontium destruction due to acute trauma, extensive caries, or severe periodontal disease. Periodontal disease is a serious health issue that can affect quality of life. One of the main therapeutic goals of today's medicine is to develop novel regenerative treatments for periodontal tissues [1, 2].

The periodontium is a complex organ consisting of both mineralized and soft connective tissues. It includes the periodontal ligament (PDL), gingiva, cementum, and alveolar bone, generally named as the "attachment apparatus" (Fig. 14.1) [3]. The attachment apparatus fastens the tooth to surrounding bone and acts as a bumper to absorb the energy and forces from mastication. Periodontitis can endanger the integrity, health, and function of periodontal tissues [4].

The periodontal ligament (PDL) is an active connective tissue that is capable of continual adaptation to preserve tissue size and width. PDL acts like an anchor that connects the tooth to the alveolar socket and as a cushion to absorb the mechanical forces and loads resulting from mastication. Hence, PDL establishes the substratum of the periodontium and determines the tooth life span [5].

Accumulation of bacteria and other pathogenic microorganisms in the subgingival biofilm can lead to tissue inflammation called periodontitis. Some risk factors that increase the probability of having periodontitis include aging, smoking [6], and

A. Iranparvar
Tehran Dental Branch, Islamic Azad University, Tehran, Iran

A. Nozariasbmarz
Department of Materials Science and Engineering, Pennsylvania State University, University Park, PA, USA

S. DeGrave · L. Tayebi (✉)
Marquette University School of Dentistry, Milwaukee, WI, USA
e-mail: lobat.tayebi@marquette.edu



L. Tayebi (ed.), *Applications of Biomedical Engineering in Dentistry*,
https://doi.org/10.1007/978-3-030-21583-5_14

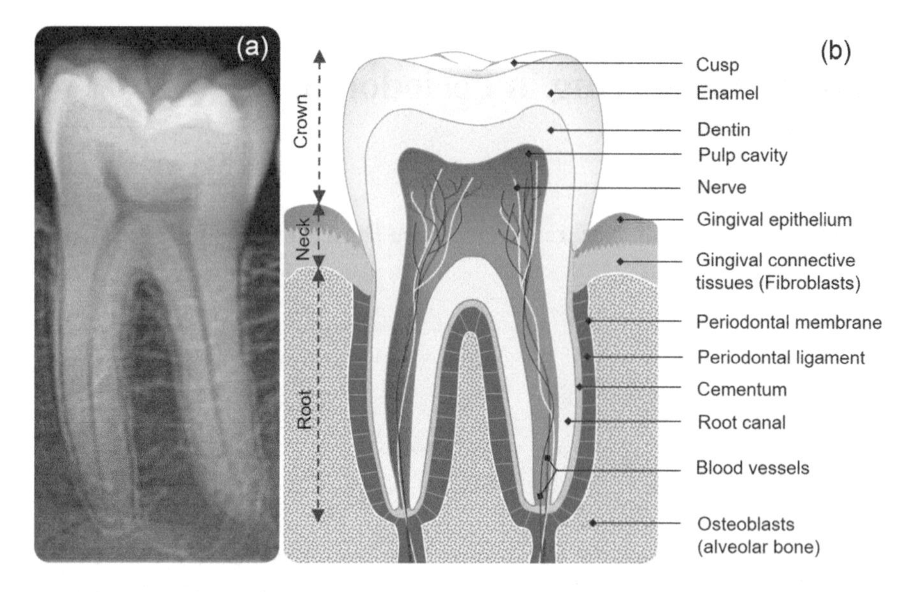


**Fig. 14.1** (**a**) Radiographic and (**b**) schematic structure of tooth and attachment apparatus

systemic disorders, such as diabetes, cardiovascular disease, rheumatoid arthritis, and adverse pregnancy outcomes [7]. Untreated periodontitis can lead to early tooth loss due to the inevitable destruction of the periodontium [6, 8].

There is an increasing demand for alternatives to replace and treat the diseased tissues and organs, such as destructed periodontal tissues. One of the major challenges in clinical periodontics has always been treating and managing periodontal defects, including intrabony defects and destructed cementum and PDL [9, 10]. Periodontal regeneration intends to repair the damaged periodontal tissues, both soft tissues (i.e., PDL) and hard tissues (i.e., alveolar bone and cementum) [2, 9].

Six tissues are typically involved to reconstruct a periodontal lesion, including the PDL, cementum, alveolar bone, gingival connective tissue, gingival epithelium, and all related vasculature [3]. Periodontal regeneration is one of the most complicated procedures to occur in the body [2].

In periodontal tissue engineering (TE), regeneration of a periodontal defect is achieved by stimulating the self-recovery capability of the periodontium. Therefore, the appropriate balance of cells and stimulating molecules, along with a durable matrix to control the regrowth of periodontal tissue, is necessary. It is important to prevent soft gingival tissue from growing into the defect so as to preserve the space for new bone formation and achieve functional regenerated tissue [4].

The regeneration ability varies for each of the mentioned tissues [11]. For instance, alveolar bone can regenerate bone that is similar to the original tissue, while the regenerative ability for the cementum and PDL is very limited and slow [12, 13]. For the first time, TE was suggested by Langer and Vacanti in 1993 as a possible technique for periodontal tissue regeneration [14].

Many regenerative treatment techniques have been established so far, such as the use of bone grafts and guided tissue/bone regeneration (GTR/GBR) [8, 15]. However, their success rates are poor and limited. Therefore, researches turned to stem cell-based techniques for periodontal regeneration. Nevertheless, these techniques also have limitations. For example, scaffold degeneration can be caused by inflammation, necrosis, unstable transplanted cells, etc. [16, 17].

In this chapter, a perspective into the fundamental principles of TE and its application in periodontal disease treatments is discussed based on the recent studies in TE and regenerative medicine.

## 2 Conventional Approaches for Periodontal Regeneration

Since the 1980s, several approaches have been established to enhance regeneration of periodontal tissues. The results of these methods have had limited success and poor clinical predictability [17, 18]. The main conventional methods are listed as follows.

### 2.1 *Bone Grafts*

Using grafts/biomaterials containing bone-inducing substances and bone-forming cells can result in bone formation. The biological function of bone grafts can be divided into three categories: osteogenesis (formation of new bone from living stem cells in graft materials), osteoinduction (bone formation by recruitment of immature cells by graft materials to become active osteoblasts), and osteoconduction (known as bone growth on the surface of the graft material) [17, 19]. There are several types of grafts used for bone regeneration.

#### 2.1.1 Autologous Bone Grafts

Autologous bone grafts, also known as autografts, are harvested from one site on the patient's body and transplanted to another site [20, 21]. Autologous bone grafts have been regarded as the gold standard in bone defect treatment because they only contain self-bone-forming cells. These cells can induce osteogenesis and are therefore able to integrate into the host bone more quickly and completely [21–23].

#### 2.1.2 Allogeneic Bone Grafts

Allogeneic bone grafts, also known as allografts, are bone tissues harvested from a genetically distinct source of the same species [24, 25]. Considering the limitation of autologous bone grafts, such as limited amount of obtained graft and surgical processes, allografts are considered the best substitute to autografts. However, it should be noted that allografts are more immunogenic in comparison to autografts and have a higher risk of failure [23, 26].

#### 2.1.3 Alloplastic Grafts

Alloplastic grafts are usually made from hydroxyapatite (prepared from bioactive glass) or calcium carbonate. Hydroxyapatite (HA) graft is the most used graft today due to its biocompatibility and osteoconduction potential. Calcium carbonate grafts are used less due to rapid resorption of the material and subsequent risk of fragile bone [27]. The major disadvantages of using bone grafts in periodontal regeneration include the risk of infection, surgical challenges, donor site morbidity, limited amount of graft in autologous and allogeneic grafts [28–30], and the risk of fibrous encapsulation associated with alloplastic materials [31, 32]. In addition, they generally result in tissue repair rather than true regeneration and cannot be used in all clinical situations [33, 34].

### *2.2 Guided Tissue Regeneration (GTR)*

The GTR technique aims to enhance the natural healing potential of the PDL and alveolar bone [4, 35–37]. If a periodontal defect is left empty after flap debridement, oral epithelium cells and fibroblasts grow down into the site of the defect, forming an unwanted fibroepithelial tissue that prevents the formation of a functional periodontal tissue [38–42].

It was considered that if the PDL and alveolar bone cells initially colonized the root surface and adjacent alveolar bone instead of gingival cells, the formation of a long junctional epithelium would be prevented, and a functional periodontium would be formed [4, 43].

In this method, a membrane with variable porosity is employed to cover the root surface, acting as a barrier to oral epithelium cells and fibroblasts, and promote the natural growth of bone and PDL cells (Fig. 14.2) [22]. GTR has been the gold standard approach for regeneration of intrabony and interradicular defects for more than a decade [40, 44]. However, several studies demonstrate that the outcomes of GTR therapies have been limited and unpredictable [1, 45–47].

## 3 Cell-Based Approaches for Periodontal Regeneration

Figure 14.3 shows three indispensable elements in cell-based regeneration in periodontal tissue engineering, including progenitor cells, signaling molecules, and scaffolds. They will be discussed in detail as follows.

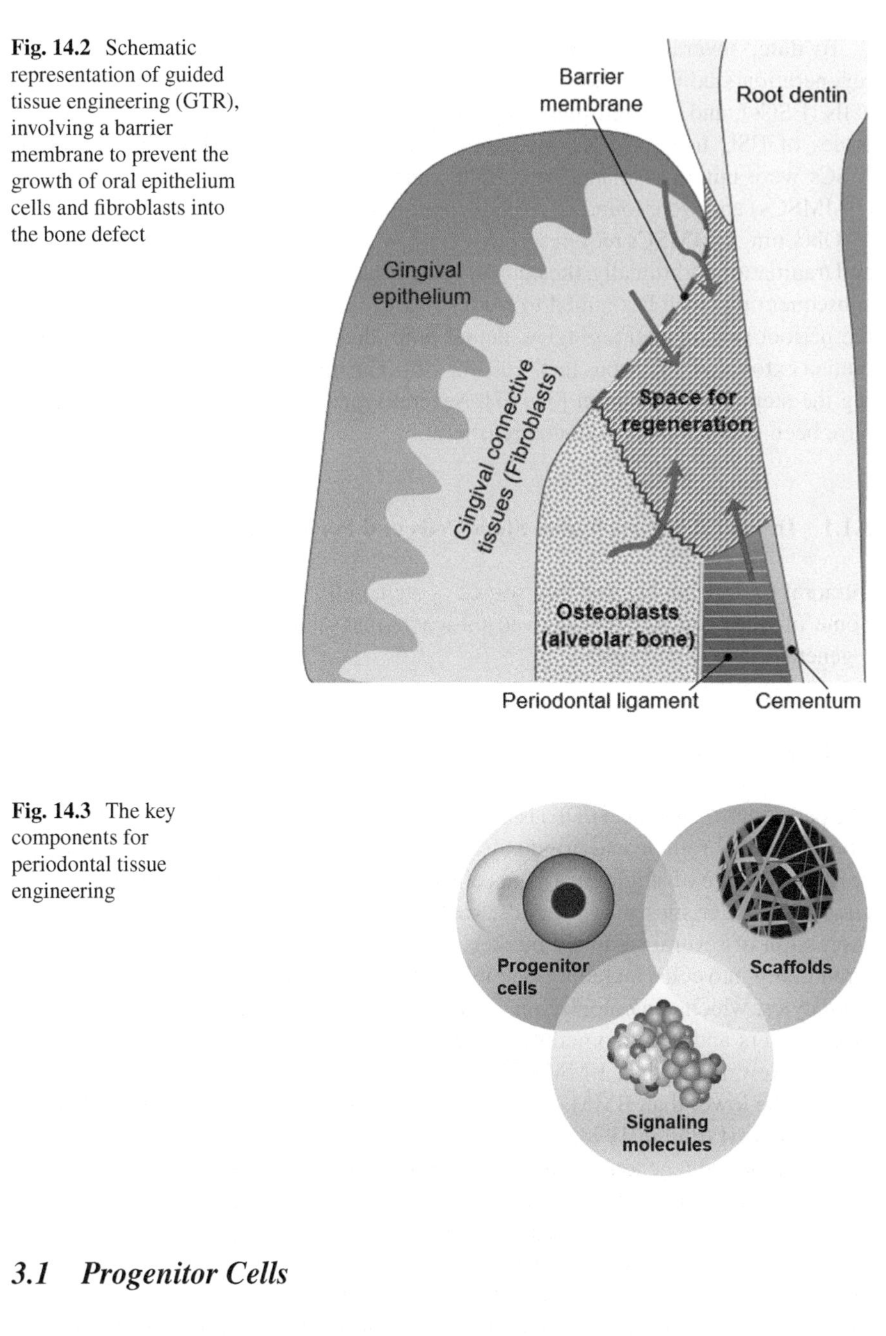


**Fig. 14.2** Schematic representation of guided tissue engineering (GTR), involving a barrier membrane to prevent the growth of oral epithelium cells and fibroblasts into the bone defect

**Fig. 14.3** The key components for periodontal tissue engineering

## *3.1 Progenitor Cells*

Stem cells are undifferentiated cells that have the potential for self-renewal, giving rise to more stem cells, and differentiation into various cell types in reaction to external signals [48].

To date, several types of stem cells have been introduced for periodontal regeneration studies, including mesenchymal stem cells (MSCs), embryonic stem cells (ESCs), and induced pluripotent stem cells (iPSCs). Considering the ethical issues of ESC usage, MSCs are more accepted for regeneration purposes [49]. MSCs were initially isolated from bone marrow-derived mesenchymal stem cells (BMMSCs) and were found to promote periodontal bone defects [50, 51].

Obtaining BMMSCs requires a bone marrow aspiration process, which is painful and traumatic. Additionally, the number of cells harvested is limited [51]. Therefore, subsequent research has aimed to harvest MSCs from oral-derived tissues such as the periodontal ligament, gingiva, dental pulp, dental follicles, apical papilla, and human exfoliated deciduous teeth [50, 52–56]. The most critical step in TE is selecting the stem cell population [32, 57]. Several types of mesenchyme-derived cells have been studied for periodontal regeneration.

### 3.1.1 Intraoral Mesenchymal Stem Cells and Periodontal Regeneration

Intraoral tissues can be used as a source of stem cells for periodontal regeneration. Some of the main intraoral-derived mesenchymal stem cells used in periodontal regeneration are listed below.

### 3.1.2 Periodontal Ligament Stem Cells (PDLSCs)

The periodontal ligament (PDL) is a specialized, dynamic connective tissue derived from the dental follicle and originating from neural crest cells [5, 58]. PDLSCs can be a good source of autologous stem cells for bone tissue engineering. They possess classic characteristics of stem cells, such as small size, slow cellular cycle, and expression of several stem cell markers [53, 59, 60]. They are also capable of differentiating into cells, including osteoblast-like cells, adipocytes, chondrocytes, and neurocytes, which can colonize on scaffolds [61–63]. PDLSCs can express all surface markers and immunomodulatory ability like BMMSCs [5, 50, 64]. They are able to grow faster than BMMSCs, although their osteogenic potential has been found to be lower than BMMSCs and dental pulp stem cells (DPSCs) [53, 59, 65].

For the first time in 1998, transplanted autologous PDL cells were used to promote periodontal regeneration in an animal study. The results suggested that autologous PDL cells can promote regeneration in vivo [3, 66]. Isaka et al. [67] placed PDL cells in a surgically created defect in an autologous dog model. Their results showed the formation of new cementum, while formation of alveolar bone was limited. Dogan et al. [68, 69] showed that seeding PDL cells in an autologous blood clot under a Teflon membrane supported regeneration of surgically created furcation and fenestrations. Seo et al. [70] harvested PDLSCs from human impacted third molar and found that these cells successfully could differentiate into PDL, cementum, alveolar bone, nerves, and blood vessels [50, 71–73]. A more recent study by Dan et al. [74] showed that PDL cells have more periodontal regenerative capacity compared to other periodontal-derived counterparts such as gingival fibroblasts and alveolar bone osteoblasts. All these studies confirm that PDL cells do have a regenerative capacity.

### Dental Follicle Stem Cells (DFSCs)

The dental follicle is a mesenchymal tissue. During the tooth development process, the dental follicle encircles the tooth germ. During root formation, dental follicle progenitors create the periodontal components, such as the PDL, alveolar bone, and cementum [75, 76]. DFSCs, which were first isolated from the dental follicle of human third molar, are the progenitor cells of osteoblast, cementoblasts, and fibroblasts. They can differentiate into osteoblasts, cementoblasts, adipocytes, and neurons [77] and produce cementum and bone [78, 79]. Bay et al. found that co-culturing of DFSCs with Hertwig epithelial root sheath (HERS) cells enhances the ability of DFSCs to regenerate cementum and PDL after transplantation [80]. Yokoi et al. [79] transplanted DFSCs subcutaneously to immunocompromised mice. They found that PDL-like structures with type I collagen began forming, indicating the potential of DFSCs in regenerating PDL.

### Gingival Epithelial Cells and Fibroblasts

Okuda et al. [81] cultured gingival epithelial cell sheets that were harvested from human gingival tissue for chronic desquamative gingivitis treatment. The results showed that autologous gingival epithelial sheets enhanced gingival regeneration. In another study, autologous gingival fibroblasts were used for patients with deficient attached gingiva, and this resulted in successfully increasing the keratinized tissue width [82].

GINTUITTM is an allogeneic cellular product, which is comprised of allogeneic cultured keratinocytes and fibroblasts in bovine collagen. McGuire et al. [83] indicated that the product is an effective therapy approach for repairing the keratinized gingiva.

### Periosteal Cells

The periosteum is a structure consisting of two layers. The outer layer is a fibrous layer containing fibroblasts, collagen, elastin, nerves, and a vascular network. The inner layer is a highly cellular layer comprised of osteoblast-like cells that support bone generation and bone reformation. The periosteum is considered a structure with regenerative capacity [84], as it has been found that cultured periosteum is capable of differentiation into an osteoblastic lineage. Autologous cultured periosteum sheet samples combined with HA and coagulated platelet-rich plasma (PRP) showed significant improvements in human infrabony defects and clinical attachment gain [85].

### Dental Pulp Stem Cells (DPSCs)

Dental pulp stem cells (DPSCs) were the first recognized human dental stem cells [86]. They have been harvested from human third molars [86, 87]. The dental pulp contains a variety of cells, including fibroblasts, neural cells, vascular cells, and undifferentiated stem cells. DPSCs are anatomically located on the most vascularized areas of the pulp. They possess multipotent differentiating and self-renewal ability. They can differentiate into osteoblasts, odontoblasts, neural cells, and chondrocytes in vitro [59, 88–90]. DPSCs can successfully be isolated and characterized from human extracted teeth, inflamed pulp tissue [91], supernumerary teeth [92], and natal teeth [93] by a variety of approaches. For example, D'Aquino et al. [94] showed that DPSCs isolated from human teeth, along with collagen sponge implants, have improved mandibular bone tissue regeneration in patients.

DPSCs have also been reported to have immunomodulatory properties on mice [95]. They have several similar features to BMMSCs; however, their osteogenic potentials are limited in comparison [86]. Human autologous DPSCs, along with HA or beta-tricalcium phosphate (TCP), have shown capability of forming bone and cementum [32, 86, 89, 96]. However, the effect of these stem cells on periodontal regeneration has been inconsistent to date [32].

### Stem Cells from Human Exfoliated Deciduous Teeth (SHED)

Miura et al. [55] described SHED as clonogenic cells with high proliferation capacity that can differentiate into several cell types. They transplanted SHED in vivo and found that they were able to promote bone generation. These stem cells are mainly obtained from children's tooth pulp tissue around ages 6 to 12 [97]. Obtaining SHED is simple and beneficial because of six reasons: (1) They are less mature compared to permanent teeth, so they possess a higher proliferation ratio. (2) They have the flexibility of differentiating into a variety of cells, including osteoblasts, adipocytes, odontoblasts, and neural cells. (3) They are easily achievable. (4) They are convenient for use in young patients with mixed dentition. (5) There is no need to sacrifice a tooth. (6) Obtaining process is atraumatic [76].

According to previous studies, SHED are not able to differentiate directly into osteoblasts, but they can induce in vivo bone generation by forming osteoinductive patterns to employ osteogenic cells in rats. Therefore, it has been concluded that deciduous teeth, in addition to providing a guidance for permanent tooth eruption, are associated with inducing bone generation during permanent tooth eruption [55]. Although both DPSCs and SHED are obtained from pulp tissue, they show noticeable differences in proliferative potentials [98]. SHED possess a higher proliferation ratio compared to DPSCs and can differentiate into a variety of mesenchymal lineages [55, 99].

#### Stem Cells from Apical Papilla (SCAP)

SCAPs were isolated and introduced by Sonoyama et al. from premature roots of human third molars [54]. They can differentiate into several mesenchymal lineages such as osteoblasts, odontoblasts, chondrocytes, adipocytes, smooth muscle cells, and neurons in vitro [100–102]. In comparison to DPSCs, SCAPs possess a higher proliferation rate and mineralization capacity. However, compared to BMMSCs, they have lower adipogenic capacity [54, 101]. It has been reported that SCAPs possess immunomodulatory properties [103].

In one study, SCAPs were transplanted into immunocompromised rats using HA and tricalcium phosphate particles as dentin-like carriers. Human SCAPs and PDLSCs were also transplanted into mini pigs. The results showed successful root and periodontal regeneration. In addition, an in vivo study on human SCAPs, along with porous ceramic discs that were transplanted into immunosuppressed rats, showed that hard tissues can be formed [104].

### 3.1.3 Extraoral Mesenchymal Stem Cells and Periodontal Regeneration

Extraoral tissues can be used as a source of stem cells for periodontal regeneration. The main extraoral-derived mesenchymal stem cells used in periodontal regeneration are listed below.

#### Bone Marrow-Derived Mesenchymal Stem Cells (BMMSCs)

Bone marrow-derived mesenchymal stem cells (BMMSCs) have been the most studied among mesenchymal stem cells. Human BMMSCs are pluripotent stem cells which originate from the bone marrow and can differentiate into multiple mesenchymal linages such as osteoblasts, chondrocytes, and adipocytes [105–107]. BMMSCs have been found to generate the cementum, periodontal ligament, and alveolar bone, indicating that the bone marrow can be a convenient source for periodontal regeneration [105].

Pittenger et al. [107] aspirated bone marrows from 350 donors and found differentiation of MSCs into bone, cartilage, and fat. Kuo et al. [108] reported that BMMSCs can induce the generation of PDL, odontoblasts, and cementum from DPSCs. Kawaguchi et al. [109] showed that autologous bone marrow-derived mesenchymal cells promote periodontal regeneration in surgically induced class III furcation defects in dogs. Other studies also showed that BMMSCs were able to control diabetes in animal models [110] and stimulate wound healing [111].

Adipose Tissue-Derived Stromal Cells (ATSCs)

Adipose tissue is another extraoral source of mesenchymal stem cells. Lately, adipose tissue-derived stem cells have been extensively studied as an applicable source of cells for regenerative medicine [112, 113]. They have been introduced as a convenient source of stem cells because they are abundant and easy to obtain [17]. Various studies have confirmed the capability of ATSCs' differentiation into osteogenic, neurogenic, adipogenic, myogenic, and chondrogenic cells [114–116]. ATSCs, in combination with platelet-rich plasma (PRP), have been shown to induce alveolar bone and PDL-like structures fabrication in mice [117].

## *3.2 Signaling Molecules*

Another major TE approach for periodontal regeneration is to stimulate cells near the defect area using biological signals. Table 14.1 summarizes different types of signaling molecules in addition to their effects and applications. The main signaling molecules are listed as follows.

### 3.2.1 Insulin-Like Growth Factors (IGFs)

Insulin-like growth factor (IGF) is a hormone with a similar molecular structure to insulin, which has different forms. IGF-1 is an effective chemotactic agent that enhances the formation of new blood vessels and promotes the formation of bone and cementum. It causes in vitro protein synthesis and periodontal ligament fibroblasts mitogenesis [118]. Studies on non-human primate models showed that IGF-1 cannot modify periodontal wound healing by itself [126]. Lynch et al. [127] proposed using IGF-1 along with platelet-derived growth factor-B (PDGF-B) to increase periodontal regeneration. IGF-2 is an active factor in bone formation which abounds in bone as a growth factor. Although it helps in bone formation, it is not as effective as IGF-1 [128].

### 3.2.2 Platelet-Derived Growth Factor (PDGF)

PDGF is a growth factor that controls cell differentiation and growth. It consists of two polypeptide chains encoded by two dissimilar genes, PDGF-A and PDGF-B [5]. PDGF can enhance periodontal tissue regeneration by stimulating mitosis of PDL cells and synthesis of gingival fibroblast hyaluronate [2]. Clinical studies have shown that using PDGF-B improves the treatment of periodontal bone defects. It enhances the rate of filling bone defects and improvement of attachment level, along with reduction of gingival recession [129].

**Table 14.1** Signaling molecules, theirs effects, and applications

| Signaling molecules | Effects | Applications | Ref. |
|---|---|---|---|
| Insulin-like growth factor (IGF) | Enhances the formation of new blood vessels and promotes the formation of bone and cementum | Protein synthesis, periodontal ligament fibroblasts mitogenesis | [118] |
| Platelet-derived growth factor (PDGF) | Controls cell differentiation and growth | Periodontal tissue regeneration | [2, 5] |
| Bone morphogenetic protein (BMP) | Interacts with specific receptors on the cell surface | Development of new blood vessels, bone fabrication | [2, 119] |
| Fibroblast growth factor (FGF) | Triggers development of new blood vessels and stimulates differentiation and proliferation of mesenchymal cells | Tissue regeneration, wound healing, and angiogenesis | [120] |
| Transforming growth factor-beta (TGF-β) | Adjusts and stimulates several biological processes and components such as embryonic growth and immune regulation | Induces cells to grow in soft agar | [121, 122] |
| Periodontal ligament-derived growth factor (PDL-CTX) | Periodontal regeneration without chemotactic effect on epithelial cells or gingival fibroblasts | Autocrine chemotactic agent for periodontal ligament cells | [2, 123] |
| Enamel matrix derivative (EMD) | Stimulates differentiation of mesenchymal cells including osteoblasts | Enamel formation, root and attachment apparatus development | [44, 124] |
| Platelet-rich plasma (PRP) | Developing grafting procedures, decreasing periodontal healing time, and improving bone quality | Source of growth factors such as PDGF and TGF-β | [1, 125] |

As mentioned earlier, the combination of PDGF-B and IGF-1 can improve periodontal regeneration; at initial stages of wound healing after a surgery, it increases the formation of the periodontal attachment apparatus [130].

### 3.2.3 Bone Morphogenetic Proteins (BMPs)

BMPs are growth factors that interact with specific receptors on the cell surface. There are several BMPs that originate from the human body. Three of these are bone morphogenetic protein-2, bone morphogenetic protein-3 (known as osteogenin), and bone morphogenetic protein-7. All are highly involved in periodontal regeneration [119]. BMP stimulates development of new blood vessels and bone fabrication [2]. BMPs have morphogenetic potential and are important in conducting migration and attachment of stem cells onto scaffolds to increase the response of stem cells to BMPs [131].

### 3.2.4 Fibroblast Growth Factor (FGF)

The FGF is one of the heparin-binding growth factors involved in tissue regeneration, wound healing, and angiogenesis [120]. FGF triggers development of new blood vessels and can stimulate differentiation and proliferation of mesenchymal cells [120]. It is a signaling protein that is isolated from regular tissue in two forms: acidic FGF (a-FGF) and basic FGF (b-FGF) [2].

There are several different forms of FGF. FGF2 is the most studied FGF and can attach to heparin to develop new blood vessels and induce mitosis [132]. In the wound healing process, it can adjust different cellular functions, including proliferation and migration, among others [133]. In vivo studies of FGF2 in non-human primates show that it can trigger regeneration of periodontal tissue with new cementum and alveolar bone creation [134]. Furthermore, it can improve bone formation by enhancing the rate of differentiation of osteoprogenitor cells. FGF2 is a capable candidate for regenerating soft and hard periodontal tissues because it can trigger the migration and proliferation of ligament cells [55, 70, 90, 95]. An in vivo study on skin defect of mice indicated that regeneration of soft tissue can be accelerated by b-FGF [135].

### 3.2.5 Transforming Growth Factor-Beta (TGF-β)

TGF-β is highly concentrated in human bone and platelets, and it can induce cells to grow in soft agar. TGF-β adjusts different types of biological processes such as differentiation of adult stem cells, embryonic growth, immune regulation, etc. [121]. It stimulates several biological processes and components, including fibronectin and osteocalcin biosynthesis, chemotaxis of osteoblasts, bone matrix deposition, type I collagen, and periodontal ligament fibroblast proliferative activity, as well as rising ECM production. Moreover, it decreases the connective tissue destruction due to the reduction of metalloproteinases and plasminogen activator inhibitor (PAI) synthesis [2, 122].

TGF-β is composed of three 25 kDa homodimeric mammalian isoforms, including β1, β2, and β3. TGF-β1 can result in proliferation of MSCs, wound healing, enhanced ECM formation, inhibition of inflammation, and production of pre-osteoblasts, chondrocytes, osteoblasts, and collagen [136–138]. In addition, it has been reported that TGF-β1 raises cell surface proteoglycan genes in PDL cells [139, 140], assists in DNA and fibronectin synthesis, and produces protein acids [141, 142].

### 3.2.6 Periodontal Ligament-Derived Growth Factor (PDL-CTX)

Periodontal ligament-derived growth factor (PDL-CTX) is a novel polypeptide growth factor from human periodontal cells [143]. It is a specific autocrine chemotactic agent for periodontal ligament cells, which is one thousand times more effective than other growth factors, including IGF, PDGF, and TGF [2]. Furthermore, PDL-CTX can have a favorable effect on periodontal regeneration because it does not have a chemotactic effect on epithelial cells or gingival fibroblasts [123].

#### 3.2.7 Enamel Matrix Derivative (EMD)

Enamel matrix proteins are produced by ameloblasts and are responsible for growth of HA crystals and enamel mineralization [144]. In addition to their role in enamel formation, they are also involved in root and attachment apparatus development [44]. EMD is available commercially in an injectable gel solution form known as Emdogain, which consists of enamel proteins amelogenin, ameloblastin, amelotin, tuftelin, and enamelin [3]. Emdogain was the first signaling product that could successfully regenerate periodontal tissue [22]. It has been reported that EMD can stimulate differentiation of mesenchymal cells including osteoblasts. Hejil et al. [124] applied EMD in intrabony defects; the results showed 66% bone fill in defected areas.

#### 3.2.8 Platelet-Rich Plasma (PRP)

PRP is a concentration of autologous plasma isolated by centrifugation of patient's blood. PRP acts as a source of growth factors and contains growth factors such as PDGF and TGF-β [125]. Various commercial PRP kits are available to facilitate chair-side PRP isolation for clinicians. Although there is not enough convincing information about PRP benefits for periodontal regeneration, it seems that PRP can be advantageous for developing grafting procedures, decreasing periodontal healing time, and improving bone quality [1].

### 3.3 *Scaffolds*

To utilize the maximum potential of stem cells, an isolated three-dimensional (3D) environment should be provided to allow the cells to proliferate in three dimensions and be transferred into the defected area [145]. Scaffolds can be in the form of a sponge, gel, or complex network of pores and channels. All the scaffolds used in TE are designed to degrade gradually after implantation in the targeted site, being replaced by new tissue [1, 146]. The major challenge in TE is to develop regeneration in three dimensions and promote angiogenesis over the entirety of the scaffold.

The main roles of scaffold include as follows [132]: (1) It serves as a framework to supply physical support for the regenerating area, to preserve the shape of the defect and to prevent surrounding tissue from collapsing into the defect. (2) It provides a 3D substratum for ECM production, cell adhesion, and migration. (3) It serves as a barrier with selective permeability to confine the migration of cells. (4) It serves as a growth factor delivery vehicle for cells [2].

Additionally, the key features of an ideal scaffold are (1) biocompatibility, biodegradability, and nontoxicity; (2) being able to preserve migration, attachment, proliferation of the cells, and production of new ECM; (3) having enough mechanical strength to endure physical stress and being able to preserve the surrounding bone from stress; (4) having an intrinsic network of interconnected pores; and (5) providing appropriate conditions for neovascularization [147].

### 3.3.1 Biomaterials Used as Scaffolds

To date, a variety of biocompatible materials have been used to fabricate scaffolds, including polymers, metals, ceramics, and proteins [148]. The following is the list of main biomaterials used as scaffolds.

#### Ceramics

Bioceramics have a long history of use for joint and tooth implants [149]. Ceramics used in bone TE are natural and synthetic hydroxyapatite (HA) and beta-tricalcium phosphate (TCP). They are biocompatible and osteoinductive and, due to being protein free, are not able to induce immunological reactions [2]. HA is a natural bioceramic found in hard tissues such as dentine and enamel [149] and was one of the first materials used as scaffolds. It can be synthetic or derived from natural sources like bovine bone or coraline [2].

Some studies suggest nanostructured HA as a potent material due to its good biocompatibility and bone integration ability [150, 151]. TCP is a natural material consisting of calcium and phosphorous and is used as a ceramic bone substitute [2].

#### Metals and Alloys

Titanium and its alloys, cobalt-chromium alloys, and stainless steel are used in fabrication of scaffolds [149]. Titanium is the most common material used for implants due to its decent biocompatibility, osteointegration potential, and ability to be laminated with various polymers [152]. However, metals and ceramics have very limited potential to be used as effective scaffolds because they are not biodegradable and cannot be processed easily [148].

#### Polymers

Polymers have been widely used for TE due to their biodegradability and capability of being processed [153–156]. There are two types of polymer materials: synthetic polymers and natural polymers [148]. The most biodegradable polymers are polyesters, polycaprolactone, polyanhydride, polycarbonate, polyfumarate, and polyorthoester [157–162]. The most widely used polymers in TE include polyesters like polyglycolic acid (PGA), polylactic acid (PLA), and their copolymer poly(lactic-co-glycolic acid) (PLGA) [163–166].

#### Synthetic Polymers

Polyglycolic acid (PGA), a simple and linear polymer of glycolic acid, is the first polymer scaffold used in TE. For the first time in the 1980s, PGA was used alone as a scaffold in the form of mesh for renal injury treatment. It is also used as a bone fracture fixation implant and suture material [2, 149].

Polylactic acid (PLA) is a polymer of lactic acid and is more hydrolysis resistant and hydrophobic than PGA. The copolymer of PLA with PGA is PLGA. It was first used as a suture material (Vicryl) in 1974 and degrades in 8 weeks [167]. It was the first FDA-approved copolymer and has been the first candidate for use in dental tissue regenerations due to its biocompatibility, structural strength, controllable degradation, and ability to deliver growth factors. PLGA can also be used in combination with other polymers like gelatin [155].

Polymethylmethacrylate (PMMA) is a highly biocompatible, but nondegradable, polymer. Due to its excellent biocompatibility, it has been widely used for mandibular reconstruction and repairing skull defects and bone cements in clinical procedures [168, 169]. Nevertheless, PMMA promotes fibrotic tissue formation [169].

#### Naturally Derived Polymers

Naturally derived polymers include proteins derived from natural ECM or polysaccharides. They have been widely used in TE [170–172].

Chitosan is a biocompatible, nontoxic, and non-immunogenic carbohydrate polymer derived from chitin, which is found in crustacean shells [173] and has shown improvement in bone regeneration and wound healing, as well as antibacterial activity [174, 175] and bioadhesive character [176]. Chitosan is capable of being made into different shapes and structures such as membranes [177], fibers [178], sponges [179], paste [180], microspheres [181], and porous scaffolds [182]. These characteristics make it suitable to be used as a scaffold for tissue regeneration. Chitosan can also be used as a copolymer with other materials [165, 183].

Collagens are made by several cell types [184]. Collagens can be formed into various forms and structures such as sheets, gels, sponges, fibers, and films [1, 185, 186]. However, collagen scaffolds have not shown enough mechanical strength, and their degradation rate is not convincing. Therefore, crosslinking agents such as formaldehyde, polyepoxy, and glutaraldehyde compounds have been used to enhance the thermal, mechanical, and biological properties of collagen [1, 187].

Fibrin is a blood component critical for hemostasis. It is produced from fibrinogen and thrombin during hemostasis and enhances wound healing [1, 149]. After tooth extractions, blood clots have been used as natural scaffolds for promoting bone healing process [149]. Fibrin is widely used as a biopolymer scaffold in periodontal TE due to its biocompatibility, biodegradability, and simple preparation and handling process [149]. Fibrin scaffolds are also available in combination with other polymers, such as fibrin-PEG blend [172, 188]. Fibrin hydrogels are used as a heparin-binding delivery system and cell seeding during inkjet printing process [172].

Hydrogels are a new type of biomaterials that are injectable into the periodontium. They are made of viscous polymers, which are composed of synthetic or natural macromolecules [189–191].

Alginate is a hydrogel isolated from brown seaweed and bacteria [192]. It is biocompatible and nontoxic and can have a slow gelling time depending on temperature and concentration [193]. Its limitations include uncontrollable degradation and low viscoelasticity. These can be improved by using alginate incorporation with HA [194].

## 4 Cell Sheet Technique

Cell sheet technique is a novel approach for harvesting and delivering cells in TE [195]. Conventionally, in TE proteolytic enzymes are utilized to fragment the ECM and release the cells, which could impair cell functions and damage the cell membrane because the proteolytic enzymes hydrolyze cell membrane proteins [32]. This technique prevents the enzymatic digestion of proteins, keeping the normal cell and ECM interactions [196]. In other words, it is possible to harvest a complete cellular sheet with intact ECM and cell-cell junctions [3]. This technique has been used recently to regenerate periodontal defects [197, 198].

Cell sheet engineering involves thermo-responsive systems including poly(N-isopropylacrylamide) (PIPAAm) polymer for cell culturing [3]. This polymer is hydrophilic at temperatures greater than 32 °C and hydrophobic when temperatures are lower than 32 °C. In addition, cells are prone to attach to hydrophobic surfaces. These properties are beneficial for detaching the cell sheets from cultures [32].

Harvested cell sheets are delicate and fragile. Thus, manipulation and implantation of them can be challenging. Therefore, 3D biocompatible scaffolds such as hyaluronic acid, fibrin gel, and ceramic bovine bone have been developed to increase stabilization and strength, also facilitating the manipulation and results [32].

Cell sheet technology has been utilized for various TE applications, such as cornea transplantation using corneal epithelial cell sheets and myocardial tissue regeneration using cardiomyocyte cell sheets [199, 200]. They have been extensively applied to improve periodontal regeneration in animal studies using dogs and rats [201].

# 5 Conclusions

During the last few decades, a rapid development has been reported in periodontal regeneration methods. Recent studies have emphasized the importance of wound stability and space preservation for a predictable and optimal tissue regeneration, but they are not achievable by current clinically applied techniques. Successful results can be feasible by utilizing a combination of cells, signaling molecules, and scaffolds to construct the anatomy based on the complex structure of periodontal tissues and defects. Three-dimensional scaffolds are the key for complete periodontal regeneration. Application of tissue engineering on periodontal regeneration is still in its initial stages and requires more investigation. Recent advances in material science, tissue engineering, and microscopy techniques provide a brighter perspective for more predictable regenerative therapies for periodontal defects in the near future.

# References


1. Chen, F.-M., & Jin, Y. (2010). Periodontal tissue engineering and regeneration: Current approaches and expanding opportunities. *Tissue Engineering: Part B, 16*, 219–225.
2. Dabra, S., Chhina, K., Soni, N., & Bhatnagar, R. (2012). Tissue engineering in periodontal regeneration: A brief review. *Dental Research Journal, 9*, 671–680.
3. Ivanovski, S., Bartold, P. M., Gronthos, S., & Hutmacher, D. W. (2017). Periodontal tissue engineering. In R. J. Waddington & A. J. Sloan (Eds.), *Tissue engineering and regeneration in dentistry: Current strategies*. West Sussex, UK, Wiley.
4. Babo, P. S., Reis, R. L., & Gomes, M. E. (2017). Periodontal tissue engineering: Current strategies and the role of platelet rich hemoderivatives. *Journal of Materials Chemistry B, 5*, 3617.
5. Maeda, H., Wada, N., Fujii, S., Tomokiyo, A., & Akamine, A. (2011). Periodontal ligament stem cells. In A. Gholamrezanezhad (Ed.), *Stem cells in clinic and research*. London, InTech.
6. Pihlstrom, B. L., Michalowicz, B. S., & Johnson, N. W. (2005). Periodontal diseases. *Lancet, 366*, 1809.
7. Al-Shammari, K. F., Al-Khabbaz, A. K., Al-Ansari, J. M., Neiva, R., & Wang, H. L. (2005). Risk indicators for tooth loss due to periodontal disease. *Journal of Periodontology, 76*, 1910.
8. Chen, F.-M., & Shi, S. (2014). Periodontal tissue engineering, in *Principles of Tissue Engineering* (pp. 1507–1540). 4th edn, ed. by R. Vacanti, R. Lanza and J. Langer. Boston, MA, Academic Press.
9. Grover, V., Malhorta, R., Kapoor, A., Verma, N., & Sahota, J. K. (2010). Future of periodontal regeneration. *Journal of Oral Health Community Dentistry, 4*, 38–47.
10. Hood, L., Heath, J. R., Phelps, M. E., & Lin, B. (2004). Systems biology and new technologies enable predictive and preventive medicine. *Science, 306*, 640–643.
11. Galler, K. M., & D'Souza, R. N. (2011). Tissue engineering approaches for regenerative dentistry. *Regenerative Medicine, 6*, 111–124.
12. Abou Neel, E. A., Chrzanowski, W., Salih, V. M., Kim, H. W., & Knowles, J. C. (2014). Tissue engineering in dentistry. *Journal of Dentistry, 42*, 915–928.
13. Silva, C. R., Gomez-Florit, M., Babo, P. S., Reis, R. L., & Gomes, M. E. (2017). 3D functional scaffolds for dental tissue engineering. In Y. Deng & J. Kuiper (Eds.), *Functional 3D tissue engineering scaffolds*.

14. Langer, R., & Vacanti, J. P. (1993). Tissue engineering. *Science, 260*, 920–926.
15. Chen, F. M., Zhang, J., Zhang, M., An, Y., Chen, F., & Wu, Z. F. (2010). A review on endogenous regenerative technology in periodontal regenerative medicine. *Biomaterials, 31*, 7892–7927.
16. Yang, J., Yamato, M., Kohno, C., Nishimoto, A., Sekine, H., Fukai, F., & Okano, T. (2005). Cell sheet engineering: Recreating tissues without biodegradable scaffolds. *Biomaterials, 26*, 6415–6422.
17. Iwata, T., Yamato, M., Ishikawa, I., Ando, T., & Okano, T. (2014). Tissue engineering in periodontal tissue. *The Anatomical Record, 297*, 16–25.
18. Esposito, M., Grusovin, M. G., Papanikolaou, N., Coulthard, P., & Worthington, H. V. (2009). Enamel matrix derivative (Emdogain(R)) for periodontal tissue regeneration in intrabony defects. *Cochrane Database Syst Rev*, CD003875.
19. Mellonig, J. T. (1992). Autogenous and allogeneic bone grafts in periodontal therapy. *Critical Reviews in Oral Biology and Medicine, 3*, 333–352.
20. King, J. A., & Miller, W. M. (2007). Bioreactor development for stem cells expansion and controlled differentiation. *Current Opinion in Chemical Biology, 11*, 394–398.
21. Hosokawa, K., Arai, F., Yoshihara, H., Nakamura, Y., Gomei, Y., Iwasaki, H., Ito, K., & Suda, T. (2007). Function of oxidative stress in the regulation of hematopoietic stem cell-niche interaction. *Biochemical and Biophysical Research Communications, 363*, 578–583.
22. Shimauchi, H., Nemoto, E., Ishihata, H., & Shimomura, M. (2013). Possible functional scaffolds for periodontal regeneration. *Japanese Dental Science Review, 49*, 118–130.
23. Wang, W., & Yeung, K. W. K. (2017). Bone grafts and biomaterials substitutes for bone defect repair: A review. *Bioactive Materials, 2*, 224–247.
24. Roberts, T. T., & Rosenbaum, A. J. (2012). Bone grafts, bone substitutes and orthobiologics: The bridge between basic science and clinical advancements in fracture healing. *Organogenesis, 8*, 114–124.
25. Goldberg, V. M., & Akhavan, S. (2005). Biology of bone grafts. In J. R. Lieberman & G. E. Friedlaender (Eds.), *Bone regeneration and repair* (pp. 57–65). Totowa, NJ. Springer.
26. Stevenson, S., & Horowitz, M. (1992). The response to bone allografts. *The Journal of Bone and Joint Surgery, 74*, 939–950.
27. Kumar, P., Vinitha, B., & Fathima, G. (2013). Bone grafts in dentistry. *Journal of Pharmacy & Bioallied Sciences, 5*(Suppl 1), S125–S127.
28. Hjørting-Hansen, E. (2002). Bone grafting to the jaws with special reference to reconstructive preprosthetic surgery: A historical review. *Mund-, Kiefer- und Gesichtschirurgie, 6*(1), 6–14.
29. Burchardt, H. (1983). The biology of bone graft repair. *Clinical Orthopaedics and Related Research, 174*, 28–42.
30. Cordaro, L., Amade, D. S., & Cordaro, M. (2002). Clinical results of alveolar ridge augmentation with mandibular block bone grafts in partially edentulous patients prior to implant placement. *Clinical Oral Implants Research, 13*(1), 103–111.
31. Garraway, R., Young, W. G., Daley, T., Harbow, D., & Bartold, P. M. (1998). An assessment of the osteoinductive potential of commercial demineralized freeze dried bone in the murine thing muscle implantation model. *Journal of Periodontal, 69*(12), 1325–1336.
32. Thomas, G. V., Thomas, N. G., John, S., & Ittycheria, P. G. (2015). The scope of stem cells in periodontal regeneration. *Journal of Dental Oral Disorders and Therapy, 3*(2), 1–9.
33. Kinaia, B. M., Chogle, S. M. A., Kinaia, A. M., & Goodis, H. E. (2012). Regenerative therapy: A periodontal-endodontic perspective. *Dental Clinics of North America, 56*(3), 537–547.
34. Ledesma-Martínez, E., Mendoza-Núñez, V. M., & Santiago-Osorio, E. (2016). Mesenchymal stem cells derived from dental pulp: A review. *Stem Cells International, 2016, 4709572*.
35. Melcher, A. H., McCulloch, C. A., Cheong, T., Nemeth, E., & Shiga, A. (1987). Cells from bone synthesize cementum-like and bone-like tissue in vitro and may migrate into periodontal ligament in vivo. *Journal of Periodontal Research, 22*, 246–247.

36. Karring, T., Nyman, S., Gottlow, J., & Laurell, L. (1993). Development of the biological concept of guided tissue regeneration-animal and human studies. *Periodontology, 2000*(1), 26–35.
37. Buser, D., Warrer, K., & Karring, T. (1990). Formation of a periodontal ligament around titanium implants. *Journal of Periodontology, 61*, 597–601.
38. Clem, D. S., & Bishop, J. P. (1991). Guided tissue regeneration in periodontal therapy. *Journal of the California Dental Association, 19*, 67.
39. Caffesse, R. G., & Becker, W. (1991). Principles and techniques of guided tissue regeneration. *Dental Clinics of North America, 35*, 479.
40. Needleman, I., Tucker, R., Giedrys-Leeper, E., & Worthington, H. (2005). Guided tissue regeneration for periodontal intrabony defects-a Cochrane systematic review. *Periodontology 2000, 2000*(37), 106.
41. Phillips, J. D., & Palou, M. E. (1992). A review of the guided tissue regeneration concept. *General Dentistry, 40*, 118.
42. Murphy, K. G., & Gunsolley, J. C. (2003). Guided tissue regeneration for the treatment of periodontal intrabony and furcation defects. A systematic review. *Annals of Periodontology, 8*, 266.
43. Gottlow, J., Nyman, S., Karring, T., & Lindhe, J. (1984). New attachment formation as the result of controlled tissue regeneration. *Journal of Clinical Periodontology, 11*, 494–503.
44. Siaili, M., Chatzopoulou, D., & Gillam, D. G. (2018). An overview of periodontal regenerative procedures for the general dental practitioner. *Saudi Dental Journal, 30*, 26–37.
45. Aichelmann-Reidy, M. E., & Reynolds, M. A. (2008). Predictability of clinical outcomes following regenerative therapy in intrabony defects. *Journal of Periodontology, 79*, 387.
46. Zeichner-David, M. (2006). Regeneration of periodontal tissues: Cementogenesis revisited. *Periodontology 2000, 2000*(41), 196.
47. Grzesik, W. J., & Narayanan, A. S. (2002). Cementum and periodontal wound healing and regeneration. *Critical Reviews in Oral Biology and Medicine, 13*, 474.
48. Lin, N. H., Menicacin, D., Mrozik, K., Gronthos, S., & Bartold, P. M. (2008). Putative stem cells in regenerating human periodontium. *Journal of Periodontal Research, 53*, 514–523.
49. Hynes, K., Menicanin, D., Gronthos, S., & Bartold, P. M. (2012). Clinical utility of stem cells for periodontal regeneration. *Periodontology 2000, 59*(1), 203–227.
50. Zhu, W., & Liang, M. (2015). Periodontal ligament stem cells: Current status, concerns, and future prospects. *Stem Cells International, 972313*, 1–11.
51. Yamada, Y., Ueda, M., Hibi, H., & Baba, S. (2006). A novel approach to periodontal tissue regeneration with mesenchymal stem cells and platelet-rich plasma using tissue engineering technology: A clinical case report. *International Journal of Periodontics and Restorative Dentistry, 26*(4), 363–369.
52. Huang, G. T. J., Gronthos, S., & Shi, S. (2009). Mesenchymal stem cells derived from dental tissues vs. those from other sources: Their biology and role in regenerative medicine. *Journal of Dental Research, 88*(9), 792–806.
53. Seo, B. M., Miura, M., Gronthos, S., Bartold, P. M., Batouli, S., Brahim, J., Young, M., Robey, P. G., Wang, C. Y., & Shi, S. (2004). Investigation of multipotent stem cells from human periodontal ligament. *The Lancet, 364*(9429), 149–155.
54. Sonoyama, W., Liu, Y., Yamaza, T., Tuan, R. S., Wang, S., Shi, S., & Huang, G. T.-J. (2008). Characterization of the apical papilla and its residing stem cells from human immature permanent teeth: A pilot study. *Journal of Endodontics, 34*(2), 166–171.
55. Miura, M., Gronthos, S., Zhao, M., Lu, B., Fisher, L. W., Robey, P. G., & Shi, S. (2003). SHED: Stem cells from human exfoliated deciduous teeth. *Proceedings of the National Academy of Sciences of the United States of America, 100*(10), 5807–5812.
56. Zhang, Q., Shi, S., Liu, Y., Uyanne, J., Shi, Y., & Le, A. D. (2009). Mesenchymal stem cells derived from human gingiva are capable of immunomodulatory functions and ameliorate inflammation related tissue destruction in experimental colitis. *The Journal of Immunology, 183*(12), 7787–7798.

57. Hynes, K., Menicanin, D., Gronthos, S., & Bartold, P. M. (2012). Clinical utility of stem cells for periodontal regeneration. *Periodontology 2000, 59*, 203–227.
58. Chai, Y., Jiang, X., Ito, Y., Bringas, P. J., Han, J., Rowitch, D. H., Soriano, P., McMahon, A. P., & Sucov, H. M. (2000). Fate of the mammalian cranial neural crest during tooth and mandibular morphogenesis. *Development, 127*, 1671–1679.
59. Bossù, M., Pacifici, A., Carbone, D., Tenore, G., Ierardo, G., Pacifici, L., & Polimeni, A. (2014). Today prospects for tissue engineering therapeutic approach in dentistry. *The Scientific World Journal, 2014*, 151252, 1–151252, 9.
60. Nagatomo, K., Komaki, M., Sekiya, I., Sakaguchi, Y., Noguchi, K., Oda, S., Muneta, T., & Ishikawa, I. (2006). Stem cell properties of human periodontal ligament cells. *Journal of Periodontal Research, 41*(4), 303–310.
61. Amrollahi, P., Shah, B., Seifi, A., & Tayebi, L. (2016). Recent advancements in regenerative dentistry: A review. *Materials Science and Engineering C, 69*, 1383–1390.
62. Bhandari, R. N., Riccalton, L. A., Lewis, A. L., Fry, J. R., Hammond, A. H., Tendler, S. J., & Shakesheff, K. M. (2001). Liver tissue engineering: A role for co-culture systems in modifying hepatocyte function and viability. *Tissue Engineering, 7*(3), 345–357.
63. Beltrán-Aguilar, E. D., Barker, L., Canto, M., Dye, B., Gooch, B., Griffin, S., et al. (2005). Centers for Disease Control and Prevention (CDC). Surveillance for dental caries, dental sealants, tooth retention, edentulism, and enamel fluorosis—United States, 1988–1994 and 1999–2002. *MMWR Surveillance Summaries, 54*(3), 1–43.
64. Wada, N., Menicanin, D., Shi, S., Bartold, P. M., & Gronthos, S. (2009). Immunomodulatory properties of human periodontal ligament stem cells. *Journal of Cellular Physiology, 219*(3), 667–676.
65. Gay, I. C., Chen, S., & MacDougall, M. (2007). Isolation and characterization of multipotent human periodontal ligament stem cells. *Orthodontics and Craniofacial Research, 10*(3), 149–160.
66. Lang, H., Schuler, N., & Nolden, R. (1998). Attachment formation following replantation of cultured cells into periodontal defects: A study in minipigs. *Journal of Dental Research, 77*, 393–405.
67. Isaka, J., Ohazama, A., Kobayashi, M., Nagashima, C., Takiguchi, T., Kawasaki, H., Tachikawa, T., & Hasegawa, K. (2001). Participation of periodontal ligament cells with regeneration of alveolar bone. *Journal of Periodontology, 72*, 314–323.
68. Dogan, A., Ozdemir, A., Kubar, A., & Oygur, T. (2002). Assessment of periodontal healing by seeding of fibroblast like cells derived from regenerated periodontal ligament in artificial furcation defects in a dog: A pilot study. *Tissue Engineering, 8*, 273–282.
69. Dogan, A., Ozdemir, A., Kubar, A., & Oygur, T. (2003). Healing of artificial fenestration defects by seeding of fibroblast-like cells derived from regenerated periodontal ligament in a dog: A preliminary study. *Tissue Engineering, 9*, 1189–1196.
70. Seo, B. M., Miura, M., Gronthos, S., Bartold, P. M., Batouli, S., Brahim, J., Young, M., Robey, P. G., Wang, C. Y., & Shi, S. (2004). Investigation of multipotent postnatal stem cells from human periodontal ligament. *Lancet, 364*, 149–155.
71. Park, J.-Y., Jeon, S. H., & Choung, P.-H. (2011). Efficacy of periodontal stem cell transplantation in the treatment of advanced periodontitis. *Cell Transplantation, 20*(2), 271–285.
72. Liu, Y., Zheng, Y., Ding, G., Fang, D., Zhang, C., Bartold, P. M., Gronthos, S., Shi, S., & Wang, S. (2008). Periodontal ligament stem cell mediated treatment for periodontitis in miniature swine. *Stem Cells, 26*(4), 1065–1073.
73. Huang, C. Y., Pelaez, D., Dominguez-Bendala, J., Garcia-Godoy, F., & Cheung, H. S. (2009). Plasticity of stem cells derived from adult periodontal ligament. *Regenerative Medicine, 4*(6), 809–821.
74. Dan, H., Vaquette, C., Fisher, A., Hamlet, S. M., Xiao, Y., Hutmacher, D. W., & Ivanovski, S. (2014). The influence of cellular source on periodontal regeneration using calcium phosphate coated polycaprolactone scaffold supported cell sheets. *Biomaterials, 35*, 113–122.
75. Morsczeck, C., Gotz, W., Schierholz, J., Zeilhofer, F., Kuhn, U., Mohl, C., et al. (2005). *Matrix Biology, 24*, 155–165.

76. Sethi, M., Dua, A., & Dodwad, V. (2012). Stem cells: A window to regenerative dentistry. *International Journal of Pharmaceutical Biomedical Research, 3*(3), 175–180.
77. Yao, S., Pan, F., Prpic, V., & Wise, G. E. (2008). Differentiation of stem cells in the dental follicle. *Journal of Dental Research, 87*, 767–771.
78. Morsczeck, C., Gotz, W., Schierholz, J., Zeilhofer, F., Kuhn, U., Mohl, C., & Hoffmann, K. H. (2005). Isolation of precursor cells (PCs) from human dental follicle of wisdom teeth. *Matrix Biology, 24*, 155–165.
79. Yokoi, T., Saito, M., Kiyono, T., Iseki, S., Kosaka, K., Nishida, E., Tsubakimoto, T., Harada, H., Eto, K., Noguchi, T., & Teranaka, T. (2007). Establishment of immortalized dental follicle cells for generating periodontal ligament in vivo. *Cell and Tissue Research, 327*(2), 301–311.
80. Bai, Y., Bai, K., Matsuzaka, S., Hashimoto, S., Fukuyama, T., Wu, L., Miwa, T., Liu, X., Wang, X., & Inoue, T. (2011). Cementum-and periodontal ligament–like tissue formation by dental follicle cell sheets co-cultured with Hertwig's epithelial root sheath cells. *Bone, 48*, 1417–1426.
81. Okuda, K., Momose, M., Murata, M., Saito, Y., Inoie, M., Shinohara, C., Wolff, L. F., & Yoshie, H. (2004). Treatment of chronic desquamative gingivitis using tissue-engineered human cultured gingival epithelial sheets: A case report. *The International Journal of Periodontics Restorative Dentistry, 24*, 119–125.
82. Mohammadi, M., Shokrgozar, M. A., & Mofid, R. (2007). Culture of human gingival fibroblasts on a biodegradable scaffold and evaluation of its effect on attached gingiva: A randomized, controlled pilot study. *Journal of Periodontology, 78*, 1897–1903.
83. McGuire, M. K., Scheyer, E. T., Nevins, M. L., Neiva, R., Cochran, D. L., Mellonig, J. T., Giannobile, W. V., & Bates, D. (2011). Living cellular construct for increasing the width of keratinized gingiva: Results from a randomized, within-patient, controlled trial. *Journal of Periodontology, 82*, 1414–1423.
84. Allen, M. R., Hock, J. M., & Burr, D. B. (2004). Periosteum: Biology, regulation, and response to osteoporosis therapies. *Bone, 35*, 1003–1012.
85. Yamamiya, K., Okuda, K., Kawase, T., Hata, K., Wolff, L. F., & Yoshie, H. (2008). Tissue-engineered cultured periosteum used with platelet-rich plasma and hydroxyapatite in treating human osseous defects. *Journal of Periodontology, 79*, 811–818.
86. Gronthos, S., Mankani, M., Brahim, J., Robey, P. G., & Shi, S. (2000). Postnatal human dental pulp stem cells (DPSCs) in vitro and in vivo. *Proceedings of the National Academy of Sciences of the United States of America, 97*(25), 13625–13630.
87. Shi, S., Robey, P. G., & Gronthos, S. (2001). Comparison of human dental pulp and bone marrow stromal stem cells by cDNA microarray analysis. *Bone, 29*, 532–539.
88. Arthur, A., Shi, S., Zannettino, A. C. W., Fujii, N., Gronthos, S., & Koblar, S. A. (2009). Implanted adult human dental pulp stem cells induce endogenous axon guidance. *Stem Cells, 27*(9), 2229–2237.
89. Gronthos, S., Brahim, J., Li, W., et al. (2002). Stem cell properties of human dental pulp stem cells. *Journal of Dental Research, 81*(8), 531–535.
90. Ishkitiev, N., Yaegaki, K., Calenic, B., et al. (2010). Deciduous and permanent dental pulp mesenchymal cells acquire hepatic morphologic and functional features in vitro. *Journal of Endodontics, 36*(3), 469–474.
91. Alongi, D. J., Yamaza, T., Song, Y., et al. (2010). Stem/progenitor cells from inflamed human dental pulp retain tissue regeneration potential. *Regenerative Medicine, 5*(4), 617–631.
92. Huang, A. H., Chen, Y. K., Lin, L. M., Shieh, T. Y., & Chan, A. W. (2008). Isolation and characterization of dental pulp stem cells from a supernumerary tooth. *Journal of Oral Pathology and Medicine, 37*(9), 571–574.
93. Karaoz, E., Dogan, B. N., Aksoy, A., et al. (2010). Isolation and in vitro characterization of dental pulp stem cells from natal teeth. *Histochemistry and Cell Biology, 133*(1), 95–112.
94. D'Aquino, R., De Rosa, A., Lanza, V., et al. (2009). Human mandible bone defect repair by the grafting of dental pulp stem/progenitor cells and collagen sponge biocomplexes. *European Cells and Materials, 18*(7), 75–83.

95. Zhao, Y., Wang, L., Jin, Y., & Shi, S. (2012). Fas ligand regulates the immunomodulatory properties of dental pulp stem cells. *Journal of Dental Research, 91*, 948–954.
96. Grzesik, W. J., Kuzentsov, S. A., Uzawa, K., Mankani, M., Robey, P. G., & Yamauchi, M. (1998). Normal human cementum-derived cells: Isolation, clonal expansion, and in vitro and in vivo characterization. *Journal of Bone and Mineral Research, 13*(10), 1547–1554.
97. Huang, G. T.-J., El Ayachi, I., & Zou, X.-Y. (2016). Induced pluripotent stem cell technologies for tissue engineering. In R. J. Waddington & A. J. Sloan (Eds.), *Tissue engineering and regeneration in dentistry*.
98. Nakamura, S., Yamada, Y., Katagiri, W., Sugito, T., Ito, K., & Ueda, M. (2009). Stem cell proliferation pathways comparison between human exfoliated deciduous teeth and dental pulp stem cells by gene expression profile from promising dental pulp. *Journal of Endodontics, 35*(11), 1536–1542.
99. Wang, X., Sha, X.-J., Li, G.-H., et al. (2012). Comparative characterization of stem cells from human exfoliated deciduous teeth and dental pulp stem cells. *Archives of Oral Biology, 57*(9), 1231–1240.
100. Sonoyama, W., Liu, Y., Fang, D., et al. (2006). Mesenchymal stem cell mediated functional tooth regeneration in swine. *PLoS One, 1*(1), e79.
101. Bakopoulou, A., Leyhausen, G., Volk, J., et al. (2011). Comparative analysis of in vitro osteo/odontogenic differentiation potential of human dental pulp stem cells (DPSCs) and stem cells from the apical papilla (SCAP). *Archives of Oral Biology, 56*(7), 709–721.
102. Abe, S., Hamada, K., Miura, M., & Yamaguchi, S. (2012). Neural crest stem cell property of apical pulp cells derived from human developing tooth. *Cell Biology International, 36*(10), 927–936.
103. Ding, G., Liu, Y., An, Y., et al. (2010). Suppression of T cell proliferation by root apical papilla stem cells in vitro. *Cells, Tissues, Organs, 191*(5), 357–364.
104. Yagyuu, T., Ikeda, E., Ohgushi, H., et al. (2010). Hard tissue-forming potential of stem/progenitor cells in human dental follicle and dental papilla. *Archives of Oral Biology, 55*(1), 68–76.
105. Bianco, P., Riminucci, M., Gronthos, S., & Robey, P. G. (2001). Bone marrow stromal stem cells: Nature, biology and potential applications. *Stem Cells, 19*(3), 180–192.
106. Mehta, D. S., Jyothy, T. M., & Kumar, T. (2005). Stem cells in dentofacial research-at the cross roads. *J. Indian. Soc. Periodontol., 9*, 91–108.
107. Pittenger, M. F., Mackay, A. M., Beck, S. C., Jaiswal, R. K., Douglas, R., Mosca, J. D., et al. (1999). Multilineage potential of adult human mesenchymal stem cells. *Science, 284*(5411), 143–147.
108. Kuo, T. F., Lin, H. C., Yang, K. C., Lin, F. H., Chen, M. H., Wu, C. C., et al. (2011). Bone marrow combined with dental bud cells promotes tooth regeneration in miniature pig model. *Artificial Organs, 35*, 113–121.
109. Kawaguchi, H., Hirachi, A., Hasegawa, N., Iwata, T., Hamaguchi, H., Shiba, H., et al. (2004). Enhancement of periodontal tissue regeneration by transplantation of bone marrow mesenchymal stem cells. *Journal of Periodontology, 75*, 1281–1287.
110. Fiorina, P., Jurewicz, M., Augello, A., Vergani, A., Dada, S., La Rosa, S., et al. (2009). Immunomodulatory function of bone marrow-derived mesenchymal stem cells in experimental autoimmune type 1 diabetes. *Journal of Immunology, 183*, 993–1004.
111. Wu, Y., Chen, L., Scott, P. G., & Tredget, E. E. (2007). Mesenchymal stem cells enhance wound healing through differentiation and angiogenesis. *Stem Cells, 25*, 2648–2659.
112. Locke, M. B., & J, V. (2015). Human, adipose-derived stem cells (ASC): Their efficacy in clinical applications. In *Regenerative medicine: Springer* (pp. 135–149).
113. Bassir, S. H., Wisitrasameewong, W., Raanan, J., Ghaffarigarakani, S., Chung, J., Freire, M., Andrada, L. C., & Intini, G. (2016). Potential for stem cell-based periodontal therapy. *Journal of Cellular Physiology, 231*(1), 50–61.
114. Gimble, J., & Guilak, F. (2003). Adipose-derived adult stem cells: Isolation, characterization, and differentiation potential. *Cytotherapy, 5*(5), 362–369.

115. Lee, R. H., Kim, B., Choi, I., Kim, H., Choi, H. S., Suh, K., Bae, Y. C., & Jung, J. S. (2004). Characterization and expression analysis of mesenchymal stem cells from human bone marrow and adipose tissue. *Cellular Physiology and Biochemistry: International Journal of Experimental Cellular Physiology, Biochemistry, and Pharmacology, 14*(4–6), 311–324.
116. Planat-Benard, V., Silvestre, J. S., Cousin, B., Andre, M., Nibbelink, M., Tamarat, R., Clergue, M., Manneville, C., Saillan-Barreau, C., Duriez, M., Tedgui, A., Levy, B., Penicaud, L., & Casteilla, L. (2004). Plasticity of human adipose lineage cells toward endothelial cells: Physiological and therapeutic perspectives. *Circulation, 109*(5), 656–663.
117. Tobita, M., Uysal, A. C., Ogawa, R., Hyakusoku, H., & Mizuno, H. (2008). Periodontal tissue regeneration with adipose-derived stem cells. *Tissue Engineering. Part A, 14*, 945–953.
118. Bennett, N. T., & Schultz, G. S. (1993). Growth factors and wound healing: Biochemical properties of growth factors and their receptors. *American Journal of Surgery, 165*, 728–737.
119. Alluri, S. V., Bhola, S., Gangavati, R., Shirlal, S., & Belgaumi, U. (2012). Tissue engineering in periodontics -a novel therapy. *Annals of Dental Research, 2*(1), 01–07.
120. Murakami, S. (2011). Periodontal tissue regeneration by signaling molecule(s): What role does basic fibroblast growth factor (FGF-2) have in periodontal therapy. *Periodontology 2000, 56*(1), 188–208.
121. Kastin, A. (2013). *Handbook of biologically active peptides*. San Diego, CA. Academic Press.
122. Sigurdsson, T. J., Lee, M. B., & Kubota, K. (1995). Periodontal repair in dogs: Recombinant bone morphogenetic protein 2 significantly enhances periodontal regeneration. *Journal of Periodontology, 66*, 131–138.
123. Wozney, J. M. (1995). The potential role of bone morphogenetic proteins in periodontal reconstruction. *Journal of Periodontology, 66*(6), 506–510.
124. Heijl, L., Heden, G., Svärdström, G., & Ostgren, A. (1997). Enamel matrix derivative (EMDOGAIN) in the treatment of intrabony periodontal defects. *Journal of Clinical Periodontology, 24*, 705–714.
125. Del Fabbro, M., Bortolin, M., Taschieri, S., & Weinstein, R. (2011). Is platelet concentrate advantageous for the surgical treatment of periodontal diseases? A systematic review and meta-analysis. J. *Periodontology 2000, 82*, 1100–1111.
126. Giannobile, W. V., Hernandez, R. A., Finkelman, R. D., Ryan, S., Kiritsy, C. P., D'Andrea, M., & Lynch, S. E. (1996). Comparative effects of platelet derived growth factor-BB and insulin-like growth factor-I, individually and in combination, on periodontal regeneration in *Macaca fascicularis. Journal of Periodontal Research, 31*, 301–312.
127. Lynch, S. E., Williams, R. C., Polson, A. M., Howell, T. H., Reddy, M. S., Zappa, U. E., & Antoniades, H. N. (1989). A combination of platelet-derived and insulin-like growth factors enhances periodontal regeneration. *Journal of Clinical Periodontology, 16*, 545–548.
128. Matsuda, N., Lin, W. L., Kumar, N. M., Cho, M. I., & Genco, R. J. (1992). Mitogenic, chemotactic and synthetic response of rat periodontal ligament fibroblastic cells to polypeptide growth factors in vitro. *Journal of Periodontology, 63*, 515–525.
129. Nevins, M., Giannobile, W. V., McGuire, M. K., et al. (2005). Platelet-derived growth factor stimulates bone fill and rate of attachment level gain: Results of a large multicenter randomized controlled trial. *Journal of Periodontology, 76*, 2205–2215.
130. Cho, M., Lin, W. L., & Genco, R. J. (1995). Platelet-derived growth factor modulated guided tissue regenerative therapy. *Journal of Periodontology, 66*, 522–530.
131. Nakashima, M., & Reddi, A. H. (2003). The application of bone morphogenetic proteins to dental tissue engineering. *Nature Biotechnology, 21*(9), 1025–1032.
132. Kao, R. T., Murakami, S., & Beirne, O. R. (2009). The use of biologic mediators and tissue engineering in dentistry. *Periodontology 2000, 50*, 127–153.
133. Shimabukuro, Y., Terashima, H., Takedachi, M., Maeda, K., Nakamura, T., Sawada, K., et al. (2011). Fibroblast growth factor-2 stimulates directed migration of periodontal ligament cells via PI3K/AKT signaling and CD44/hyaluronan interaction. *Journal of Cellular Physiology, 226*, 809–821.

134. Murakami, S. (2011). Periodontal tissue regeneration by signaling molecule(s): What role does basic fibroblast growth factor (FGF-2) have in periodontal therapy. *Periodontology 2000, 56*, 188–208.
135. Nishino, Y., Ebisawa, K., Yamada, Y., Okabe, K., Kamei, Y., & Ueda, M. (2011). Human deciduous teeth dental pulp cells with basic fibroblast growth factor enhance wound healing of skin defect. *The Journal of Craniofacial Surgery, 22*, 438–442.
136. Lieberman, J. R., Daluiski, A., & Einhorn, T. A. (2002). The role of growth factors in the repair of bone. Biology and clinical applications. *J Bone Joint Surg Am, 84-A*, 1032–1044.
137. Janssens, K., Ten Dijke, P., Janssens, S., & Van Hul, W. (2005). Transforming growth factor-β1 to the bone. *Endocrine Reviews, 26*, 743–774.
138. Bostrom, M. P. (1998). Expression of bone morphogenetic proteins in fracture healing. *Clin. Orthopead. Rel. Res., 355*, S116–S123.
139. Worapamorn, W., Haase, H. R., Li, H., & Bartold, P. M. (2001). Growth factors and cytokines modulate gene expression of cell-surface proteoglycans in human periodontal ligament cells. *Journal of Cellular Physiology, 186*, 448–456.
140. Fujii, S., Maeda, H., Tomokiyo, A., Monnouchi, S., Hori, K., Wada, N., & Akamine, A. (2010). Effects of TGF-β1 on the proliferation and differentiation of human periodontal ligament cells and a human periodontal ligament stem/progenitor cell line. *Cell and Tissue Research, 342*, 233–242.
141. Fujita, T., Shiba, H., & Van Dyke, T. E. (2004). Differential effects of growth factors and cytokines on the synthesis of SPARC, DNA, fibronectin and alkaline phosphatase activity in human periodontal ligament cells. *Cell Biology International, 28*, 281–286.
142. Takeuchi, H., Kubota, S., Murakashi, E., et al. (2009). Effect of transforming growth factor-beta1 on expression of the connective tissue growth factor (CCN2/CTGF) gene in normal human gingival fibroblasts and periodontal ligament cells. *Journal of Periodontal Research, 44*, 161–169.
143. Nishimura, F., & Terranova, V. P. (1996). Comparative study of the chemotactic responses of periodontal ligament cells and gingival fibroblasts to polypeptide growth factors. *Journal of Dental Research, 75*(4), 986–992.
144. Hammarström, L. (1997). Enamel matrix, cementum development and regeneration. *Journal of Clinical Periodontology, 24*, 658–668.
145. Grover, V., Malhotra, R., Kapoor, A., Verma, N., & Sahota, J. K. (2010). Future of periodontal regeneration. *Journal of Oral Health Community Dentistry, 4*, 38–47.
146. Griffith, L. G., & Naughton, G. (2002). Tissue engineering-current challenges and expanding opportunities. *Science, 295*, 1009.
147. Yaszemski, M. J., Oldham, J. B., Lu, L., & Currier, B. L. (2000). In J. E. Davies (Ed.), *Bone engineering* (p. 541). Toronto: em2 Inc..
148. Patil, A. S., Merchant, Y., & Nagarajan, P. (2013). Tissue engineering of craniofacial tissues – A review. *Journal of Regenerative Medicine & Tissue Engineering*. 2, 1–6.
149. Horst, O. V., Chavez, M. G., Jheon, A. H., Desai, T., & Klein, O. D. (2012). Stem cell and biomaterials research in dental tissue engineering and regeneration. *Dental Clinics of North America, 56*, 495–520.
150. Tripathi, G., & Basu, B. (2012). A porous hydroxyapatite scaffold for bone tissue engineering: Physico-mechanical and biological evaluations. *Ceramics International, 38*(1), 341–349.
151. Shalini, M., & Gajendran, P. (2017). The role of scaffolds in periodontal regeneration. *International Journal of Pharmaceutical Sciences Review and Research, 45*(1), 135–140.
152. Mooney, D. J., Powell, C., Piana, J., & Rutherford, B. (1996). Engineering dental pulp-like tissue in vitro. *Biotechnology Progress, 12*, 865–868.
153. Kim, B. S., & Mooney, D. J. (1998). Development of biocompatible synthetic extracellular matrices for tissue engineering. *Trends in Biotechnology, 16*, 224–230.
154. Freed, L. E., Vunjak-Novakovic, G., Biron, R. J., Eagles, D. B., Lesnoy, D. C., Barlow, S. K., & Langer, R. (1994). Biodegradable polymer scaffolds for tissue engineering. *Biotechnology, 12*, 689–693.

155. Thomson, R. C., Yaszemski, M. J., Powers, J. M., & Mikos, A. G. (1995). Fabrication of biodegradable polymer scaffolds to engineer trabecular bone. *Journal of Biomaterials Science. Polymer Edition, 7*, 23–38.
156. Temenoff, J. S., & Mikos, A. G. (2000). Injectable biodegradable materials for orthopedic tissue engineering. *Biomaterials, 21*, 2405–2412.
157. Hutmacher, D. W., Schantz, T., Zein, I., Ng, K. W., Teoh, S. H., & Tan, K. C. (2001). Mechanical properties and cell cultural response of polycaprolactone scaffolds designed and fabricated via fused deposition modeling. *Journal of Biomedical Materials Research, 55*, 203–216.
158. Ma, P. X., & Choi, J. W. (2001). Biodegradable polymer scaffolds with well defined interconnected spherical pore network. *Tissue Engineering, 7*, 23–33.
159. Agrawal, C. M., & Ray, R. B. (2001). Biodegradable polymeric scaffolds for musculoskeletal tissue engineering. *Journal of Biomedical Materials Research, 55*, 141–150.
160. Dormer, K. J., & Gan, R. Z. (2001). Biomaterials for implantable middle ear hearing devices. *Otolaryngologic Clinics of North America, 34*, 289–297.
161. Langer, R. (2000). Biomaterials in drug delivery and tissue engineering: One laboratory's experience. *Accounts of Chemical Research, 33*, 94–101.
162. Burg, K. J., Porter, S., & Kellam, J. F. (2000). Biomaterial developments for bone tissue engineering. *Biomaterials, 21*, 2347–2359.
163. Nehrer, S., Breinan, H. A., Ramappa, A., Young, G., Shortkroff, S., Louie, L. K., Sledge, C. B., Yannas, I. V., & Spector, M. (1997). Matrix collagen type and pore size influence behaviour of seeded canine chondrocytes. *Biomaterials, 18*, 769.
164. Suh, J. K., & Matthew, H. W. (2000). Application of chitosan-based polysaccharide biomaterials in cartilage tissue engineering: A review. *Biomaterials, 21*, 2589–2598.
165. Van Osch, G. J., Van Der Veen, S. W., Burger, E. H., & Verwoerd-Verhoef, H. L. (2000). Chondrogenic potential of in vitro multiplied rabbit perichondrium cells cultured in alginate beads in defined medium. *Tissue Engineering, 6*, 321–330.
166. Rowley, J. A., Madlambayan, G., & Mooney, D. J. (1999). Alginate hydrogels as synthetic extracellular matrix materials. *Biomaterials, 20*, 45–53.
167. Singhal, A. R., Agrawal, C. M., & Athanasiou, K. A. (1996). Salient degradation features of a 50:50 PLA/PGA scaffold for tissue engineering. *Tissue Engineering, 2*, 197–207.
168. Lye, K. W., Tideman, H., Wolke, J. C., Merkx, M. A., Chin, F. K., & Jansen, J. A. (2013). Biocompatibility and bone formation with porous modified PMMA in normal and irradiated mandibular tissue. *Clinical Oral Implants Research, 24*, 100–109.
169. Punet, X., Mauchauffé, R., Rodríguez Cabello, J. C., Alonso, M., Engel, E., & Mateos-Timoneda, M. A. (2015). Biomolecular functionalization for enhanced cell–material interactions of poly(methyl methacrylate) surface. *Regenerative Biomaterials, 2*, 167–175.
170. Chen, F. M., Zhao, Y. M., Wu, H., Deng, Z. H., Wang, Q. T., Zhou, W., Liu, Q., Dong, G. Y., Li, K., Wu, Z. F., & Jin, Y. (2006). Enhancement of periodontal tissue regeneration by locally controlled delivery of insulin-like growth factor-I from dextran-co-gelatin microspheres. *Journal of Controlled Release, 114*, 209.
171. Chen, F. M., Zhao, Y. M., Zhang, R., Jin, T., Sun, H. H., Wu, Z. F., & Jin, Y. (2007). Periodontal regeneration using novel glycidyl methacrylate dextran (Dex-GMA)=gelatin scaffolds containing microspheres loaded with bone morphogenetic proteins. *Journal of Controlled Release, 121*, 81.
172. Ahmed, T. A., Dare, E. V., & Hincke, M. (2008). Fibrin: A versatile scaffold for tissue engineering applications. *Tissue Engineering. Part B, Reviews, 14*, 199.
173. Kim, I. Y., Seo, S. J., Moon, H. S., Yoo, M. K., Park, I. Y., Kim, B. C., & Cho, C. S. (2008). Chitosan and its derivatives for tissue engineering applications. *Biotechnology Advances, 26*, 1–21.
174. Muzzarelli, R., Tarsi, R., Filippini, O., Giovanetti, E., Biagini, G., & Varaldo, P. E. (1990). Antimicrobial properties of N-carboxybutyl chitosan. *Antimicrobial Agents and Chemotherapy, 34*, 2019–2023.

175. No, H. K., Park, N. Y., Lee, S. H., & Meyers, S. P. (2002). Antibacterial activity of chitosans and chitosan oligomers with different molecular weights. *International Journal of Food Microbiology, 74*, 65–72.
176. Bertram, U., & Bodmeier, R. (2006). In situ gelling, bioadhesive nasal inserts for extended drug delivery: In vitro characterization of a new nasal dosage form. *European Journal of Pharmaceutical Sciences, 27*, 62–71.
177. Muzzarelli, R., Baldassarre, V., Conti, F., Ferrara, P., Biagini, G., Gazzanelli, G., & Vasi, V. (1988). Biological activity of chitosan: Ultrastructural study. *Biomaterials, 9*, 247–252.
178. Costa-Pinto, A. R., Correlo, V. M., Sol, P. C., Bhattacharya, M., Charbord, P., Delorme, B., Reis, R. L., & Neves, N. M. (2009). Osteogenic differentiation of human bone marrow mesenchymal stem cells seeded on melt based chitosan scaffolds for bone tissue engineering applications. *Biomacromolecules, 10*, 2067–2073.
179. Seol, Y. J., Lee, J. Y., Park, Y. J., Lee, Y. M., Young, K., Rhyu, I. C., Lee, S. J., Han, S. B., & Chung, C. P. (2004). Chitosan sponges as tissue engineering scaffolds for bone formation. *Biotechnology Letters, 26*, 1037–1041.
180. Maruyama, M., & Ito, M. (1996). In vitro properties of a chitosan-bonded self hardening paste with hydroxyapatite granules. *Journal of Biomedical Materials Research, 32*, 527–532.
181. Jameela, S. R., Misra, A., & Jayakrishnan, A. (1994). Cross-linked chitosan microspheres as carriers for prolonged delivery of macromolecular drugs. *Journal of Biomaterials Science. Polymer Edition, 6*, 621–632.
182. Costa-Pinto, A. R., Salgado, A. J., Correlo, V. M., Sol, P., Bhattacharya, M., Charbord, P., Reis, R. L., & Neves, N. M. (2008). Adhesion, proliferation, and osteogenic differentiation of a mouse mesenchymal stem cell line (BMC9) seeded on novel melt-based chitosan/polyester 3D porous scaffolds. *Tissue Engineering. Part A, 14*, 1049–1057.
183. Kleinman, H. K., & Martin, G. R. (2005). Matrigel: Basement membrane matrix with biological activity. *Seminars in Cancer Biology, 15*, 378–386.
184. Rosso, F., Marino, G., Giordano, A., Barbarisi, M., Parmeggiani, D., & Barbarisi, A. (2005). Smart materials as scaffolds for tissue engineering. *Journal of Cellular Physiology, 203*, 465–470.
185. Vasita, R., & Katti, D. S. (2006). Growth factor-delivery systems for tissue engineering: A materials perspective. *Expert Review of Medical Devices, 3*, 29.
186. Barboza, E. P., Duarte, M. E., Geola, S. L., Sorensen, R. G., Riedel, G. E., & Wikesjo, U. M. (2000). Ridge augmentation following implantation of recombinant human bone morphogenetic protein-2 in the dog. *Journal of Periodontology, 71*, 488.
187. Cen, L., Liu, W., Cui, L., Zhang, W., & Cao, Y. (2008). Collagen tissue engineering: Development of novel biomaterials and applications. *Pediatric Research, 63*, 492.
188. Galler, K. M., C, A., Cavender, U., Koeklue, et al. (2011). Bioengineering of dental stem cells in a PEGylated fibrin gel. *Regenerative Medicine, 6*, 191–200.
189. Drury, J. L., & Mooney, D. J. (2003). Hydrogels for tissue engineering: Scaffold design variables and applications. *Biomaterials, 24*, 4337.
190. Hall, H. (2007). Modified fibrin hydrogel matrices: Both, 3D scaffolds and local and controlled release systems to stimulate angiogenesis. *Current Pharmaceutical Design, 13*, 3597.
191. Buxton, P. G., & Cobourne, M. T. (2007). Regenerative approaches in the craniofacial region: Manipulating cellular progenitors for oro-facial repair. *Oral Diseases, 13*, 452.
192. Smidsrod, O., & Skjak-Braek, G. (1990). Alginate as immobilization matrix for cells. *Trends in Biotechnology, 8*, 71–78.
193. Drury, J. L., Dennis, R. G., & Mooney, D. J. (2004). The tensile properties of alginate hydrogels. *Biomaterials, 25*, 3187–3199.
194. Yuan, Z., Nie, H., Wang, S., et al. (2011). Biomaterial selection for tooth regeneration. *Tissue Engineering. Part B, Reviews, 17*, 373–388.
195. Matsuura, K., Utoh, R., Nagase, K., & Okano, T. (2014). Cell sheet approach for tissue engineering and regenerative medicine. *Journal of Controlled Release, 190*, 228–239.

196. Yang, J., Yamato, M., Shimizu, T., Sekine, H., Ohashi, K., Kanzaki, M., Ohki, T., Nishida, K., & Okano, T. (2007). Reconstruction of functional tissues with cell sheet engineering. *Biomaterials, 28*, 5033–5043.
197. Zhang, H., Liu, S., Zhu, B., Xu, Q., Ding, Y., & Jin, Y. (2016). Composite cell sheet for periodontal regeneration: Crosstalk between different types of MSCs in cell sheet facilitates complex periodontal-like tissue regeneration. *Stem Cell Research & Therapy, 7*(168), 1–15.
198. Tsumanuma, Y., Iwata, T., Washio, K., Yoshida, T., Yamada, A., Takagi, R., Ohno, T., Lin, K., Yamato, M., Ishikawa, I., Okano, T., & Izumi, Y. (2011). Comparison of different tissue-derived stem cell sheets for periodontal regeneration in a canine 1-wall defect model. *Biomaterials, 32*, 5819–5825.
199. Sawa, Y., & Miyagawa, S. (2013). Present and future perspectives on cell sheet-based myocardial regeneration therapy. *BioMed Research International, 2013*, 583912.
200. Zavala, J., Jaime, G. R. L., Barrientos, C. A. R., & Valdez-Garcia, J. (2013). Corneal endothelium: Developmental strategies for regeneration. *Eye (London, England), 27*, 579–588.
201. Wang, J., Zhang, R., Shen, Y., Xu, C., Qi, S., Lu, L., Wang, R., & Xu, Y. (2014). Recent advances in cell sheet technology for periodontal regeneration. *Current Stem Cell Research & Therapy, 9*, 162–173.

# Chapter 15
# Oral Mucosal Grafting in Ophthalmology

**Parisa Abdi, Golshan Latifi, and Hamed Ghassemi**

## 1 Introduction

There are many ocular surface syndromes that can cause sight-threatening conditions, including cicatricial diseases such as Stevens-Johnson syndrome (SJS) and ocular cicatricial pemphigoid (OCP) and chemical burns [1]. These conditions may lead to scarring complications in the lid margin, tarsus, and fornix while also causing keratinization, trichiasis, entropion, and symblepharon, which result in visual morbidity. Autologous oral mucosal graft (OMG) can be an approach to overcome such complications [1].

The oral mucosa consists of keratinized or nonkeratinized stratified squamous avascular epithelium with underlying lamina propria that is a vascular connective tissue. Its interface has many connective tissue projections into the epithelium, which leads to an increased surface area and ability to resist forces. The epithelium is also rich in elastin, which makes it resistant to shearing, stretching, and compression forces [2].

The lamina propria has extensive blood vessels and nerve fibers that allow for excellent grafting that facilitates angiogenesis. In contrast to gastrointestinal mucosa, there is no muscularis mucosal layer between the epithelium and lamina propria in the oral cavity [2]. The oral mucosa has many advantages that make it optimal as a graft for the ocular surface including:

1. Good flexibility and minimal contraction in the recipient bed [2].
2. Not containing hair follicles [3].
3. Tolerating wet environment [4].
4. High histocompatibility.

P. Abdi · G. Latifi · H. Ghassemi (✉)
Cornea Service, Farabi Eye Hospital, Tehran University of Medical Sciences, Tehran, Iran
e-mail: h_ghassemi@sina.tums.ac.ir



L. Tayebi (ed.), *Applications of Biomedical Engineering in Dentistry*,
https://doi.org/10.1007/978-3-030-21583-5_15

5. High resistance to microbial agents due to (a) secretion of antimicrobial peptides (defensing and cytokines) [5, 6], (b) the presence of mucosa-associated lymphoid tissue (MALT) [5, 6], (c) its function as a barrier to microbial invasion, and (d) the presence of lymphocytes, PMNs, macrophages, plasma cells, and mast cells [5, 6].
6. Capability of rapid healing and reepithelialization faster than a dermal wound, due to the presence of growth factors and tissue factors [7].

The presence of epithelial stem cells in the oral tissue has also been proven, which helps reepithelialization [8]. OMG has gained widespread popularity in ophthalmology and is commonly used during ocular reconstruction surgeries to replace the conjunctiva and corneal surface, along with reconstruction of the fornices [9], eyelid margin [1], and ophthalmic socket [10]. OMG is readily accessible and available in most patients. The surgical technique is fast, inexpensive, and not complex. The transplantation is safe with few recipient and donor site complications [11].

In this chapter, after introducing different types of oral mucosal grafts and describing the procedure and complications of OMG, we will discuss its applications in ophthalmology to show how biomedical engineers can play key roles in such applications.

## 2 Types of Oral Mucosal Grafts

OMGs are 1–5 mm in size and can be harvested from the buccal mucosa, labial mucosa, or lingual mucosa [11].

### *2.1 Buccal Mucosa-Based OMG*

The buccal mucosa refers to the mucosa overlying the inner cheek of the oral cavity. It is bordered by the outer commissures of the lips in the anterior, anterior tonsillar pillar in the posterior, maxillary vestibular fold superiorly, and mandibular vestibular fold inferiorly [2, 11]. Vascular supply is derived mainly from branches of the maxillary artery—the buccal artery, middle and posterior superior alveolar arteries, and the anterior superior alveolar branch of the infraorbital artery [2, 11]. The buccal mucosa is innervated by the long buccal nerve, a branch of the third division of the trigeminal nerve (CNV3), and the anterior, middle, and posterior superior alveolar branches of the second division of the trigeminal nerve (CNV2). The sensory innervation is through the facial nerve [2, 11].

The buccal mucosa should be dissected off the submucosal fat and minor salivary glands (MSGs) covering the buccinator muscle. The buccinator muscle is a muscle of facial expression, and trauma to it may lead to limitation of mouth opening [2, 11]. During the harvesting, the surgeon must pay attention to anatomical structures, including the buccal fat pad, Stensen's duct of the parotid gland, the facial artery and nerve anteriorly, the buccal artery posteriorly, and lymphatic vessels and buccal branches of the facial and trigeminal nerves [2, 11]. The buccal mucosa is tough, flexible, easy to harvest, easily recoverable, and simple to handle and leaves no visible scar after OMG [2].

### 2.2 *Labial Mucosa-Based OMG*

The labial mucosa refers to the mucosa overlying the inner lower lip. The mandibular labial alveolar mucosa is delineated by the vermilion border superiorly, the vestibular fold inferiorly, and the outer commissures of the lower lip laterally [2, 11]. Vascular supply is derived from the buccal and mental branches of the maxillary artery and the inferior labial branch of the facial artery [2, 11].

Sensory innervation is by the mental nerve, a terminal branch of the inferior alveolar nerve which is rising from the mandibular branch of CNV3. The mental nerve arises from the mental foramen, which is located between the first and the second premolar teeth. Thus, in harvesting the mucosa, the initial incision should be medial to the center of the canines to avoid mental nerve injury. Additionally, the incision should maintain at least a 1.0–1.5 cm margin from the lip vermilion to prevent lip contracture [12]. On the other hand, injury to the orbicularis oris muscle can cause limitation in lip motility and smiling. MSGs are easily accessible in the labial mucosa and form a continuous layer of tightly packed lobules between the quadratus labii and the labial mucosa [13]. MSG secretions are predominantly seromucinous [14].

### 2.3 *Lingual Mucosa-Based OMG*

The lingual mucosa refers to the mucosa overlying the tongue. The mucosa covering the undersurface and lateral surface of the tongue is indistinguishable from and the same in structure as the mucosa lining the rest of the oral cavity. It has no particular functional feature and is easily accessible and easy to harvest [15]. It is mostly used in complications of urethroplasty, which requires a large supply of graft tissue in patients with a small mouth or difficult mouth opening.

## 3 Procedure and Complications of Oral Mucosal Grafting

### 3.1 *Graft Harvesting and Surgical Procedures*

In the preoperative period, any inflammation should be controlled. To estimate the graft size, the conjunctival defect is measured. The shape and size of the graft is marked on the mucosa (Fig. 15.1a). The graft size should be larger than the defect,

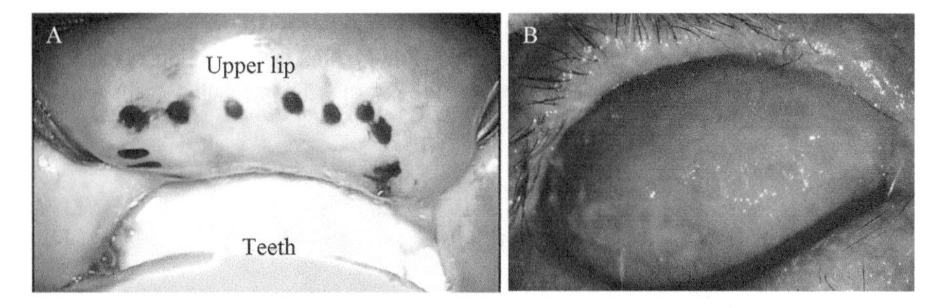


**Fig. 15.1** (**a**) Marking the shape and size of the graft on the mucosa to be used for the OMG procedure. Due to the possible 20% contracture, the size of the graft is larger than the actual defect size. (**b**) OMG in an eye after the surgery (courtesy of Dr. Mehran Zarei-Ghanavati, MD)

taking into account an average of 20% contracture. For the buccal mucosa, the parotid duct must be avoided (which is usually located opposite the second upper molar). For the lip, the incisions should not extend too close to the vermilion or attached gingiva [16]. Injection of saline or local anesthetic solution with adrenaline (bupivacaine 0.25% mixed with 1/200,000 epinephrine) helps to elevate the graft from the submucosal tissue and reduce hemorrhage [17].

The graft should be excised as thinly as possible by a blade and scissors. Submucosal dissection should be above the adipose layer, superficial to the buccinator muscle. The graft is trimmed and the edges secured under the conjunctival margins with Vicryl sutures. The subconjunctival fibrovascular cicatrix should be dissected at the recipient bed [2, 11]. The graft bed can be left to granulate, or it can be sutured if the edges of the wound can be approximated without deforming the lip or the tissue [16]. The graft is then spread over a surface, and the excess fat is cleared from the undersurface of the graft. The graft is then spread on the defect at the recipient site and secured with suturing or fibrin glue (Fig. 15.1b).

## *3.2 Complications*

Donor harvest site morbidities include persistent pain and wound contracture, which result in limitation of mouth opening and oral tightness. Moreover, other morbidities—such as buccal hematoma, inclusion cysts, numbness in the cheek and lip, parotid duct injury, lip contracture and inversion of the lip vermilion, and poor cosmesis—should be considered as well [18]. Common complications affecting OMG after implantation include as follows:

A. *Graft shrinkage or contracture*: It has been reported about 20–45% shrinkage in size for the buccal mucosa and about 10% for the hard palate. This contracture commonly appears within 6 months after implantation [11].

B. *Mucosal necrosis*: It has been reported 8–50% of eyes after osteo-odonto-keratoprosthesis undergo mucosal necrosis, which can lead to exposure of the underlying ocular surface or implant [19].
C. *Mucosal overgrowth*: In Basu's study, the rate of overgrowth was 13%, and all of them were managed by debulking and trimming [19].
D. *Excessive MSG secretions*: Excessive MSG secretions can be treated by graft excision, cryotherapy, or botulinum toxin injection [11].

# 4 Applications of Oral Mucosal Grafting in Ophthalmology

OMGs have been used for different purposes in ophthalmology, including ocular surface reconstruction, socket reconstruction, correction of eyelid abnormalities, glaucoma surgery, and lacrimal drainage surgery.

## *4.1 Ocular Surface Reconstruction*

OMGs can be used in different scenarios for ocular surface reconstructions as described below:

A. Symblepharon (adhesion of the palpebral conjunctiva to the bulbar conjunctiva) can be a sight-threatening condition and may cause other ocular abnormalities, such as reduction of goblet cells, tear film and tear meniscus abnormalities, lid disorder like entropion and trichiasis, limitation in ocular motility, and failure of ocular surface reconstruction and corneal transplantation [16]. Many different materials have been employed to reconstruct the fornices, like conformers and rings; however, their effect is often temporary. To maintain the fornices, it is required to include epithelial tissue or basement membrane that can be populated by normal host epithelial cells [16]. Available graft materials include conjunctival autograft, OMG, and amniotic membrane graft (AMG) [16].

   The ideal material for fornix reconstruction is conjunctival or tarsal autograft, but there are limitations in their availability, especially in bilateral diseases. In such cases, a full-thickness oral mucosal membrane is the simplest available graft to use. Split-thickness mucosal grafts are less suitable for fornix reconstruction, as they contract more; but since they are less bulky and pink, they are used on the globe. Among OMGs, hard palate grafts are the thickest and the most difficult to harvest, but contract the least for ocular surface reconstruction [16]. OMG can also be employed for fornix reconstruction in the eyes with low-grade symblepharon. However, in severe cases, cases with difficulty in controlling inflammation, poor lacrimal function, or near-total lack of healthy conjunctiva, an oral mucosal graft may be more appropriate than an AMG [16]. In a study by Kheirkhah et al., 84.4% of eyes with severe (grade 3 or 4) symblepharon had a deep fornix with no scar or motility restriction after 16.4 ± 7.6 months of follow-up. In this study, a combined approach was employed: symblepharon lysis, intraoperative mitomycin C application, OMG in tarsal conjunctival defect, and amniotic membrane transplantation (AMT) in bulbar conjunctival defect [20].

B. Pterygium (a triangular tissue growth of thickened conjunctiva that grows over portion of the cornea) recurrence rate after simple excision is 24–67%, but with adjuvant therapy like conjunctival autograft, the rate is 0–47% [21]. OMG has been employed to cover the defects in pterygium surgery. It is especially useful in recurrent pterygium with conjunctival scarring, fornix shortening, inadequate conjunctiva, and limitation of ocular motility [21].
C. Osteo-odonto-keratoprosthesis is a procedure to restore vision in the most severe cases of corneal and ocular surface patients. In this procedure, a tooth is removed, a lamina of it is cut and drilled, and then the hole is fitted with optics. The lamina is grown in the patient's cheek for a period of months, and then prosthesis is implanted in the eye. In osteo-odonto-keratoprosthesis, OMGs have been used for ocular resurfacing and to provide a stable epithelium instead of a dry keratinized one [19]. However, complications have been reported, such as mucosal overgrowth over the optical cylinder, which decreases vision and causes necrosis [19]. On the other hand, melting of the cornea may occur, causing keratoprosthesis extrusion, particularly in patients with chronic conjunctival inflammation. In these patients with conjunctival deficiency, OMG is helpful to repair the defect [22].
D. OMGs have been employed to protect delicate corneas in cases of fitting cosmetic scleral shells. Traditionally, a Gunderson flap (a type of conjunctival flap that covers the total corneal surface) is used in such conditions. However, in some cases with conjunctival scarring or a large corneal diameter, OMGs are superior to flaps with a lesser risk of retraction [23].
E. OMGs combined with tenoplasty have been used to repair sclerocorneal melts in patients with chemical burns [24].

## *4.2 Socket Reconstruction*

After enucleation, the conjunctival contraction is common in the anophthalmic socket, leading to cosmetic deformity and difficulty in filling the prosthesis. This condition is more common after irradiation of the ophthalmic socket, for instance, in patients with uveal melanoma. An OMG can be used in these patients, as it is thin and easily accessible and maintains moisture of the prosthesis [25]. OMGs can augment the conjunctival surface, especially in fornices, to have sufficient depth for the prosthesis [26]. OMGs have been used in combination with hard palate grafts to make a stable fornix and provide rigidity and support in the palpebral surface [26].

Another post-enucleation complication is orbital volume loss. It can be corrected with orbital floor wedge implant, but it may shorten the fornix, which can be managed by OMG simultaneously. Another approach is using a buccal mucous membrane-fat graft to correct the volume and the surface simultaneously [27]. OMGs have also been used to manage hydroxyapatite orbital implant exposures [28].

### *4.3 Correction of Eyelid Abnormalities*

Eyelid abnormalities are commonly seen in cicatricial disorders, such as mucous membrane pemphigoid (MMP), Stevens-Johnson syndrome (SJS), toxic epidermal necrolysis (TEN), trachoma, and chemical burns. These abnormalities are lid margin scarring, trichiasis, distichiasis and entropion [26]. OMGs are commonly used to reconstruct these eyelid abnormalities, particularly before other procedures, such as limbal stem cell grafts and penetrating or lamellar keratoplasties [29]. OMG also has been used in correcting congenital distichiasis by resecting a strip of tarsus in the eyelid margin with the roots of lashes and replacing it with an OMG [30]. OMGs with more stromal fat have been used to increase the tarsal height and correct the cicatricial lagophthalmos [1]. A complex skin-muscle-mucosa graft from the lower lip can be employed as a one-stage procedure to repair lid margin defects after tumor resection [31]. OMGs have been used to repair congenital eyelid defects like cryptophthalmos [32]. In ichthyosis, the oral mucosa is not affected by the disease and is used to lengthen the anterior lamella and correct the ectropion. After transplantation, this tissue undergoes metaplasia into keratinized skin [26].

### *4.4 Glaucoma Surgery*

One of the complications of glaucoma drainage devices is erosion and exposure of the plate or the tube through the conjunctiva. It is usually repaired with conjunctival flaps or autologous conjunctival grafts. OMGs are used in cases with scarred or insufficient conjunctiva to cover the eroded tube or plate [33].

### *4.5 Retinal Surgery*

Scleral buckles are used in retinal detachment surgery. One of the complications is the explant exposure through the overlying tissue or conjunctiva. In these cases, the explant is usually covered with a scleral patch graft. OMGs have been used to cover this scleral graft, especially in patients with scarred conjunctiva due to multiple retinal procedures [34].

### 4.6 Lacrimal Drainage Surgery

Conjunctivodacryocystorhinostomy (CDCR) is a procedure that is performed in patients with total canalicular block. In this procedure, a Jones tube is placed in the canalicule. However, if the tube becomes dislodged or lost, the channel will be closed. OMGs have been used to line the CDCR tract to epithelize the channel and obviate closure in these cases. OMGs also have been used to reconstruct the medial canthal area and canalicules secondary to chemical burn. On the other hand, OMGs have been used in challenging cases of rE-DCR (dacryocystorhinostomy) with extensive scarring and mucosal shortage, to maintain the patency of the DCR tract [35, 36].

## 5 Summary

OMG can be used to promote ocular surface barrier function when it is defective. It is one of the finest substitutes for the conjunctiva in different ocular reconstruction procedures when autologous conjunctiva is unavailable. It can be harvested from the mucosa overlying the inner cheek of the oral cavity (buccal mucosa-based OMG), mucosa overlying the inner lower lip (labial mucosa-based OMG), or, less frequently, mucosa overlying the tongue (lingual mucosa-based OMG). Some of the most popular indications of OMG in ophthalmology are fornix reconstruction, fixing contracted anophthalmic socket, ocular resurfacing in osteo-odonto-keratoprosthesis, and prevention of channel closure in CDCR.

## References


1. Fu, Y., Liu, J., & Tseng, S. C. (2011). Oral mucosal graft to correct lid margin pathologic features in cicatricial ocular surface diseases. *American Journal of Ophthalmology, 152*(4), 600–608.
2. Markiewicz, M. R., Margarone, J. E., III, Barbagli, G., & Scannapieco, F. A. (2007). Oral mucosa harvest: An overview of anatomic and biologic considerations. *EAU-EBU update series, 5*(5), 179–187.
3. Cohen, S. D., Armenakas, N. A., Light, D. M., Fracchia, J. A., & Glasberg, S. B. (2012). Single-surgeon experience of 87 buccal mucosal graft harvests. *Plastic and Reconstructive Surgery, 130*(1), 101–104.
4. Akyüz, M., Güneş, M., Koca, O., Sertkaya, Z., Kanberoğlu, H., & Karaman, M. İ. (2014). Evaluation of intraoral complications of buccal mucosa graft in augmentation urethroplasty. *Turkish Journal of Urology, 40*(3), 156.
5. Rudney, J. D., & Chen, R. (2006). The vital status of human buccal epithelial cells and the bacteria associated with them. *Archives of Oral Biology, 51*(4), 291–298.
6. Walker, D. M. (2004). Oral mucosal immunology: An overview. *Annals-academy of Medicine Singapore, 33*, 27–30.

7. Wong, E., Fernando, A., Alhasso, A., & Stewart, L. (2014). Does closure of the buccal mucosal graft bed matter? Results from a randomized controlled trial. *Urology, 84*(5), 1223–1227.
8. Sotozono, C., Inatomi, T., Nakamura, T., Koizumi, N., Yokoi, N., Ueta, M., Matsuyama, K., Kaneda, H., Fukushima, M., & Kinoshita, S. (2014). Cultivated oral mucosal epithelial transplantation for persistent epithelial defect in severe ocular surface diseases with acute inflammatory activity. *Acta Ophthalmologica, 92*(6), e447–e453.
9. Kheirkhah, A., Blanco, G., Casas, V., Hayashida, Y., Raju, V. K., & Tseng, S. C. (2008). Surgical strategies for fornix reconstruction based on symblepharon severity. *American Journal of Ophthalmology, 146*(2), 266–275.
10. Klein, M., Menneking, H., & Bier, J. (2000). Reconstruction of the contracted ocular socket with free full-thickness mucosa graft. *International Journal of Oral and Maxillofacial Surgery, 29*(2), 96–98.
11. Grixti, A., & Malhotra, R. (2018). Oral mucosa grafting in periorbital reconstruction. *Orbit, 37*(6), 411–428.
12. Muruganandam, K., Dubey, D., Gulia, A. K., Mandhani, A., Srivastava, A., Kapoor, R., & Kumar, A. (2009). Closure versus nonclosure of buccal mucosal graft harvest site: A prospective randomized study on post operative morbidity. *Indian journal of urology: IJU: journal of the Urological Society of India, 25*(1), 72.
13. Geerling, G., Raus, P., & Murube, J. (2008). Minor salivary gland transplantation. In *Surgery for the dry eye* (Vol. 41, pp. 243–254). Karger Publishers.
14. Holsinger, F. C., & Bui, D. T. (2007). Anatomy, function, and evaluation of the salivary glands. In *Salivary gland disorders* (pp. 1–16). Berlin, Heidelberg: Springer.
15. Song, L. J., Xu, Y. M., Lazzeri, M., & Barbagli, G. (2009). Lingual mucosal grafts for anterior urethroplasty: A review. *BJU International, 104*(8), 1052–1056.
16. Bertolin, M., Breda, C., Ferrari, S., Van Acker, S. I., Zakaria, N., Di Iorio, E., Migliorati, A., Ponzin, D., Ferrari, B., Lužnik, Z., & Barbaro, V. (2019). Optimized protocol for regeneration of the conjunctival epithelium using the cell suspension technique. *Cornea, 38*(4), 469–479.
17. Goel, A., Dalela, D., Sinha, R. J., & Sankhwar, S. N. (2008). Harvesting buccal mucosa graft under local infiltration analgesia—Mitigating need for general anesthesia. *Urology, 72*(3), 675–676.
18. Dublin, N., & Stewart, L. H. (2004). Oral complications after buccal mucosal graft harvest for urethroplasty. *BJU International, 94*(6), 867–869.
19. Basu, S., Pillai, V. S., & Sangwan, V. S. (2013). Mucosal complications of modified osteo-odonto keratoprosthesis in chronic Stevens-Johnson syndrome. *American Journal of Ophthalmology, 156*(5), 867–873.
20. Kheirkhah, A., Ghaffari, R., Kaghazkanani, R., Hashemi, H., Behrouz, M. J., & Raju, V. K. (2013). A combined approach of amniotic membrane and oral mucosa transplantation for fornix reconstruction in severe symblepharon. *Cornea, 32*(2), 155–160.
21. Forbes, J., Collin, R., & Dart, J. (1998). Split thickness buccal mucous membrane grafts and β irradiation in the treatment of recurrent pterygium. *British Journal of Ophthalmology, 82*(12), 1420–1423.
22. Ziai, S., Rootman, D. S., Slomovic, A. R., & Chan, C. C. (2013). Oral buccal mucous membrane allograft with a corneal lamellar graft for the repair of Boston type 1 keratoprosthesis stromal melts. *Cornea, 32*(11), 1516–1519.
23. Ma'luf, R. N., & Awwad, S. T. (2005). Mucous membrane graft versus Gunderson conjunctival flap for fitting a scleral shell over a sensitive cornea. *Ophthalmic Plastic & Reconstructive Surgery, 21*(5), 356–358.
24. Wang, S., Tian, Y., Zhu, H., Cheng, Y., Zheng, X., & Wu, J. (2015). Tenonplasty combined with free oral buccal mucosa autografts for repair of sclerocorneal melt caused by chemical burns. *Cornea, 34*(10), 1240–1244.
25. Nasser, Q. J., Gombos, D. S., Williams, M. D., Guadagnolo, B. A., Morrison, W. H., Garden, A. S., Beadle, B. M., Canseco, E., & Esmaeli, B. (2012). Management of radiation-induced

severe anophthalmic socket contracture in patients with uveal melanoma. *Ophthalmic Plastic and Reconstructive Surgery, 28*(3), 208.
26. Mai, C., & Bertelmann, E. (2013). Oral mucosal grafts: Old technique in new light. *Ophthalmic Research, 50*(2), 91–98.
27. Kim, H. E., Jang, S. Y., & Yoon, J. S. (2014). Combined orbital floor wedge implant and fornix reconstruction for postenucleation sunken socket syndrome. *Plastic and Reconstructive Surgery, 133*(6), 1469–1475.
28. Yoon, K. C., Yang, Y., Jeong, I. Y., & Kook, M. S. (2011). Buccal mucosal graft for hydroxyapatite orbital implant exposure. *Japanese Journal of Ophthalmology, 55*(3), 318–320.
29. Iyer, G., Pillai, V. S., Srinivasan, B., Guruswami, S., & Padmanabhan, P. (2010). Mucous membrane grafting for lid margin keratinization in Stevens–Johnson syndrome: Results. *Cornea, 29*(2), 146–151.
30. White, J. H. (1975). Correction of distichiasis by tarsal resection and mucous membrane grafting. *American Journal of Ophthalmology, 80*(3. Pt 2), 507.
31. Sakai, S. (1993). Marginal eyelid reconstruction with a composite skin-muscle-mucosa graft from the lower lip. *Annals of Plastic Surgery, 30*(5), 445–447.
32. Weng, C. J. (1998). Surgical reconstruction in cryptophthalmos. *British Journal of Plastic Surgery, 51*(1), 17–21.
33. Rootman, D. B., Trope, G. E., & Rootman, D. S. (2009). Glaucoma aqueous drainage device erosion repair with buccal mucous membrane grafts. *Journal of Glaucoma, 18*(8), 618–622.
34. Murdoch, J. R., Sampath, R., Lavin, M. J., & Leatherbarrow, B. (1997). Autogenous labial mucous membrane and banked scleral patch grafting for exposed retinal explants. *Eye, 11*(1), 43.
35. Tao, J. P., Luppens, D., & McCord, C. D. (2010). Buccal mucous membrane graft-assisted lacrimal drainage surgery. *Ophthalmic Plastic & Reconstructive Surgery, 26*(1), 39–41.
36. Benlier, E., Bozkurt, M., & Kulahci, Y. (2008). An alternative procedure for conjunctivodacryocystorhinostomy: Supratrochlear artery-based island flap combined with buccal mucosal graft. *Annals of Plastic Surgery, 60*(1), 55–57.

# Chapter 16
# Microfluidic Technologies Using Oral Factors: Saliva-Based Studies

**Hassan Salehipour Masooleh, Mehrsima Ghavami-Lahiji, Annamarie Ciancio, and Lobat Tayebi**

## 1 Introduction

Medical devices are essential for a proper diagnosis by healthcare providers. Advances in medical devices and diagnoses in recent years have increased life expectancy by up to 5 years and reduced many common diseases [1]. However, people in developing countries do not have access to many new and expensive medical diagnostic technologies. For people who live far from medical laboratories, in developed countries as well as developing countries, it is difficult to go to a well-equipped lab for continuous (periodic) checkups. Microfluidic systems are designed to process the measurements of small volumes of liquids without the need for an expert, with relatively high sensitivity and speed. These unique features require creation of portable point-of-care (POC) medical diagnostic tools [2]. The advancement of microfluidic devices, in conjunction with lower price for POC applications, may provide instruments that can better serve the general population.

Microfluidic technologies, which are used in lab-on-a-chip (LOC) or miniaturized-total-analysis systems, allow for many different laboratory operations to be carried out on a small-scale portable chip [3]. Some microfluidic studies provide methods for shifting traditional macroscale assays to microscale portable

H. Salehipour Masooleh
MEMS and NEMS Laboratory, School of Electrical and Computer Engineering, University of Tehran, Tehran, Iran

M. Ghavami-Lahiji
Department of Dental Biomaterials, School of Dentistry, Tehran University of Medical Sciences, Tehran, Iran

Research Center for Science and Technology in Medicine, Tehran University of Medical Sciences, Tehran, Iran

A. Ciancio · L. Tayebi (✉)
Marquette University School of Dentistry, Milwaukee, WI, USA
e-mail: lobat.tayebi@marquette.edu



L. Tayebi (ed.), *Applications of Biomedical Engineering in Dentistry*,
https://doi.org/10.1007/978-3-030-21583-5_16

assays [4]. Microfluidics has revolutionized POC diagnostic tools in the realms of medical products, biology, bioengineering, microbiology, and chemistry. Revolution in these fields can be considered similar to the revolution of integrated circuits in the electronics industry, a keystone of modern electronics [5]. Microfluidics is currently attempting to be implemented for use in monitoring devices for patients, detection of bacteria, disease diagnostics, drug delivery systems, and microbial studies.

There are many advantages of implementing microfluidics. Some major advantages include, but are not limited to, reducing sample volume, reducing consumption of reagent, reducing consumption of dangerous materials and infectious sample, decreasing risk of contamination, possibility of performing experiments in parallel, controlling the flow rate and providing a dynamic environment, being timesaving, and having low cost. Ultimately, microfluidic devices bring the capabilities of advanced analytical techniques to deprived areas of the developing world where common analytical labs do not exist [5, 6]. Microfluidic systems bring the laboratory to the patient and enable in situ monitoring of analytes.

Microfluidics has advantages over more traditional methods, such as enzyme-linked immunosorbent assay (ELISA) and polymerase chain reaction (PCR); these are used for the detection of proteins and small molecules and deoxyribonucleic acid (DNA), respectively. These methods are costly, laborious, and time-consuming. The ELISA requires multiple steps of washing and incubation, while PCR requires thermal cycling. Both techniques should be performed by trained personnel and require a large sample size [7].

This chapter aims to provide a review of microfluidics that has been developed using oral factors. Most studies that have benefited from microfluidics in this field have used saliva as a diagnostic fluid. Using saliva as a diagnostic fluid is advantageous because it does not require highly trained personnel and its collection is noninvasive. Saliva samples can be easily stored, and salivary biomarkers can be used to evaluate some diseases and physiological conditions and/or progression of diseases [8]. The primary focus of this paper is saliva-based studies, and this has been subdivided according to the microfluidic technique: on microfluidic chip, paper-based microfluidic devices, and smartphone-based microfluidic devices. The last part of this study explores the application of microfluidics in early diagnosis of cancer and biofilm studies.

## 2 Saliva as a Diagnostic Tool

The technology of using saliva instead of blood for the diagnosis of diseases is rapidly developing. Interestingly, most studies that use saliva as a diagnostic fluid are typically associated with systemic diseases, rather than localized oral diseases [9, 10]. If the relationship between systemic diseases and the oral cavity is better understood, it will strengthen the collaboration between medicine and dentistry. Since the oral cavity is readily accessible, saliva and mucosal biopsy (transudate) are used for oral diagnostics [11, 12]. Most of the analytes found in the blood are also secreted into the salivary fluid, specifically inorganic and organic materials (carbohydrates, glycoproteins, lipids, etc.), drugs, and their metabolites. Moreover, the collection method of saliva is easy, inexpensive, noninvasive, and safe for patients and healthcare professionals [10]. In addition to its other advantages, this approach requires small amount of saliva. It is rapid, portable, and appropriate for POC testing [8, 13].

## 2.1 Detection of Disease on Microfluidic Chips

Herr et al. [13] demonstrated a microfluidic device to detect biomarkers that are responsible for the progression of periodontal disease. In this study, they first bound special antigens that exist primarily in saliva samples with antibodies labeled by fluorescent receptors. Then, they separated antibody-bound antigens using electrophoretic assays. Detection was made using diode lasers.

Malamud [11] offered the feasibility of employing microfluidic devices with saliva samples for detection of diseases like tuberculosis (TB), HIV, and malaria.

Chen et al. [14] made a platform for nucleic acid extraction from bacteria and miniaturized the PCR process into a microfluidic device. In the final step, DNA was labeled with upconverting phosphor to detect on the lateral flow strip.

Chen et al. [12], in an additional study, utilized a similar platform for the diagnosis of HIV infection as a model to investigate the simultaneous detection of both viral RNA and human antibodies against HIV. Highly sensitive reporter upconverting phosphor and high salt lateral flow (HSLF) assays were employed for antibody detection. Three years later, Chen et al. designed a microfluidic device for early detection of HIV disease in the "seroconversion window." During the seroconversion period, the viral load of HIV is highest, meaning the antibody is present but not detectable [15].

Since thiocyanate is considered an important biomarker in human health evaluation, finding a fast and reproducible way to analyze thiocyanate in bodily fluids is of interest. Wu et al. [16] developed a droplet microfluidic device for thiocyanate detection in real human saliva or serum using the surface-enhanced Raman scattering (SERS) technique. However, Pinto et al. [17] combined the immunoassay on a polydimethylsiloxane (PDMS) microfluidic chip and employed the complementary metal-oxide-semiconductor (CMOS) optical absorption system to detect the amount of cortisol in human saliva (Fig. 16.1).

Table 16.1 summarizes the studies of saliva on chip-based microfluidics for detection of infectious diseases. Other studies in this area have been done using filter paper or smartphone technology, which is explained in Sects. 2.2 and 2.3 in greater detail.

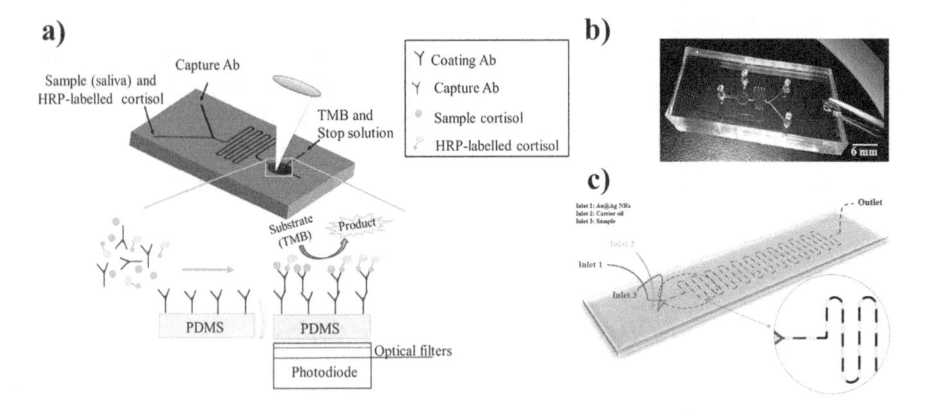


**Fig. 16.1** (**a**) Schematic image of the microfluidic immunosensor to detect salivary cortisol. (**b**) PDMS microfluidic device [17]. (**c**) Schematic image of a droplet microfluidic device for detection of salivary thiocyanate [16]

**Table 16.1** Summary of detection of infectious diseases based on saliva on microfluidic chips

| Analyte of interest in saliva | Method of processing (comment) | Method of detection | Reference |
|---|---|---|---|
| Biomarkers of periodontal disease (TNF-β and IL-6) | Electrophoretic immunoassays | Laser-induced fluorescence detector | [13] |
| *B. cereus* | Microfluidic chip for PCR-based testing | Laser scanner on the lateral flow strip | [14] |
| Human antibodies against HIV and viral RNA | Mixed/diluted with HSLF assay buffer<br>Silica-based nucleic acid purification<br>RT-PCR amplification | Lateral flow assay (LFA) | [12] |
| Human antibodies against HIV and viral RNA | Mixed/diluted with HSLF assay buffer<br>A magnetic bead-based process<br>Loop-mediated isothermal amplification (LAMP) | Lateral flow assay | [15] |
| Thiocyanate | Mixed with gold-silver core-shell nanorods<br>Droplet microfluidics | Surface-enhanced Raman scattering (SERS) technique | [16] |
| Salivary cortisol | PDMS microfluidic immunosensor | Colorimetric detection with CMOS | [17] |

## 2.2 *Microfluidic Paper-Based Analytical Devices (µPADs)*

Paper-based systems are considered an alternative rather than the main analytical tools, which are practical for POC testing. These devices have gained popularity due to their ease of use, ease of fabrication, and low cost.

µPADs are built on a filter paper, which explains how they got the name lab-on-a-paper devices, whereas lab-on-a-chip (LOC) devices are usually made of polydimethylsiloxane (PDMS). Furthermore, µPADs do not require any external forces because of capillary phenomenon, while LOC devices require external forces for the movement of fluids. This system has been of interest due to the hydrophilic nature of filter paper, passive fluid movement, biocompatibility, and disposability. Various methods have been introduced for the fabrication of paper-based devices, such as lithography, three-dimensional (3D) printing, wax jetting, wax smearing, PDMS screen printing, permanent marker pen, wax printing, ink-jet printing, eye-liner pencil, cutter printer, hydrophobic sol-gel fabrication, and scholar glue spray method [18]. µPADs employ different detection methods, such as colorimetric, luminescence, and electrochemical detection. The most common way of detection in these microfluidic systems is colorimetric readouts.

Colorimetric detection is based on visual comparison and determines the concentration of analytes by means of color reagents. There are various types of luminescence. Both fluorescence and chemiluminescence (CL) are common types of luminescence that have been successful in paper-based devices. Unlike fluorescence, CL relies on producing photons as a by-product of a chemical reaction without requiring a light source [19, 20].

Electrochemical detection is based on the measurement of electrical parameters in the sample [21]. In this method, electrochemical analytical devices should be connected to a smartphone to measure changes from one of the input/output ports, such as the micro-USB.

Bhakta et al. [22] developed a µPAD with the wax printing method to identify and quantify levels of nitrite in saliva. It has been proven that nitrite concentration in saliva is associated with clinical symptoms of periodontitis (bleeding, swelling, and redness) [23]. In this approach, the main channel of the µPAD is placed vertically in contact with the saliva sample. The sample is taken up by capillary action and driven into the four branched channels and testing zones (Fig. 16.2). The nitrite in the saliva is combined with the Griess reagent, and this leads to magenta azo compound formation. The Griess reagent is made by mixing sulfanilamide in 5% (v/v) phosphoric acid solution and 0.1% (w/v) naphthylethylenediamine dihydrochloride in water. Color intensity is associated with the concentration of nitrite in the sample and can be representative of the progression of periodontitis [22].

Nitrite is also known as a helpful biomarker for patients with end-stage renal disease to detect progression of hemodialysis. It has been reported that the concentration of nitrite in the patient's saliva reflects the amount of nitrite in the blood and is suitable for POC application [24]. Salivary nitrite concentrations were measured

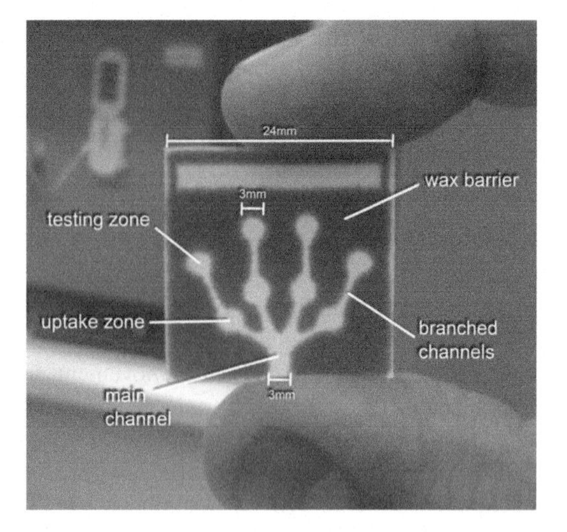


**Fig. 16.2** μPAD designed for nitrite detection in human saliva [22]

in a study by Blicharz et al. with test strips. They showed nitrite concentrations decreased after dialysis and found this method to be a noninvasive and beneficial way of monitoring renal disease status [25].

Formaldehyde and acetaldehyde are well known as carcinogenic agents. Smoking is one of the most important sources of aldehyde contamination in the indoor air. Additionally, it has been shown that consuming alcoholic beverages has the same carcinogenic effect due to the transformation of ethanol into acetaldehyde [26]. Ramdzan et al. [27] employed a two-layer configuration paper-based microfluidic device for determining salivary aldehydes. This study revealed that this paper-based technique could be a successful alternative to the costly and large-scale analytical tools [e.g., high-performance liquid chromatography (HPLC) or gas chromatography (GC)] that determine aldehydes in biological fluids, such as salivary fluid. In addition, the sensitivity of this technique is comparable to that of the aforementioned methods [27].

One of the more basic of the "paper-based devices" is lateral flow immunoassay (LFI). LFI has been employed with smartphones as a new developing field in recent literature. This situation is discussed in the next section.

## 2.3 Smartphone-Based Microfluidic Devices

Integration between microfluidic devices and smartphones introduces a new world and has the potential to revolutionize the smartphone industry. Smartphone-based diagnostics provides a user-friendly, easily accessible, miniaturized, and portable technology [28].

In this approach, the phone is the main device that performs the entire analytical process, including data acquisition, analysis, and result readout. Smartphone, like a computer, has a processor (CPU) and hardware for receiving, sending, and processing a variety of signals. Therefore, it has the ability to receive data from sensors and control various actuators or send data to and receive data from other devices, by wire or wirelessly. This allows a variety of applications on the smartphone to run in order to analyze data and check the biological samples.

Many studies in this area utilize smartphone cameras to receive information from samples. Different principles for the development of biosensors have been used. Biosensors in these systems work based on color, luminescence, or electrochemical detection. Smartphone microfluidic systems that employ saliva as a diagnostic fluid often use colorimetric and luminescence techniques.

It is almost impossible for the human eye to quantize the color variation or the light emitted from the luminescence samples [29]. Therefore, an accessory is needed to standardize the effective factors to eliminate quantization errors. In these methods, a dark chamber is required to avoid ambient light interfering with measurements. Different techniques are considered to standardize the camera flashlight. A holder is needed for connecting the dark chamber to the smartphone [20]. Another detection method that has been mentioned in the articles using smartphones is electrochemical sensors (amperometric, impedimetric, and potentiometric sensors). This method uses different sample mediums, such as saliva, blood, water, food, and urine [19].

Monitoring pH in saliva is important for investigating the person's diet and its relationship with enamel decalcification. Monitoring pH in sweat helps explain the risk of dehydration during physical activities. Oncescu et al. [30] designed a software and a hardware accessory installed on a smartphone. After collecting a saliva or sweat sample, the test strip was inserted into the device, and the pH analysis was carried out using a mobile platform. The flash on the smartphone's camera was used to illuminate the back of the test strip, exposing the pH indicator. Colorimetry was used to understand the pH of either saliva or sweat sample.

Other studies reported using a smartphone for detection of bile acid in serum and oral fluid [31], salivary cortisol [32–35], L-lactate [20, 36, 37], glucose [38, 39], Zika virus (ZIKV) [40, 41], drugs related to driving under influence (DUI) cases [42–46], ovulation time [47], and others [48, 49] in human saliva (Table 16.2). However, there are some published papers that utilize blood as the diagnostic fluid with smartphone technology.

Nowadays, stress is one of the major causes of psychiatric disease. Stressful daily routines can lead to additional mental health problems, such as depression, anxiety, low self-esteem, and more. Thus, many efforts have been made to design stress monitoring tools [17, 32]. Cortisol is one of the most well-known biomarkers of stress. The main advantages of using saliva as a diagnostic fluid to measure cortisol levels are its easy, noninvasive, and rapid collection method. This itself reduces a potential stress response and allows continuous monitoring of stress level. Cortisol has two active states: free active state and protein-bonded state. Cortisol in the saliva is in the free active state, meaning that it is detectable, unlike what exists in the blood—where about 90% of it is protein-bonded [17, 50]. This is a major advantage of using saliva over blood for detection of cortisol.

**Table 16.2** Summary of detection of analytes in saliva by smartphone-based microfluidic devices

| Target/Analyte | Method of sample processing/ detection | Data acquisition methods | Reference |
|---|---|---|---|
| pH in sweat and saliva | Test strip Includes an indicator strip, a reference strip, and a flash diffuser | Colorimetry with smartphone camera | [30] |
| Bile acid in serum and oral fluid Total cholesterol in serum | Minicartridge | Biochemiluminescence (BL-CL) with smartphone camera | [31] |
| Salivary cortisol | Lateral flow immunoassay | Colorimetry with smartphone camera | [32] |
| Lactate levels in oral fluid and sweat | Analytical cartridge | Chemiluminescence with smartphone camera or thermoelectrically cooled CCD camera | [20] |
| Salivary cortisol | Lateral flow immunoassay (CL-LFI) | Chemiluminescence with smartphone camera | [33] |
| Microbial pathogens | LAMP technique with a microfluidic network named "airlock" | Using Gene-Z device with a smartphone camera or a digital camera, which only requires a green LED for excitation and orange filter lenses for emissions | [52] |
| Alcohol | Alco-Screen test strips were provided by Chematics, Inc. | Colorimetry, with smartphone camera | [42] |
| α-Amylase | Sensing chip including electrodes and a capillary channel | Potentiometric measurement connected to the smartphone via a USB port | [48] |
| Drug-of-abuse detection (six drugs + alcohol in saliva) | Lateral flow immunoassay | Image processing with neural network machine learning using smartphone camera | [43] |
| Marijuana or cannabis containing main psychoactive substance, tetrahydrocannabinol (THC) | Giant magnetoresistive biosensors with a reaction well | A measurement reader connected to smartphone via Bluetooth module | [44] |
| Cocaine | Upconversion nanoparticle-based paper device | Luminescence with smartphone camera using an external diode laser (980 nm) light source | [45] |

(continued)

**Table 16.2** (continued)

| Target/Analyte | Method of sample processing/ detection | Data acquisition methods | Reference |
|---|---|---|---|
| Salivary L-lactate | The functionalized paper-based assay | Colorimetry with smartphone camera | [36] |
| Zika virus | Reverse transcription-loop-mediated isothermal amplification (RT-LAMP) | Colorimetry with smartphone camera using an external RGB excitation source | [40] |
| Salivary glucose | Test strip | Colorimetry with smartphone camera | [38] |
| Lactate in saliva | Cloth-based devices | Electrochemiluminescence, imaging by the smartphone camera, transfering to PC by Wi-Fi network | [37] |
| Alcohol | Test strips | Colorimetry with smartphone camera using different machine learning algorithms (linear discriminant analysis, support vector machine, and artificial neural network) | [46] |
| Salivary cortisol | A paper-based lateral flow assay (LFA) strip | Colorimetry with smartphone camera | [34] |
| Salivary glucose | Graphene oxide modified μPADs (reservoir array-based and lateral flow designs) | Colorimetry with smartphone camera | [39] |
| Zika virus (ZIKV) in saliva and urine and HIV in blood | Bioluminescent assay in real time and loop-mediated isothermal amplification (BART-LAMP) | Bioluminescence with the smartphone camera | [41] |
| Salivary cortisol | Lateral flow assay | A portable imaging device with a CMOS camera which enables sending image via Wi-Fi to a smartphone, tablet, or laptop computer | [35] |
| Urea | A filter paper-based strip | Color change detection based on RGB profiling with smartphone camera | [49] |
| Nitrite | A paper-based device using electrokinetic stacking (ES) mechanism | Colorimetry with a smartphone fixing on stereomicroscope or macro lens using ImageJ | [53] |

(continued)

**Table 16.2** (continued)

| Target/Analyte | Method of sample processing/ detection | Data acquisition methods | Reference |
|---|---|---|---|
| Valproic acid (VPA) | Vertical flow immunoassay (VFIA) | Thermochemiluminescence (TCL), imaging by the smartphone camera | [54] |
| Ovulation-specific hormones LH + estrogen | A microfluidic channel to make saliva smear block | Detection of salivary ferning patterns using AI with smartphone camera | [47] |

Choi et al. [32] and Zangheri et al. [33] have demonstrated a smartphone-based system with lateral flow immunoassay for quantitative measurement of salivary cortisol. Choi et al. [32] compared the changes in the hue (color) and brightness (lightness or darkness) values with cortisol concentration. Zangheri et al. [33] immobilized anti-cortisol antibodies in rabbits (T-line) and anti-peroxidase antibodies in rabbits (C-line). These antibodies were placed on nitrocellulose membranes to make LFI test strips for their experiment. They measured the intensity of the chemiluminescence signal of the T-line for quantification of the amount of cortisol. It was found that the intensity of the chemiluminescence and cortisol in the sample were inversely correlated. Chemiluminescence signal of the C-line was also used to evaluate the validity of the test (Fig. 16.3).

At first, Zika virus appeared to only cause mild disease, but the outbreak in Brazil in 2015 showed the relationship between the virus and severe fetal abnormalities, called congenital Zika syndrome. In search of diagnostic technologies, Priye et al. [40] designed a study to detect the virus using similar cases. Unlike most papers, in this research, a microcontroller was used to monitor and control the temperature of a dark plastic enclosure containing the samples. This microcontroller, an Arduino, was wirelessly connected to the smartphone and was able to control the RGB LED light source placed in this box. The smartphone application with a simple graphical user interface (GUI) was created to actuate the LED excitation source and the isothermal heater through the microcontroller and display a live camera feed. It also provided other features and facilities for the user. Finally, the test results were displayed on the final screen after processing.

Internet of Medical Things (IoMT)—a new technology to connect the medical devices to the healthcare providers—is revolutionizing the medical world. This technology offers new paradigms of diagnosis, treatment, and healthcare services in a timely and cost-effective manner. In addition, it may be helpful in epidemiology studies [51]. However, current IoMT devices are limited to monitor physiological information, such as heart rate and blood pressure. Song et al. [41] demonstrated a IoMT POC device based on a smartphone for molecular diagnostics, providing quantitative detection for Zika virus (ZIKV) and HIV, transferring test results to the doctor's office, and allowing communication of data.

Calabria et al. [36] demonstrated "wafer-like" structures as a functionalized paper of cellulose that contained reagents and enzymes to measure accurate L-lactate

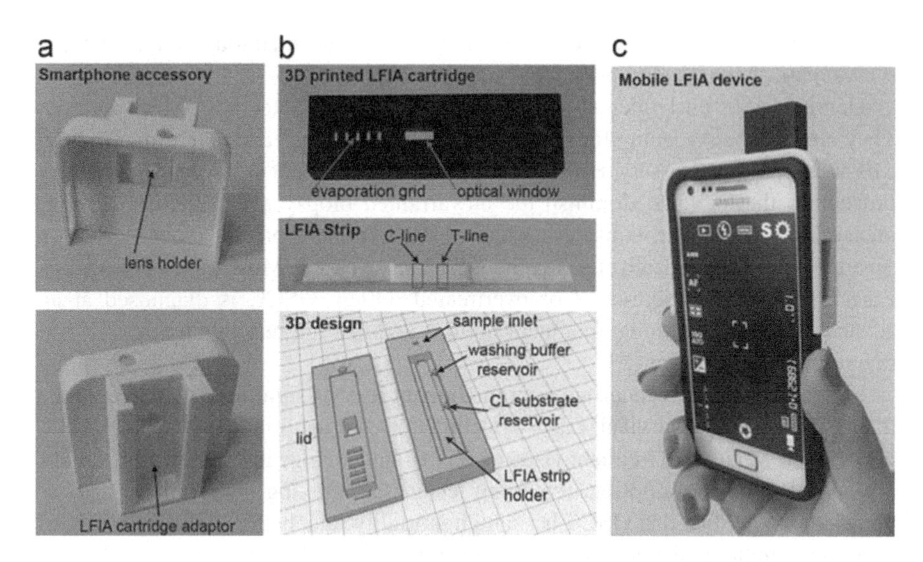


**Fig. 16.3** (**a**) 3D printed smartphone accessory. (**b**) 3D printed cartridge hosting the LFI strip with control (C-line) and test lines (T-line). (**c**) Smartphone-based microfluidic device for measuring salivary cortisol [33]

levels in saliva. It was shown that smartphones could also detect L-lactate based on the hue saturation value (HSV) for rapid colorimetric measurement.

In another study by Roda et al. [20], a chemiluminescence biosensor was introduced, which is comprised of a disposable minicartridge with two reaction chambers. Inside these chambers are nitrocellulose disks that contain the enzymes needed for reaction. Each of chambers were connected to two reservoirs containing reagents using channel.

In 2019, Potluri et al. [47] introduced a low-cost smartphone-based device beneficial for couples interested in planning pregnancy. Studies have shown that during the follicular phase of the menstrual cycle, increased level of estradiol in the blood results in an increase in the salivary electrolytes, which can cause a crystallized pattern like fern leaves in air-dried saliva. This pattern may be used for ovulation detection. They utilized a neural network which is trained with salivary ferning images. Artificial intelligence (AI) was employed for detection of ovulation period from air-dried saliva samples.

## 3 Detection of Oral Cancer

Cancers of the oral cavity comprise approximately 40% of head and neck cancers and affect several areas, such as the tongue, gums, lips, palate, floor of the mouth, and buccal mucosa [55]. Despite recent advances in diagnostics, therapeutics, and surgical procedures, the success rate of treating oral squamous cell carcinoma (OSCC) still remains very poor [56].

Dentists and oral hygienists play a key role in early detection of oral cancers. They ought to be screening for suspicious malignant lesions and determine whether a tissue biopsy is necessary. However, while they do not want delay in any necessary procedure, they tend to diminish the unwarranted biopsy and patients' inconvenience [57]. Moreover, considering aggressive treatment of OSCC can lead to a severe deformity or death, its treatment is controversial. Most patients with this cancer are either undertreated or overtreated. Often, OSCC is diagnosed at an advanced stage. This limits treatment options and is a big reason why the survival rate of patients is so low [5].

Early diagnosis of cancerous or premalignant lesions significantly increases the likelihood of patient survival. Early detection does not automatically mean success. However, it can lead to frequent visits by the patient, change in diet, stopping smoking and alcohol consumption, removing lesions, and taking the required medications. Due to the fact that OSCC has a high mortality rate, better screening methods need to be implemented to detect this cancer early [5, 58].

Some studies demonstrated cell-based microfluidic sensors to detect cancer biomarkers. Cytology, which is the easiest way to screen premalignant and cancerous lesions, was employed to capture cells from the targeted tissues. Expression of cancer-specific biomarkers could be used to discriminate cancer cells from normal cells [56, 59, 60]. This review focuses on saliva-based microfluidic devices for screening of cancers.

In a study conducted by De et al. [61], a LOC microfluidic system was employed for hypermethylated DNA extraction and enrichment, which was suitable for processing small biological samples such as saliva and urine. This device was demonstrated to identify the patterns of hypermethylation parts in tumor-suppressor genes with the potential for the early detection and diagnosis of cancers.

Zilberman et al. [62, 63] introduced a new platform to assist stomach cancer diagnosis. The underlying cause of the stomach cancer is the infection by a gram-negative bacterium *Helicobacter pylori.* This bacterium converts urea into ammonia ($NH_3$) and carbon dioxide ($CO_2$) by secreting the urease enzyme, resulting in high levels of these substances in the body fluids and breath. They demonstrated a microfluidic optoelectronic sensor to detect the amount of salivary $NH_3$ and $CO_2$. Using saliva for screening cancers is a convenient and noninvasive approach compared to traditional endoscopy method. Using the proposed method of Zilberman et al. can eliminate the need for trained personnel and high costs of endoscopy.

Biomarkers, which represent normal biological and pathological procedures, may provide helpful information for detection, diagnosis, and prognosis of the diseases. More than 100 biomarkers (DNA, RNA, mRNA, protein markers) have already been recognized in oral fluid, including cytokines (IL-8, IL-1b, TNF-a), p53, Cyfra 21-1, defensin-1, and tissue polypeptide-specific antigen [64].

Lin et al. [65] developed an automated microfluidic chip using magnetic bead-based immunoassays, well suited for anti-p53 quantification in saliva. The proposed

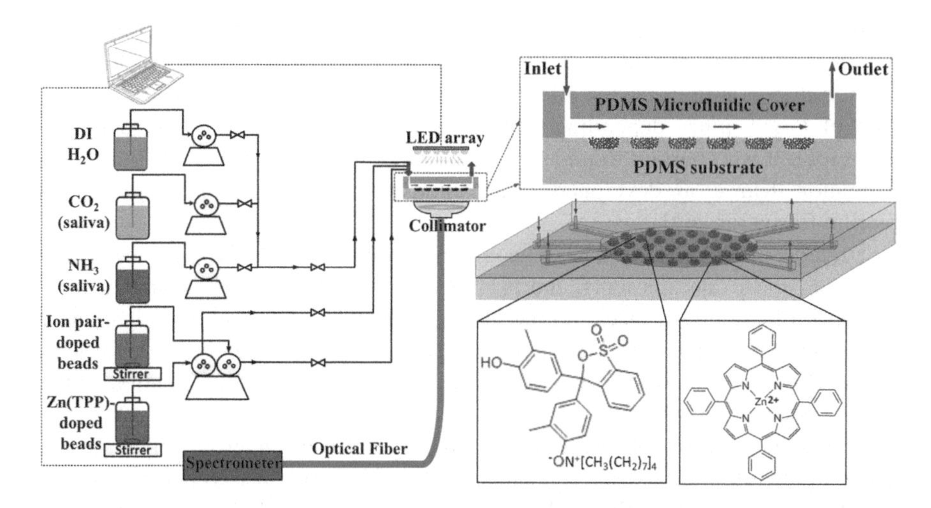


**Fig. 16.4** Schematic representation of a microfluidic device including inlets and outlets, which embeds microwells occupied with organic dye-doped ion-exchange polymer microbeads. The response of this optoelectronic sensor is monitored by a USB spectrometer [63]

device can considerably reduce the time for conventional immunoassay, which takes about 3 hours, to approximately 60 minutes.

In a study by Dong et al. [66], an optical microfluidic biosensor has demonstrated good analytical performance for salivary protein biomarkers (IL-8, IL-1β, and MMP-8) to differentiate patients with oral cancer from healthy people.

A microfluidic paper-based electrochemical DNA biosensor was fabricated by Tian et al. [67] to detect epidermal growth factor receptor (EGFR) mutations in DNA extracted from non-small cell lung cancer patients' saliva samples (Fig. 16.4).

# 4 Biofilm Formation

Most of the bacteria tend to switch from a free-floating planktonic state to a sticky organized biofilm state. Forming the biofilm protects the bacteria from harmful conditions (e.g., nutrient deficiency, pH alterations, antibacterial agents, and shear stress) in the host, and the bacteria benefit from cooperating with each other.

The microfluidic systems provide a closed system where bacteria can exist in biofilms and interact with hydrodynamic environments. Microfluidic systems can be beneficial for studying biofilm formation mechanisms and solving problems associated with biofilm. Importantly, they allow for the flow of fluids to be controlled. The small scale of these devices makes it easy to cultivate bacteria and form biofilms because it is easy to set up a variety of conditions. In addition, their transparency makes it possible to observe the development of biofilms [68].

It has been reported that most bacteria utilize a form of cell-to-cell communication named quorum sensing (QS) for their initial colonization and development of biofilm communities. This allows each bacterial species to adjust the expression of target genes depending on the environment and physiological needs. Therefore, it is important to understand the role of various QS signals in biofilm formation. Kim et al. developed a microfluidic device to investigate QS in oral biofilm formation [69].

*Streptococcus mutans* is the main cause of dental caries [70]. Environmental factors (e.g., shear rate, nutrients, and pH) greatly affect the biofilm formation of *S. mutans* on the tooth surface, and monitoring of these factors and investigation of their effects are of interest to researchers [71]. *S. mutans* plays an important role in the development of the exopolysaccharide (EPS) matrix in biofilm formation on the tooth surface of the tooth [70].

Quantitative analysis of EPS can be investigated using microliter plate-based assay, which is recognized as a reliable technique. However, this assay is performed in static conditions. Microfluidic devices have the advantage of providing a dynamic flow system that mimics the environment of the oral cavity [72].

In a study conducted by Shumi et al., the effect of the environmental factors on biofilm formation of *S. mutans* was examined in a microfluidic device with glass beads. In this study, glass beads mimicked the interproximal space between teeth. They found production of EPS and attachment of *S. mutans* to the surface of the glass beads happened in the presence of sucrose [71]. In another study, Shumi et al. designed a microfluidic platform with a funnel that provided various ranges of shear stresses.

Sucrose-dependent and sucrose-independent aggregates of *S. mutans* were evaluated under different flow rates and times. The findings showed *S. mutans* colonies that were sucrose-dependent strongly adhered to the funnel wall. Detachment of sucrose-dependent colonies from the funnel wall was possible only with high shear stress, while in the case of sucrose-independent colonies, they were easily separated from the funnel by a slight shear stress [73].

The dental plaque on the tooth's surface is a multispecies biofilm, containing over 500 species of bacteria. The bacteria in biofilms are less susceptible to antibacterial agents than planktonic cells [74, 75]. To evaluate the effects of antibacterial agents on bacteria, it is important to create biofilms that contain the species present in the oral cavity. Nance et al. and Samarian et al. simulated the condition of the oral cavity with a commercially available BioFlux microfluidic system (Fluxion Biosciences, Inc., Alameda, CA 94502, USA) [6, 75]. This system is useful for overcoming limitations, such as using less materials and not requiring artificial lab media, especially since it can be costly and time-consuming to run culture-based studies. A lot of media are required in tests that are conducted in flow cell studies. Using this high-throughput system allows multiple experiments to be done in parallel. Finally, this system is able to combine imaging systems to allow precise investigation of biofilm testing [6, 76, 77].

Nance et al. investigated the effect of different concentrations of antimicrobial agent (cetylpyridinium chloride) using confocal laser scanning microscope (CLSM) and 3D imaging software. Some studies have utilized a germane environmental situation to resemble the real-world environment. The use of human saliva in this method has become popular for investigating biofilms. Cell-free saliva (CFS) plays the role of growth medium, and the untreated bacterial cell-containing saliva (CCS) plays the role of inoculum that contains bacterial species in the oral cavity. The formed multispecies biofilm is washed and stained for in situ confocal laser scanning microscopy [6, 75, 77].

Most studies examine biofilms in a static state. In the oral cavity, designing continuous fluid flow is preferred to mimic formed biofilm in the body. In the case of peri-radicular lesions (non-ideal root canal therapy or pulpal necrosis), there is a fluid exchange inside and outside the root canal space that provides feeding and flow for the growth of bacteria. Cheng et al. compared the bactericidal effect of several root canal irrigants against *Enterococcus faecalis* biofilm, recognized as the most important persistent endodontic infection. They evaluated *E. faecalis* biofilm in flow state as well as static state [78].

In the study conducted by Lam et al., a high-throughput microfluidic system with the name of "artificial teeth" was introduced. This device had different layers of channels (e.g., water jackets, gas control, upper and lower flow control), which could provide complex and dynamic environmental situations and acquire quantitative characteristics about thickness and cell viability of dental bacteria [79]. The summary of microbial studies using a microfluidic device is provided in Table 16.3 (Fig. 16.5).

## 5 Summary

Microfluidics is an attractive, rapidly developing, and promising technology that may enable detection of certain diseases, such as diabetes and periodontal disease. Microfluidics can also be exploited as a diagnostic tool for early detection of complex diseases, such as cancers and viral infections, like HIV. Among the microfluidic systems used in the biomedical field, μPADs have become the most commercially available system due to their low manufacturing cost, as well as not requiring complex accessories during tests. This developing approach faces many challenges requiring standardization to verify its reproducibility and reliability.

For future development, it is expected to involve other technological devices—such as smartphones or tablets with microfluidics—to analyze the physiological state of humans using a drop of saliva or other biological fluids. Considering how advanced smartphones have become and how rapidly they are developing, the combination of these technologies will allow continuous and easy health monitoring of individuals or target groups. The results can then be sent directly to the patient's physician or healthcare provider. The ramifications of this technology are powerful; it has the potential to make major improvements in the quality of life of people in modern and developing societies.

**Table 16.3** Summary of microbial studies based on saliva using microfluidic devices

| Source of bacteria | Microfluidic device/aim | Equipment of investigation | Reference |
|---|---|---|---|
| *S. mutans* strains | Fabrication of microfluidic device evaluating the effect of signaling molecule autoinducer 2 (AI-2) on *S. mutans* strains | CLSM, Imaris software | [69] |
| Pre-culture of *S. mutans* + fresh TSB (trypticase soy broth) + with or without sucrose washed with TSB | Microfluidic device with glass beads evaluating the effect of the environmental factors (metal ions and sucrose) on biofilm formation of *S. mutans* | Staining of live cells, CLSM imaging, AFM imaging | [71] |
| Washed with TSB + conditioned with saliva + culture of *S. mutans* | Designing a simple microfluidic funnel device *S. mutans* aggregates (sucrose-dependent and sucrose-independent) were evaluated under different flow rates and times | CLSM and ImageJ software | [73] |
| Pooled human saliva: inoculum/nutrient | Developing a high-throughput dental biofilm system using a commercially available microfluidic system Different concentrations of antimicrobial agent (cetylpyridinium chloride) | Live/dead stain, CLSM and 3D imaging software | [6] |
| Pooled human saliva: inoculum/nutrient | Using a commercially available microfluidic system | CLSM, Imaris, and ImageJ software | [75] |
| Human saliva | Fabrication of microfluidic device composed of multiple incubation chambers (128) capable of controlling different fluid flows of each chamber separately Evaluating the growth of dental bacteria in the biofilm under different concentrations of sucrose and different dissolved oxygen and nitrogen gas conditions | Inverted fluorescence microscope equipped with a motorized XYZ stage, sCMOS camera | [79] |
| *Enterococcus faecalis* suspension | Using a commercially available microfluidic system Evaluating the bactericidal effect of sodium hypochlorite (NaOCl, 5.25%), strong acid electrolyzed water (SAEW), and normal saline (0.9%) against *Enterococcus faecalis* biofilm as a root canal irrigant | CLSM and ImageJ software, SEM | [78] |

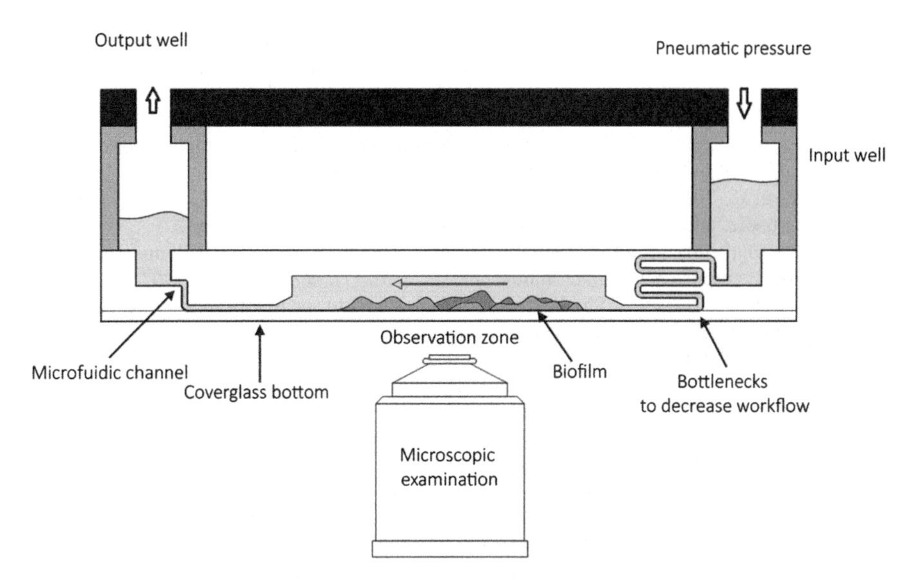


**Fig. 16.5** Cross section of the BioFlux microfluidic device showing the formed biofilm. The concept of this image is provided by references [6, 76]

# References


1. Guan, A., et al. (2017). Medical devices on chips. *Nature Biomedical Engineering, 1*(3), 1–10.
2. Yager, P., et al. (2006). Microfluidic diagnostic technologies for global public health. *Nature, 442*(7101), 412–418.
3. Gupta, S., et al. (2016). Lab-on-chip technology: A review on design trends and future scope in biomedical applications. *International Journal of Bio-Science and Bio-Technology, 8*(5), 311–322.
4. Sackmann, E. K., Fulton, A. L., & Beebe, D. J. (2014). The present and future role of microfluidics in biomedical research. *Nature, 507*(7491), 181–189.
5. Ziober, B. L., et al. (2008). Lab-on-a-chip for oral cancer screening and diagnosis. *Head & Neck, 30*(1), 111–121.
6. Nance, W. C., et al. (2013). A high-throughput microfluidic dental plaque biofilm system to visualize and quantify the effect of antimicrobials. *Journal of Antimicrobial Chemotherapy, 68*(11), 2550–2560.
7. Lim, W. Y., Goh, B. T., & Khor, S. M. (2017). Microfluidic paper-based analytical devices for potential use in quantitative and direct detection of disease biomarkers in clinical analysis. *Journal of Chromatography B, 1060*, 424–442.
8. Meagher, R., & Kousvelari, E. (2018). Mobile oral heath technologies based on saliva. *Oral Diseases, 24*(1–2), 194–197.
9. Arunkumar, S., et al. (2014). Developments in diagnostic applications of saliva in oral and systemic diseases-A comprehensive review. *Journal of Scientific and Innovative Research, 3*(3), 372–387.
10. Chojnowska, S., et al. (2018). Human saliva as a diagnostic material. *Advances in Medical Sciences, 63*(1), 185–191.
11. Malamud, D. (2013). The oral-systemic connection: role of salivary diagnostics. In Sensing Technologies for Global Health, Military Medicine, and Environmental Monitoring III. International Society for Optics and Photonics.

12. Chen, Z., et al. (2013). Development of a generic microfluidic device for simultaneous detection of antibodies and nucleic acids in oral fluids. *BioMed Research International, 2013*, 1–12.
13. Herr, A. E., et al. (2007). Integrated microfluidic platform for oral diagnostics. *Annals of the New York Academy of Sciences, 1098*(1), 362–374.
14. Chen, Z., et al. (2007). A microfluidic system for saliva-based detection of infectious diseases. *Annals of the New York Academy of Sciences, 1098*(1), 429–436.
15. Chen, Z., et al. (2016). A rapid, self-confirming assay for HIV: Simultaneous detection of anti-HIV antibodies and viral RNA. *Journal of AIDS & Clinical Research, 7*(1), 1–8.
16. Wu, L., et al. (2014). Rapid and reproducible analysis of thiocyanate in real human serum and saliva using a droplet SERS-microfluidic chip. *Biosensors and Bioelectronics, 62*, 13–18.
17. Pinto, V., et al. (2017). Microfluidic immunosensor for rapid and highly-sensitive salivary cortisol quantification. *Biosensors and Bioelectronics, 90*, 308–313.
18. Sriram, G., et al. (2017). Paper-based microfluidic analytical devices for colorimetric detection of toxic ions: A review. *TrAC Trends in Analytical Chemistry, 93*, 212–227.
19. Roda, A., et al. (2016). Smartphone-based biosensors: A critical review and perspectives. *Trends in Analytical Chemistry, 79*, 317–325.
20. Roda, A., et al. (2014). A 3D-printed device for a smartphone-based chemiluminescence biosensor for lactate in oral fluid and sweat. *Analyst, 139*(24), 6494–6501.
21. Snober, A., Minh-Phuong, N., & Abdennour, A. (2016). Paper-based chemical and biological sensors: Engineering aspects. *Biosensors and Bioelectronics, 77*, 249–263.
22. Bhakta, S. A., et al. (2014). Determination of nitrite in saliva using microfluidic paper-based analytical devices. *Analytica Chimica Acta, 809*, 117–122.
23. Allaker, R., et al. (2001). Antimicrobial effect of acidified nitrite on periodontal bacteria. *Molecular Oral Microbiology, 16*(4), 253–256.
24. Klasner, S. A., et al. (2010). Based microfluidic devices for analysis of clinically relevant analytes present in urine and saliva. *Analytical and Bioanalytical Chemistry, 397*(5), 1821–1829.
25. Blicharz, T. M., et al. (2008). Use of colorimetric test strips for monitoring the effect of hemodialysis on salivary nitrite and uric acid in patients with end-stage renal disease: A proof of principle. *Clinical Chemistry, 54*(9), 1473–1480.
26. Demkowska, I., Polkowska, Ż., & Namieśnik, J. (2010). Formaldehyde in human saliva as an indication of environmental tobacco smoke exposure. *Polish Journal of Environmental Studies, 19*(3), 573–577.
27. Ramdzan, A. N., et al. (2016). Development of a microfluidic paper-based analytical device for the determination of salivary aldehydes. *Analytica Chimica Acta, 919*, 47–54.
28. Yang, K., et al. (2016). Novel developments in mobile sensing based on the integration of microfluidic devices and smartphones. *Lab on a Chip, 16*(6), 943–958.
29. Deeb, S. (2005). The molecular basis of variation in human color vision. *Clinical Genetics, 67*(5), 369–377.
30. Oncescu, V., O'Dell, D., & Erickson, D. (2013). Smartphone based health accessory for colorimetric detection of biomarkers in sweat and saliva. *Lab on a Chip, 13*(16), 3232–3238.
31. Roda, A., et al. (2014). Integrating biochemiluminescence detection on smartphones: Mobile chemistry platform for point-of-need analysis. *Analytical Chemistry, 86*(15), 7299–7304.
32. Choi, S., et al. (2014). Real-time measurement of human salivary cortisol for the assessment of psychological stress using a smartphone. *Sensing and Bio-Sensing Research, 2*, 8–11.
33. Zangheri, M., et al. (2015). A simple and compact smartphone accessory for quantitative chemiluminescence-based lateral flow immunoassay for salivary cortisol detection. *Biosensors and Bioelectronics, 64*, 63–68.
34. Choi, S., et al. (2017). Relationship analysis of speech communication between salivary cortisol levels and personal characteristics using the Smartphone Linked Stress Measurement (SLSM). *BioChip Journal, 11*(2), 101–107.
35. Rey, E., et al. (2018). Personalized stress monitoring: A smartphone-enabled system for quantification of salivary cortisol. *Personal and Ubiquitous Computing, 22*(4), 867–877.

36. Calabria, D., et al. (2017). Smartphone–based enzymatic biosensor for oral fluid L-lactate detection in one minute using confined multilayer paper reflectometry. *Biosensors and Bioelectronics, 94*, 124–130.
37. Yao, Y., et al. (2017). An electrochemiluminescence cloth-based biosensor with smartphone-based imaging for detection of lactate in saliva. *Analyst, 142*(19), 3715–3724.
38. Soni, A., & Jha, S. K. (2017). Smartphone based non-invasive salivary glucose biosensor. *Analytica Chimica Acta, 996*, 54–63.
39. Jia, Y., et al. (2018). Based graphene oxide biosensor coupled with smartphone for the quantification of glucose in oral fluid. *Biomedical Microdevices, 20*(4), 89.
40. Priye, A., et al. (2017). A smartphone-based diagnostic platform for rapid detection of Zika, chikungunya, and dengue viruses. *Scientific Reports, 7*, 44778.
41. Song, J., et al. (2018). Smartphone-based mobile detection platform for molecular diagnostics and spatiotemporal disease mapping. *Analytical Chemistry, 90*(7), 4823–4831.
42. Jung, Y., et al. (2015). Smartphone-based colorimetric analysis for detection of saliva alcohol concentration. *Applied Optics, 54*(31), 9183–9189.
43. Carrio, A., et al. (2015). Automated low-cost smartphone-based lateral flow saliva test reader for drugs-of-abuse detection. *Sensors, 15*(11), 29569–29593.
44. Lee, J.-R., et al. (2016). Small molecule detection in saliva facilitates portable tests of marijuana abuse. *Analytical Chemistry, 88*(15), 7457–7461.
45. He, M., et al. (2016). Portable upconversion nanoparticles-based paper device for field testing of drug abuse. *Analytical Chemistry, 88*(3), 1530–1534.
46. Kim, H., et al. (2017). Colorimetric analysis of saliva–alcohol test strips by smartphone-based instruments using machine-learning algorithms. *Applied Optics, 56*(1), 84–92.
47. Potluri, V., et al. (2019). An inexpensive smartphone-based device for point-of-care ovulation testing. *Lab on a Chip, 19*(1), 59–67.
48. Zhang, L., et al. (2015). Smartphone-based point-of-care testing of salivary α-amylase for personal psychological measurement. *Analyst, 140*(21), 7399–7406.
49. Soni, A., Surana, R. K., & Jha, S. K. (2018). Smartphone based optical biosensor for the detection of urea in saliva. *Sensors and Actuators B: Chemical, 269*, 346–353.
50. Kaushik, A., et al. (2014). Recent advances in cortisol sensing technologies for point-of-care application. *Biosensors and Bioelectronics, 53*, 499–512.
51. Haghi, M., Thurow, K., & Stoll, R. (2017). Wearable devices in medical internet of things: Scientific research and commercially available devices. *Healthcare Informatics Research, 23*(1), 4–15.
52. Stedtfeld, R. D., et al. (2015). Static self-directed sample dispensing into a series of reaction wells on a microfluidic card for parallel genetic detection of microbial pathogens. *Biomedical Microdevices, 17*(5), 89.
53. Zhang, X.-X., et al. (2018). Sensitive paper-based analytical device for fast colorimetric detection of nitrite with smartphone. *Analytical and Bioanalytical Chemistry, 410*(11), 2665–2669.
54. Roda, A., et al. (2019). A simple smartphone-based thermochemiluminescent immunosensor for valproic acid detection using 1,2-dioxetane analogue-doped nanoparticles as a label. *Sensors and Actuators B: Chemical, 279*, 327–333.
55. Massano, J., et al. (2006). Oral squamous cell carcinoma: Review of prognostic and predictive factors. *Oral Surgery, Oral Medicine, Oral Pathology, Oral Radiology and Endodontics, 102*(1), 67–76.
56. Abram, T. J., et al. (2016). Cytology-on-a-chip' based sensors for monitoring of potentially malignant oral lesions. *Oral Oncology, 60*, 103–111.
57. Lydiatt, D. D. (2002). Cancer of the oral cavity and medical malpractice. *The Laryngoscope, 112*(5), 816–819.
58. Pandya, D., et al. (2015). Lab-on-a-chip-oral cancer diagnosis at your door step. *Journal of International Oral Health, 7*(11), 122–128.

59. Patel, V., et al. (2013). DSG3 as a biomarker for the ultrasensitive detection of occult lymph node metastasis in oral cancer using nanostructured immunoarrays. *Oral Oncology, 49*(2), 93–101.
60. Weigum, S. E., et al. (2010). Nano-bio-chip sensor platform for examination of oral exfoliative cytology. *Cancer Prevention Research, 3*(4), 518–528.
61. De, A., et al. (2014). Rapid microfluidic solid-phase extraction system for hyper-methylated DNA enrichment and epigenetic analysis. *Biomicrofluidics, 8*(5), 054119.
62. Zilberman, Y., Chen, Y., & Sonkusale, S. R. (2014). Dissolved ammonia sensing in complex mixtures using metalloporphyrin-based optoelectronic sensor and spectroscopic detection. *Sensors and Actuators B: Chemical, 202*, 976–983.
63. Zilberman, Y., & Sonkusale, S. R. (2015). Microfluidic optoelectronic sensor for salivary diagnostics of stomach cancer. *Biosensors and Bioelectronics, 67*, 465–471.
64. Najeeb, S., Slowey, P. D., & Rehmanjj, I. U. (2018). Role of salivary biomarkers in oral cancer detection. *Advances in Clinical Chemistry, 86*, 23.
65. Lin, Y.-H., et al. (2018). Detection of anti-p53 autoantibodies in saliva using microfluidic chips for the rapid screening of oral cancer. *RSC Advances, 8*(28), 15513–15521.
66. Dong, T., & Pires, N. M. M. (2017). Immunodetection of salivary biomarkers by an optical microfluidic biosensor with polyethylenimine-modified polythiophene-C70 organic photodetectors. *Biosensors and Bioelectronics, 94*, 321–327.
67. Tian, T., et al. (2017). Based biosensor for noninvasive detection of epidermal growth factor receptor mutations in non-small cell lung cancer patients. *Sensors and Actuators B: Chemical, 251*, 440–445.
68. Kim, J., Park, H.-D., & Chung, S. (2012). Microfluidic approaches to bacterial biofilm formation. *Molecules, 17*(8), 9818–9834.
69. Kim, S. H. (2008). *Role of AI-2 in oral biofilm formation using microfluidic devices*. College Station: Texas A & M University.
70. Koo, H., et al. (2010). Exopolysaccharides produced by Streptococcus mutans glucosyltransferases modulate the establishment of microcolonies within multispecies biofilms. *Journal of Bacteriology, 192*(12), 3024–3032.
71. Shumi, W., et al. (2010). Environmental factors that affect Streptococcus mutans biofilm formation in a microfluidic device mimicking teeth. *BioChip Journal, 4*(4), 257–263.
72. Kolenbrander, P., Andersen, R., & Moore, L. (1989). Coaggregation of Fusobacterium nucleatum, Selenomonas flueggei, Selenomonas infelix, Selenomonas noxia, and Selenomonas sputigena with strains from 11 genera of oral bacteria. *Infection and Immunity, 57*(10), 3194–3203.
73. Shumi, W., et al. (2013). Shear stress tolerance of Streptococcus mutans aggregates determined by microfluidic funnel device (μFFD). *Journal of Microbiological Methods, 93*(2), 85–89.
74. Ten Cate, J., & Zaura, E. (2012). The numerous microbial species in oral biofilms: How could antibacterial therapy be effective? *Advances in Dental Research, 24*(2), 108–111.
75. Samarian, D. S., et al. (2014). Use of a high-throughput in vitro microfluidic system to develop oral multi-species biofilms. *Journal of Visualized Experiments*, (94), e52467.
76. Benoit, M. R., et al. (2010). New device for high-throughput viability screening of flow biofilms. *Applied and Environmental Microbiology, 76*(13), 4136–4142.
77. Foster, J. S., & Kolenbrander, P. E. (2004). Development of a multispecies oral bacterial community in a saliva-conditioned flow cell. *Applied and Environmental Microbiology, 70*(7), 4340–4348.
78. Cheng, X., et al. (2016). Bactericidal effect of strong acid electrolyzed water against flow enterococcus faecalis biofilms. *Journal of Endodontics, 42*(7), 1120–1125.
79. Lam, R. H., et al. (2016). High-throughput dental biofilm growth analysis for multiparametric microenvironmental biochemical conditions using microfluidics. *Lab on a Chip, 16*(9), 1652–1662.

# Chapter 17
# Injectable Gels for Dental and Craniofacial Applications

**Mohamed S. Ibrahim, Noha A. El-Wassefy, and Dina S. Farahat**

## 1 Introduction

Dental and craniofacial tissue loss due to disease, injury, or congenital anomalies can have serious and even detrimental effects on the quality of life. Dental and craniofacial structures, including bone, teeth, cartilage, ligaments, and muscles, form complex systems that are responsible for many critical tasks in the living body—mastication, speech, and craniofacial support, to name a few. Therefore, a lot of effort has been dedicated toward the regeneration of these lost or diseased tissues to restore, maintain, or improve function. The main goal of tissue engineering is to develop functional replacements for diseased or damaged tissues, usually using a combination of cells, scaffolds, and growth factors. The scaffolds are designed to closely mimic the extracellular matrix and act as templates for tissue regeneration and three-dimensional environments for cell support [1]. Injectable scaffolds or in situ forming scaffolds have attracted attention due to their unique characteristics, which make them the scaffolds of choice over preformed scaffolds in specific indications such as sites with limited accessibility, irregularly shaped defects, and areas with frail tissues or associated morbidity that can't withstand the implantation process of preformed scaffolds [2]. The use of injectable scaffolds enables minimally invasive administration of the scaffolds using needles or catheters without the need for surgery, consequently avoiding its complications, such as patient discomfort, infection, scarring, longer convalescence times, and high surgery costs [3]. Utilizing

M. S. Ibrahim (✉)
Marquette University, School of Dentistry, Milwaukee, WI, USA

Mansoura University, Faculty of Dentistry, Mansoura, Egypt
e-mail: mohamed.ibrahim@marquette.edu

N. A. El-Wassefy · D. S. Farahat
Mansoura University, Faculty of Dentistry, Mansoura, Egypt



L. Tayebi (ed.), *Applications of Biomedical Engineering in Dentistry*,
https://doi.org/10.1007/978-3-030-21583-5_17

injectable hydrogels can also help overcome any troubles associated with cell adhesion or bioactive molecule incorporation, as they are simply mixed with the scaffold solution prior to administration [4]. There are some requirements a scaffold must fulfil to be considered for use as an injectable scaffold for tissue regeneration. First, the scaffold should be acceptably flowable before injection, but rapidly become immobile after injection into the target site [5]. The injectable scaffold should not be toxic to encapsulated cells or to the surrounding tissue; if it undergoes gelation in situ, as in cases of hydrogels, it should occur under mild conditions to avoid damage of incorporated or surrounding biologic structures [3]. The mechanical properties of a scaffold should help it withstand biomechanical forces and offer early support for cells in stress-bearing and non-stress-bearing sites [5]. Finally, the scaffold should degrade to provide space for the newly formed tissue at a rate that matches that of tissue formation [6].

This chapter reviews the different hydrogel materials used in dental and craniofacial tissue engineering followed by a comprehensive discussion of the different types of injectable scaffolds, including hydrogels and microspheres. Furthermore, different types of hydrogels, categorized according to their method of cross-linking, nanocomposite hydrogels and self-assembled peptide amphiphiles, which are chemical compounds that can be assembled into nanofibrillar hydrogels that mimic the extracellular matrix, are also discussed. Finally, injectable microspheres and the different techniques used in their manufacturing are reviewed.

## 2 Hydrogel Materials Used in Tissue Engineering

Different kinds of biomaterial scaffolds have been developed to create novel engineered tissues or organs. These scaffolds may act as a replacement for the extracellular matrix (ECM) and have the capability to guide cell attachment and proliferation [7, 8]. Ideal scaffold criteria include suitable physical properties, mechanical strength, controlled degradation, chemical stability, and biocompatibility for cells' adhesion function and their proliferation. Different biomaterials are used as scaffold materials including polymers. Polymers are composed of covalently bonded small repeated building blocks to form long-chain molecules. Polymers can assume multiple conformations by the rotation of their valence bonds [9]. Natural polymeric materials can simulate the physiological reactions and microenvironment suitable for tissue regeneration. Natural polymers are biocompatible and have a coordinated biodegradation rate that can be beneficial, as compared to synthetic polymers [7, 10].

Hydrogels are natural origin polymers often used as the main components of injectable scaffolds. This section is dedicated to briefly introduce these materials.

## 2.1 Collagen/Gelatin

Collagen is a plentiful protein in mammalian tissues, a major part of natural ECM, and an attractive material for tissue engineering applications [11]. Collagen is a ropelike structure of triple polypeptide chains [12]. Collagen degradation is locally controlled by engineered tissue cells, as it naturally occurs by collagenase and serine proteases [13]. Collagen can be hydrolyzed into a single-strand molecule named gelatin [14]. Collagen, gelatin, and glutaraldehyde can all be used for producing hydrogel, while chemical cross-links can enhance their mechanical properties. Collagen scaffolds can maintain cells' proliferation and differentiation and can also promote calcified tissue formation [15]. However, one in vivo study denoted that dental pulp stem cells (DPSCs) seeded in a collagen sponge produced more connective tissue than a dentin-like tissue and called for further studies on 3D scaffolds seeded with DPSCs [16].

## 2.2 Chitin/Chitosan

Chitin, which is detected in insects' cuticles, shrimps' shells, and fungal cell walls, is a highly abundant natural polymer. Chitin polymer can promote regeneration and has bacteriostatic and fungistatic actions; however, being insoluble in organic solvents and water has limited its applications [17]. The deacetylation reaction of chitin in alkaline media produces a biocompatible polysaccharide polymer named chitosan. Chitosan has antibacterial, antiviral, and antifungal properties; it can promote wound healing and has biodegradable behavior. For biomedical applications, chitosan nanocomposites have been molded into various forms as fibers, sponges, or hydrogels, providing beneficial roles in regenerative medicine [18].

An injectable temperature-responsive hydrogel scaffold was produced from chitosan for cartilage tissue regeneration [19]. It was shown that this injectable composite scaffold maintained the chondrocytes' existence and conserved their morphology [20]. Another study made porous chitosan-collagen scaffolds through a freeze-drying method and stacked them with TGF-1 and then assessed the in vivo cell behavior. It was shown that the human periodontal ligament cells proliferated and grew in the scaffold with the recruitment of the adjacent tissue. This means that the chitosan/collagen scaffold can function as a substrate for the regeneration of periodontal tissue, together with the TGF-1 [21].

## 2.3 Hyaluronic Acid (HA)

Hyaluronic acid (HA) is a water-soluble naturally occurring polysaccharide significantly spread in the animal connective tissue with many important biological roles [22]. Hyaluronic acid and its derivatives have excellent gel-forming properties, biocompatibility, and biodegradability by hyaluronidase; thus, they can be used as hydrogels for tissue engineering [23]. The effects of hyaluronic acid sponge on the odontoblastic cell responses in vitro, as well as responses of the amputated dental pulp of rat molar in vivo, were both examined by Inuyama et al. In vitro results showed that cells adhered to the HA sponge's stable structure, while cell-rich reorganizing tissue was observed in the dentin defect near the HA scaffold in vivo. They suggested that because of its appropriate properties, hyaluronic acid sponge can be used for dental pulp regeneration [24]. Chondroitin sulfate can be used as a cartilaginous scaffold in tissue engineering because it can enhance cell proliferation and matrix formation. It was revealed that the use of gelatin, chondroitin sulfate, and HA scaffolds seeded with chondrocytes supported the survival of chondrocytes, as they were constantly distributed and functioned in secreting collagen and ECM [25].

### 2.4 Alginate

Alginate is a copolymer derived from sea algae, composed of mannuronic and guluronic acid. Alginate can form stable hydrogels with the existence of divalent cations as strontium or calcium at room temperature [26]. Alginate has a good potential for regenerative functions; thus, it is indicated in skin, cartilage, and bone tissue repair [27]. However, alginate does not comply with all the required properties, with such limitations regarding bioactivity, mechanical properties, and biodegradation [28]. A nano-scaled fiber matrix alginate scaffold is similar to fibrous ECM proteins (i.e., ECM mimetic material) [29]. Studies are being conducted to improve alginate properties that support the natural tissue growth. Modified alginate with cationic properties, such as small interfering RNAs or functional DNAs, is important in constructing bioactive alginate [27]. In a study, an alginate scaffold was seeded with human dental pulp stem cells, and it was subcutaneously implanted to the backs of mice. Six weeks later, radiopaque calcified bodies were observed in the mouse back tissue, with the seeded cells having differentiated into odontoblasts and triggered calcification in the alginate scaffold [30, 31].

## 3 Injectable Scaffolds Used in Dental and Craniofacial Applications

### 3.1 Injectable Hydrogels

Hydrogels consist of cross-linked polymer chains, which form a three-dimensional hydrophilic network capable of absorbing substantial amounts of fluids or water. The hydrophilic nature of the hydrogels, their high resemblance to the microenvironment of the extracellular matrix, and the ease of combination of cells and drugs into the aqueous solution resulted in their broad use as cell and drug delivery systems [32]. The injectable forms of these materials are made of aqueous solutions of gel precursors that undergo gelation in situ, mostly under mild settings such as changes in pH or temperature or chemical reactions, like a Schiff base reaction [33]. For a hydrogel to be used in injectable applications, it should be in a satisfactorily liquid state or undergo shear thinning during administration to boost injectability. Additionally, the gelation process should commence, or at least is not complete, until after injection. The hydrogel should also possess specific characteristics according to the intended use. For example, it should contain cellular adhesive capabilities if used in tissue engineering or provide sustained release if used for drug delivery [34, 35]. Injectable hydrogels in the liquid state undergo gelation in situ via cross-linking. According to the method used, they are categorized into chemical and physical hydrogels. Chemical hydrogels result when polymer chains are cross-linked by stable covalent bonds, whereas physical hydrogels result from cross-linking of the chains with secondary bonds, such as hydrogen and ionic bonding or hydrophobic forces. The secondary bonds are inherently weak and respond to alterations in pH, solution ionic strength, and temperature, which makes most physical hydrogels reversible, unlike chemical hydrogels that are generally irreversible [36, 37]. Chemical hydrogels may be associated with harsh cross-linking conditions, such as heat liberation during the reaction which may affect any encapsulated cells, loaded proteins, or surrounding tissue at the injection site, the need for photo-irradiation, the use of organic solvents, or the toxicity of the cross-linking agents. Physical hydrogels do not require such factors for gelation, which makes them attractive candidates for biomedical applications. However, physical hydrogels were reported to be less stable than chemical ones [32].

### 3.1.1 Types of Injectable Hydrogels According to the Method of Cross-Linking

Chemically Cross-Linked Hydrogels

*Photopolymerizable Injectable Hydrogels*

In this kind of material, the hydrogel precursors are cross-linked in vivo by photopolymerization resulting in their gelation. A photoinitiator, which is a compound that is sensitive to light with a specific wavelength, is incorporated in the hydrogel solution and is responsible for initiating the polymerization reaction. When the hydrogel macromers are injected into the target site, they are exposed to a specific external light source (ultraviolet or visible light), which causes the photoinitiator to break down and form free radicals. The free radicals induce cross-linking by reacting with double bonds present in the hydrogel precursors [38]. To enable the polymerization reaction, the hydrogel precursors are functionalized with polymerizable groups, such as acrylate or methacrylate groups [39]. For example, Nicodemus et al. utilized photopolymerizable polyethylene glycol hydrogels as scaffolds to regenerate the cartilage of the condylar process present in the temporomandibular joint with and without dynamic loading. The results indicated that these scaffolds are appropriate choices for the encapsulation of condylar chondrocytes in the absence of loading. However, dynamic compression inhibited gene expression and cellular proliferation [40]. An important advantage of this methodology is the easy control of the gelation rate, since the presence of light is a critical factor for beginning the reaction. Adjusting the light intensity, the photoinitiator concentration, the number of available cross-linking moieties, and the molecular weight of the polymer macromers helps to control the polymerization rate, mechanical properties, and degradation rate of the resulting hydrogel [41].

*Injectable Hydrogels Prepared by Click Chemistry*

Click chemistry does not denote a specific type of reaction, but rather a synthetic concept that is inspired by nature. For a reaction to be categorized as click chemistry, it must comply with the strict prerequisites defined by K. B. Sharpless. For example, it should result in high product yield, be wide in scope, produce nonharmful products, be easy to perform, be stereospecific, use no solvent or a harmless solvent that can be simply removed, and utilize already available reagents. Furthermore, if the product requires purification, it should be done using easy nonchromatographic methods, like crystallization [42, 43]. In click chemistry, complex compounds are produced by joining smaller building blocks using heteroatom links (C-X-C) [42, 44]. Park et al. synthesized a BMP-2 immobilized injectable hydrogel capable of inducing osteogenic differentiation of human periodontal ligament stem cells. First, O-propargyl-tyrosine (OpgY) was incorporated into BMP-2 to prepare BMP-2-OpgY with an alkyne group. Then, a methoxy polyethylene glycol-polycaprolactone block copolymer hydrogel was prepared via a click reaction between the alkyne group on BMP-2-OpgY and an azide group in the diblock copolymer [45].

*Injectable Hydrogels Cross-Linked by Michael Addition Reaction*

The Michael addition reaction has been commonly exploited to cross-link hydrogel precursors in situ to form injectable scaffolds. The reaction involves the addition of a nucleophile, a reactant that offers a pair of electrons in a reaction to form a bond (e.g., thiol groups), to an electrophilic (having affinity for electrons) α,β-unsaturated carbonyl-containing compound (e.g., vinyls and acrylates) [46]. For instance, Li et al. synthesized an in situ forming collagen/hyaluronan composite hydrogel via rapid Michael addition reaction between thiol-derivatized hyaluronan and maleilated collagen. The resulting hydrogel supported proliferation of the seeded cells, and the incorporated collagen showed no signs of denaturation due to the reaction [47]. Michael addition reactions are preferred in biological applications, since they are fast reactions that take place at room temperature without the need for toxic nonbiocompatible reagents [46, 48].

*Enzymatically Cross-Linked Injectable Hydrogels*

Using enzymes as cross-linking agents to produce in situ forming hydrogels has recently gained broad attention due to the mild settings of the reaction. Plenty of the enzymes that can be used for hydrogel cross-linking are similar to the enzymes that naturally catalyze different reactions in the body. For example, transglutaminase, which is an enzyme that has a significant role in wound healing and blood clotting and is present in nearly every living organism, can introduce covalent bonds between primary amines and the $\gamma$-carboxamide group of a protein or peptide-bound glutamine. This can help form stable polymeric networks and thus can be used to cross-link injectable hydrogels [49, 50]. Other enzymes that can be used to cross-link hydrogels include tyrosinases, peroxidases, lysyl oxidases, plasma amine oxidases, phosphatases, thermolysin, and phosphopantetheinyl transferases [51]. The occurrence of these reactions at neutral pH, normal temperatures, and a fast rate, in addition to their low cytotoxicity, makes this cross-linking method an attractive choice for synthesizing injectable hydrogels. Another important advantage is the substrate specificity of the enzyme, which helps avoid any adverse reactions with nontarget surrounding tissues [48].

*Injectable Hydrogels Prepared by Schiff Base Reaction*

A Schiff base is a chemical structure that results from the reaction of nucleophilic amines with electrophilic aldehydes or ketones to form an imine compound containing a carbon-nitrogen double bond with a general composition of $R_2C{=}NR'$ [39]. An example of this reaction used to produce injectable hydrogels is the work by Tan et al., who fabricated a composite scaffold by reacting N-succinyl-chitosan and aldehyde hyaluronic acid. The formed hydrogel supported the survival of bovine articular chondrocytes, and the cells maintained their chondrocyte morphology [20]. Schiff base reaction does not require the use of chemical cross-linkers or catalysts and takes place under normal physiologic conditions. Therefore, it has been significantly used in the fabrication of injectable hydrogels [48]. The reactivity of the Schiff base is considerably influenced by the pH of the solution. In an alkaline solution, it is fairly stable; however, the Schiff base can be damaged by extremely low solution pH. This feature enables the control of the reaction rate, and the Schiff base can be used as a stimulus-responsive entity [52]. Residual aldehyde groups may react with amino groups present in tissues surrounding the injected hydrogel at the site of administration, which has resulted in the introductions of novel bioadhesive systems for use in the human body [53, 54].

Physical Hydrogels

*Temperature-Sensitive Injectable Hydrogels*

These hydrogels undergo gelation and changes in solubility in response to changes in temperature. They garnered substantial interest in biomedical applications due to their simple administration and almost instantaneous gelling at physiologic temperatures without the need for external cross-linkers. Generally, temperature-sensitive hydrogels are amphiphilic in nature, having both hydrophilic and hydrophobic domains. The balance between these domains determines the solubility of the hydrogel [39]. These hydrogels are in the aqueous state at room temperature and solidify when the temperature increases. The threshold at which the hydrogel experiences this phase transition is known as lower critical solution temperature (LCST). Below the LCST, the hydrogel is in sol state and transforms into hydrogel when its temperature surpasses the LCST. The process is reversible, and the formed gel will redissolve upon cooling below the LCST. If the polymer has been chemically cross-linked, it will experience changes in its dimensions with temperature changes; in other words, it will be swollen, but not soluble below the LCST, and it will contract above its LCST [55].

#### *pH-Sensitive Hydrogels*

pH-sensitive hydrogels are hydrogels that experience changes in their volume in response to changes in the surrounding pH. Basically, these materials contain basic structures, such as tertiary amine groups, acidic entities like carboxylic acids, or sulfonamides that undergo ionization. The change in the configuration and the volume of these hydrogels results from protonation and deprotonation of the functional groups [59]. For instance, chitosan hydrogels, which are cationic hydrogels, are sensitive and responsive to low pH. They undergo swelling in acidic media due to protonation of amino/imine groups with the subsequent repulsion between these positively charged moieties on the polymer chains [60]. pH-sensitive hydrogels have been comprehensively used as drug carriers, because the release of drugs can be controlled by external pH [61]. Since the pH differs from one location to another in the body, these hydrogels only release loaded drugs at a specific site, which makes them attractive choices for site-specific drug delivery [62].

#### *Injectable Hydrogels Prepared by Ionic Cross-Linking*

A common example of injectable hydrogels that undergo gelation by ionic cross-linking and are significantly used in dental applications are alginate hydrogels. Alginates are polysaccharides consisting of β-(1,4)-linked D-mannuronic acid and α-(1,4)-linked L-guluronic acid residues [63, 64]. Gelation occurs in the presence of divalent cations, such as calcium ions ($Ca^{+2}$), where an ionic electrostatic interaction occurs between divalent ions and blocks of guluronic units, bridging different chains together. The gelation rate is affected by the type of the cation used, as the affinity of alginate with divalent cations differs according to the type of the ion [64]. The increase in the concentration of the cations and guluronic units increases the rate of the reaction. However, increasing the concentration of alginate decreases the rate of gelation, which produces hydrogels with a more homogenous structure and better mechanical properties [39]. A problem that may affect the use of these materials in biomedical applications is their long-term instability. Ionic molecules in the hydrogel may diffuse into the body fluid or get exchanged with other monovalent cations from the surrounding environment, influencing the stability and strength of the hydrogel [65]. Nevertheless, efforts have been directed to enhance the hydrogel's longevity by incorporating additional covalent cross-linking or photopolymerizable groups or by increasing the concentration of calcium cations [35, 66, 67].

### 3.1.2 Nanocomposite Injectable Hydrogels

Hydrogels have been extensively utilized in biomedical applications due to their superior qualities, such as their porous nature, biocompatibility, and close resemblance to the extracellular matrix. However, their inferior strength, bioinertness, and restricted functionality limited their use in various applications. Nanocomposites were introduced in an effort to enhance the performance of hydrogels where nano-sized particles are added to serve as reinforcing agents or to impart functionality to the hydrogels [68]. Various types of nanoparticles can be used to produce nanocomposite hydrogels, such as metal nanoparticles (e.g., silver nanoparticles), inorganic nanoparticles (e.g., hydroxyapatite, silica, and calcium phosphate), and carbon nanotubes [69]. Composite injectable hydrogels incorporating inorganic nanoparticles are the most commonly used in dental and maxillofacial applications. Nejadnik et al. reported the synthesis of a nanocomposite hydrogel consisting of bisphosphonated hyaluronic acid and calcium phosphate nanoparticles. The nanocomposite showed adhesion to mineralized surfaces like enamel and newly formed trabecular-like bone, while a homogenous disbursement throughout the material was also detected 4 weeks after injecting the hydrogel into bony defects in Westar rats [70]. Martinez-Sanz et al. investigated the use of hyaluronic acid hydrogel containing nano-hydroxyapatite and BMP-2 in mandibular augmentation. An enhanced bone formation and osteoinductive ability of nano-hydroxyapatite were evident with higher bone formation in hydrogels with the nano-hydroxyapatite particles as compared to hydrogels alone [71]. Gaharwar et al. synthesized a tough polyethylene glycol nanocomposite hydrogel incorporating silicate (Laponite) nanoparticles. Addition of the nanoparticles enhanced elasticity, bioactivity, and cellular adhesion of the hydrogel providing mechanically strong and elastic tissue matrices for orthopedic, craniofacial, and dental applications [72].

## *3.2 Self-Assembled Peptide Amphiphiles*

Self-assembly is a bottom-up approach in which stable ordered supramolecular structures are formed due to spontaneous arrangement and organization of individual molecules by preprogrammed non-covalent bonds [73, 74]. The most frequently studied self-assembling materials in dental and craniofacial tissue engineering are the peptide amphiphiles. Peptide amphiphiles with specific sequences can self-assemble into nanofibrillar hydrogels creating scaffolds that strongly mimic the extracellular matrix since protein fibrils represent most of the extracellular matrix composition. Peptide amphiphiles are chemical compounds that contain both hydrophobic and hydrophilic structures. They consist of a hydrophobic non-peptide tail that is covalently bonded to a peptide sequence [75]. The ease of inclusion of functional motif sequence (e.g., short peptides) that can stimulate cellular adhesion and differentiation in the peptides is a major advantage of this approach in tissue regeneration [73]. In aqueous solutions, hydrophobic parts tend to organize to shield themselves from water. The collapse of the hydrophobic tail and the hydrogen bonding formed along the peptide axis results in the formation of cylindrical nanofibers [75]. Gelation of the formed fibers into a three-dimensional network necessitates charge screening that can be achieved by altering the pH or adding electrolytes or by ions present in physiologic media. Rosa et al. investigated whether stem cells from human exfoliated deciduous teeth (SHED) could generate a functional pulp when mixed with PuraMatrix (a nanofibrous peptide hydrogel) and injected into full-length human root canals. SHED differentiated into functional odontoblasts, which suggested that that approach can be used in immature necrotic permanent teeth to complete root formation [76]. Cavalcanti et al. evaluated the compatibility of PuraMatrix with dental pulp stem cells (DPSCs) and its effect on their growth and differentiation. After 21 days of seeding, the cells expressed markers of odontoblastic differentiation, which suggested that this scaffold can be a good candidate for use in regenerative endodontics [77]. Galler et al. cultured SHED and DPSCs in peptide amphiphile hydrogels with different osteogenic supplements. After 4 weeks, SHED showed collagen production and soft tissue formation, whereas DPSCs expressed osteoblast marker genes and mineral deposition was reported. The results indicated that the utilized scaffold can be used in regenerating both soft and hard matrices for dental tissue engineering [78].

### *3.3 Injectable Microspheres*

Microspheres are spherical shaped particles synthesized from organic or inorganic materials with a diameter that ranges from 1 to 1000 μm [79]. Microspheres have been broadly utilized as controlled drug and bioactive molecule delivery systems due to their large volume to area ratio, their adjustable physicochemical characteristics that enable temporal and spatial control of the release of the loaded agents, and their uniform small sizes that facilitate their transport to target locations [79, 80]. The use of microspheres in cellular applications has also been extensively reported. Microspheres can be used for cell culturing in vitro or as a platform for transfer and delivery of cells to target locations in cell replacement therapy and tissue regeneration in vivo [81]. When used as cell delivery systems, cells are either attached to the surface of the microspheres, usually known as microcarriers, or the cells are encapsulated within the spheres and thus known as microcapsules. Microcarriers are commonly synthesized with cell adhesion motifs to facilitate attachment of anchorage-dependent cells [82, 83]. Microcapsules are formed by cross-linking a suspension of cells and a polymer to encapsulate the cells inside the microsphere [81]. The microencapsulation process enables isolation and protection of cells from being rejected or destroyed by the immune system without the need of immunosuppressive drugs [84].

Microspheres may comprise just one constituent of a scaffold, or they may represent its basic component. Accordingly, scaffolds involving microspheres may be classified into two main types: microsphere-incorporating scaffolds or microsphere-based scaffolds. In microsphere-incorporating scaffolds, microspheres are disseminated into another matrix (e.g., hydrogels), to form a composite construct for complex tissue formation [79]. In such structures, microspheres act as carriers for drugs, cells, and other bioactive molecules. They might also function as a porogen for tailoring the porosity of the scaffolds or as a reinforcing agent in scaffolds used in load-bearing applications [85, 86]. Microsphere-based scaffolds contain microspheres as their main building blocks that form integral scaffolds by a bottom-up approach. They are categorized into two main forms: sintered or injectable scaffolds. Sintered scaffolds are not used as injectable scaffolds, since they are prepared by manufacturing discrete microspheres and then fusing them together to form a three-dimensional assembly that can be implanted in intended sites [87]. On the other hand, injectable microsphere-based scaffolds are prepared as liquid suspensions, gels, or colloids that attain the configuration of a defect when administered in a minimally invasive surgery [79]. When using these scaffolds for tissue engineering, the cells are mostly mixed with the microspheres in a suspension culture before being injected into the target location [88]. To ensure adhesion of cells, adhesive factors can be blended, coated, or conjugated to the microspheres [81, 88].

Various techniques have been adopted for the fabrication of microspheres. The emulsion solvent evaporation technique involves dissolution of the microsphere-forming material in a water-immiscible solvent, usually an organic solvent, to form the oil phase. The resulting solution is emulsified in an aqueous phase of water comprising an emulsifier such as polyvinyl alcohol (PVA). Different methods, such as sonication and homogenization, are used to create the oil/water emulsion with the subsequent formation of discrete fine-sized droplets. Finally, the evaporation of the organic solvent from the droplets is induced by continuous stirring or reduced pressure resulting in the formation of the desired microspheres [89, 90]. Precision particle fabrication technique enables better control of the size and size distribution of the microspheres. In this technique, a jet of microsphere-forming solution is pumped through a small orifice and is interrupted by a piezoelectric transducer at a predetermined frequency, breaking the jet down into uniform droplets. The stream of droplets is driven by a non-solvent carrier stream into 1% solution of PVA and then stirred to allow evaporation of the solvent to produce the microspheres [91, 92]. Spray drying is also a common procedure to produce organic and inorganic microspheres. It involves spraying a solution, suspension, or emulsion of the microsphere-forming material into a drying gas (e.g., nitrogen) by atomization to form fine droplets. When the solvent evaporates, the droplets harden, and the formed microspheres are recovered from the drying gas and collected [93, 94]. Thermally induced phase separation has recently been utilized for the production of porous microspheres. This technique encompasses adding an emulsion or solution of the microsphere-forming material, mostly a polymer, in a drop-wise fashion into liquid nitrogen. The extremely low temperature induces phase separation into a polymer-rich phase and a polymer-lean phase with solvent crystallization. The solvent crystals are removed by lyophilization with the subsequent production of porous microspheres [95, 96]. Liu et al. prepared nanofibrous hollow microspheres by synthesizing star-shaped poly(L-lactic acid) followed by an oil-in-oil emulsification process and phase inversion and separation to stimulate the self-assembling of the polymer solution into nanofibrous hollow microspheres [97]. Kuang et al. utilized nanofibrous spongy microspheres as carriers for human dental pulp stem cells to regenerate dental pulp tissues. In comparison to control carriers (nanofibrous microspheres and smooth microspheres) used in the study, nanofibrous spongy microspheres improved cellular attachment, proliferation, odontogenic differentiation, and angiogenesis. Increased tissue and blood vessel formation was also reported when cell-seeded microspheres were subcutaneously injected into mice, compared to control microspheres. The results were attributed to the nanofibrous porous nature of the microspheres that simulated the extracellular matrix and offered a favorable microenvironment to the cells [98].

## 4 Conclusion

Various materials and approaches for fabrication of injectable gels for dental and craniofacial applications have been reviewed in this chapter. Chemically and physically cross-linked hydrogels have been reviewed regarding their types and methods of processing. Nanocomposite hydrogels as well as peptide amphiphiles which can self-assemble into nanofibrillar hydrogels creating scaffolds and mimic the extracellular matrix have been explained. The chapter also includes the review of microsphere-incorporating scaffolds that form a composite construct for complex tissue formation and act as carriers for drugs, cells, and other bioactive molecules. Injectable microsphere-based scaffolds that are prepared as suspensions mixed with cells and administered in a minimally invasive surgery have been discussed in this chapter with descriptions about their methods of fabrication.

## References

1. O'Brien, F. J. (2011). Biomaterials & scaffolds for tissue engineering. *Materials Today, 14*, 88–95.
2. Guyot, C., & Lerouge, S. (2018). Can we achieve the perfect injectable scaffold for cell therapy? *Future Science OA, 4*, FSO284.

3. Hou, Q., De Bank, P. A., & Shakesheff, K. M. (2004). Injectable scaffolds for tissue regeneration. *ChemInform, Journal of Materials Chemistry, 14,* 1915–1923.
4. Kretlow, J. D., Klouda, L., & Mikos, A. G. (2007). Injectable matrices and scaffolds for drug delivery in tissue engineering. *Advanced Drug Delivery Reviews, 59,* 263–273.
5. Chang, B., Ahuja, N., Ma, C., & Liu, X. (2017). Injectable scaffolds: Preparation and application in dental and craniofacial regeneration. *Materials Science & Engineering R: Reports, 111,* 1–26.
6. Drury, J. L., & Mooney, D. J. (2003). Hydrogels for tissue engineering: Scaffold design variables and applications. *Biomaterials, 24,* 4337–4351.
7. Taylor, P. M. (2007). Biological matrices and bionanotechnology. *Philosophical Transactions of the Royal Society of London. Series B, Biological Sciences, 362,* 1313–1320.
8. Langer, R., & Tirrell, D. A. (2004). Designing materials for biology and medicine. *Nature, 428,* 487–492.
9. Ratner, B. D., Hoffman, A. S., Schoen, F. J., & Lemons, J. E. (2012). *Biomaterials science: An introduction to materials in medicine*. Amsterdam: Academic Press.
10. Silva, S. S., Mano, J. F., & Reis, R. L. (2010). Potential applications of natural origin polymer-based systems in soft tissue regeneration. *Critical Reviews in Biotechnology, 30,* 200–221.
11. Tan, H., Wan, L., Wu, J., & Gao, C. (2008). Microscale control over collagen gradient on poly(L-lactide) membrane surface for manipulating chondrocyte distribution. *Colloids and Surfaces. B, Biointerfaces, 67,* 210–215.
12. Guarino, V., Gloria, A., De Santis, R., & Ambrosio, L. (2010). Composite hydrogels for scaffold design, tissue engineering, and prostheses. In *Biomedical applications of hydrogels handbook* (pp. 227–245). New York: Springer.
13. Mueller, S. M., et al. (1999). Meniscus cells seeded in type I and type II collagen-GAG matrices in vitro. *Biomaterials, 20,* 701–709.
14. Tan, H., Huang, D., Lao, L., & Gao, C. (2009). RGD modified PLGA/gelatin microspheres as microcarriers for chondrocyte delivery. *Journal of Biomedical Materials Research. Part B, Applied Biomaterials, 91,* 228–238.
15. Sumita, Y., et al. (2006). Performance of collagen sponge as a 3-D scaffold for tooth-tissue engineering. *Biomaterials, 27,* 3238–3248.
16. Zhang, W., et al. (2006). The performance of human dental pulp stem cells on different three-dimensional scaffold materials. *Biomaterials, 27,* 5658–5668.
17. Khor, E. (2010). Medical applications of chitin and chitosan. In *Chitin, chitosan, oligosaccharides and their derivatives* (pp. 405–413). Boca Raton: CRC Press.
18. Qasim, S., et al. (2018). Electrospinning of chitosan-based solutions for tissue engineering and regenerative medicine. *International Journal of Molecular Sciences, 19,* 407.
19. Hao, T., et al. (2010). The support of matrix accumulation and the promotion of sheep articular cartilage defects repair in vivo by chitosan hydrogels. *Osteoarthritis and Cartilage, 18,* 257–265.
20. Tan, H., Chu, C. R., Payne, K. A., & Marra, K. G. (2009). Injectable in situ forming biodegradable chitosan-hyaluronic acid based hydrogels for cartilage tissue engineering. *Biomaterials, 30,* 2499–2506.
21. Zhang, Y., et al. (2006). Novel chitosan/collagen scaffold containing transforming growth factor-β1 DNA for periodontal tissue engineering. *Biochemical and Biophysical Research Communications, 344,* 362–369.
22. Kogan, G., Soltés, L., Stern, R., & Gemeiner, P. (2007). Hyaluronic acid: A natural biopolymer with a broad range of biomedical and industrial applications. *Biotechnology Letters, 29,* 17–25.
23. Fraser, J. R. E., & Laurent, T. C. (2007). Turnover and metabolism of hyaluronan. In *Novartis Foundation Symposia* (pp. 41–59). Chichester: Wiley.
24. Inuyama, Y., et al. (2010). Effects of hyaluronic acid sponge as a scaffold on odontoblastic cell line and amputated dental pulp. *Journal of Biomedical Materials Research. Part B, Applied Biomaterials, 92B,* 120–128.

25. Chang, C.-H., et al. (2006). Tissue engineering-based cartilage repair with allogenous chondrocytes and gelatin-chondroitin-hyaluronan tri-copolymer scaffold: A porcine model assessed at 18, 24, and 36 weeks. *Biomaterials, 27*, 1876–1888.
26. Seal, B. (2001). Polymeric biomaterials for tissue and organ regeneration. *Materials Science & Engineering R: Reports, 34*, 147–230.
27. Sun, J., & Tan, H. (2013). Alginate-based biomaterials for regenerative medicine applications. *Materials, 6*, 1285–1309.
28. Boontheekul, T., Kong, H.-J., & Mooney, D. J. (2005). Controlling alginate gel degradation utilizing partial oxidation and bimodal molecular weight distribution. *Biomaterials, 26*, 2455–2465.
29. Kang, E., et al. (2012). Microfluidic spinning of flat alginate fibers with grooves for cell-aligning scaffolds. *Advanced Materials, 24*, 4271–4277.
30. Kumabe, S., et al. (2006). Human dental pulp cell culture and cell transplantation with an alginate scaffold. *Okajimas Folia Anatomica Japonica, 82*, 147–155.
31. Fujiwara, S., Kumabe, S., & Iwai, Y. (2006). Isolated rat dental pulp cell culture and transplantation with an alginate scaffold. *Okajimas Folia Anatomica Japonica, 83*, 15–24.
32. Nguyen, M. K., & Lee, D. S. (2010). Injectable biodegradable hydrogels. *Macromolecular Bioscience, 10*, 563–579.
33. Li, Y., Rodrigues, J., & Tomás, H. (2012). Injectable and biodegradable hydrogels: Gelation, biodegradation and biomedical applications. *Chemical Society Reviews, 41*, 2193–2221.
34. Yu, L., & Ding, J. (2008). Injectable hydrogels as unique biomedical materials. *Chemical Society Reviews, 37*, 1473–1481.
35. Bidarra, S. J., Barrias, C. C., & Granja, P. L. (2014). Injectable alginate hydrogels for cell delivery in tissue engineering. *Acta Biomaterialia, 10*, 1646–1662.
36. Yang, J.-A., Yeom, J., Hwang, B. W., Hoffman, A. S., & Hahn, S. K. (2014). In situ-forming injectable hydrogels for regenerative medicine. *Progress in Polymer Science, 39*, 1973–1986.
37. Caló, E., & Khutoryanskiy, V. V. (2015). Biomedical applications of hydrogels: A review of patents and commercial products. *European Polymer Journal, 65*, 252–267.
38. Nguyen, K. T., & West, J. L. (2002). Photopolymerizable hydrogels for tissue engineering applications. *Biomaterials, 23*, 4307–4314.
39. Nguyen, Q. V., Huynh, D. P., Park, J. H., & Lee, D. S. (2015). Injectable polymeric hydrogels for the delivery of therapeutic agents: A review. *European Polymer Journal, 72*, 602–619.
40. Nicodemus, G. D., Villanueva, I., & Bryant, S. J. (2007). Mechanical stimulation of TMJ condylar chondrocytes encapsulated in PEG hydrogels. *Journal of Biomedical Materials Research. Part A, 83*, 323–331.
41. Davis, K. A., Burdick, J. A., & Anseth, K. S. (2003). Photoinitiated crosslinked degradable copolymer networks for tissue engineering applications. *Biomaterials, 24*, 2485–2495.
42. Thirumurugan, P., Matosiuk, D., & Jozwiak, K. (2013). Click chemistry for drug development and diverse chemical–biology applications. *Chemical Reviews, 113*, 4905–4979.
43. Kolb, H. C., Finn, M. G., & Sharpless, K. B. (2001). Click chemistry: Diverse chemical function from a few good reactions. *Angewandte Chemie (International Ed. in English), 40*, 2004–2021.
44. Nandivada, H., Jiang, X., & Lahann, J. (2007). Click chemistry: Versatility and control in the hands of materials scientists. *Advanced Materials, 19*, 2197–2208.
45. Park, S. H., et al. (2017). BMP2-modified injectable hydrogel for osteogenic differentiation of human periodontal ligament stem cells. *Scientific Reports, 7*, 6603.
46. Mather, B. D., Viswanathan, K., Miller, K. M., & Long, T. E. (2006). Michael addition reactions in macromolecular design for emerging technologies. *Progress in Polymer Science, 31*, 487–531.
47. Li, R., et al. (2017). Synthesis of in-situ formable hydrogels with collagen and hyaluronan through facile Michael addition. *Materials Science & Engineering. C, Materials for Biological Applications, 77*, 1035–1043.

48. Liu, M., et al. (2017). Injectable hydrogels for cartilage and bone tissue engineering. *Bone Research, 5*, 17014.
49. Teixeira, L. S. M., Feijen, J., van Blitterswijk, C. A., Dijkstra, P. J., & Karperien, M. (2012). Enzyme-catalyzed crosslinkable hydrogels: Emerging strategies for tissue engineering. *Biomaterials, 33*, 1281–1290.
50. Sperinde, J. J., & Griffith, L. G. (2000). Control and prediction of gelation kinetics in enzymatically cross-linked poly(ethylene glycol) hydrogels. *Macromolecules, 33*, 5476–5480.
51. Parhi, R. (2017). Cross-linked hydrogel for pharmaceutical applications: A review. *Advanced Pharmaceutical Bulletin, 7*, 515–530.
52. Xin, Y., & Yuan, J. (2012). Schiff's base as a stimuli-responsive linker in polymer chemistry. *Polymer Chemistry, 3*, 3045–3055.
53. Hoffmann, B., et al. (2009). Characterisation of a new bioadhesive system based on polysaccharides with the potential to be used as bone glue. *Journal of Materials Science. Materials in Medicine, 20*, 2001–2009.
54. Wu, Y., et al. (2017). A soft tissue adhesive based on aldehyde-sodium alginate and amino-carboxymethyl chitosan preparation through the Schiff reaction. *Frontiers of Materials Science, 11*, 215–222.
55. Klouda, L. (2015). Thermoresponsive hydrogels in biomedical applications: A seven-year update. *European Journal of Pharmaceutics and Biopharmaceutics, 97*, 338–349.
56. Boustta, M., Colombo, P.-E., Lenglet, S., Poujol, S., & Vert, M. (2014). Versatile UCST-based thermoresponsive hydrogels for loco-regional sustained drug delivery. *Journal of Controlled Release, 174*, 1–6.
57. Haq, M. A., Su, Y., & Wang, D. (2017). Mechanical properties of PNIPAM based hydrogels: A review. *Materials Science & Engineering. C, Materials for Biological Applications, 70*, 842–855.
58. Jain, K., Vedarajan, R., Watanabe, M., Ishikiriyama, M., & Matsumi, N. (2015). Tunable LCST behavior of poly (N-isopropylacrylamide/ionic liquid) copolymers. *Polymer Chemistry, 6*, 6819–6825.
59. Xie, J., Li, A., & Li, J. (2017). Advances in pH-sensitive polymers for smart insulin delivery. *Macromolecular Rapid Communications, 38*, 1700413.
60. Rizwan, M., et al. (2017). pH sensitive hydrogels in drug delivery: Brief history, properties, swelling, and release mechanism, material selection and applications. *Polymers, 9*, 137.
61. Liu, Y.-Y., et al. (2006). pH-responsive amphiphilic hydrogel networks with IPN structure: A strategy for controlled drug release. *International Journal of Pharmaceutics, 308*, 205–209.
62. Wang, K., Fu, Q., Chen, X., Gao, Y., & Dong, K. (2012). Preparation and characterization of pH-sensitive hydrogel for drug delivery system. *RSC Advances, 2*, 7772–7780.
63. Draget, K. I., Skjåk-Braek, G., & Smidsrød, O. (1997). Alginate based new materials. *International Journal of Biological Macromolecules, 21*, 47–55.
64. Russo, R., Malinconico, M., & Santagata, G. (2007). Effect of cross-linking with calcium ions on the physical properties of alginate films. *Biomacromolecules, 8*, 3193–3197.
65. Donati, I., Asaro, F., & Paoletti, S. (2009). Experimental evidence of counterion affinity in alginates: The case of nongelling ion $Mg^{2+}$. *The Journal of Physical Chemistry. B, 113*, 12877–12886.
66. Sun, J.-Y., et al. (2012). Highly stretchable and tough hydrogels. *Nature, 489*, 133–136.
67. Wang, M. S., Childs, R. F., & Chang, P. L. (2005). A novel method to enhance the stability of alginate-poly-L-lysine-alginate microcapsules. *Journal of Biomaterials Science. Polymer Edition, 16*, 91–113.
68. Song, F., Li, X., Wang, Q., Liao, L., & Zhang, C. (2015). Nanocomposite hydrogels and their applications in drug delivery and tissue engineering. *Journal of Biomedical Nanotechnology, 11*, 40–52.
69. Gaharwar, A. K., Peppas, N. A., & Khademhosseini, A. (2014). Nanocomposite hydrogels for biomedical applications. *Biotechnology and Bioengineering, 111*, 441–453.

70. Nejadnik, M. R., et al. (2014). Self-healing hybrid nanocomposites consisting of bisphosphonated hyaluronan and calcium phosphate nanoparticles. *Biomaterials, 35*, 6918–6929.
71. Martínez-Sanz, E., et al. (2012). Minimally invasive mandibular bone augmentation using injectable hydrogels. *Journal of Tissue Engineering and Regenerative Medicine, 6*, s15–s23.
72. Gaharwar, A. K., Rivera, C. P., Wu, C.-J., & Schmidt, G. (2011). Transparent, elastomeric and tough hydrogels from poly(ethylene glycol) and silicate nanoparticles. *Acta Biomaterialia, 7*, 4139–4148.
73. Dvir, T., Timko, B. P., Kohane, D. S., & Langer, R. (2011). Nanotechnological strategies for engineering complex tissues. *Nature Nanotechnology, 6*, 13–22.
74. Thomas, D., Gaspar, D., & Sorushanova, A. (2016). Scaffold and scaffold-free self-assembled systems in regenerative medicine. *Biotechnology, 113*, 1155–1163.
75. Matson, J. B., & Stupp, S. I. (2012). Self-assembling peptide scaffolds for regenerative medicine. *Chemical Communications, 48*, 26–33.
76. Rosa, V., Zhang, Z., Grande, R. H. M., & Nör, J. E. (2013). Dental pulp tissue engineering in full-length human root canals. *Journal of Dental Research, 92*, 970–975.
77. Cavalcanti, B. N., Zeitlin, B. D., & Nör, J. E. (2013). A hydrogel scaffold that maintains viability and supports differentiation of dental pulp stem cells. *Dental Materials, 29*, 97–102.
78. Galler, K. M., et al. (2008). Self-assembling peptide amphiphile nanofibers as a scaffold for dental stem cells. *Tissue Engineering. Part A, 14*, 2051–2058.
79. Gupta, V., Khan, Y., Berkland, C. J., Laurencin, C. T., & Detamore, M. S. (2017). Microsphere-based scaffolds in regenerative engineering. *Annual Review of Biomedical Engineering, 19*, 135–161.
80. Hossain, K., Patel, U., & Ahmed, I. (2015). Development of microspheres for biomedical applications: A review. *Progress in Biomaterials, 4*, 1–19.
81. Leong, W., & Wang, D. A. (2015). Cell-laden polymeric microspheres for biomedical applications. *Trends in Biotechnology, 33*, 653–666.
82. Wang, H., Leeuwenburgh, S., & Li, Y. (2011). The use of micro-and nanospheres as functional components for bone tissue regeneration. *Engineering Part B: Reviews, 18*, 24–39.
83. Hernández, R. M., Orive, G., Murua, A., & Pedraz, J. L. (2010). Microcapsules and microcarriers for in situ cell delivery. *Advanced Drug Delivery Reviews, 62*, 711–730.
84. Rokstad, A., Lacík, I., de Vos, P., & Strand, B. L. (2014). Advances in biocompatibility and physico-chemical characterization of microspheres for cell encapsulation. *Advanced Drug Delivery Reviews, 67*, 111–130.
85. Tang, G., et al. (2012). Preparation of PLGA scaffolds with graded pores by using a gelatin-microsphere template as Porogen. *Journal of Biomaterials Science. Polymer Edition, 23*, 2241–2257.
86. Matsuno, T., Hashimoto, Y., Adachi, S., & Omata, K. (2008). Preparation of injectable 3D-formed β-tricalcium phosphate bead/alginate composite for bone tissue engineering. *Dental Materials, 27*, 827–834.
87. Huang, W., Li, X., Shi, X., & Lai, C. (2014). Microsphere based scaffolds for bone regenerative applications. *Biomaterials Science, 2*, 1145.
88. Zhang, Z., Eyster, T. W., & Ma, P. X. (2016). Nanostructured injectable cell microcarriers for tissue regeneration. *Nanomedicine, 11*, 1611–1628.
89. McGinity, J. W., & O'Donnell, P. B. (1997). Preparation of microspheres by the solvent evaporation technique. *Advanced Drug Delivery Reviews, 28*, 25–42.
90. Nava-Arzaluz, M. G., Piñón-Segundo, E., Ganem-Rondero, A., & Lechuga-Ballesteros, D. (2012). Single emulsion-solvent evaporation technique and modifications for the preparation of pharmaceutical polymeric nanoparticles. *Recent Patents on Drug Delivery & Formulation, 6*, 209–223.
91. Xia, Y., & Pack, D. W. (2015). Uniform biodegradable microparticle systems for controlled release. *Chemical Engineering Science, 125*, 129–143.

92. Berkland, C., King, M., Cox, A., Kim, K., & Pack, D. W. (2002). Precise control of PLG microsphere size provides enhanced control of drug release rate. *Journal of Controlled Release, 82*, 137–147.
93. Paudel, A., Worku, Z. A., Meeus, J., Guns, S., & Van den Mooter, G. (2013). Manufacturing of solid dispersions of poorly water soluble drugs by spray drying: Formulation and process considerations. *International Journal of Pharmaceutics, 453*, 253–284.
94. Cal, K., & Sollohub, K. (2010). Spray drying technique. I: Hardware and process parameters. *Journal of Pharmaceutical Sciences, 99*, 575–586.
95. Blaker, J. J., Knowles, J. C., & Day, R. M. (2008). Novel fabrication techniques to produce microspheres by thermally induced phase separation for tissue engineering and drug delivery. *Acta Biomaterialia, 4*, 264–272.
96. Feng, W., et al. (2015). Synthesis and characterization of nanofibrous hollow microspheres with tunable size and morphology via thermally induced phase separation technique. *RSC Advances, 5*, 61580–61585.
97. Liu, X., Jin, X., & Ma, P. X. (2011). Nanofibrous hollow microspheres self-assembled from star-shaped polymers as injectable cell carriers for knee repair. *Nature Materials, 10*, 398–406.
98. Kuang, R., et al. (2016). Nanofibrous spongy microspheres for the delivery of hypoxia-primed human dental pulp stem cells to regenerate vascularized dental pulp. *Acta Biomaterialia, 33*, 225–234.

# Chapter 18
# Animal Models in Dental Research

**Hanieh Nokhbatolfoghahaei, Zahrasadat Paknejad, Mahboubeh Bohlouli, Maryam Rezai Rad, and Arash Khojasteh**

## 1 Introduction

Comparative biomedical sciences are founded on the concept that animal species share physiological, behavioral, or other characteristics with humans. Animal models are often superior to in vitro or clinical studies. Since human studies cannot always be coupled with harvesting the tissues or body parts necessary for microscopic analyses and defining the biologic impact of the regenerative methods and materials, animal studies are critical in addressing mechanistic questions and serving as an essential link between hypotheses and treatments. A high-quality designed animal experiment provides fundamental information for the future randomized clinical trials in human.

H. Nokhbatolfoghahaei · M. Rezai Rad
Dental Research Center, Research Institute of Dental Sciences, Shahid Beheshti University of Medical Sciences, Tehran, Iran

Z. Paknejad
Medical Nanotechnology and Tissue Engineering Research Center, Shahid Beheshti University of Medical Sciences, Tehran, Iran

Department of Tissue Engineering and Applied Cell Sciences, School of Advanced Technologies in Medicine, Shahid Beheshti University of Medical Sciences, Tehran, Iran

M. Bohlouli
Department of Tissue Engineering and Applied Cell Sciences, School of Advanced Technologies in Medicine, Shahid Beheshti University of Medical Sciences, Tehran, Iran

A. Khojasteh (✉)
Department of Tissue Engineering and Applied Cell Sciences, School of Advanced Technologies in Medicine, Shahid Beheshti University of Medical Sciences, Tehran, Iran

Department of Oral and Maxillofacial Surgery, Dental School, Shahid Beheshti University of Medical Sciences, Tehran, Iran
e-mail: arashkhojasteh@sbmu.ac.ir



L. Tayebi (ed.), *Applications of Biomedical Engineering in Dentistry*,
https://doi.org/10.1007/978-3-030-21583-5_18

In dental research, animal experimentation is essential in order to understand the basic biology underling dentomaxillofacial anomalies and diseases, as well as evaluating the various medications and treatment approaches. Since there is no single animal model that represents all aspects of dental anomalies, dental tissue architecture, and disease process and healing, the goal should be the use of various models that provide insights into the mechanisms of disease and treatments. In dental research, animal models, including monkeys, dogs, rabbit, sheep, mini-pigs, rats, and mice, are frequently used in interventions. The selection of an experimental model is determined according to research objectives, as well as constraints such as housing of large or nonstandard animals. In most cases, small animal models would be sufficient to assess the role of disease procedure at the histological level and provide enough statistical significance and preclinical relevance. The use of large animals with ethical and social issues, such as monkeys and dogs, should be considered for last phase of validation of new treatments, prior to use in human clinical practice.

This chapter composes of the general information of different animal models used in various specialties of dentistry. Also, an emphasis has been given to the required ethical guideline in order to design an animal model.

## 2 Animal Model Classifications

Animal models can be classified based on the aspects of the different studies, which are described below.

In the first classification, the animal models may be classified according to the aim of studies [1]. The models may be exploratory, which tends to help the discovery of a biological process, including either an operative and normal biological mechanism or an abnormal biological mechanism. The next model is called explanatory, which helps to interpret more or less complex biologic problems. In order to achieve the results, in addition to the animal model, other study models could be used, including the in vitro studies, bioinformatics databases, and computer simulations.

The most common and important model is predictive models. These models are used to evaluate the function of a drug or a treatment approach in a physiologic environment [1, 2].

To select an appropriative animal model, similarity between animal species and human in terms of biological and physiological structures is very important—this is termed fidelity. Therefore, high-fidelity models are the best models to study a biological process. Moreover, if the symptoms shown by animals are similar to those of human, this is called homology. However, homologous models are relatively few, and most of the models are partial models, in which they can show symptoms that are somewhat similar to humans.

Animal models are generally used to evaluate the cause, process, and treatment of human models. Thus, another classification, called the classification of disease models, includes four groups that are described below [1].

Induced (experimental) disease models: In this group, the healthy animal is used to induce a disease or an abnormal mechanism, and then, the disease process and the selected treatment approach are evaluated, for example, the induction of bone regeneration by a calvarial bone defect [3, 4] and induction periodontitis by inoculation or injection of human oral bacteria into animal's gingival tissues [5]. To achieve the best results, animal models should be high-fidelity or homologous models. Nevertheless, most induced models are partial because the etiology and physiology of the disease are different in animals.

Spontaneous disease models: Genetic mutations cause many human disorders [6]. In this group, a genetic mutation is created in the animal model, and then the progression of the disorder and its treatment are studied. These models can be helpful to study various disorders in humans. Outstanding examples of spontaneous models are nude mice, which can receive many different types of tissue and tumor grafts, and Snell's dwarf mice, without a functional pituitary. The experimental models are often partial models because an impaired gene or sequence of the gene results in the activation of other genes and physiologic processes, which results in differences between human beings and animal models [1].

Transgenic disease models: Considering the advances in genetic engineering and embryo manipulation technology, transgenic disease models are an important category of animal disease models. The many physiological responses are controlled by more than one gene. These models are created by the insertion of DNA sequences into the genome or deletion of specific genes from the animal's embryo, and they help to compare normal and abnormal physiological conditions at the level of gene and protein expressions up to the level of biological and behavioral changes [1]. For example, transgenic mice that resemble Amelogenesis imperfecta misexpress the ameloblastin gene [7]. Transgenic models are similar to spontaneous disease models from many aspects.

Negative animal models: This model includes animals that do not respond to external stimuli, such as pathogenic organisms or allergens. The main application of this animal model is to understand mechanism of resistance through study physiology and biology of animals. A famous example of negative animal models is resistance to gonococcal infection in rabbits [1].

The third classification of animal models is introduced by Page and Schroeder [8]. In this classification, more attention is focused on the size and species of animals. In this regard, three main groups are outlined: the first group includes small rodent animals which include mice, rat, hamster, and mink. Dog and sheep are placed in the second group, which is assigned as large animals division. The third group is nonhuman primates, such as baboon, *Macaca*, chimpanzee, and gorilla [8].

# 3 Animal Selection for Different Field of Dentistry

## 3.1 Endodontics

Dental pulp tissue is often damaged by infection, such as cariogenic and periodontal bacteria, dental trauma, and clinical operative procedures [9]. Once the pulp tissue is exposed to bacteria, it begins a process of irreversible pulpitis, which cannot be healed at all; subsequent proceeding of inflammation would cause necrosis [10]. A routine clinical treatment for infected, necrotic pulp tissue, or even teeth with some degree of pulpitis, is root canal therapy (RCT), which involves the extirpation of injured pulp and filling of the root canal systems with bioinert synthetic materials. The main aim of an RCT is to prevent bacterial spread via the infectious root into peri-apex neighboring bone. However, endodontically treated teeth are prone to fracture and periapical infections resulting from inadvertently left pulp remnants, which are good substrata for bacterial growth. Also, patients experience the absence of sensitivity with endodontic treated teeth [9]. Strategies to overcome these limitations have been established. Although usage of superior filling materials and sealers has extensively promoted the long-term outcome of RCT, pulp tissue regeneration is still the treatment of choice for involved teeth for which tissue vitality and sensation can be maintained (Table 18.1).

Primary assessment of dentin-pulp complex regeneration by means of new treatments, materials, and cell sources is feasible by ectopic evaluations in animal models, instead of orthotropic assessments. Ectopic transplantation is chosen for investigations due to its advantages, including being rapid and reproducible, requiring easy surgical access, and providing minimal labor for animal. Formation of pulp and dentin-like tissue is expected for endodontic regeneration when a tooth or tooth slice undertaking the new treatment modality is transplanted into ectopic sites [11]. Although a variety of researches have confirmed the regeneration of mineralized tissue within a transplanted tooth, a few reported detection of dentin-like tissue and mostly found tissue that instead reflects the bone-like morphology [12]. Subcutaneous tissue, renal capsule, and in-jaw sites have been used for ectopic implementation of tooth [10, 11]. It is claimed that differentiation of stem cells within transplanted teeth is likely assigned to the different microenvironments of transplanted sites rather than the cell origin. For instance, rat calvarias have showed to offer a more appropriate condition for the formation of pulp-like tissue than dorsal tissues in these animals [13]. Small animals such as mice or rats are preferred over large animals, since the experiment is more cheap and the breeding management and ethical considerations are less concerned. Mice are the most frequently employed species for ectopic implementation. In addition to easier and inexpensive manipulation, the mouse genome is highly similar to that in humans and its anatomy is well known [10].

Disease modeling prior to pulp regeneration requires a pretreatment conditioning of root, which is applied by exposure of the pulp chamber via creation of access cavity. This procedure is followed by either total removal of the pulp tissue or

**Table 18.1** Tooth formula of permanent teeth and eruption time in some species

| | Animals | Permanent formula<br>Maxillary ICPM<br>Mandibular ICPM | Total teeth | Eruption time | References |
|---|---|---|---|---|---|
| 1 | Rodents | 1003<br>1003 | 16 | $I_1$: 8–10 d [47, 48]<br>$M_1$: 19 d, $M_2$: 21 d, $M_3$: 35–40 d [48] | [47, 48] |
| 2 | Ruminants | 0033<br>3133 | 32 | $I_1$: 13–16 m, $I_2$: 25–28 m,<br>$I_3$: 33–36 m<br>C: 45–48 m<br>$P_2$: 27–32 m, $P_{3,4}$: 25–30 m<br>$M_1$: 1–4 m, $M_2$: 8–13 m,<br>$M_3$: 22–40 m | [49] |
| 3 | Rabbit | 2033<br>1023 | 28 | 0–5 w | [50] |
| 4 | Ferret | 3131<br>3132 | 34 | 50–74 d | [51] |
| 5 | Cat | 3131<br>3121 | 30 | $I_{1,2,3}$: 3.5–5.5 m<br>C: 5.5–6.5 m<br>$P_{2,3,4}$: 4–5 m<br>$M_1$: 5–6 m | [52] |
| 6 | Dog | 3142<br>3143 | 42 | $I_{1,2,3}$: 3–5 m<br>C: 5–7 m<br>$P_1$: 4–5 m, $P_{2,3,4}$: 5–6 m<br>$M_1$: 4–5 m, $M_2$: 5–6 m, $M_3$: 6–7 m | [52] |
| 7 | Pig | 3143<br>3143 | 40 | $I_1$: 12–16 m. $I_2$: 16–20 m.<br>$I_3$: 8–10 m<br>C: 8–10 m<br>$P_{1(man)}$: 18–24 m. $P1_{(max)}$: >28. $P_{2,3,4}$: 12–15 m<br>$M_1$: 4–6 m. $M_2$: 9–12 m.<br>$M_3$: 24–28 m | [53] |
| 8 | Primates (Mostly) | 2123<br>2123 | 32 | $I_1$: 48–84 m, $I_2$: 54–97 m<br>C: 78–121 m<br>$M_1$: 67–102 m, $M_2$: 73–109 m | [54] |

*C* canine, *d* day, *I* incisor, *M* molar, *m* month, *P* premolar, *w* week

disruption of the pulp chamber without extirpation of root pulp [14–21]. Some researchers tend to evaluate the pulpal response to the new treatment modalities in the absence of bacterial interferences. For this aim they apply their treatments after root conditioning [22]. In opposition, some studies assess the confounding effects of bacteria on pulp regenerative therapies and confirm the microbial contamination by observation of periapical lesion. Bacterial invasion can be induced under aerobic conditions, which is performed by leaving the access cavity open for 1–3 weeks [17, 18]. Anaerobic technique is applicable by coronal sealing of teeth after its exposure to oral environment [19, 23–25] or intentional placement of plaque suspension inside the root canals that can be transferred by sponge, cotton balls carrier, or even alone [15, 16, 20, 21, 26–29] (Fig. 18.1). It seems that application of the latter method, which assesses the bacterial confounding factor, is more easily extrapolated to clinical treatments. But, it should be considered that delivery of bacterial suspension inside the canals in some species, such as canine, is more preferable since the higher pH of saliva is not in favor of bacterial colonization that is proposed to occur in case of exposure to oral cavity [30].

Proper establishment of disease modeling for better judgment of pulp responses, along with a comprehensive knowledge about tooth and root anatomy of various species, is crucial. The shape of animal teeth depends greatly on its diet. Herbivores possess molars and premolars with broad chewing surfaces for continuous grinding and grazing of the plant and grain matter. Dental crown attrition has been matched by the development of hypsodonts or high-crowned teeth in herbivorous mammals

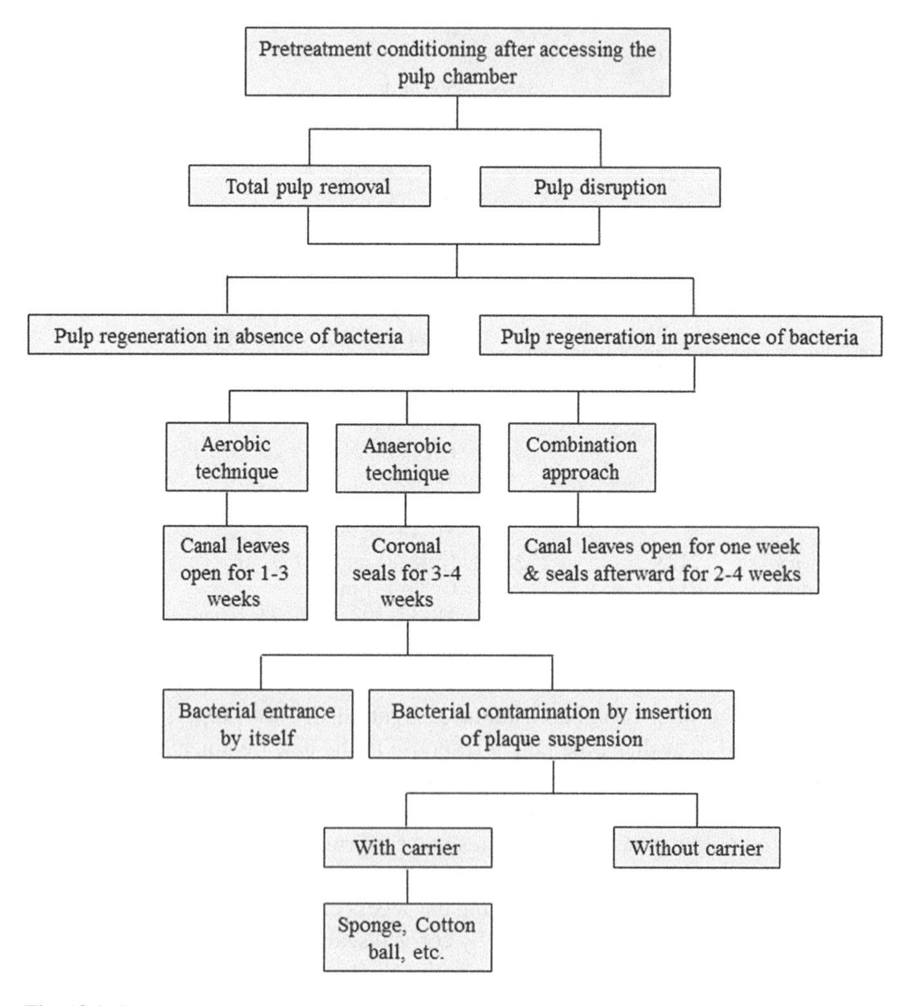


**Fig. 18.1** Endodontic disease modeling chart

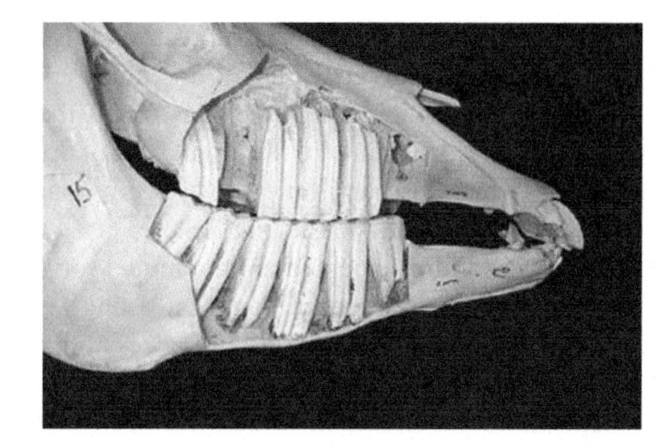

**Fig. 18.2** Hypsodont teeth of horse. (Reuse with permission) [55]

and has been explained as an adaptation to the wear-inducing diet of high fiber (Fig. 18.2) [31]. This is a kind of tooth that grows continuously throughout the animal's life to compensate for the attrition of respective tooth. It has a long anatomic crown, in which the subgingival part is regarded as reserve crown. The entire length of crown below and above the gum line is covered by enamel and cementum, which surrounds the enamel surface [32]. Hypsodont teeth can be either radicular, eventually forming an anatomical root, or aradicular, which never makes an anatomical root. Similar to herbivores, lagomorphs and rodents represent hypsodont features. The incisor of all rodents, incisor and cheek teeth of lagomorphs, cheek teeth of ruminants, and whole dentition of horses show these characteristics. The constant growing and wide-open apical foramen of hypsodonts have made them an inappropriate model for any purpose in field of dental research.

In contrast to rat incisors, rat molars are brachydonts, and overlooking their small size for performing the access and treatment, they serve as a suitable model for endodontics. Also, germ-free rats are advantageous for evaluating the role of non-infective factors in the establishment of periapical lesions [33]. Among small animals, ferrets have been suggested as an appropriate animal model for pulp regeneration experiments due to its closer phylogenetic relationship to humans. Endodontic procedure is better to be carried out on its large single-rooted canine, which has adequate pulp size and proper root anatomy [34].

Dogs have been introduced as a proper model for experimental endodontics and have been utilized widely for this purpose. They have teeth with large enough size, making endodontic treatments easier, and their premolar is the tooth of choice due to its similarity to human molars [35–38]. But the pulp anatomy restricts its manipulation for study of mature teeth [33], since the apical portion of the canal varies from that in human, consisting of a delta with a complex system of cavities for passage of blood vessels and nerve branches to the root apex [39]. Masson et al. revealed that 100% of teeth extracted from dog more than 1 year old represented apical delta [40]. The apical arborization is associated with either cleaning or filling deficiency, which results in persistence of apical lesion and treatment hampering. Similarly cats and ferrets have the apical delta and consequent chronic lesions have been reported [39, 41]. These animals are suitable for the design of experiments in immature teeth, which is elaborated in the pediatric section. It is notable that creation of access cavity for the endodontic goals in cats and dogs requires further attention. The enamel in these two animals is thinner than that of the human (i.e., 0.2 mm in cats and 0.5 mm in dogs, compared with a thickness of up to 2.5 mm in human) [42]. In addition, dog furcation in multiple-rooted teeth is highly close to CEJ line, so there is potential for perforation risk (Fig. 18.3).

Swine is another accepted animal model for study of endodontics and periapical lesions, albeit not the entire dentition. Long and curvy anterior teeth and molars with complex anatomy and difficult accessibility are not potentially suitable teeth for experiments. Swine premolars are relatively easier samples for such studies, except for the ones that have multiple split roots like maxillary fourth premolars [22].

Sheep appears to be an appropriate animal model for endodontic regeneration research [35] due to their incisor teeth being similar to humans in many anatomical and histological aspects [43]. A prominent feature of ruminant dental anatomy is the lack of upper incisors and presence of dental pad.

Due to both psychopathological and anatomical similarities of primates to human, they have been used in many endodontic regeneration studies [44–46]. However, special consideration should be taken when applying treatment to their premolar and molars because of the multi-rooted features [33].

## 3.2 Pediatric Dentistry

Today, both children and parents place a considerable value to pediatric dentistry, and there is a growing interest toward the preservation of primary teeth. The deciduous dentition plays a crucial role in the fate of successive teeth, since they maintain the required space for eruption of permanent teeth. Also, infection in primary teeth can easily harm the bud of succeeding teeth due to close proximity to the deciduous tooth root. Besides, the most important aspect for unhealthy dentition turns to the child's self-confidence: the speech, esthetics, and smiling of the baby can be negatively influenced. There are two major concerns that have drawn dentistry pediatrician's attention.

### 3.2.1 Immature Pulp Regeneration

The main challenge is the vital pulp salvation and regeneration of damaged or infectious teeth. Although a tooth can be maintained in the oral cavity without vitality, it is appealing to keep the pulp vital since the immature teeth walls need to thicken and elongate until the apex is thoroughly closed.

The possibility of revitalization treatment of immature infected teeth is a recent progress providing considerable biological advantages [13, 56]. The first approach to regenerate dental pulp dates back to the experiment conducted by Ostby in the

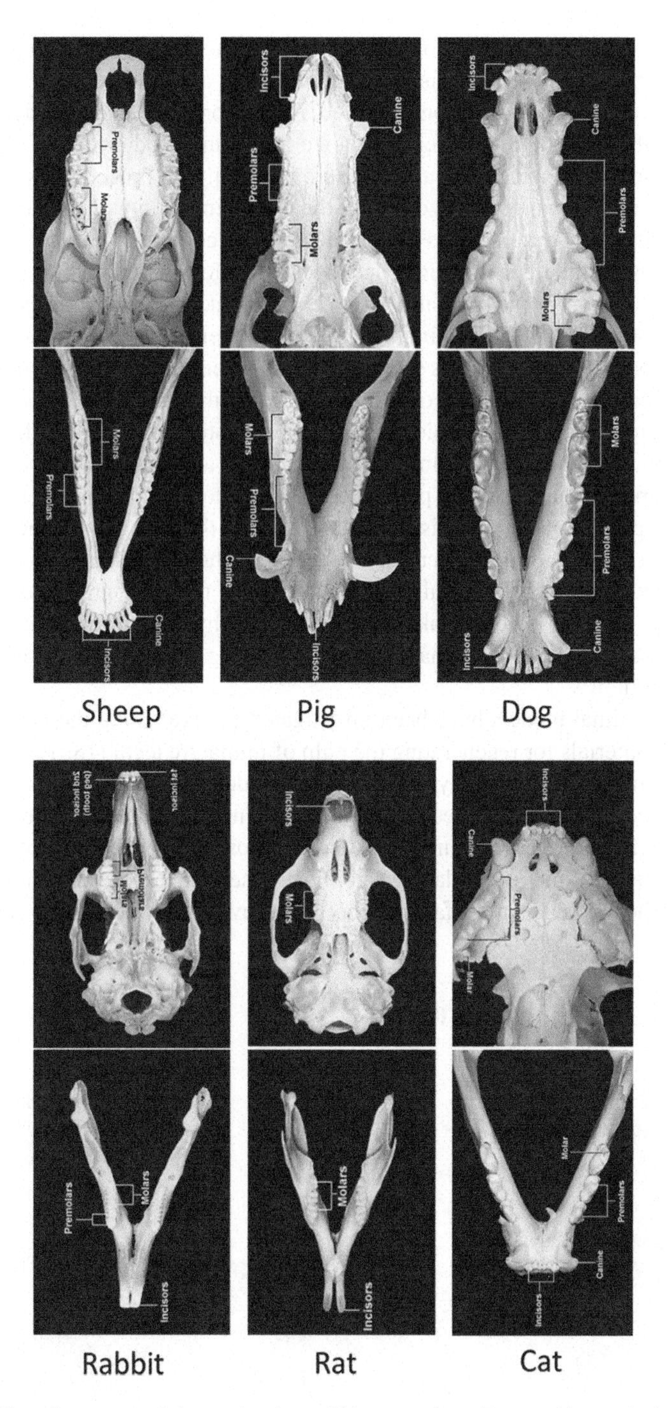


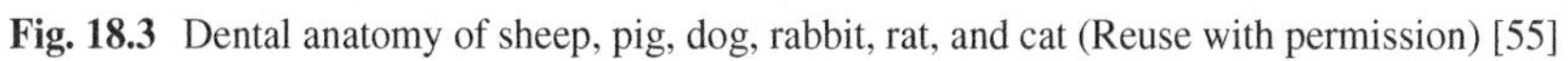
**Fig. 18.3** Dental anatomy of sheep, pig, dog, rabbit, rat, and cat (Reuse with permission) [55]

1960s, who discovered the role of blood clot in regenerative therapy using a dog as an animal model [57, 58]. This foundation led to apexification method, which focused on achieving disinfection, followed by creation of an apical barrier [59, 60]. Vital pulp therapy is the treatment of choice for traumatized or carious teeth with vital pulp and open apices on pulp exposure [61–63]. The procedure is performed by amputating coronal pulp and covering the remaining pulp with suitable capping biomaterials [62]. Apexogenesis is one of the most common approaches for vital pulp therapy. Unlike apexification, apexogenesis allows continuation of the root formation, leading to apical closure, stronger root structure, and a greater structural integrity [64] (Fig. 18.4). Continuing the development of apexogenesis and vital therapy of pulp tissue, nowadays scientists have concentrated mostly on introducing a better method or production of a novel material that can promote outstanding pulpal regeneration, which should be primarily be tested on animal models.

Creation of pulpal necrosis in immature teeth of animal models is identical to adult mature teeth and can be produced by either tooth exposure or subsequent removal of pulp tissue or pulp disruption and leaving the pulp open to the oral environment for a predetermined period. The latter method is designed to induce the pulpal necrosis by means of oral bacteria and seems to be the preferred technique for this aim. Many researchers take the oral radiography after the exposure period to ensure that a periapical lesion has emerged following the bacterial invasion to the chamber [65].

Various animal models have been investigated for evaluating the new methods and novel materials for regenerating the pulp of immature teeth [18, 19, 25, 29, 65, 66]. In this field, although many studies have been devoted on rat models [65], treatment protocols for immature teeth still have been inspected mainly in dogs [18, 20, 25–28, 65]. Monkeys have been used extensively for pulp regeneration of immature teeth because of the exemplary anatomical resemblance to human dentition. However, the monkey is not a favored choice for investigation of pulp regeneration,

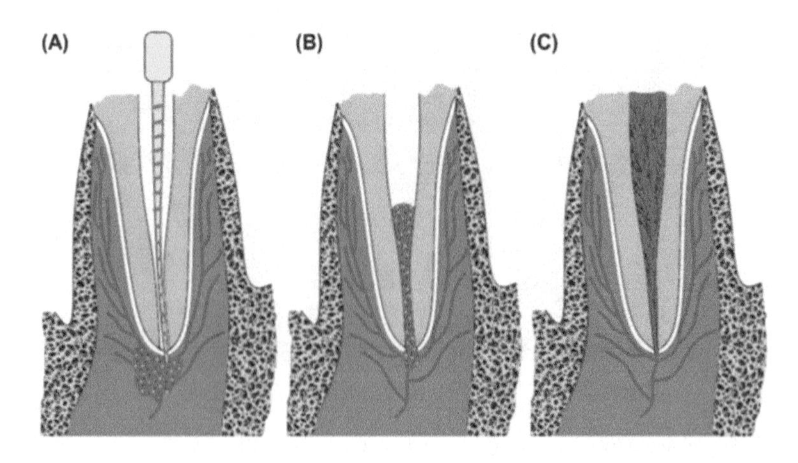


**Fig. 18.4** Root canal revascularization procedure. (Reuse with permission) [78]

since their pulp tissues have greater recovering ability compared to human teeth. Also, they are extremely resistant to the impact of oral contamination, which is capable of hard tissue repair in the form of dentin, cementum, and bone, even in the presence of severe inflammatory disease. Therefore, the monkey is not a favored choice for investigation of pulp regeneration. In contrast, canine teeth are more sensitive to damages and infection due to higher permeability of dentin and cementum. So, it is expected that successful treatments in the more sensitive teeth of dogs are more likely to provide satisfactory results in human. This has made dogs an ideal animal model for immature vital pulp therapy.

The key factor to consider when performing treatment on immature teeth is the knowledge of apical closure timing. Rat immature molars are chosen for pulp regeneration in this species, since the incisors do not develop an anatomical root and possess continuous growing capability throughout life that limits the experimental procedures [67]. Therefore, regarding the studies carried out by Scarparo and Duarte, rat molars represented an open apex in 4–5 weeks of age [65]. Ascertaining the age at which the dog root is completed has been verified by radiographic evaluation—the apices of the upper first and second incisors, lower premolars, and molars are closed at 7 months of age. The root apices of the upper third incisor and premolars are completed at 8 months of age, while the apex of the upper canine is closed later at 9.5 months of age [68]. Histological evaluation has revealed that apical closure occurred with approximately 1-month discrepancy, in which most of the teeth are closed at 7 month and all teeth, including canines, are completed at 8 month of age [69]. A notable matter is that all investigations on pulp regeneration of immature teeth should be performed on the permanent dentition, since the roots of primary teeth are expected to resorb and the efforts to maintain the root development processes are not dialectical. In this regard, it should be elaborated that different species exhibit various dentition types. Animals with two successions of teeth (i.e., deciduous and permanent teeth) are labeled as diphyodonts and include dogs, rats, rabbits, and most of other mammalians that are involved in experimental study of dentistry (Table 18.2). In contrast, the dentition of some animals, like rats, displays only one set of teeth throughout life and is defined as monophyodont [70].

**Table 18.2** Biquadrant dental formula of deciduous teeth for different species

| Tooth species | Incisors | Canine | Premolar | Molar | Total number | References |
|---|---|---|---|---|---|---|
| Beagle dog | 3/3 | 1/1 | – | 3/3 | 28 | [76] |
| Cat | 3/3 | 1/1 | 3/2 | – | 26 | [52] |
| Sheep | 0/3 | 0/1 | 3/3 | – | 20 | [52] |
| Rhesus monkey | 2/2 | 1/1 | – | 2/2 | 20 | [77] |
| Pig | 3/3 | 1/1 | 3/3 | – | 28 | [52] |

### 3.2.2 Avulsed Teeth Replantation

Traumatic injuries to the teeth mostly cause tooth displacement in its alveolar socket. If the tooth is totally displaced from its own socket, avulsion has occurred, in which the pulp neurovascular supply and the periodontal ligaments would cut off [71]. Replantation at the socket of avulsed tooth can provide the best long-term results, if the pulp is regenerated properly and the healthy PDL reattaches to the tooth wall. These complications can cause inflammatory or replacement root resorption. Pulp revascularization is more prospective in immature teeth, since the apical foramen is not completely formed and the blood supply is favorable for pulp regeneration. Moreover, the presence or absence of bacteria in the pulp lumen is the other confounding factor that affects the pulp revascularization success. The prognosis of a replanted avulsed tooth is influenced by the extra-alveolar time, storage medium prior to replanting, root conditioning before replantation, careful manipulation of tooth during transfer, intracanal medication, and systemic antibiotic administration [72]. These factors should be considered to reduce the bacterial accumulation inside the pulp cavity and mainly to maintain the maximum possible viable cells of PDL on the root, leading to tooth reattachment to the socket bone and eliminating the osteoclast invasion after replantation. Hence, many studies have been designed to optimize the interfering factors, including the determination of the ideal time for replantation or the best transferring medium [72, 73]. To mimic the avulsion accident in animal studies, the purposed teeth should be extracted atraumatically (Fig. 18.5), unless the research is designed to evaluate the replantation accomplishments in a fractured alveolar bone.

The choice of animal model and the extracted tooth in investigation of avulsed teeth is still controversial. Basically, determined teeth are better to be selected from the animal's single-root teeth or sectioned teeth. However, some studies have been conducted on double or multiple-root teeth [74]. The maxillary central incisors are the most commonly involved teeth [75], that almost always have a single root, so treatment modalities for avulsion of single-root teeth in animals can be more easily extrapolated to human condition. Rats and dogs are the two species that have been mainly used. However, rat incisors are continuously growing and have an extreme curvature [67], which hamper the atraumatic extraction of teeth. Also, rat molars have double roots, and removal of teeth without root fracture or damage is somewhat

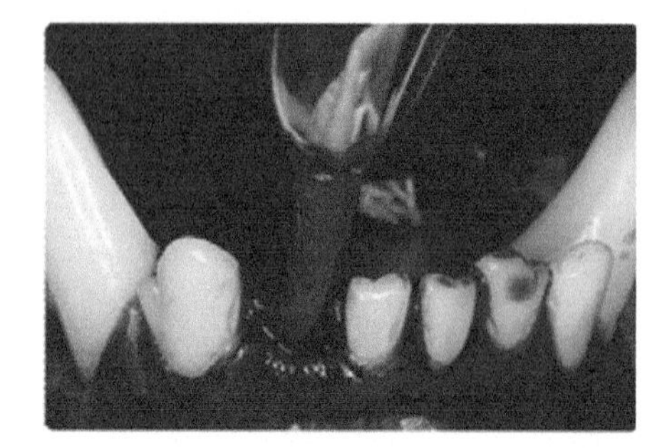

**Fig. 18.5** Atraumatic tooth extraction in a canine model. (Reuse with permission) [79]

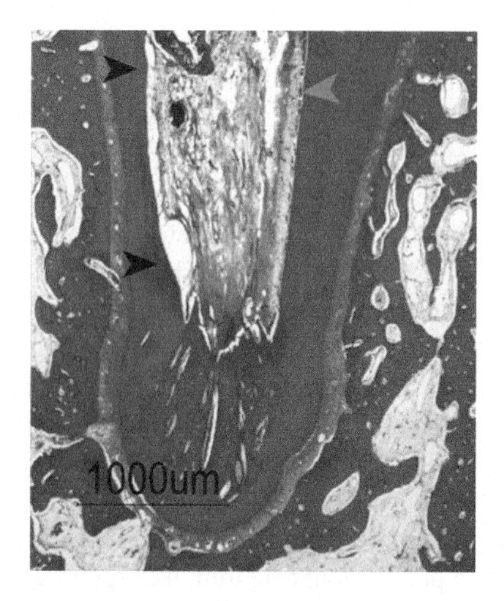


**Fig. 18.6** Apical delta in a dog tooth. (Reuse with permission) [80]

difficult. Therefore, rats are not considered as a proper animal model for this experiment. Although presence of apical delta in canine mature teeth has the possibility to deviate the animal responses to replantation from human teeth (Fig. 18.6) [67], dog incisors are the more suitable models for avulsion studies because the healing processes of teeth and supporting tissues, along with the curvature of the incisor, are similar to that of humans.

### *3.3 Periodontics and Implant Dentistry*

Dental plaque has been proven to initiate and elevate gingival inflammation. Gingivitis, the gentlest form of periodontal disease, is frequently established by the bacterial biofilm accumulation on teeth surfaces, adjacent to the gingiva, and is the result of an interaction between microorganisms and inflammatory reactions of host responses. However, gingivitis is reversible, since it does not destruct the supporting structures of the teeth and is confined to the soft tissues [81]. Following the accumulation of subgingival plaque with greater microbial density and the prolonged retention of the specific microorganisms, further disinsertion of periodontal ligaments and destruction of alveolar bone provokes and results in increased pocket depth, recession, or both. Invasion of the host inflammatory infiltrate in the periodontium is the major pathological characteristic of periodontitis, which can be altered by the effects of local factors or systemic conditions [82, 83]. The clinical signs that discriminate between periodontitis and gingivitis are attachment loss, alveolar bone resorption, and periodontal pocketing.

As an analogy to periodontal disease, accumulation of plaque on the mucosal margin of implants is the contributing element for inflammatory response of peri-implant tissue that can result in implant failure. These processes are delineated as peri-implant mucositis and peri-implantitis are the main complications of implant treatment. Peri-implant mucositis is the inflammation of implant-surrounding mucosa without the breakdown of the supporting bone [84]. On the other hand, peri-implantitis leads to deprivation of bone at osseointegrated implants [85]. Peri-implantitis and periodontitis have several biological and clinical similarities except in peri-implantitis, the presence of larger and deeper lesions, higher inflammatory cell infiltration, and greater osteoclast number occurs [86, 87].

Treatment of these adverse conditions is mainly based on accurate hygiene regimen that is aimed at the stabilization of disease progression or alleviation of the inflammation [88]. However, periodontium has a minimal capability for regeneration since the prolonged chronic inflammation reduces the number of resident stem cells within the periodontal niche and attenuates the potential of tissue repopulation [89]. Therefore, considering other procedures is crucial to restore the damaged dental supporting apparatus of the cementum, periodontal ligaments, and alveolar bone, such as bone grafting, guided tissue regeneration, or tissue engineering approaches. In periodontal research, human longitudinal studies encounter many complications, such as various unpredictable host immune responses and determining the stages of disease activity. In addition to disease complexity, the inflammatory reaction of the host is not linear due to an increase in the number of microbial species associated with periodontal breakdown as a function of inflammation and immune system activity. So, in addition to in vitro experiments, it is necessary to choose laboratory animal models prior to testing the safety and efficacy of new treatments in human [90].

Given the simultaneous role of living microorganisms and host inflammation, animal models were primarily used to determine the association of the bacterial etiology and host responses to uncover the pathogenesis of periodontal disease mechanism. In this regard, production of genetically modified transgenic or knockout variants, especially in small animals, gives the opportunity for discovering the single biological aspect of periodontal disease [91]. Utilization of gnotobiotic or germ-free animals, such as germ-free rats of the Sprague Dawley strain, seems to be beneficial to demonstrate the ability of various bacterial species to form plaque and propagate periodontal lesions in the absence of other microorganisms or to scrutinize the mono-infections by periodontopathogens [92].

Also, animal experiments are designed for the trial of possible regenerative and tissue engineering periodontal remedies to provide acceptable evidence for translation of these modalities into clinical setting. Within the context of periodontal disease and regenerative treatments, numerous animals from different species comprising small animals and large models have been employed. In certain species, periodontitis can occur naturally, like beagle dogs and nonhuman primates in late life with asymmetric pattern, whereas in others, periodontal lesions require experimental induction [93]. For intentional induction of periodontal disease and peri-implant lesions, great emphasis has been put on producing chronic inflammatory responses in addition to defect creation in order to mimic the naturally occurring periodontitis. This aim is achievable by placing plaque-accumulating devices, including resin blocks [94], non-resorbable sutures, impression materials [95], orthodontic elastics [96], and ligature wires [97, 98] around teeth in the gingival sulcus for 4–24 weeks depending on the type of animal studies. These foreign bodies are

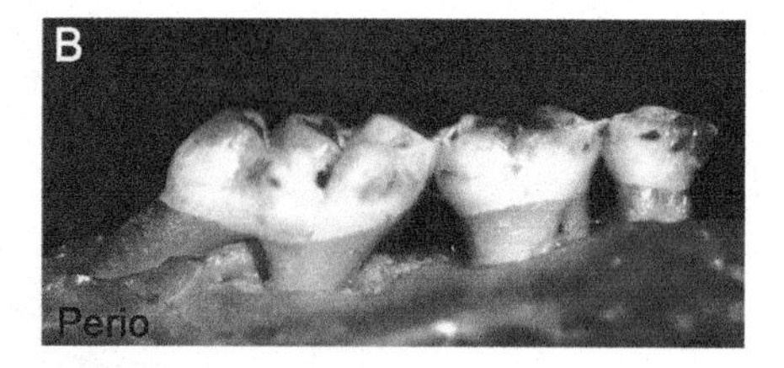


**Fig. 18.7** Maxillary molar region of a mice model monoinfected with *Porphyromonas gingivalis* infected. (Permission is not required under the terms of the Creative Commons Attribution License (CC BY)) [192]

fixed around the teeth to initiate sulcular epithelium ulceration, which accelerates the invasion of connective tissue. Chronic stimulation of periodontitis can be also obtained by introduction of virulent bacterial species into the oral microbiota, known as gavage method, injection of bacterial species, or their virulence factors, such as the lipopolysaccharide, into periodontal tissues (Fig. 18.7). The common bacterial species utilized for propagation of periodontitis are *Porphyromonas gingivalis*, *Actinobacillus actinomycetemcomitans*, and *Streptococcus mutans* [99]. Bacterial inoculation disturbs the native oral microbiota and changes the oral environment in favor of periodontal pathogen proliferation. Alteration of animal feeding to a sucrose-rich diet or even a soft-minced diet can develop a rapid proliferation of bacteria and would facilitate the plaque accumulation and subsequent inflammation cascades [100, 101]. Exposure of the animals to chronic cold stress is another approach for induction of periodontal destruction [102]. However, extent and configuration of the consequent periodontal lesions are not always predictable by these naturally inducing methods, since the inflammatory tissue destruction may change the expected designed resorption morphologies and mostly cause irregularly shaped defects [103]. Although surgical creation of periodontal defects does not mimic the inflammatory process of periodontal disease alone, it has attracted much attention due to the homogeneity and reproducibility in defect height and morphology. Combination of the abovementioned approaches [104] allows inducted defects to be generated in one of the following categories [93]:

1. Periodontal pocket defects in which the mesial/distal interdental alveolar bone, the adjacent periodontal ligament, and cementum are removed and generate a one-, two-, or three-wall defect (Fig. 18.8). The lesion dimension differs between various animals (e.g., lesion with 5 × 7 × 3 mm in pig [89, 105] and 5 × 5 × 4 mm in dog [106]).
2. Furcation defects are characterized by the removal of the bone filling and the furcation between roots in multi-rooted teeth, mostly in a buccolingual direction.
3. Dehiscence or fenestration defects in which the bone on the facial, or less common on the lingual, aspect of a tooth is removed. Then, the root is exposed to the gingiva or alveolar mucosa. These defects are frequently applied on single-rooted teeth.

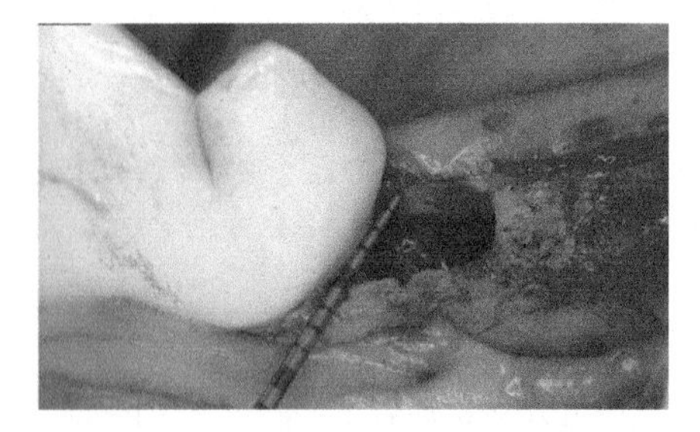

**Fig. 18.8** A surgically created three-wall defect on the mesial side of mandibular first molar of a dog model [193]

4. Recession defects that are generated by excision of the facial gingiva and exposure of the root surfaces to the oral environment.
5. Irregular-shaped defects are usually produced by utilization of chronic stimulating periodontal inductors.
6. Combined defects. (Fig. 18.9)

Experimental induction of peri-implant lesions is approximately identical to that conducted for periodontitis. Establishment of peri-implant mucositis is feasible by assisting in undisturbed accumulation of bacterial plaque via termination of oral hygiene and plaque control cessation. The total duration for induction of disease varies among species over a period of 21 days up to 9 months [107]. The ligature-induced model is a standard chronic experimental model for assessment of pathogenesis and treatment aspects of peri-implantitis lesions (Fig. 18.10). The submerged implants that are widely implemented for investigation of new material capability in promotion of osseointegration are not the choice for peri-implantitis assessment. Since they are not in contact with oral pathogenic microflora, commencement of peri-implant disease is less expected. In the active breakdown period, in which the ligature is located around implant, undisturbed plaque accumulation takes place that leads to tissue damage. Various species exhibit different periods for onset of periodontal lesion post-ligature placement. Table 18.3 summarizes the experimental period of ligature induction for various species. When this predetermined period ligature is removed, the lesion will progress with no spontaneous regeneration. During progression, periodic plaque control should be performed to eliminate the confounding effect of bacteria [107]. Surgical creation of peri-implant bony lesions is also practical for generation of reproducible and homogenous periodontal defects (Fig. 18.11). Further information on peri-implant disease modeling is demonstrated in Fig. 18.12.

The impact of host systemic condition and metabolic status on periodontal lesions and disease progression rate is well-established. Modeling this interplay is feasible by induction of periodontium damage in unhealthy animals, such as diabetic mice/rat or mice/rat with a certain predisposition to cardiovascular disease [104, 108]. Rabbit also represents a good animal model for investigation of non-dental inflammation processes, since it is commonly used as a model for cardiovascular disease. They are highly responsive to lipid manipulation, and the high-cholesterol diet is a functional method to induce experimental atherosclerosis [109].

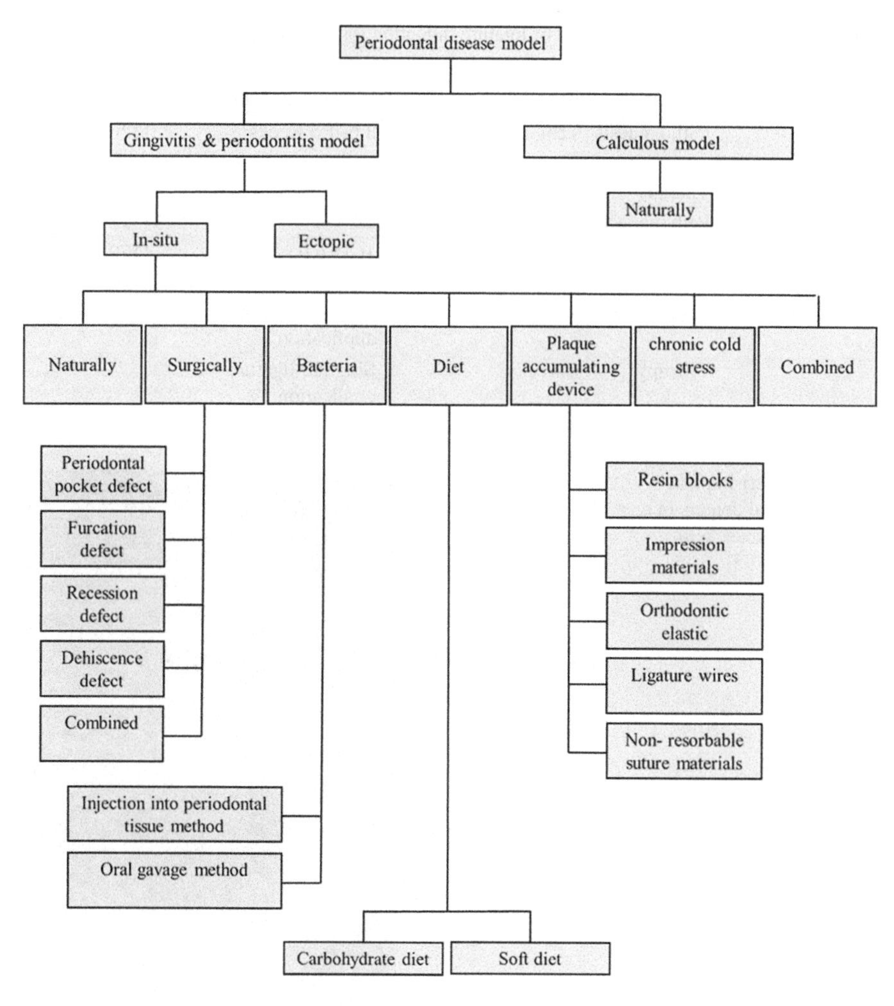


**Fig. 18.9** Periodontal disease modeling

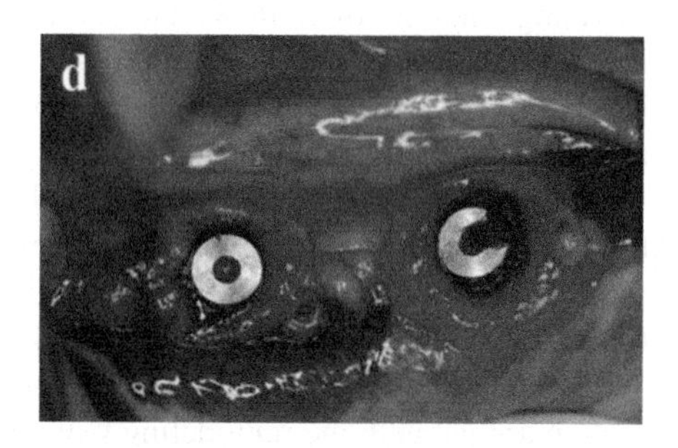


**Fig. 18.10** Ligature-induced peri-implantitis defect model in a dog model. (Reuse with permission) [194]

**Table 18.3** The experimental period of ligature induction for various species

| Animal modeling | Objectives | Active breakdown period | Ligature exchange | References |
|---|---|---|---|---|
| Canine | Pathogenesis | 12.0–5.0 weeks | 3.6–1.5 weeks | [120, 132–151] |
| | Therapy | 14.4–6.2 weeks | 2.4–2.5 | [152–176] |
| Nonhuman primate | Pathogenesis | 30.0–13.2 weeks | 2.8–3.3 | [177–185] |
| | Therapy | 59.0–19.0 weeks | 16.0–6.0 | [179, 186–189] |
| Swine | Pathogenesis | 45 days | Singular ligature application | [190, 191] |
| | Therapy | 6 weeks | Singular ligature application | |

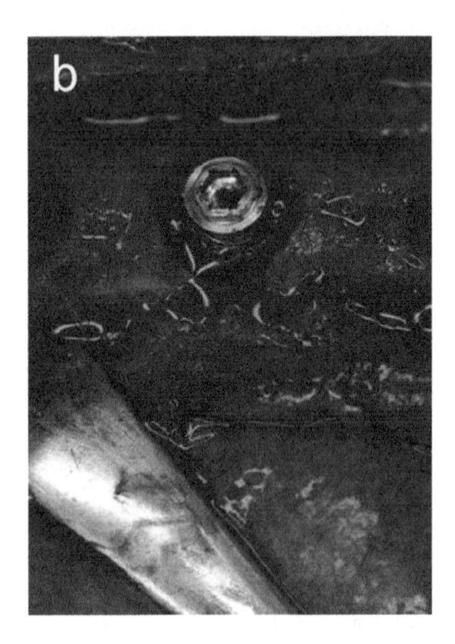


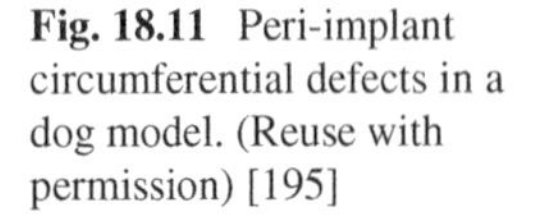

**Fig. 18.11** Peri-implant circumferential defects in a dog model. (Reuse with permission) [195]

A large amount of valuable data has been provided by animal models. However, it is difficult to adjudicate whether these outcomes can be transferred to human clinics due to differences in pathogenesis of periodontal disease and its response to treatment modalities, albeit more human similarities can be observed in large animals. Although small animals have revealed precious information on molecular and biological aspects of periodontal and peri-implant lesions, the poor similarity of their dentition to human and difficulty of surgical procedures in their small jaws have restricted their application in periodontology [90].

In implant investigation studies, the determining factors that influence osseointegration are native bone remodeling features and adequate bone volume that allows implant placement [110]. In this regard, scientists prefer to insert implants in large animals that offer enough bone volume for placement of customized implants.

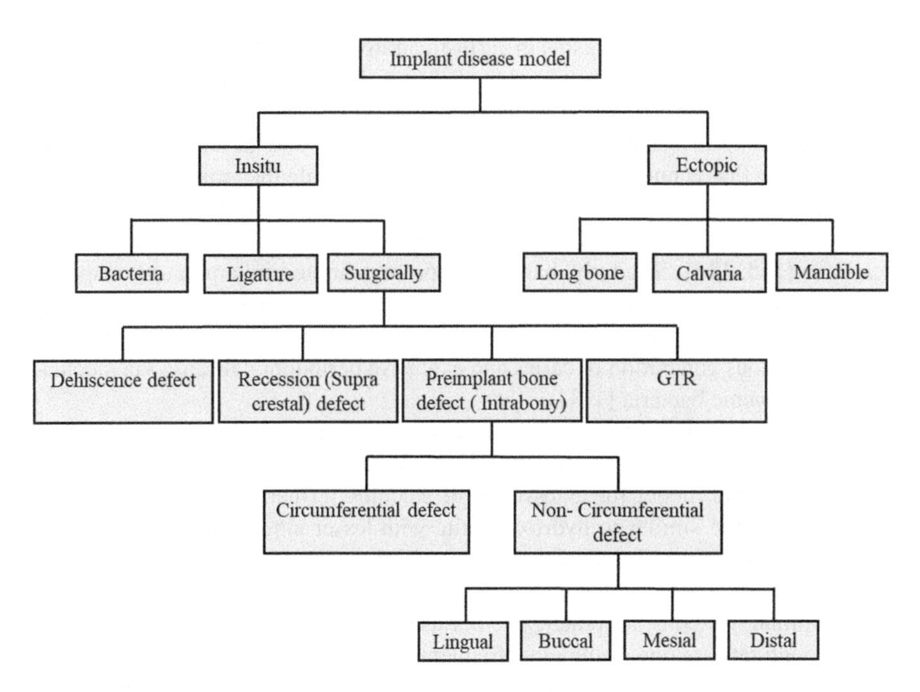


**Fig. 18.12** Implant disease modeling

Although rabbit, as a small animal model, is the most studied species for implant researches due to its easier accessibility and parameters like bone remodeling rate, large animals, such as dogs, have greater resemblance to human bone turnover [111]. The following section will discuss the drawbacks and advantages of each commonly used species.

Laboratory rats have demonstrated an acceptable model for caries assessment, but they have limitations to serve as model for periodontal disease. The structure of their dental gingiva resembles to human with a shallow gingival sulcus and presence of sulcular and junctional epithelium [112]. Most histologic characteristics of periodontal epithelium and connective tissue in the rats are identical to that observed in human, except for several major differences which differs to the occurrence of periodontal disease in this species: the first is the keratinization of sulcular epithelium in rats [113]. Keratinized cells have made rats extremely resistant to periodontal disease. The second is the gingival response that is comprised of an acute, not chronic, immune infiltrate. So, while the infection occurs, the destruction of periodontal apparatus occurs quite rapidly. The next dissimilarity is narrow interdental septum, which limits development of infrabony defects and causes horizontal bone loss as a consequence of periodontal destruction. In rat species, the most apical extent of periodontal lesion is on the central zone of interdental tissues, in contrast to human which migrates apically along the root surface. This fact causes bone loss in the absence of apical migration of junctional epithelium [114, 115].

Inoculation of microorganisms in germ-free rats has revealed that rapid progression of periodontal destruction possibly alleviates the need for inducing the disease with ligatures [115]. In addition, monocontamination in rats by gram-negative species failed to form bacterial plaque on tooth surfaces and developed a minimal inflammation that is not similar to human responses, while the gram-positive infection was capable of inducing periodontal destruction. So, periodontal damage caused by gram-negative bacteria in rat is not based on cell-mediated immune response [115, 116]. Similarly, hamsters represent limited inflammatory response and show development of periodontal lesions identical to rats with horizontal bone loss and crater-like gingival pocketing [115]. An interesting feature of hamsters is the synchronous generation of caries and extensive periodontal disease via inoculation of cariogenic bacteria [117].

Rat has been studied for evaluation of calculus formation in which diet represents the most dependable factor [100]. However, among small animals, ferrets are the most suitable model for assessment of calculus formation, since it manifests physical structure similar to hydroxyapatite with lesser amount of calcification in ferret deposits compared to human calculus. Furthermore, formation of calculus in ferret is not influenced by diet alteration and scoring the calculus is possible in the awake animal, which is not practicable in rats [118].

Although rats are one of the most frequently studied animals for medical objectives, it is not a suitable model for evaluation of dental implants, due to healing, anatomical and bone composition dissimilarities to human. In addition, the small size of this animal restricts the simultaneous placement of several implants as experimental and control groups [119].

Rabbit is known as an appropriate animal for investigation and creation of periodontal bone defects. However, they are not considered as a suitable candidate for studies on periodontal ligament due to the special adaptation of PDL with continuous growth of teeth [5]. The exclusive periodontal feature of rabbits is that ligature introduction into periodontal crevice alone does not induce soft or hard tissue damage [90]. Hence, presence of periodontitis-specific microorganisms is required for disease modeling, if ligature placement is intended.

As mentioned above, in vivo investigations require species with proper bone remodeling and adequate bone volume for implant placement. Rabbit fulfill these two main prerequisites, and considering their easy management and economical concerns, it is a suitable model for first implant design evaluation [110]. Moreover, rabbit has rapid bone remodeling and skeletal alteration in comparison to some species, such as primates and even some rodents [119].

Since dental implants mainly affect their adjacent tissues, it is of great significance to select proper site for implant insertion in the rabbit skeleton. Various anatomical regions with different physiological conditions including skull, mandible, femur, and tibia are available for analysis of dental implants in rabbit body. Although intraoral and calvarial bone represent an ossification process and presence of extrinsic muscle force similar to human condition, extraoral bone sites provide much more bone volume and application of more comfortable surgery, due to more easily accessible locations than the jaw [119]. In addition, blood supply and flow to the mandible resemble the amount of rabbit's long bones, and the remodeling rate of the mandible is comparable to the tibia bone, which occurs more rapidly than the same amount of skull and maxilla [110]. Rat calvaria has about 3.5 mm thickness, which limits the insertion of conventional implant with approximately 10 mm length within calvaria, so it is not a common zone for implantation. In contrast, dimension of rabbit tibia and femur allows placement of cylindrical implants with 8–10 mm length and 4 mm diameter [110]. However, insertion of implants larger than 6 mm in length and 2 mm in diameter is not recommended [119]. Nevertheless, implant insertion in rabbit tibia and femur which is standardized for bony condition of test site is relevantly equivalent. Proximal tibia consists of a thick cortical bone layer that contributes to the formation of bone-to-implant contact. Distal femur also can support implant stability, since it represents a limited amount of trabecular bone. Hence, it is recommended to test implants in these two locations [110].

It is noteworthy that the international standard for the biological evaluation of medical devices recommends a maximum number of implants for each test and control groups. This is defined to be the total number of six implants in each rabbit that exhibit the half amount of recommended implant number for larger animals such as sheep, dogs, and pigs [119].

Dogs are of great value as a model for assessment of periodontal disease. They demonstrate comparable characteristics in terms of periodontal tissues and teeth size to humans [90]. Their periodontal supragingival and subgingival microbiota is similar to human and is mainly composed of gram-positive cocci and virulent anaerobic gram-negative cocci and rods, respectively [120]. However, subgingival microflora of dogs has higher percentage of gram-negative bacteria, which would decrease in disease [121]. In healthy dog that has been maintained plaque-free by hygienic control, gingival sulcus is not apparent. But, gingivitis and pocket formation occur as a consequence of plaque accumulation, and periodontitis follows gingivitis [115]. Dogs represent naturally occurring gingivitis and periodontitis with clinical manifestation of human periodontal disease (i.e., bleeding on probing, gingival recession, bone loss, and even as common tooth loss). Nonetheless, disease progress 5 times more rapidly in dogs than human [122]. Histologically, dense inflammatory cellular infiltrate is seen in dog periodontal involvement [90]. Although, the prevalence and severity of periodontal disease enhances with aging, differences exist between various breeds. The first and second premolars and the bifurcation region are more frequently involved than interdental spaces, since the alveolar bone resorption occurs in the pattern of narrow lesion, which extends vertically around single rooted-teeth and does not damage interdental tissues [90, 93]. Despite the etiologic predisposing factors of periodontal disease in canine being identical to human, major differences, such as the lack of lateral jaw movement, occlusal contacts at the premolar level, and presence of open contacts between their teeth, do exist that can alter the interpretation of in vivo findings [93, 116].

Calculus deposition in aged dogs is commonly evident and leads to gingivitis and periodontitis. Therefore, canine is a suitable model for efficacy assessment of different approaches in subgingival calculus removal and has been mainly utilized for researches on calculus [116, 123].

The canine model is the most commonly used large animal for investigation of implant suitability and peri-implantitis pathogenesis, and has been proven to be a beneficial model in surveys on regeneration around implants [90, 107]. Although vast utilization of dog for research is probably attributed to their docile character, the composition of dog bone (ash weight, hydroxyproline, and extractable proteins) and wound-healing kinetics is also quite similar to that of human, as well as pig bone [107, 119, 124]. In addition the specific anatomy of jaw bone allows the insertion of conventional dental implants (10 mm length and 3–4 mm diameter) [107]. Ligature-induced peri-implantitis model requires plaque control and postoperative hygiene procedure, which is more easily managed in dog than pig or some other animals [125]. Furthermore, these defects in canine resemble naturally occurring lesions in human in terms of associated microflora, defect size, and configuration [85]. Despite all similarities, some major differences exist between human and dog bone features; canine possesses faster turnover rate (1.5–2.0 μm/day for dog vs. 1.0–1.5 μm/day for human) [107, 126], and bone modeling/remodeling of extracted socket is 3–5 times more rapid in dogs compared to that of human [124]. It is important to note that the remodeling ability of bone is influenced by site, animal age, and breed. Dog bone has remarkably greater mineral density than human bone [119].

Aside from disobedient temperament of pigs, miniature pigs share many analogous periodontal characteristics to human. Gross anatomy of their periodontal tissue as well as pathophysiology of periodontium breakdown is identical to human. In addition, in intact periodontium, gingival sulcus is present and has a probing depth of 2–3 mm with a long junctional epithelium. Miniature pigs are susceptible to naturally occurring gingivitis from 6 months of age that can lead to periodontitis from 16 months as a result of plaque accumulation. The following inflammatory changes and disease progression represent the same patterns as that in human: gingival swelling, plaque accumulation and calculus formation, bleeding on probing, gingival recession [127], periodontal pocketing up to 5 mm, and periodontal tissue loss with poor capability for spontaneous regeneration, like human [53, 90, 93].

The mini-pig has also been studied for compatibility in peri-implantitis explorations and serves as a good model for this aim. With regard to micro- and macrostructure of bone, pig has shown relative similarity to human bone, and both its bone composition and bone remodeling are approximately close to what is seen in human except for the denser trabecular network of porcine [107, 119, 128]. The most attractive feature of pig bone that makes them a suitable model for implant dentistry is the specific anatomy of the jaw that further facilitates the implantation of customized dental implants [107].

Sheep, a commonly manipulated small ruminant, has very short-rooted incisors that are mobile physiologically. These teeth can experience spontaneous periodontitis with pocketing and marked bone loss [116]. Their premolar and molars also can be affected by naturally occurring periodontitis. However, the grinding teeth possess similar periodontal structure to human with the presence of human periodontal pathogens in subgingival microflora [93].

Adult sheep offer a good animal model for insertion of human implants within the long bones due to their suitable dimension and macroscopic relevance to human bone, which is not obtainable in smaller species. However, sheep have a considerable higher bone density and greater strength in comparison to human. Since the bone location and animal age modify the bone composition and bone remodeling rate in sheep, the immature sheep demonstrates weaker bone with less density and more porosity, which is comparable to human bone. Nevertheless, the impact of different bone density should be considered in the interpretation of implant stability and bone-implant contact interface prior to data translation to clinics [119].

Nonhuman primates possess oral and periodontal structure similar to human. In addition, in terms of periodontal disease, they show naturally occurring dental plaque, calculus and subsequent gingivitis, and destructive periodontal disease [116]. However, a small increase in the pocket depth is associated with periodontal disease [115]. The major drawback of using nonhuman primates in periodontal researches is their susceptibility to certain infections, mainly tuberculosis [129].

A vast number of nonhuman primate species are maintained under laboratory condition that provides selection of species with suitable features for each periodontal study. In certain species, like cynomolgus monkeys, the inflammatory response of periodontal disease is quite similar to man as well as the gram-positive composition of plaque in supragingival zone and gram-negative bacteria in subgingival plaque. However, squirrel monkeys and marmosets display limited inflammatory infiltrate, making these species improper models for periodontal investigations [115, 116]. Furthermore, besides their small oral cavity, marmoset dentition expresses severe occlusal abrasion and bony lesions that are mostly attributed to plunger cusps [130]. Marmoset, as a small nonhuman primate, has small oral cavity. In contrast, mature adult cynomolgus and rhesus monkeys with similar periodontal wound healing [131], proper furcation sites [126], and possibility of defect creation that does not repair spontaneously serve as acceptable models for periodontitis trials [115].

Nonhuman primate is known as a desirable model for investigation of implant safety and efficacy, since their jaw bone anatomy allows the insertion of diameter-reduced dental implants and also their close approximate to human biology and physiology.

## 3.4 *Maxillofacial Surgery*

Bone defects in the maxillofacial area, due to the congenital abnormalities, trauma, or cancer surgery, are associated with major functional, sociological, and psychological problems [196–198].

The advantages of using animal models for this field are not only to evaluate the safety and efficacy of various treatments but to understand the underlying biological processes using methods that may be considered too invasive for human application, such as repeated harvesting of biological samples, biopsies, etc. [199]. Small animal models, including rodents and rabbits, are the starting points for proof-of-principle or feasibility studies [200, 201], whereas large animal model studies, including dogs, pigs, sheep, and primates, attempt to simulate clinical conditions more closely and predict therapeutic efficacy [202–204]. Animal models used for study in the field of surgery were generally covered following treatment purposes: bone defects and bone augmentation.

### 3.4.1 Bone Defect

Reconstruction of alveolar defects, due to aging, trauma, ablative surgery, or pathology, remains a clinical challenge [205]. Although autologous bone transplantation is still considered the gold standard for maxillofacial bone regeneration [206, 207], large defects may require volumes of bone that are locally unavailable. Moreover, the morbidity associated with bone harvesting is a major limiting factor [208]. There is no consensus currently available over the application of alternatives such as allogeneic, xenogeneic, and alloplastic bone substitutes [209, 210].

Generally, bone represents good regeneration ability and majority of bony lesions can heal spontaneously under well-balanced biological and physiological situations. However, unfavorable biomechanical properties of wound environment or actual large defects can result in reduced regeneration potential of bone and lead to the formation of critical-size defects, which extremely affect patients' quality of life [211]. Such lesions pose a great challenge for researchers and clinicians. Critical-size defects are the smallest osseous wound that does not heal spontaneously without an intervention. A more precise definition is clarified to involve any defect that has less than 10% of bony regeneration during the entirety of animal life. For practical purposes, if there is less than 30% of mineralized area after 52 weeks, it is unlikely that mineralization will ever take place. Although the minimum size of critical-size defects is not defined exactly, defects with length deficiency exceeding 2–2.5 times its diameter are shown to illustrate critical defect characteristics [212, 213]. Since each species has its own features of bone metabolism, the sizes of critical defects vary. Table 18.4 demonstrates the dimension of critical-size defects in different species that has been investigated.

Creation of critical-size defects in vivo is mainly generated by surgical procedure and is based upon the defect type and the location where the lesion is generated (Fig. 18.13). Ectopic models with lower cost and less invasive procedure are principally designed to distinguish between the proliferative and inductive capabilities of new materials, while orthotopic models are chosen for evaluating the safety and success of new surgical methods or products [199]. In terms of defect configuration, bony lesion can be either created in a segmental or non-segmental form. Application of the later defect is feasible in jaw bone by tooth extraction and allows the alveolar bone to resorb. Ridge augmentation is the treatment option for regeneration of non-segmental jaw defects that will be discussed in the next section. Interrupted and continuous bone defects are the two shapes of segmental defects, which are categorized by removal of partial- or full-thickness of bone, respectively.

The choice of a particular species for assessment of bone regeneration on critical-size defects is of great importance and several factors should be considered.

**Table 18.4** Critical-size defects in different species

| Animal | Site | | Critical-size defect (mm) | References |
|---|---|---|---|---|
| Rabbit | Extra maxillofacial region | Tibia | 5 × 15<br>6 (D)<br>5 (S) | [271–273] |
| | | Femur | 7 × 10 $mm^2$(C)<br>15 (L)<br>6 (D) × 5 (C) | [274–276] |
| | | Ulna | 12 (S)<br>15 (S) | [277, 278] |
| | Maxillofacial region | Calvaria | 10 (D) × 1.2<br>9 (D) | [279, 280] |
| | | Mandible | 15 × 6<br>12 × 8<br>10 × 4 × 3<br>10 × 6<br>6 × 4 × 3<br>10 × 15<br>10 × 5 × 4<br>8 (D) | [281–285] |
| Dog | Extra maxillofacial region | Femur | 15<br>21 | [286, 287] |
| | | Radial | 15<br>25<br>20 | [288, 289] |
| | | Tibia | 20 | [290] |
| | | Ulna | 25<br>15<br>20 | [289, 291, 292] |
| | | Fibula | 10 | [293] |
| | Maxillofacial region | Mandible | 20 × 6.5<br>10 × 10<br>10 (D)<br>20 × 10 × 10<br>9 (D)<br>20 × 10<br>30 (L) | [237, 294–298] |
| | | Maxilla | 10 × 5 × 15<br>15 | [299] |
| Rodent | Extra maxillofacial region | Distal femur | 2 (D) × 2 (d)<br>2 (D) × 3 (L) | [300, 301] |
| | | Mid-femur | 2 (L)<br>5 (L) | [302–304] |
| | Maxillofacial region | Calvaria | 4 (D)<br>8 (D) | [305, 306] |
| | | Mandible | 4 (D)<br>5 (D)<br>4 × 4 × 3<br>3 (D) | [307–309] |

(continued)

**Table 18.4** (continued)

| Animal | Site | | Critical-size defect (mm) | References |
|---|---|---|---|---|
| Pig | Extra maxillofacial region | Tibia | 11 (D) × 25 (d) | [310] |
| | Maxillofacial region | Calvaria | 10 (D) × 10 (d)<br>20 × 40<br>40 (D)<br>35 × 25 | [311, 312] |
| | | Mandible | 25 × 15 × 15<br>3.5 × 8<br>20 × 20<br>6 (D)<br>12 × 10 × 12 × 5–6<br>6 (d) × 8 (D)<br>20 × 10<br>7 (D) × 4 (d)<br>10 (D)<br>8 (d) × 3.5 (D)<br>20 (d) × 30 (D)<br>1.7 × 0.8 × 1.4 | [243, 313–318] |
| | | Maxilla | 30 × 12 | [319] |
| Sheep | Extra maxillofacial region | Mid-diaphyseal metatarsal | 25 (L)<br>20 | [320, 321] |
| | | Tibia | 35<br>48<br>30<br>20<br>40<br>45<br>16<br>18 | [322–325] |
| | | Femur | 25 | [326] |
| | | Radial | 12 | [327] |
| | Maxillofacial region | Mandible | 35 (L) | [328] |
| Goat | Extra maxillofacial region | Femur | 20<br>25 | [329, 330] |
| | | Tibia | 26 | [331] |
| Monkey | Extra maxillofacial region | Tibia | 20 | [332] |
| | | Femur | 20 | [333] |
| | Maxillofacial region | Mandible | 15 (L) | [236] |

*D* diameter, *d* depth, *L* length, *S* segment

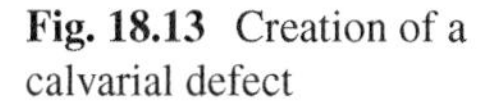
**Fig. 18.13** Creation of a calvarial defect

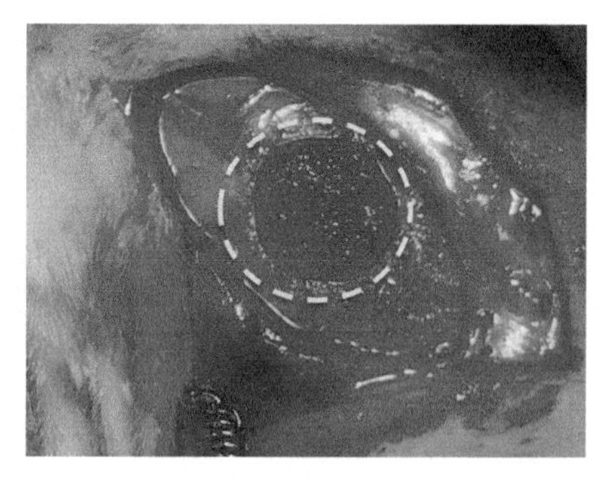

The chosen animal should represent similar microstructural and biomechanical characteristics to human bone, as well as healing and regeneration potential. Differences in gross anatomy, distribution and amount of cortical and trabecular portions, density, thickness, and remodeling of bone exist among various species and have rendered different regeneration potentials. Although nonhuman primates are definitely the best characterized large animal model in terms of bone biology for skeletal research due to the utmost bone similarities to human [199], knowledge of bone structure in frequently used animals is essential.

Out of laboratory animals, mice and rats have the least similarity to human bone biology. Having small long bones, permanent open growth plates, absence of Haversian system, thin cortical plates, and limited amount of cancellous bone at epiphyses of long bones have rendered them as unfavorable species for skeleton-based studies [196]. Nevertheless, calvarial bone defects are established for regenerative bone assessment due to bone marrow deficiency and poor blood supply of this region [214]. Optimal rat calvarial defect is recommended to be bilateral, 5 mm trephined, and full-thickness bone defects, and precautions should be taken to minimize the risk of damage to sagittal sinus [215].

Rabbit, in small animals, and dog, in large animals, are the most frequently used species for bone defect models. Rabbit skeleton does not possess the major drawbacks of rodent models (i.e., lack of Haversian system and open growth plates). In addition, they have similarities in bone density to human and short time for bone maturation. Various anatomical locations can be manipulated for experiments. The most common implantation sites include bilateral tibiae and distal femur, since bone mineral density and the fracture toughness of mid-diaphyseal rabbit bone resemble that of human [199, 213]. The amount of trabecular bone (bone volume/total volume) has been reported to be 99.50% and 93.49% for tibia and maxillary bone of rabbit, respectively. In performing experiments on skull bone of rabbits, one should consider that defect thickness plays an important role in healing [216]. Since the endosteal compartment is a rich source for bone-forming cells, defects that reach this layer by penetration of outer cortical plate have higher regenerative potential compared to the ones that have persisting cortical plate [110].

Canine and pig are established appropriate animal models for bone regeneration trials [119, 217, 218]. Porcine bone anatomy and turnover rate are analogous to

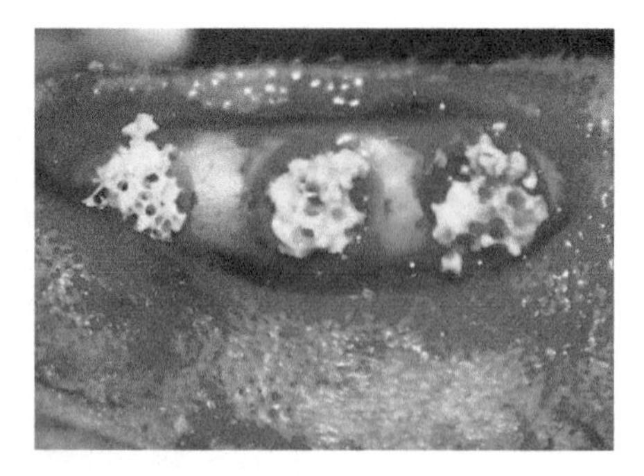

**Fig. 18.14** Circular defects in the inferior border of the dog mandible filled by beta-tricalcium phosphate scaffolds coated with polylactic-co-glycolic acid microspheres that gradually release vascular endothelial growth factor. (Reuse the figure of author's own article; no permission is required) [220]

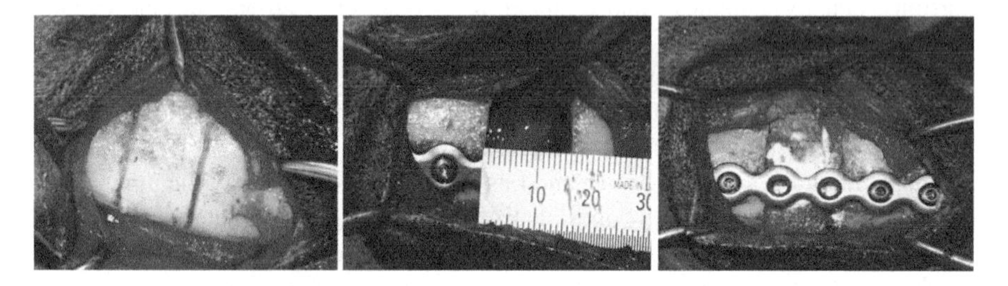

**Fig. 18.15** Intraoperative clinical photography of segmental osteotomy and repair with an organic bovine bone mineral collagen, functionalized with anti-BMP-2 monoclonal antibodies. (Reuse the figure of author's own article; no permission is required) [222]

those of human. Particularly, bone remodeling in human is 1.0–1.5 μm/day, while the reported rate for porcine (1.2–1.5 μm/day) is slightly closer than that for canine (1.5–2.0 μm/day) [219]. Although dog has a greater bone density than human, the cortical thickness of porcine bone is generally higher than in human and other species like dog. Dogs are frequently used in regenerative studies as a second species [220] (Fig. 18.14). Mandibular bone turnover of alveolar process is 10 times greater than in the mid-shaft of the tibia in dog model [221]. Therefore, orthotopic investigation of bone defects in jaw of dogs is more common [222] (Fig. 18.15) considering that the trabecular volume of maxilla and mandible is approximately identical (average of 97.8% for mandible and 98.2% for maxilla) [223]. Introduction of minipigs has overcome the limitations of using pigs in skeletal studies to some extent: quick growth and extreme body weight of them. The tibia of mini-pigs has been considered to be the suitable zone for production and assessment of bone defects [217], as well as its jaw bone. Experimentation of calvarial defect in pig is usually performed on the frontal or parietal bones [224].

Sheep tibia models are reliable for assessing the bone regeneration potential having long bone dimension and being as a maximal weight bearing limb. The bone maturation takes a long time in sheep, but the mineral density and bone strength of adult sheep is promoted relative to human [199]. Also, sheep has represented larger amount of bone ingrowth to the defect site [225]. It is noteworthy that being seasonal breeders alter the bone metabolism in sheep during the year [199].

The first alveolar bone model using an animal, attempted by Harvold in the 1950s, involved the induction of bone resorption by creating a 2 mm defect at the alveolar and hard palate of rhesus monkeys [226]. Since then, numerous studies using cat, dog, and rabbit models have been conducted [227–229].

The calvarial critical-size defect is a widely used experimental model for screening bone biomaterials in small and large animals. However, calvarial defects poorly reflect the clinical scenario of alveolar bone defects, given the variation in development and healing pattern between different skeletal sites [230, 231] and the additional influence of dental and masticatory factors on alveolar bone physiology [232, 233]. For this reason, critical-size defect models have been developed involving the maxillary and mandibular bones of small and large animals. Studies reported the use of critical-size defect more frequently in the mandible (83.3%) than the maxilla [198].

For mandible defects, rat, canine, goat, swine, and monkey models have been used to evaluate the effect of bone regeneration [4, 234–237]. The difference of the mandible defects in size, position, and shape has different clinical value. Bone defect commonly created in the body and alveolar bone of mandible [198]. Bone defects created in the ramus and angle of mandible can also be applied in many animal models.

In maxillary bone defect models, lots of studies focus on the maxillary sinus floor elevation [238–240], which is treated as an effective way to resolve the inadequate bone height in the posterior region of the maxilla in order to promote stability of endosseous implants [196].

The mini-pig, or swine, has been used frequently due to its similarities to humans in terms of platelet count, clotting parameters, metabolic rate, and bone structure [241, 242]. Besides, the surgical procedure is simple, with a limited risk of infection, and a similar intervention by grafting is advocated clinically. A true critical-sized mandibular defect in the mini-pig model is more than 5 mm [243].

Maxillary alveolar cleft is one of the bone defects with specific etiology, known as a congenital malformation, which occurs during fetal development, leading to a compromised dental arch anatomy and disrupted sequence teeth eruption [244]. In this context, the establishment of a proper in vivo biological model simulating alveolar clefts is essential. Several animal models have been developed in mice, rats, rabbits, cats, dogs, swine, goats, sheep, and monkeys [244–250]. Modeling can be produced by transgenic modification of animals such as rats or mouse [251, 252] or by intentional removal of a predetermined zone of palate by surgery (Fig. 18.16) [244, 253].

Goat model is suitable to study alveolar cleft defect repair [254], since the size of defect is similar to human, and the goat metabolism is more equivalent to the human situation than phylogenetically related rodents, in which bone metabolism is higher and defect sizes are much smaller [255, 256].

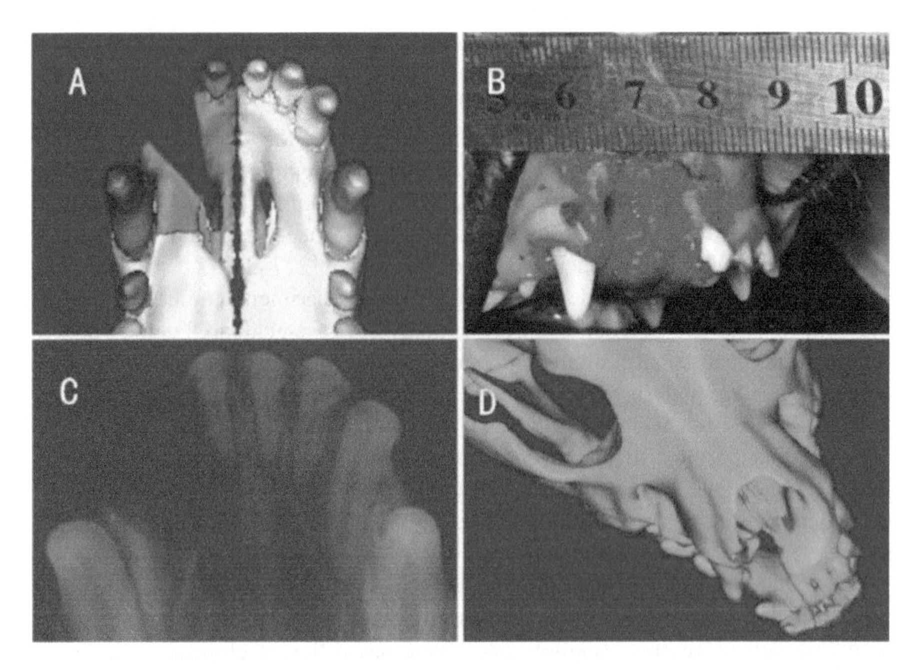


**Fig. 18.16** Alveolar cleft in a dog model. (**a**) Scheme designed to show the size and shape of the alveolar cleft that would be created by surgery. (**b**) Photograph of the surgically created alveolar cleft after surgery. (**c**) Occlusal view of the alveolar cleft was taken immediately after operation by X-ray. (**d**) Reconstructed three-dimensional tomogram by computer tomography immediately after surgery operation. (Reuse with permission) [334]

Due to the wide array of genes involved in craniofacial morphogenesis, defect-specific mechanisms have been difficult to delineate. However, the identification of specific effects exerted by the genome is becoming possible due to recent advances in recombinant DNA technology and transgenesis [257, 258]. Mouse models have been particularly important for new insights into the etiology of orofacial clefting and now became the basis for novel future molecular and transgenic approaches [257, 259]. The transgenic mouse models have been used to determine the primary and secondary causes of palatal clefting and the mechanisms for activation and regulation of essential developmental processes [257]. (Fig. 18.17)

### 3.4.2 Bone Augmentation

Bone augmentation includes sinus augmentation and ridge augmentation. Maxillary sinus floor augmentation, nowadays a routine procedure, aims at creating bone of adequate quantity and quality to facilitate the installation, osseointegration, and functional loading of implants [202]. Although several animal platforms, including rabbit [260], dog [261], mini-pig [262], goat/sheep [263], and primates [179], have been employed to evaluate sinus augmentation protocols, functional loading of

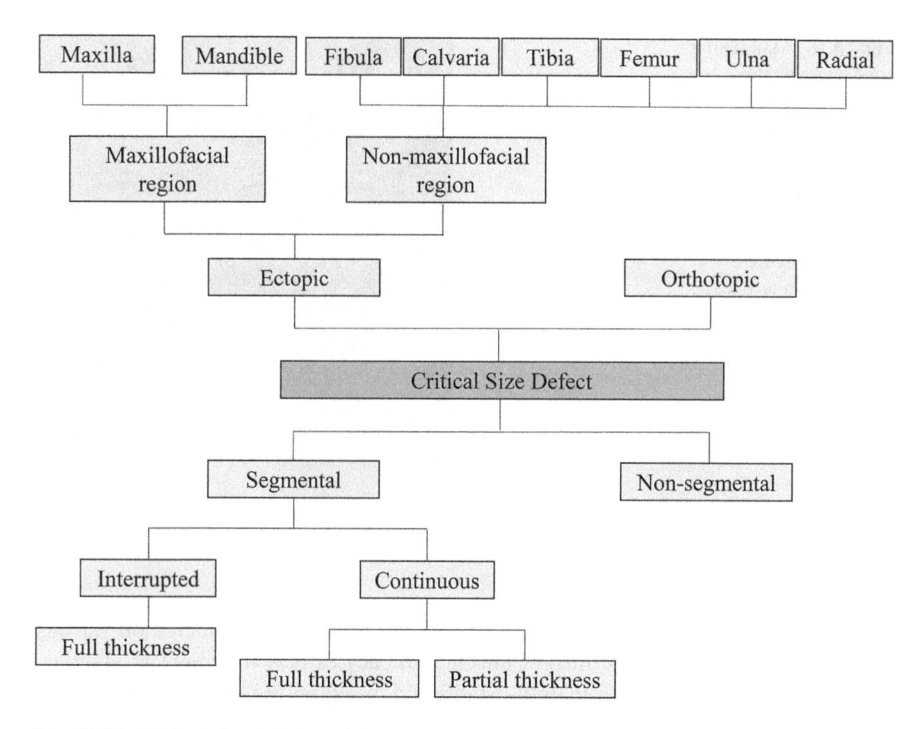


**Fig. 18.17** Critical-size defect model

implants can be properly simulated only with skeletally large animals. The mini-pig model presents several advantages [264]. Due to the convenient size and disposition of the maxillary sinus, the mini-pig features skeletal proportions that allow the use of dental implants of clinically meaningful dimensions. Evaluation of the potential of a biomaterial to enhance bone formation within the sinus cavity can be relatively realistically simulated in rabbits [265–267]. Rabbit maxillary sinuses have a well-defined ostium opening to their nasal cavities and air-pressure measurements that are similar to those in humans [268]. Rabbit was used in maxillary sinus augmentation model in many studies [239, 240, 269]. However, the maxillary sinus of rabbit is small, and its bone physiology and structure differ from that of humans. So bigger animal models, such as beagle dog [66] and sheep [270], were used (Fig. 18.18). Sheep model is a proper model to establish a maxillary sinus augmentation, since it has an easy working disposition, adequate maxillary sinus size, and bone physiology and structure similar to that of humans [196].

Regeneration of atrophied alveolar bone prior to insertion of dental implants is also a major challenge for oral and maxillofacial surgery. In the mandible, the volume of the alveolar ridge may also be reduced to a varying degree as a result of congenital malformations, loss of teeth, or aging [217]. Disease modeling for pathological situation in humans for atrophic jaws can be either simulated by extraction of teeth or/and removal of the buccal bone to create narrow alveolar ridge [217].

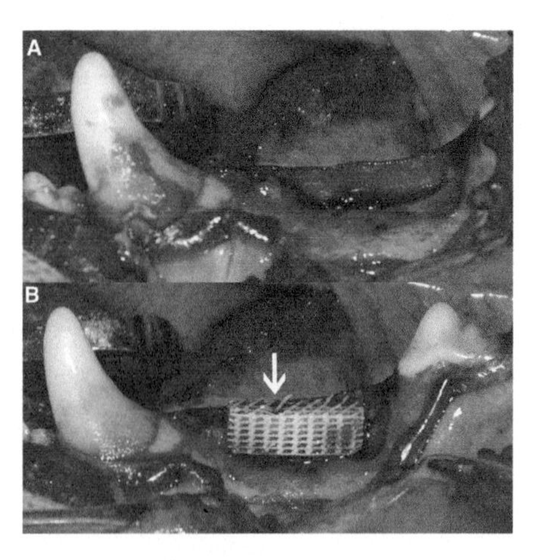


**Fig. 18.18** Mandibular bone augmentation. (**a**) Creating a critical-size vertical defect in posterior mandible area of the dogs; (**b**) fixation of the PCL-TCP blocks to the bone with mini-screw. (Reuse the figure of author's own article; no permission is required) [218]

## *3.5 Orthodontics*

Although the vast number of experimental studies have been conducted on various animal models to gain more insight into the efficacy of new treatment modalities, the orthodontic concepts are mainly established based on the clinical experiences rather than in vivo trials [335]. This is due to the fact that the growth patterns in animals and humans are substantially different [336]. Also, some orthodontics therapies, such as prescription of removable functional appliances, are not applicable in animal models. Besides, the maintenance of appliance for prolonged time in animals is challenging. The orthodontics researched on animal models can be broadly classified into three main categories.

### 3.5.1 Tooth Movement

Orthodontic tooth movement is achieved by remodeling of surrounding alveolar bone during the force application [337]. Bone resorption and bone formation are components of bone remodeling, which take place on the alveolar wall by newly induced osteoblasts on the tension site as well as the activity of osteoclasts in compression site [338]. Modification of the body metabolic state such as diabetes malfunctions or general and local administration of pharmaceutical agents can alter the normal bone remodeling, which consequently influences the rate of tooth movement in animal and clinical studies [339–344]. Besides these factors, some approaches, including photobiomodulation [345], pulsed electromagnetic fields [346], laser irradiation [347], and surgical methods such as corticotomy, cortical bone damage [348], or piezocision [349], have been inspected in terms of bone movement acceleration or inhibition. Such information is imperative for clinicians as the agents could interfere with the biological processes of tooth movement acceleration during

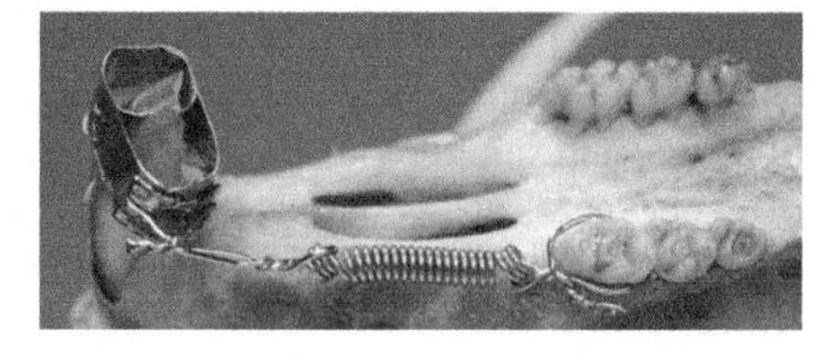

**Fig. 18.19** Lateral view of coil spring located between the molar and incisors of a rat model. (Reuse with permission) [397]

orthodontic treatment or inhibition that is required for anchorage stability or during retention period.

Animal models have been widely used for assessment of bone regeneration during tooth movement. An ideal animal should have the biology and anatomy resembling human body to allow researchers to extrapolate data for patient treatments. Sprague Dawley rats, Wistar rats, and beagle dogs are the most commonly used animal models to investigate tooth movement. In rodent models, the most studied tooth movement is mesial movement of molars and incisor separation (Fig. 18.19). In dogs, the most studied sites are mesiodistal movement of premolars [350].

Disease modeling in animals undergoing tooth drifting can be created by extraction of adjacent teeth to prepare the demanded space for tooth movement [351]. However, in rats or rabbits, molars are located far enough from the incisors, and there are no premolars in between, so there is no need to perform the extract [342, 343]. Rats are broadly utilized for laboratorial experiments due to its practical benefits including being inexpensive and accessible, short time space generation, pasture with omnivorous diet, and availability of antibodies required for cellular and molecular assessments. However, there are some differences in terms of biological responses following tooth movement [352]. Moreover, rat has tiny teeth and its molar is about 50 times smaller than human molars. Therefore, manufacturing and providing smaller device that can be fitted to rat teeth and apply low load with calibrated force is still challenging [350]. Ideal force level in rodent model should not exceed 25 cN, and higher forces are not considered physiologic [353]. It has been stated that force of 10 cN produced in rodents is equivalent to the stress of 80 cN in human canine [354]. Alveolar bone of rats also displays distinct features; it possesses greater bone density without Haversian canals and fewer marrow spaces that undergo massive bone volume (60–70%) reduction subsequent to tooth movement [355]. Besides, rat molars have natural distal drifting with age, and the mesial shifting of molars, which is forced during tooth movement, might be misinterpreted and therefore should be considered [335].

Canine model is also widely used for tooth movement. Compared to the rat, the anatomy, biology, and dentition of canines are more closely resembled to humans. In contrast, rabbits have distinct root structures and jaw bones compared to canine and human [350]. However, they are not accepted for bone investigations since their bone remodeling period is shorter than human bone turnover and changes quickly, i.e., bone remodeling takes place within 6 weeks in rabbits, while in human, it takes 3–6 months [119]. Porcine is the other animal model that serves to aid in learning of tooth movement interferences.

Although primates are the most related species to human in terms of genetics and anatomy, differences such as larger marrow spaces of interradicular and interproximal bone and smaller marrow space of crest alveolar bone, as well as the higher cost of experiment, are generally preclusive and limit their application in preclinical studies [352]. Besides, the application of primates is associated with ethical considerations.

### 3.5.2 Distraction Osteogenesis

Distraction osteogenesis (DO) is a minimally invasive technique in which new bone formation occurs via gradually separated bone segments using incremental traction by an external lengthener. DO has enabled surgeons to achieve great bone movement without the need for soft or hard tissue grafting [356].

There are three phases of DO, which lead to formation of mature bone: (a) latency period in which the generated gap is filled with callus tissue, (b) distraction phase where the traction force is applied, and (c) consolidation phase in which the callus tissue is replaced by mature bone [357].

The main drawback of DO pertains to the prolonged consolidation periods in which the site is susceptible to various complications such as device breakage, infection of device-inserted region, and dislocation of bone segments [358]. Many investigations have been carried out to delineate the optimal methods of accelerating the maturation of bone during consolidation phase and to enhance the quality of regenerated bone using animal models [359].

Rat [358, 360], rabbit [357, 361–366], dog [367–369], sheep, pig [370], and primate [371] have been used for DO. Various methods have been applied in order to evaluate the osteogenesis acceleration or reduction in the corticotomy gap, such as addition of growth factors, stem cells, and scaffolds, administration of pharmaceutical agents systemically or locally to the defect site, or irradiation of laser beam or ultrasonic stimulation [356, 367, 368, 370, 372–375].

In spite of the fact that DO of alveolar bone is indicated for atrophic mandibular or maxillary ridge in the vertical or horizontal directions according to the ridge morphology, most of the in vivo trials have been conducted on animals without deficiency, except for those who created the defect intentionally [371] (Fig. 18.20). Since the DO procedure appears to be more complicated and challenging in maxilla than that of the mandible, majority of animal investigations have been performed on the mandible. In particular, in mandibular areas, the body region for horizontal augmentation has been commonly used, and it is less common to repair the ramus or angle of the lower jaw [368, 376].

The application of DO for membranous bone was initially inspected in the canine model [377], but the rabbit model is the well-established model for exploration of mandibular DO. Rabbits have been introduced as a proper model for learning the physiology of human bone, because they have similar patterns of bone formation and peak mass profile [378].

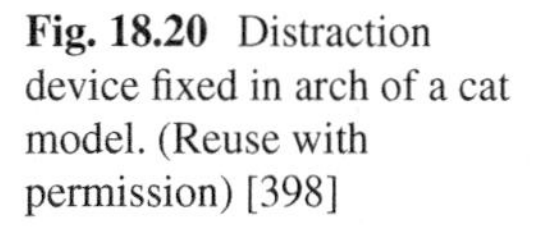

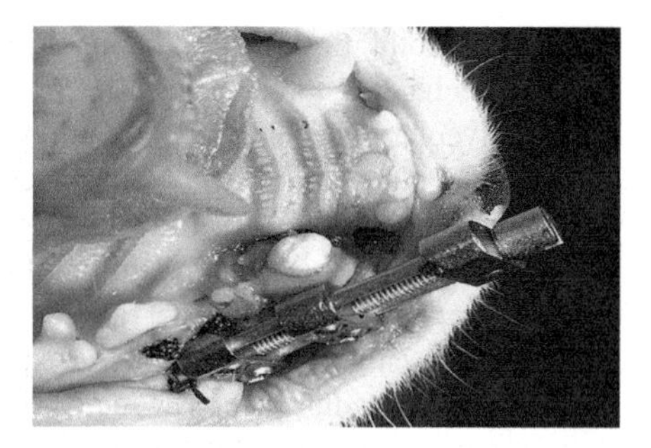

**Fig. 18.20** Distraction device fixed in arch of a cat model. (Reuse with permission) [398]

### 3.5.3 Trans-sutural Expansion of Maxilla

Correction of maxillary constriction in transverse dimension is preferably obtained by expansion of maxilla with rapid palatal expansion and semi-rapid or slow expansion protocols [379]. These treatments are characterized by opening of the midpalatal suture in response to implementation of tension force using a suture expander. The mechanical strain can be applied on the suture through the anchorage of molar teeth or bone, via mini-implants or mini-screw, to activate the biologic chain of events for bone formation, resorption, and fiber rearrangement until the goal is achieved [380]. Secondary cartilage in the midpalatal suture is responsible of the changes following mechanical forces in which the proliferation and differentiation of mesenchymal cells presented in the inner surface of cartilaginous tissue into osteoblasts would be triggered [381, 382]. Rapid maxillary expansion is one of the most popular techniques for maxillary deficit therapies, which has the same mechanism as distraction osteogenesis entitled as trans-sutural distraction osteogenesis and has the same pitfalls such as prolonged retention period to ensure the complete ossification of the suture and to decline the relapse risk of arch width [383]. Many researchers have tried various methods on animal models to overcome the drawbacks prior to translating the data to clinics and to hasten bone regeneration in the suture lesion including agent administrations such as vitamins [384, 385], antioxidants [386, 387], growth factors [388, 389], laser irradiation [383, 390], stem cell-based applications [391], and surgical-assisted therapies [392].

Although most of the preclinical experiments have been performed on animals with normal palatal bone, a practical disease modeling for maxillary constriction has been introduced. Modeling is conducted by mucoperiosteal denudation of palatal bone, which affects the transverse growth of alveolar bone by the formation of scar tissue. Scar tissue causes wound contraction with the contractile tension of myofibroblasts located in the granulation tissue and subsequently inhibits the lateral palatal growth [393].

The rat model is the most popular in animal studies designed for maxillary expansion [394] since it can provide an explicit image of bony and sutural reactions under mechanical forces [390]. As previously mentioned, forces lower than 25 cN can cause tooth movement without affecting the maxillary suture. Continuous heavier mechanical forces lead to necrosis of periodontal ligament and hyalinized zone of alveolar bone and prevent tooth movement, which results in the detachment of the lateral plates of maxilla with the remaining force [395].

Compared with those in rodents, dogs have larger oral cavity volume, which provides easier insertion and retention of expansion screw or devices. This priority and the simpler follow-up observation of these animals have made them an ideal model for investigation of maxillary expansion [334] (Fig. 18.21). Similarly, the size of maxilla in adult sheep is wider and more proper than rodents. Also, the dental arch is more identical to human for schemed treatment [392]. Although different animal models have illustrated beneficial data for clinical application of maxillary expanders, considerations should be taken into account, as the human palate lacks a premaxilla and cartilaginous premaxillary suture, and the tension is only exerted to the mid-palatine suture. Also the posterior part of maxilla is buttressed with zygomaticotemporal complex, which impresses the opening feature of palates [396] and offers comfort and welfare to the animals during the experiments. Although familiarity with the principles of laboratory animal surgery is necessary for researchers, attendance and guidance of pertinent veterinarian are strongly recommended. The following are the momentous notes which should be considered for animal surgeries (Fig. 18.22).

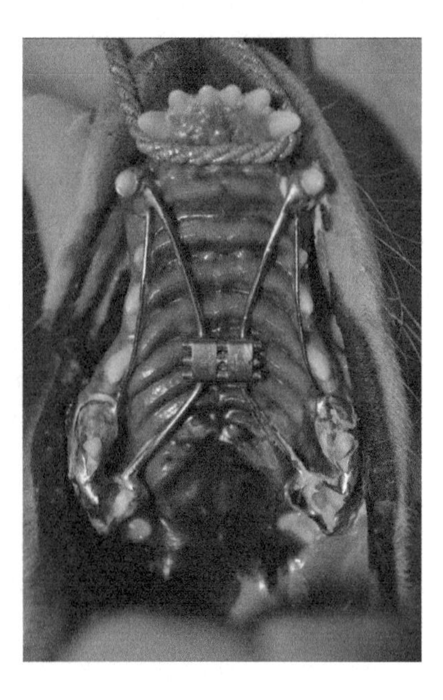

**Fig. 18.21** Magnetic appliance for rapid maxillary expansion in a dog model. (Reuse with permission) [399]

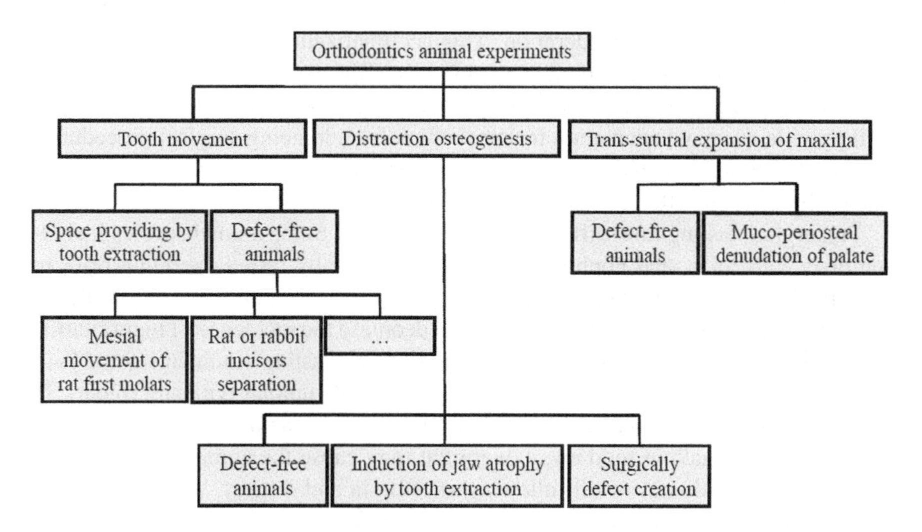


**Fig. 18.22** Animal modeling of orthodontics experiments

# 4 Experimental Procedure and Guidelines

Research involving animal surgery not only focuses on the surgical techniques but also looks at pre- and postoperative managements. In addition to sufficient surgical skills, knowledge of all procedures is essential to guarantee the aseptic results for promoting the success rate of surgery.

## *4.1 Presurgical Preparation*

Only healthy, disease-free animals should be included in an experimental surgery program. So, prior to incorporation of animals in an experimental procedure or surgical plan, their health status should be evaluated. Health evaluation is commonly performed during quarantine period when the animals are set apart from conditioned animals of their own species. In some cases, vaccination or medical histories of individual animals can be beneficial for assessment of animals undergoing surgery. The use of specific pathogen-free (SPF) rodents and rabbits that are available commercially has eliminated the health examinations prior to experiments. In contrast, acquiring random-source animals necessitate their immunization against common infectious diseases and excess conditioning period under the veterinarian recommendations [400, 401]. Following health status assessments, information should be recorded for all animals, especially their precise weight prior to surgery and should be written on the postsurgical cage cards.

A period of conditioning, in which the animal can adapt to the new environment prior to surgery to allow the animal's body system to stabilize to the surrounding conditions, is a crucial consideration. This acclimatization period will reduce the experienced distress by the animal and ensure that the experimental results will not be compromised by environmental impressions. A 1–4-week conditioning period will provide adequate adaptation for most animals undergoing surgical procedures. During this time, animals should be fed a standard diet with tap water ad libitum under climate-controlled conditions [342, 357, 392].

Presurgical fasting time differs for various species. Some animal species including dogs, cats, pigs, and nonhuman primates are usually fasted overnight prior to surgery, and food should not be deprived for more than 12 hours before anesthesia induction. Feed withdrawal for 12 hours will decrease the incidence of regurgitation and aspiration of vomit during general anesthesia. Fasting ruminants for 24–48 hours prior to anesthesia alleviates the occurrence of ruminal tympany (bloat). In contrast, feed deprivation is not requisite for rodents and rabbits since they are nocturnal eaters and taking food away overnight may cause the animal fasting for 24 hours. Also, they do not vomit following anesthesia and surgery. Water should not be withheld prior to surgery in any species to eliminate the risk of dehydration [401, 402].

## *4.2 Surgical Considerations*

Aseptic procedures and sterility are required for all survival surgeries in which animals are expected to recover from anesthesia. Also, prolonged non-survival surgeries that take more than 6 hours in duration must be performed using aseptic techniques. But, since non-survival surgery is infrequent for dentistry experiments, specific issues will not be discussed in the section. Four main areas should be considered for a surgical procedure including surgical work spaces, instruments, surgeon, and animal. Surgery must be conducted in a clean, disinfected, and uncluttered room that is isolated from the preparation or support area.

Surgical instruments should be sanitized and sterilized prior to surgery commencement using pressurized steam (heat sterilization), gas (ethylene oxide), or chemical (cold sterilization) methods. Also, objects inserted into the animal body, such as implants, vascular access ports, and any other devices, must be sterile. Surgeon should have appropriate surgical attire such as shoe covers, surgical face mask, a cap cover, sterile lab coat or gown, and sterile gloves. Although all species undergoing surgery should receive the principals of aseptic technique, special considerations pertain to some species. For instance, surgery on rodents does not always demand full surgical attire. Non-sterile garments could be worn for rodent surgery, albeit, it should be clean and the sleeves should not contact sterile surfaces. Also, sterile instruments and gloves may be reused when performing “multiple-run surgeries” in the same session in which multiple rodents within a related group are undergoing the same procedure. If instruments are planned to be used more than once, they must be disinfected by immersing them in a germicidal solution between animals [401].

Animals are prepared prior to surgery by clipping their hair from the operative site via shaving or administration of depilatory agent to ensure the complete disinfection of surgical zone. It is worthy to note that this procedure should be performed in an area separate from the surgical room, and it is recommended that the loose hair be removed by a vacuum cleaning device [400]. Afterward, the surgical site is scrubbed with appropriate disinfectants such as iodophors or chlorhexidine solutions. Special care must be taken when shaving and disinfecting the operative site of small animals, since they are prone to hypothermia from a wide hair-free zone and by being overwet.

Animal anesthesia and alleviation of surgical pain are crucial concerns of experimental animal surgeries. Accurate dose of anesthesia should be administered to ensure pain sensation blockage and unconsciousness without possessing dangerous effects on animal well-being. Drugs designated for general anesthesia can be delivered as inhalant or injectable anesthetics. Administration of inhaled anesthetics by mask or endotracheal tube is suggested for all species undergoing dentistry researches except for procedures where placement of mask or tube interferes with the surgical interventions. Isoflurane and sevoflurane are commonly used inhalant anesthetic agents delivered in a determined percentage in oxygen via a precision vaporizer. This technique provides rapid induction and fast recovery besides its safety for modulating the depth of anesthesia by just adjusting the percentage of anesthetic gas instead of redosing drug injection which is performed for injectable anesthetics. But pre-emptive analgesia is mandatory when using inhaled anesthetics. For administration of injectable anesthetic drug dose, route administration and injected volume should be carefully decided and calculated due to the animal species, individual weight, and the surgical procedure. Combination of ketamine and α2-agonists, namely, xylazine-dexmedetomidine, is efficiently and routinely administered for induction of general anesthesia in animal models and can provide surgical level of anesthesia up to one and a half hour. To maintain the extent of anesthesia in prolonged surgeries, further doses of ketamine can be imposed during the operation with 30-minute intervals [372]. Injectable anesthetics are regularly injected via intraperitoneal route in small animals such as mice, hamsters, rabbits, and rats since intramuscular injection is restricted due to their small muscle mass. Also, administration of ketamine outside the vein and in muscle can cause tissue necrosis and animal discomfort because of the sting sensation during injection.

Preemptive supplementation of analgesic agents is beneficial to lessen animal pain as the general anesthesia is wearing off. This will help to lower the total amount of required general anesthesia and will prevent sensitization of sensory mechanisms known as ramp-up or wind-up phenomenon. Opioids (buprenorphine and butorphanol) and NSAIDs (meloxicam, carprofen, ketoprofen) are effective analgesics for surgical pain which are administered immediately when the animal has been anesthetized to eliminate the postsurgical pain. Local anesthetics (lidocaine, bupivacaine) can be infiltrated adjuncts to general anesthetic agents to prepare additional analgesic effects for surgery and postoperative period and reduce the redosing need of anesthetics.

Appropriate surgical protocol requires frequent assessment of the physiological condition of the animals to ensure their stable status during surgery. Basic monitoring of cardiovascular system, respiratory system, and body temperature is important, and the depth of anesthesia should be checked at least every 15 minutes. Also, prior to first incision, evaluation of the anesthesia depth is recommended by assessing the animal's responses to a painful stimulus, such as pedal withdrawal reflex (toe pinch) in which the toe or foot is forcefully squeezed with two fingers. Evaluating the respiration pattern is critical, since anesthesia causes slowing of respiratory rate and it is facilitated by the application of transparent drapes. Observing the color of skin parts, such as ear or toe and mucous membrane of conjunctiva or gum, is also useful for monitoring the animal and is considered as an alarm bell for reduced blood oxygenation if the skin becomes bluish. Moreover, the animals under anesthesia lose their thermoregulating ability and are prone to hypothermia. So, maintenance of body temperature throughout surgery and in the recovery time with an external heat support, such as water-supplied heating pads or reusable thermal pads, should be considered. Surgeon should also pay significant attention to fluid demand of animals; since longer-lasting surgeries in which significant blood loss occurs require the electrolyte replacement or blood transfusion in order to prevent hypovolemic shock or dehydration.

## *4.3 Postsurgical Care*

Recovery from anesthesia needs repeated or even continuous monitoring. During immediate postoperative period (acute phase), the animal should move to a warm and dry place; administration of analgesic and supplemental fluid and frequent rotation of animal to avoid lung congestion or bruising should be considered [401]. Animals must be assessed at least every 15 minutes until they are fully recovered (i.e., the animal can keep itself in sternal recumbency, the body temperature and physiological parameters are back to normal and are stabilized, and normal eating and drinking resume). After complete recovery, which animals were kept in an isolated quite room for intensive care, they are moved to an animal-holding room. In the long-term postoperative period (chronic phase), the animals should be monitored daily until the body weight, condition, and activity are stable [401]. Depending on the suture type, it will be removed 7–14 days after surgery when the wound healing is confirmed.

For surgeries that prevent animals from feeding with standardized food in the postoperative period, such as surgeries manipulated in oral cavity or which place appliances in the oral lesion, palatable foods like wet chew or Nutri-Cal gel must be available for the animal.

# 5 Ethical Considerations

The increasing number of animals used in research has drawn an attention to their ethical consideration. One of the important issues is that a researcher properly cares and uses the animals in order to avoid or minimize their pain or distress. Animal research may not be conducted until the research protocol has been reviewed and approved by a local Institutional Animal Care and Use Committee (IACUC). The mission of IACUC is to ensure that the procedures are appropriate and are performed according to the highest standard, animal research complies with animal welfare laws and regulations, and animals are not subject to unnecessary pain and distress [403].

Considering the growing concerns involving the use of animals in biomedical researches, the first step in animal studies is to provide explanation that the research will increase the scientific knowledge in different aspects of medical sciences and could improve the quality of health or welfare of humans or other animals. It is assumed that the scientific purpose of the research has sufficient potential significance to justify the use of animals [403, 404]. Also, the following parameters should be considered in order to design the experiment properly and in accordance with the ethical considerations.

## *5.1 Number of the Animals*

The good experimental design helps to minimize the number of animals used in research. However, a sufficient number of animals must be used to enable precise statistical analysis and results, preventing the repetition of experiments and the consequent need to use more animals [405]. A statistical analysis should be used to justify animal numbers; the goal is not to minimize the number of animals used but to determine the right number of animals for obtaining valid results [403].

## *5.2 Veterinarian Consult*

Consulting with a local veterinarian not only can be helpful in advising the investigators on administration of proper anesthetics, analgesics, and procedures but also can be a legal requirement in some institutions [403].

### 5.3 The Three R's Concepts

In 1959, two pioneers of laboratory animal welfare, William Russell and Rex Burch, defined the principle of the three R's [406]—refinement, reduction, and replacement of animal experiments—and urged all animal researchers to follow this policy in order to minimize animal use and pain or distress while still achieving critical scientific objectives [405, 407–410].

Replacement: Replacing the use of animals with non-animal techniques such as computer models, in vitro culture systems, and microfluidic models.

Reduction: Reducing the number of animals used by using appropriate size to obtain statistically significant data. This may include performing multiple experiments simultaneously so that the same control group can be used.

Refinement: Changing experiments or procedures to reduce pain and distress including refinements in anesthesia, surgery, and analgesia.

### 5.4 Species Choosing

The investigators should have enough justification to choose a specific species. The least sentient species capable of providing the needed data should be used. The previous work in biomedical literatures that validate the use of a particular species in an animal model of a human disease could be helpful.

### 5.5 Euthanasia

It is defined as the act of killing animals by methods that induce rapid unconsciousness and death without pain and distress [403]. Since it is necessary to euthanize most of the animals as part of the experiments, choosing appropriate euthanasia technique is very important in the experimental design. Euthanasia methods can be separated into physical and nonphysical methods. Nonphysical methods such as carbon dioxide inhalation and barbiturate overdose are the most desirable. Physical methods are normally used in conjunction with sedation and anesthesia; examples include exsanguination and decapitation [403]. Consultation with veterinarian would be beneficial to choose the appropriate methods on euthanasia.

### 5.6 Pain and Distress

Pain and distress in animals are defined as procedures that would cause pain or distress in a human [403]. Most institutions require the investigators to assign animals to categories based on the level of pain/distress. In order to prevent unnecessary pain and distress endpoint criteria including euthanizing an animal, discontinuation of painful procedures and removal of animals from a study should be considered.

### 5.7 The Pilot Study

Administration of the pilot study can be used to refine the techniques. Also, it demonstrates the feasibility of the given experiments and provides a justification with larger experiments.

### 5.8 Training

Investigators should ensure that all personnel involving an animal study receive essential instructions in experimental methods and in the care, maintenance, and handling of the species being studied. Besides they should be familiar with ethical guidelines by IACUC. Therefore, adequate training is an important aspect of the refinement of animal research and should be reviewed and improved [403]. Many institutions provide courses for animal care and use in research and education, which is designed to train important issues in animal research [403].

## 6 Future Perspectives

The conclusive goal of all biomedical researches is to understand either human development process or the physiopathology of human disease, which helps to provide new and more effective diagnosis, prevention, and therapeutic approach. Animal models are introduced to achieve this goal. However, there are major differences between animal models and humans in terms of molecular and cellular mechanisms, as well as diseases phenotype [411]. These discrepancies are the most important reasons for increasing number of animal models and even failure in many clinical trials [411].

This issue, as well as ethical concerns associated with use of animals in biomedical sciences, encouraged investigators and engineers to present a functional and effective tissue- and organ-level structure to understand human development and pathophysiology of disease and provide new method of diagnosis and prevention.

On the most acceptable structure as an alternative is microfluidic (or microfabrication) technology, which has made a remarkable progress in the past decade [412]. The combination of microfluidic technologies and biological sciences resulted in advancement of both in vitro and in vivo studies. Also by using this technology, studies can be conducted under controlled physiologically appropriate condition.

Microfluidic systems provide the ability to control multiple factors at the same time, connecting different culture chambers and evaluation in 3D microenvironment. Also, analysis can be done in a real-time manner [411, 413].

There is a type of microfluidic system called organ-an-a-chip or disease models-on-chip [414]. These systems tend to mimic in vivo scenarios and represent one of the most promising approaches for various engineered disease models, such as heart disease, asthma, inherited metabolic liver disorder, polycystic kidney disease, bone marrow niche, and atherosclerosis and cancer metastasis [415–421]. Unfortunately, the use of microfluidic systems to diagnose and treat oral and maxillofacial diseases, as well as understanding of teeth development, is associated with a little progress.

Wahhida Shumi and colleagues showed the effect of environmental factors, such as sucrose and metal ions on streptococcus mutant attachment and biofilm formation in a microfluidic device packed with glass bead to simulate the interproximal space [422] (Fig. 18.23b). Furthermore, other studies performed by this research group in 2013 evaluated the effect of shear stress in *S. mutans* aggregation in microfluidic funnel device (μFFD). They suggested that the in vitro condition was successfully mimicked and suitable for in situ monitoring of oral biofilms in both studies [423] (Fig. 18.23a).

William C. Nance et al. designed a high-throughput microfluidic system that was combined with a confocal laser scanning microscope to quantitatively evaluate the effectiveness of cetylpyridinium chloride (CPC) against oral multi-species biofilm grown in human saliva [424].

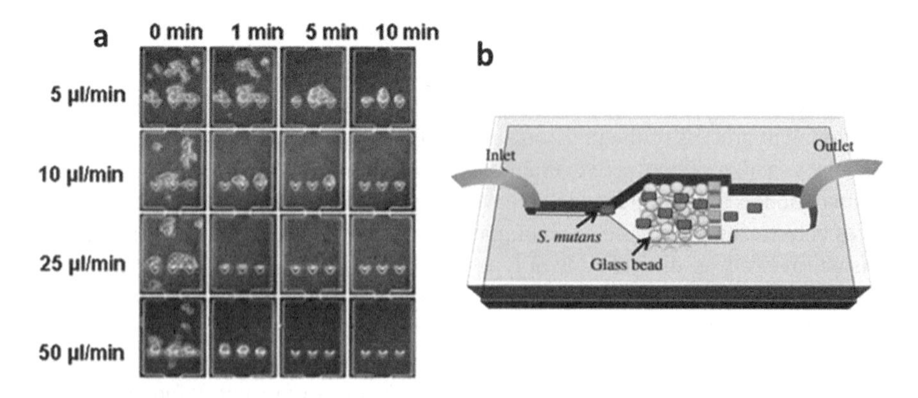


**Fig. 18.23** (**a**) Representative image of adherent aggregates on the funnels microfluidic device (μFFD). (Reuse with permission) [423]. (**b**) Microfluidic device packed with glass beads for oral biofilm formation. (Reuse with permission) [422]

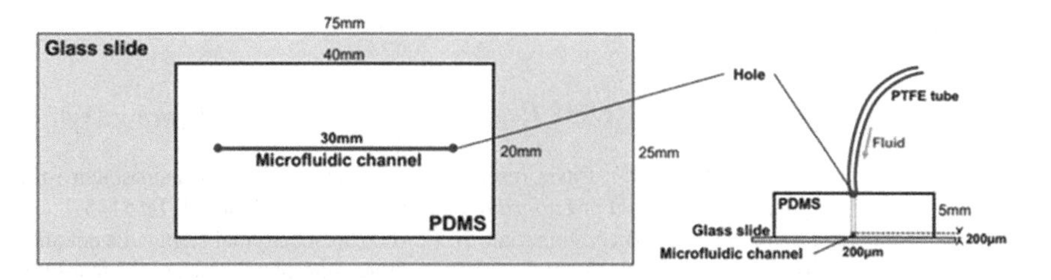


**Fig. 18.24** Dimensions of the microfluidic chip and channel. PDMS polydimethylsiloxane, PTFE polytetrafluoroethylene. (Reuse with permission) [426]

The newest high-throughput microfluidic system was introduced by Raymond H.W. Lam and colleagues, which was called artificial teeth device. This system provided extended application for general biofilm research, including screening of the biofilm properties developing under combinations of specified growth parameters, such as seeding bacteria population, growth medium compositions, medium flow rates, and dissolved gas levels [425].

One of the applications of the microfluidic systems is the introduction of the new diagnostic methods. Dobyun Kim et al. simulated arteriole blood flow within dental pulp in the microfluidic system for the measurement of pulpal blood flow in human teeth via Doppler ultrasound devices [426] (Fig. 18.24).

Also, the microfluidic system has been used for evaluation of teeth development. P. Pagella and colleagues evaluated the usefulness of a microfluidic system for co-culturing mouse trigeminal ganglia and molars. They suggested that this system provided a valuable tool to study the behavior of neurons during the development of orofacial organs [427]. The next study performed by Kyung-Jung Kang et al. determined that stem cells from human exfoliated deciduous teeth were incubated in the concentration gradient of media cultured with human gingival fibroblast and periodontal ligament stem cells in the microfluidic device system [428].

As noted above, a number of studies on the use of microfluidic systems in dentistry are limited. Microfluidic system has a great potential to mimic the normal and abnormal human tissue and organs and can provide a new form of personalized medicine, engineering tissue, and cell therapy. Moreover, numerous challenges, such as study of embryonic development of teeth, can be conducted through microfluidic system and microfabrication.

# 7 Conclusion

Animal selection for in vivo experiments in the field of dentistry is of great importance regarding the different anatomy, physiology, tissue architecture, and healing responses in various species. This chapter presents the specific features and applications of different animals that can be used for dental research.

## References


1. Melby, E. C., & Altman, N. H. (1974). *Handbook of laboratory animal science* (Vol. 2). Cleveland: CRC Press Inc.
2. Mogensen, J., & Holm, S. (1989). Basic research and animal models in neuroscience-the necessity of. *Scandinavian Journal of Laboratory Animal Science, 16*(Suppl. 1), 51–57.
3. Khojasteh, A., Eslaminejad, M. B., & Nazarian, H. (2008). Mesenchymal stem cells enhance bone regeneration in rat calvarial critical size defects more than platelete-rich plasma. *Oral Surgery, Oral Medicine, Oral Pathology, Oral Radiology, and Endodontics, 106*(3), 356–362.
4. Rezai-Rad, M., et al. (2015). Evaluation of bone regeneration potential of dental follicle stem cells for treatment of craniofacial defects. *Cytotherapy, 17*(11), 1572–1581.
5. Oz, H. S., & Puleo, D. A. (2011). Animal models for periodontal disease. *BioMed Research International, 2011*, 754857.
6. Veltman, J. A., & Brunner, H. G. (2012). De novo mutations in human genetic disease. *Nature Reviews Genetics, 13*(8), 565.
7. Paine, M. L., et al. (2003). A transgenic animal model resembling amelogenesis imperfecta related to ameloblastin overexpression. *Journal of Biological Chemistry, 278*(21), 19447–19452.
8. Page, R. C., & Schroeder, H. E. (1982). *Periodontitis in man and other animals. A comparative review*. Basel/New York: S. Karger.
9. Gong, T., et al. (2016). Current advance and future prospects of tissue engineering approach to dentin/pulp regenerative therapy. *Stem Cells International, 2016*, 9204574.
10. Kim, S., et al. (2015). In vivo experiments with dental pulp stem cells for pulp-dentin complex regeneration. *Mediators of Inflammation, 2015*, 409347.
11. Kodonas, K., et al. (2012). Experimental formation of dentin-like structure in the root canal implant model using cryopreserved swine dental pulp progenitor cells. *Journal of Endodontics, 38*(7), 913–919.
12. Yang, X., et al. (2009). Mineralized tissue formation by BMP2-transfected pulp stem cells. *Journal of Dental Research, 88*(11), 1020–1025.
13. Ruangsawasdi, N., et al. (2016). Regenerative dentistry: Animal model for regenerative endodontology. *Transfusion Medicine and Hemotherapy, 43*(5), 359–364.
14. da Silva, L. A. B., et al. (2010). Revascularization and periapical repair after endodontic treatment using apical negative pressure irrigation versus conventional irrigation plus triantibiotic intracanal dressing in dogs' teeth with apical periodontitis. *Oral Surgery, Oral Medicine, Oral Pathology, Oral Radiology and Endodontology, 109*(5), 779–787.
15. Yamauchi, N., et al. (2011). Tissue engineering strategies for immature teeth with apical periodontitis. *Journal of Endodontics, 37*(3), 390–397.
16. Yamauchi, N., et al. (2011). Immunohistological characterization of newly formed tissues after regenerative procedure in immature dog teeth. *Journal of Endodontics, 37*(12), 1636–1641.
17. Tawfik, H., et al. (2013). Regenerative potential following revascularization of immature permanent teeth with necrotic pulps. *International Endodontic Journal, 46*(10), 910–922.
18. Londero, C. L. D., et al. (2015). Histologic analysis of the influence of a gelatin-based scaffold in the repair of immature dog teeth subjected to regenerative endodontic treatment. *Journal of Endodontics, 41*(10), 1619–1625.
19. Torabinejad, M., et al. (2015). Histologic examination of teeth with necrotic pulps and periapical lesions treated with 2 scaffolds: An animal investigation. *Journal of Endodontics, 41*(6), 846–852.
20. Zuong, X.-Y., et al. (2010). Pulp revascularization of immature anterior teeth with apical periodontitis. *Hua xi kou qiang yi xue za zhi = Huaxi kouqiang yixue zazhi = West China Journal of Stomatology, 28*(6), 672–674.
21. Thibodeau, B., et al. (2007). Pulp revascularization of immature dog teeth with apical periodontitis. *Journal of Endodontics, 33*(6), 680–689.

22. Zhu, X., et al. (2018). A miniature swine model for stem cell-based de novo regeneration of dental pulp and dentin-like tissue. *Tissue Engineering - Part C: Methods, 24*(2), 108–120.
23. da Silva, L. A. B., et al. (2010). Revascularization and periapical repair after endodontic treatment using apical negative pressure irrigation versus conventional irrigation plus triantibiotic intracanal dressing in dogs' teeth with apical periodontitis. *Oral Surgery, Oral Medicine, Oral Pathology, Oral Radiology, and Endodontics, 109*(5), 779–787.
24. Zhu, W., et al. (2013). Regeneration of dental pulp tissue in immature teeth with apical periodontitis using platelet-rich plasma and dental pulp cells. *International Endodontic Journal, 46*(10), 962–970.
25. Saoud, T. M. A., et al. (2015). Histological observations of pulpal replacement tissue in immature dog teeth after revascularization of infected pulps. *Dental Traumatology, 31*(3), 243–249.
26. Khademi, A. A., et al. (2014). Outcomes of revascularization treatment in immature dog's teeth. *Dental Traumatology, 30*(5), 374–379.
27. Yoo, Y.-J., et al. (2014). Effect of conditioned medium from preameloblasts on regenerative cellular differentiation of the immature teeth with necrotic pulp and apical periodontitis. *Journal of Endodontics, 40*(9), 1355–1361.
28. Zhang, D.-D., et al. (2014). Histologic comparison between platelet-rich plasma and blood clot in regenerative endodontic treatment: An animal study. *Journal of Endodontics, 40*(9), 1388–1393.
29. Altaii, M., et al. (2017). Endodontic regeneration and tooth revitalization in immature infected sheep teeth. *International Endodontic Journal, 50*(5), 480–491.
30. Hale, F. A. (2009). Dental caries in the dog. *The Canadian Veterinary Journal, 50*(12), 1301.
31. Kaiser, T. M., et al. (2013). Hypsodonty and tooth facet development in relation to diet and habitat in herbivorous ungulates: Implications for understanding tooth wear. *Mammal Review, 43*(1), 34–46.
32. Sahara, N. (2014). Development of coronal cementum in hypsodont horse cheek teeth. *The Anatomical Record, 297*(4), 716–730.
33. Torabinejad, M., & Bakland, L. K. (1978). An animal model for the study of immunopathogenesis of periapical lesions. *Journal of Endodontics, 4*(9), 273–277.
34. Torabinejad, M., et al. (2014). Histologic examinations of teeth treated with 2 scaffolds: A pilot animal investigation. *Journal of Endodontics, 40*(4), 515–520.
35. Altaii, M., et al. (2016). Standardisation of sheep model for endodontic regeneration/revitalisation research. *Archives of Oral Biology, 65*, 87–94.
36. Del Fabbro, M., et al. (2016). Autologous platelet concentrates for pulp and dentin regeneration: A literature review of animal studies. *Journal of Endodontics, 42*(2), 250–257.
37. Albuquerque, M., et al. (2014). Tissue-engineering-based strategies for regenerative endodontics. *Journal of Dental Research, 93*(12), 1222–1231.
38. Katsamakis, S., et al. (2013). Histological responses of the periodontium to MTA: A systematic review. *Journal of Clinical Periodontology, 40*(4), 334–344.
39. Holland, G. J. (1992). Periapical innervation of the ferret canine one year after pulpectomy. *Journal of Dental Research, 71*(3), 470–474.
40. Masson, E., Hennet, P. R., & Calas, P. L. (1992). Apical root canal anatomy in the dog. *Dental Traumatology, 8*(3), 109–112.
41. Holland, G. (1984). Periapical response to apical plugs of dentin and calcium hydroxide in ferret canines. *Journal of Endodontics, 10*(2), 71–74.
42. Gorrel, C., & Derbyshire, S. (2004). Anatomy of the teeth and periodontium. In *Veterinary dentistry for the general practitioner* (pp. 29–33). Philadelphia: Saunders.
43. Taii, A., & Hamed M. T. (2016). Investigations on the suitability of sheep as a model for endodontic revitalisation research (Doctoral dissertation).
44. Nevins, A. J., et al. (1976). Revitalization of pulpless open apex teeth in rhesus monkeys, using collagen-calcium phosphate gel. *Journal of Endodontia, 2*(6), 159–165.

45. Petrovic, V., Pejcic, N., & Cakic, S. (2013). The influence of different therapeutic modalities and platelet rich plasma on apexogenesis: A preliminary study in monkeys. *Advances in Clinical and Experimental Medicine, 22*(4), 469–479.
46. Panzarini, S. R., et al. (2007). Mineral trioxide aggregate as a root canal filling material in reimplanted teeth. Microscopic analysis in monkeys. *Dental Traumatology, 23*(5), 265–272.
47. Addison, W. H., & Appleton, J., Jr. (1915). The structure and growth of the incisor teeth of the albino rat. *Journal of Morphology, 26*(1), 43–96.
48. Farris, E. J., & Griffith, J. Q., Jr. (1949). *The rat in laboratory investigation*. Philadelphia: J. B. Lippincott.
49. Hemming, J. E. (1969). Cemental deposition, tooth succession, and horn development as criteria of age in Dall sheep. *The Journal of Wildlife Management, 33*, 552–558.
50. Rod Salter, B. (2007). Rabbit and rodent dentistry. In *World Small Animal Veterinary Association World Congress Proceeding*. Melborne Veterinary Referral Centre, Glen Waverley, Australia.
51. Milella, L. (2006). Oral and dental conditions in ferrets. *Companion Animal, 11*(4), 74–77.
52. Ia, S. (1963) The ageing of domestic animals. In *Science in archaeology: A comprehensive survey of progress and research*. Basic Books. Thames and Hudson. London. p. 250–268.
53. Wang, S., et al. (2007). The miniature pig: A useful large animal model for dental and orofacial research. *Oral Diseases, 13*(6), 530–537.
54. Nissen, H. W., & Riesen, A. H. (1964). The eruption of the permanent dentition of chimpanzee. *American Journal of Physical Anthropology, 22*(3), 285–294.
55. Rouge, M. Dental anatomy. Hypertexts for Biomedical Sciences.
56. Ghoddusi, J., et al. (2017). Histological evaluation of the effect of platelet-rich plasma on pulp regeneration in nonvital open apex teeth: An animal study. *The Journal of Contemporary Dental Practice, 18*(11), 1045–1050.
57. Östby, B. N. (1961). The role of the blood clot in endodontic therapy an experimental histologic study. *Acta Odontologica Scandinavica, 19*(3-4), 323–353.
58. Nygaard-Östby, B., & Hjortdal, O. (1971). Tissue formation in the root canal following pulp removal. *European Journal of Oral Sciences, 79*(3), 333–349.
59. Damle, S. G., Bhattal, H., & Loomba, A. (2012). Apexification of anterior teeth: A comparative evaluation of mineral trioxide aggregate and calcium hydroxide paste. *The Journal of Clinical Pediatric Dentistry, 36*(3), 263–268.
60. Diogenes, A., et al. (2013). An update on clinical regenerative endodontics. *Endodontic Topics, 28*(1), 2–23.
61. Nosrat, A., & Asgary, S. (2010). Apexogenesis treatment with a new endodontic cement: A case report. *Journal of Endodontics, 36*(5), 912–914.
62. Witherspoon, D. E. (2008). Vital pulp therapy with new materials: New directions and treatment perspectives—Permanent teeth. *Journal of Endodontics, 34*(7), S25–S28.
63. Rafter, M. (2005). Apexification: A review. *Dental Traumatology, 21*(1), 1–8.
64. Katebzadeh, N., Dalton, B. C., & Trope, M. (1998). Strengthening immature teeth during and after apexification. *Journal of Endodontia, 24*(4), 256–259.
65. Scarparo, R. K., et al. (2011). Response to intracanal medication in immature teeth with pulp necrosis: An experimental model in rat molars. *Journal of Endodontics, 37*(8), 1069–1073.
66. Wang, S., et al. (2010). Systematic evaluation of a tissue-engineered bone for maxillary sinus augmentation in large animal canine model. *Bone, 46*(1), 91–100.
67. Mori, G. G., Poi, W. R., & Castilho, L. R. (2013). Evaluation of the anti-resorptive ability of an experimental acetazolamide paste for the treatment of late replanted teeth: A study in rats. *Dental Traumatology, 29*(1), 34–40.
68. Wilson, G. J. (1998). Atlas of the radiographic closure of the apices of the teeth of the dog. School of Veterinary Science, The University of Queensland.
69. Watanabe, K., et al. (2001). The formation of apical delta of the permanent teeth in dogs. *Journal of Veterinary Medical Science, 63*(7), 789–795.

70. Goldberg, M., et al. (2014). Comparative studies between mice molars and incisors are required to draw an overview of enamel structural complexity. *Frontiers in Physiology, 5*, 359.
71. Corrêa, A. P. S., et al. (2017). Histomorphometric analysis of the healing process after the replantation of rat teeth maintained in bovine milk whey and whole milk. *Dental Traumatology, 33*(6), 472–481.
72. Barbizam, J. V., et al. (2015). Histopathological evaluation of the effects of variable extraoral dry times and enamel matrix proteins (enamel matrix derivatives) application on replanted dogs' teeth. *Dental Traumatology, 31*(1), 29–34.
73. Longo, D. L., et al. (2018). Efficiency of different storage media for avulsed teeth in animal models: A systematic review. *Dental Traumatology : Official Publication of International Association for Dental Traumatology, 34*(1), 12–19.
74. Citrome, G. P., Kaminski, E. J., & Heuer, M. A. (1979). A comparative study of tooth apexification in the dog. *Journal of Endodontics, 5*(10), 290–297.
75. Heydari, A., et al. (2016). The effect of root coating with titanium on prevention of root resorption in avulsed teeth: An animal study. *Iranian Endodontic Journal, 11*(4), 309.
76. Shabestari, L., Taylor, G., & Angus, W. (1967). Dental eruption pattern of the beagle. *Journal of Dental Research, 46*(1), 276–278.
77. McNamara, J. A., Jr., Foster, D. L., & Rosenstein, B. D. (1977). Eruption of the deciduous dentition in the rhesus monkey. *Journal of Dental Research, 56*(6), 701–701.
78. Bindal, P., et al. (2017). Dental pulp tissue engineering and regenerative endodontic therapy. In *Biomaterials for oral and dental tissue engineering* (pp. 297–318). San Diego: Elsevier.
79. Zhao, Y.-H., et al. (2013). The combined use of cell sheet fragments of periodontal ligament stem cells and platelet-rich fibrin granules for avulsed tooth reimplantation. *Biomaterials, 34*(22), 5506–5520.
80. Palma, P. J., et al. (2017). Histologic evaluation of regenerative endodontic procedures with the use of chitosan scaffolds in immature dog teeth with apical periodontitis. *Journal of Endodontics, 43*(8), 1279–1287.
81. Pihlstrom, B. L., Michalowicz, B. S., & Johnson, N. W. (2005). Periodontal diseases. *The Lancet, 366*(9499), 1809–1820.
82. Newman, M. G., et al. (2011). *Carranza's clinical periodontology*. St. Louis: Elsevier Health Sciences.
83. Kinane, D. F. (2001). Causation and pathogenesis of periodontal disease. *Periodontology 2000, 25*(1), 8–20.
84. Kämmerer, P. W., et al. (2017). Guided bone regeneration using collagen scaffolds, growth factors, and periodontal ligament stem cells for treatment of peri-implant bone defects in vivo. *Stem Cells International, 2017, 1-9.*
85. Shanbhag, S., et al. (2018). Bone tissue engineering in oral peri-implant defects in preclinical in vivo research: A systematic review and meta-analysis. *Journal of Tissue Engineering and Regenerative Medicine, 12*(1), e336–e349.
86. Ramos, U. D., et al. (2017). Comparison between two antimicrobial protocols with or without guided bone regeneration in the treatment of peri-implantitis. A histomorphometric study in dogs. *Clinical Oral Implants Research, 28*(11), 1388–1395.
87. Carcuac, O., & Berglundh, T. (2014). Composition of human peri-implantitis and periodontitis lesions. *Journal of Dental Research, 93*(11), 1083–1088.
88. Hernández-Monjaraz, B., et al. (2018). Mesenchymal stem cells of dental origin for inducing tissue regeneration in periodontitis: A mini-review. *International Journal of Molecular Sciences, 19*(4), 944.
89. Liu, Y., et al. (2008). Periodontal ligament stem cell-mediated treatment for periodontitis in miniature swine. *Stem Cells, 26*(4), 1065–1073.
90. Kantarci, A., Hasturk, H., & Van Dyke, T. E. (2015). Animal models for periodontal regeneration and peri-implant responses. *Periodontology 2000, 68*(1), 66–82.

91. Graves, D. T., et al. (2008). The use of rodent models to investigate host–bacteria interactions related to periodontal diseases. *Journal of Clinical Periodontology, 35*(2), 89–105.
92. Socransky, S., Hubersak, C., & Propas, D. (1970). Induction of periodontal destruction in gnotobiotic rats by a human oral strain of Actinomyces naeslundii. *Archives of Oral Biology, 15*(10), 993–IN13.
93. Fawzy El-Sayed, K. M., & Dörfer, C. E. (2017). Animal models for periodontal tissue engineering: A knowledge-generating process. *Tissue Engineering Part C: Methods, 23*(12), 900–925.
94. Sugaya, A., et al. (1990). Effects on wound healing of tricalcium phosphate-collagen complex implants in periodontal osseous defects in the dog. *Journal of Periodontal Research, 25*(1), 60–63.
95. Lindhe, J., et al. (1995). The effect of flap management and bioresorbable occlusive devices in GTR treatment of degree III furcation defects. *Journal of Clinical Periodontology, 22*(4), 276–283.
96. Madden, T. E., & Caton, J. G. (1994). Animal models for periodontal disease. *Methods in Enzymology*, 235, 106–119. Elsevier.
97. Lindhe, J., & Ericsson, I. (1978). Effect of ligature placement and dental plaque on periodontal tissue breakdown in the dog. *Journal of Periodontology, 49*(7), 343–350.
98. Kimura, S., et al. (2000). Induction of experimental periodontitis in mice with *Porphyromonas gingivalis*-adhered ligatures. *Journal of Periodontology, 71*(7), 1167–1173.
99. Meng, H., Xie, H., & Chen, Z. (1996). Evaluation of ligature-induced periodontitis in minipig. *Zhonghua kou qiang yi xue za zhi= Zhonghua kouqiang yixue zazhi= Chinese journal of stomatology, 31*(6), 333–336.
100. Baer, P. N., Stephan, R. M., & White, C. L. (1961). Studies on experimental calculus formation in the rat I. Effect of age, sex, strain, high carbohydrate, high protein diets. *Journal of Periodontology, 32*(3), 190–196.
101. Egelberg, J. (1965). Local effect of diet on plaque formation and development of gingivitis in dogs. I. Effect of hard and soft diets. *Odontologisk Revy, 16*, 31.
102. Shklar, G. (1966). Periodontal disease in experimental animals subjected to chronic cold stress. *Journal of Periodontology, 37*(5), 377–383.
103. Haney, J. M., Zimmerman, G. J., & Wikesjö, U. M. (1995). Periodontal repair in dogs: Evaluation of the natural disease model. *Journal of Clinical Periodontology, 22*(3), 208–213.
104. Lalla, E., et al. (2000). Blockade of RAGE suppresses periodontitis-associated bone loss in diabetic mice. *The Journal of Clinical Investigation, 105*(8), 1117–1124.
105. Cao, Y., et al. (2015). Adenovirus-mediated transfer of hepatocyte growth factor gene to human dental pulp stem cells under good manufacturing practice improves their potential for periodontal regeneration in swine. *Stem Cell Research & Therapy, 6*(1), 249.
106. Suaid, F. F., et al. (2011). Autologous periodontal ligament cells in the treatment of class II furcation defects: A study in dogs. *Journal of Clinical Periodontology, 38*(5), 491–498.
107. Schwarz, F., et al. (2015). Animal models for peri-implant mucositis and peri-implantitis. *Periodontology 2000, 68*(1), 168–181.
108. Zhang, T., et al. (2010). Aggregatibacter actinomycetemcomitans accelerates atherosclerosis with an increase in atherogenic factors in spontaneously hyperlipidemic mice. *FEMS Immunology and Medical Microbiology, 59*(2), 143–151.
109. Jain, A., et al. (2003). Role for periodontitis in the progression of lipid deposition in an animal model. *Infection and Immunity, 71*(10), 6012–6018.
110. Stübinger, S., & Dard, M. (2013). The rabbit as experimental model for research in implant dentistry and related tissue regeneration. *Journal of Investigative Surgery, 26*(5), 266–282.
111. Stadlinger, B., et al. (2012). Systematic review of animal models for the study of implant integration, assessing the influence of material, surface and design. *Journal of Clinical Periodontology, 39*(s12), 28–36.
112. Yamasaki, A., et al. (1979). Ultrastructure of the junctional epithelium of germfree rat gingiva. *Journal of Periodontology, 50*(12), 641–648.

113. Listgarten, M. A. (1975). Similarity of epithelial relationships in the gingiva of rat and man. *Journal of Periodontology, 46*(11), 677–680.
114. Heijl, L., et al. (1980). Periodontal disease in gnotobiotic rats. *Journal of Periodontal Research, 15*(4), 405–419.
115. Weinberg, M. A., & Bral, M. (1999). Laboratory animal models in periodontology. *Journal of Clinical Periodontology, 26*(6), 335–340.
116. Struillou, X., et al. (2010). Experimental animal models in periodontology: A review. *The Open Dentistry Journal, 4*, 37.
117. Jordan, H., & Keyes, P. (1964). Aerobic, gram-positive, filamentous bacteria as etiologic agents of experimental periodontal disease in hamsters. *Archives of Oral Biology, 9*(4), 401–IN11.
118. Harper, D., Mann, P., & Regnier, S. (1990). Measurement of dietary and dentifrice effects upon calculus accumulation rates in the domestic ferret. *Journal of Dental Research, 69*(2), 447–450.
119. Pearce, A., et al. (2007). Animal models for implant biomaterial research in bone: A review. *European Cells & Materials, 13*(1), 1–10.
120. Lindhe, J., Hamp, S. E., & Löe, H. (1973). Experimental periodontitis in the beagle dog. *Journal of Periodontal Research, 8*(1), 1–10.
121. Kornman, K., et al. (1981). The predominant cultivable subgingival flora of beagle dogs following ligature placement and metronidazole therapy. *Journal of Periodontal Research, 16*(3), 251–258.
122. Ericsson, I., et al. (1975). Experimental periodontal breakdown in the dog. *Scandinavian Journal of Dental Research, 83*(3), 189–192.
123. Schroeder, H., & Attström, R. (1979). Effect of mechanical plaque control on development of subgingival plaque and initial gingivitis in neutropenic dogs. *European Journal of Oral Sciences, 87*(4), 279–287.
124. Sculean, A., Chapple, I. L., & Giannobile, W. V. (2015). Wound models for periodontal and bone regeneration: The role of biologic research. *Periodontology 2000, 68*(1), 7–20.
125. Schwarz, F., Sager, M., & Becker, J. (2011). Peri-implantitis defect model. Osteology guidelines for oral and maxillofacial regenerations. Preclinical models for translational research. *Quintessence*, 211(10), 1–56.
126. Giannobile, W. V., Finkelman, R. D., & Lynch, S. E. (1994). Comparison of canine and non-human primate animal models for periodontal regenerative therapy: Results following a single administration of PDGF/IGF-I. *Journal of Periodontology, 65*(12), 1158–1168.
127. Gould, T., Robertson, P., & Oakley, C. (1992). Effect of free gingival grafts on naturally-occurring recession in miniature swine. *Journal of Periodontology, 63*(7), 593–597.
128. Mosekilde, L., et al. (1993). Calcium-restricted ovariectomized Sinclair S-1 minipigs: An animal model of osteopenia and trabecular plate perforation. *Bone, 14*(3), 379–382.
129. Schou, S., Holmstrup, P., & Kornman, K. S. (1993). Non-human primates used in studies of periodontal disease pathogenesis: A review of the literature. *Journal of Periodontology, 64*(6), 497–508.
130. Ammons, W. F., Schectman, L. R., & Page, R. C. (1972). Host tissue response in chronic periodontal disease. *Journal of Periodontal Research, 7*(2), 131–143.
131. Caton, J. G., & Kowalski, C. J. (1976). Primate model for testing periodontal treatment procedures: II. Production of contralaterally similar lesions. *Journal of Periodontology, 47*(9), 506–510.
132. Martines, R. T., et al. (2008). Sandblasted/acid-etched vs smooth-surface implants: Implant mobility and clinical reaction to experimentally induced peri-implantitis in Beagle dogs. *The Journal of Oral Implantology, 34*(4), 185–189.
133. Zechner, W., et al. (2004). Histomorphometrical and clinical comparison of submerged and nonsubmerged implants subjected to experimental peri-implantitis in dogs. *Clinical Oral Implants Research, 15*(1), 23–33.

134. Leonhardt, Å., et al. (1992). Putative periodontal and teeth in pathogens on titanium implants and teeth in experimental gingivitis and periodontitis in beagle dogs. *Clinical Oral Implants Research, 3*(3), 112–119.
135. Berglundh, T., et al. (2007). Spontaneous progression of ligature induced peri-implantitis at implants with different surface roughness: An experimental study in dogs. *Clinical Oral Implants Research, 18*(5), 655–661.
136. Albouy, J. P., et al. (2009). Spontaneous progression of ligatured induced peri-implantitis at implants with different surface characteristics. An experimental study in dogs II: Histological observations. *Clinical Oral Implants Research, 20*(4), 366–371.
137. Kozlovsky, A., et al. (2007). Impact of implant overloading on the peri-implant bone in inflamed and non-inflamed peri-implant mucosa. *Clinical Oral Implants Research, 18*(5), 601–610.
138. Gotfredsen, K., Berglundh, T., & Lindhe, J. (2002). Bone reactions at implants subjected to experimental peri-implantitis and static load. *Journal of Clinical Periodontology, 29*(2), 144–151.
139. Cook, S., & Rust-Dawicki, A. (1995). In vivo evaluation of CSTi dental implants in the presence of ligature-induced peri-implantitis. *The Journal of Oral Implantology, 21*(3), 191–200.
140. Hanisch, O., et al. (1997). Experimental peri-implant tissue breakdown around hydroxyapatite-coated implants. *Journal of Periodontology, 68*(1), 59–66.
141. Lang, N., et al. (1994). Histologic probe penetration in healthy and inflamed peri-implant tissues. *Clinical Oral Implants Research, 5*(4), 191–201.
142. Martins, M. C., et al. (2004). Experimental peri-implant tissue breakdown around different dental implant surfaces: Clinical and radiographic evaluation in dogs. *The International Journal of Oral & Maxillofacial Implants*, 19(6), 839–848.
143. Martins, M. C., et al. (2005). Progression of experimental chronic peri-implantitis in dogs: Clinical and radiographic evaluation. *Journal of Periodontology, 76*(8), 1367–1373.
144. Nociti, F. H., et al. (2001). Clinical and microbiological evaluation of ligature-induced peri-implantitis and periodontitis in dogs. *Clinical Oral Implants Research, 12*(4), 295–300.
145. Schwarz, F., et al. (2007). Comparison of naturally occurring and ligature-induced peri-implantitis bone defects in humans and dogs. *Clinical Oral Implants Research, 18*(2), 161–170.
146. Sennerby, L., et al. (2005). Implant stability during initiation and resolution of experimental periimplantitis: An experimental study in the dog. *Clinical Implant Dentistry and Related Research, 7*(3), 136–140.
147. Shibli, J. A., et al. (2003). Microbiologic and radiographic analysis of ligature-induced peri-implantitis with different dental implant surfaces. *The International Journal of Oral & Maxillofacial Implants, 18*(3), 383–390.
148. Shibutani, T., et al. (2001). Bisphosphonate inhibits alveolar bone resorption in experimentally-induced peri-implantitis in dogs. *Clinical Oral Implants Research, 12*(2), 109–114.
149. Tillmanns, H. W., et al. (1998). Evaluation of three different dental implants in ligature-induced peri-implantitis in the beagle dog. Part II. Histology and microbiology. *International Journal of Oral and Maxillofacial Implants, 13*(1), 59–68.
150. Weber, H., et al. (1994). Inhibition of peri-implant bone loss with the nonsteroidal anti-inflammatory drug flurbiprofen in beagle dogs. A preliminary study. *Clinical Oral Implants Research, 5*(3), 148–153.
151. Zitzmann, N., et al. (2004). Spontaneous progression of experimentally induced periimplantitis. *Journal of Clinical Periodontology, 31*(10), 845–849.
152. Albouy, J. P., et al. (2011). Implant surface characteristics influence the outcome of treatment of peri-implantitis: An experimental study in dogs. *Journal of Clinical Periodontology, 38*(1), 58–64.
153. Deppe, H., et al. (2002). Titanium deposition after peri-implant care with the carbon dioxide laser. *The International Journal of Oral & Maxillofacial Implants*, 17(5), 707–714.

154. Deppe, H., et al. (2001). Peri-implant care of ailing implants with the carbon dioxide laser. *The International Journal of Oral & Maxillofacial Implants*, 16(5), 659–667.
155. Ericsson, I., et al. (1996). The effect of antimicrobial theram on peri-implantitis lesions. An experimental study in the dog. *Clinical Oral Implants Research, 7*(4), 320–328.
156. Grunder, U., et al. (1993). Treatment of ligature-induced peri-implantitis using guided tissue regeneration: A clinical and histologic study in the beagle dog. *The International Journal of Oral & Maxillofacial Implants, 8*(3), 282–293.
157. Hayek, R. R., et al. (2005). Comparative study between the effects of photodynamic therapy and conventional therapy on microbial reduction in ligature-induced peri-implantitis in dogs. *Journal of Periodontology, 76*(8), 1275–1281.
158. Hürzeler, M. B., et al. (1995). Treatment of peri-implantitis using guided bone regeneration and bone grafts, alone or in combination, in beagle dogs. Part 1: Clinical findings and histologic observations. *The International Journal of Oral & Maxillofacial Implants, 10*(4), 474–484.
159. Hürzeler, M. B., et al. (1997). Treatment of peri-implantitis using guided bone regeneration and bone grafts, alone or in combination, in beagle dogs. Part 2: Histologic findings. *The International Journal of Oral & Maxillofacial Implants, 12*(2), 168–175.
160. Jovanovic, S. A., et al. (1993). The regenerative potential of plaque-induced peri-implant bone defects treated by a submerged membrane technique: An experimental study. *The International Journal of Oral & Maxillofacial Implants, 8*(1), 13–18.
161. Machado, M., et al. (1999). Treatment of ligature-induced peri-implantitis defects by regenerative procedures: A clinical study in dogs. *Journal of Oral Science, 41*(4), 181–185.
162. Marinello, C., et al. (1995). Resolution of ligature-induced peri-implantitis lesions in the dog. *Journal of Clinical Periodontology, 22*(6), 475–479.
163. Nociti, F. H., Jr., et al. (2000). Evaluation of guided bone regeneration and/or bone grafts in the treatment of ligature-induced peri-implantitis defects: A morphometric study in dogs. *The Journal of Oral Implantology, 26*(4), 244–249.
164. Nociti, F. H., et al. (2001). Absorbable versus nonabsorbable membranes and bone grafts in the treatment of ligature-induced peri-implantitis defects in dogs. *Clinical Oral Implants Research, 12*(2), 115–120.
165. Parlar, A., et al. (2009). Effects of decontamination and implant surface characteristics on re-osseointegration following treatment of peri-implantitis. *Clinical Oral Implants Research, 20*(4), 391–399.
166. Persson, L. G., et al. (2001). Re-osseointegration after treatment of peri-implantitis at different implant surfaces. *Clinical Oral Implants Research, 12*(6), 595–603.
167. Persson, L., et al. (1996). Guided bone regeneration in the treatment of peri-implantitis. *Clinical Oral Implants Research, 7*(4), 366–372.
168. Persson, L., et al. (2001). Osseintegration following treatment of peri-implantitis and replacement of implant components. *Journal of Clinical Periodontology, 28*(3), 258–263.
169. Persson, L. G., et al. (2004). Carbon dioxide laser and hydrogen peroxide conditioning in the treatment of periimplantitis: An experimental study in the dog. *Clinical Implant Dentistry and Related Research, 6*(4), 230–238.
170. Schüpbach, P., Hürzeler, M., & Grunder, U. (1994). Implant-tissue interfaces following treatment of peri-implantitis using guided tissue regeneration. A light and electron microscopic study. *Clinical Oral Implants Research, 5*(2), 55–65.
171. Schwarz, F., et al. (2011). Surgical therapy of advanced ligature-induced peri-implantitis defects: Cone-beam computed tomographic and histological analysis. *Journal of Clinical Periodontology, 38*(10), 939–949.
172. Shibli, J. A., et al. (2003). Lethal photosensitization in microbiological treatment of ligature-induced peri-implantitis: A preliminary study in dogs. *Journal of Oral Science, 45*(1), 17–23.
173. Shibli, J. A., et al. (2006). Lethal photosensitization and guided bone regeneration in treatment of peri-implantitis: An experimental study in dogs. *Clinical Oral Implants Research, 17*(3), 273–281.

174. Shibli, J. A., et al. (2003). Treatment of ligature-induced peri-implantitis by lethal photosensitization and guided bone regeneration: A preliminary histologic study in dogs. *Journal of Periodontology, 74*(3), 338–345.
175. Stübinger, S., et al. (2005). Bone regeneration after pen-implant care with the CO 2 laser: A fluorescence microscopy study. *The International Journal of Oral & Maxillofacial Implants, 20*(2), 103–210.
176. You, T.-M., et al. (2007). Treatment of experimental peri-implantitis using autogenous bone grafts and platelet-enriched fibrin glue in dogs. *Oral Surgery, Oral Medicine, Oral Pathology, Oral Radiology, and Endodontics, 103*(1), 34–37.
177. Akagawa, Y., et al. (1993). Changes of subgingival microflora around single-crystal sapphire endosseous implants after experimental ligature-induced plaque accumulation in monkeys. *The Journal of Prosthetic Dentistry, 69*(6), 594–598.
178. Eke, P. I., Braswell, L. D., & Fritz, M. E. (1998). Microbiota associated with experimental peri-implantitis and periodontitis in adult Macaca mulatta monkeys. *Journal of Periodontology, 69*(2), 190–194.
179. Hanisch, O., et al. (1997). Bone formation and reosseointegration in peri-implantitis defects following surgical implantation of rhBMP-2. *The International Journal of Oral & Maxillofacial Implants, 12*(5), 785–792.
180. Hürzeler, M. B., et al. (1998). Changes in peri-implant tissues subjected to orthodontic forces and ligature breakdown in monkeys. *Journal of Periodontology, 69*(3), 396–404.
181. Lang, N., et al. (1993). Ligature-induced peri-implant infection in cynomolgus monkeys. Clinical and radiographic findings. *Clinical Oral Implants Research, 4*(1), 2–11.
182. Schou, S., et al. (1993). Ligature-induced marginal inflammation around osseointegrated implants and ankylosed teeth. Clinical and radiographic observations in cynomolgus monkeys (Macaca fascicularis). *Clinical Oral Implants Research, 4*(1), 12–22.
183. Schou, S., et al. (2002). Probing around implants and teeth with healthy or inflamed peri-implant mucosa/gingiva. *Clinical Oral Implants Research, 13*(2), 113–126.
184. Warrer, K., et al. (1995). Plaque-induced peri-implantitis in the presence or absence of keratinized mucosa. An experimental study in monkeys. *Clinical Oral Implants Research, 6*(3), 131–138.
185. Schou, S., et al. (1996). Microbiology of ligature-induced marginal inflammation around osseointegrated implants and ankylosed teeth in cynomolgus monkeys Macaca fascicularis. *Clinical Oral Implants Research, 7*(3), 190–200.
186. Fritz, M. E., et al. (1997). Experimental Peri-Implantitis in Consecutively Placed, Loaded Root-Form and Plate-Form Implants in Adult Macaca mulatta Monkeys. *Journal of Periodontology, 68*(11), 1131–1135.
187. Schou, S., et al. (2003). Anorganic porous bovine-derived bone mineral (Bio-Oss®) and ePTFE membrane in the treatment of peri-implantitis in cynomolgus monkeys. *Clinical Oral Implants Research, 14*(5), 535–547.
188. Schou, S., et al. (2003). Implant surface preparation in the surgical treatment of experimental peri-implantitis with autogenous bone graft and ePTFE membrane in cynomolgus monkeys. *Clinical Oral Implants Research, 14*(4), 412–422.
189. Schou, S., et al. (2003). Autogenous bone graft and ePTFE membrane in the treatment of peri-implantitis. I. Clinical and radiographic observations in cynomolgus monkeys. *Clinical Oral Implants Research, 14*(4), 391–403.
190. Hickey, J. S., et al. (1991). Microbiologic characterization of ligature-induced peri-implantitis in the microswine model. *Journal of Periodontology, 62*(9), 548–553.
191. Singh, G., et al. (1993). Surgical treatment of induced peri-implantitis in the micro pig: Clinical and histological analysis. *Journal of Periodontology, 64*(10), 984–989.
192. Coyac, B. R., et al. (2018). Periodontal reconstruction by heparan sulfate mimetic-based matrix therapy in Porphyromonas gingivalis-infected mice. *Heliyon, 4*(8), e00719.
193. Iwata, T., et al. (2009). Periodontal regeneration with multi-layered periodontal ligament-derived cell sheets in a canine model. *J Biomaterials, 30*(14), 2716–2723.

194. Liu, R., et al. (2018). In vitro and in vivo studies of anti-bacterial copper-bearing titanium alloy for dental application. *Dental Materials*, 34(8), 11112–1126.
195. Salata, L., et al. (2007). Osseointegration of oxidized and turned implants in circumferential bone defects with and without adjunctive therapies: An experimental study on BMP-2 and autogenous bone graft in the dog mandible. *The International Journal of Oral & Maxillofacial Surgery, 36*(1), 62–71.
196. Liu, N., et al. (2014). Animal models for craniofacial reconstruction by stem/stromal cells. *Current Stem Cell Research & Therapy, 9*(3), 174–186.
197. Bhumiratana, S., et al. (2016). Tissue-engineered autologous grafts for facial bone reconstruction. *Science Translational Medicine, 8*(343), 343ra83–343ra83.
198. Shanbhag, S., et al. (2017) Alveolar bone tissue engineering in critical-size defects of experimental animal models: a systematic review and meta-analysis. *Journal of tissue engineering and regenerative medicine, 11*(10), 2935–2949.
199. Peric, M., et al. (2015). The rational use of animal models in the evaluation of novel bone regenerative therapies. *Bone, 70*, 73–86.
200. Houshmand, B., et al. (2011). Simvastatin and lovastatin induce ectopic bone formation in rat subcutaneous tissue. *Journal of Periodontology & Implant Dentistry, 2*(1), 12–16.
201. Mortazavi, S. H., et al. (2009). The effect of fluoxetine on bone regeneration in rat calvarial bone defects. *Oral Surgery, Oral Medicine, Oral Pathology, Oral Radiology, and Endodontics, 108*(1), 22–27.
202. Stavropoulos, A., et al. (2015). Pre-clinical in vivo models for the screening of bone biomaterials for oral/craniofacial indications: Focus on small-animal models. *Periodontology 2000, 68*(1), 55–65.
203. Eslaminejad, M. B., et al. (2008). In vivo bone formation by canine mesenchymal stem cells loaded onto HA/TCP scaffolds: Qualitative and quantitative analysis. *Yakhteh, 10*(3), 205–212.
204. Eslaminejad, M. B., et al. (2007). Enhancing ectopic bone formation in canine masseter muscle by loading mesenchymal stem cells onto natural bovine bone minerals. *Iranian Journal of Veterinary Surgery (IJVS), 2*(4), 25–35.
205. Götz, C., Warnke, P. H., & Kolk, A. (2015). Current and future options of regeneration methods and reconstructive surgery of the facial skeleton. *Oral Surgery, Oral Medicine, Oral Pathology, Oral Radiology, 120*(3), 315–323.
206. Corbella, S., et al. (2016). Histomorphometric outcomes after lateral sinus floor elevation procedure: A systematic review of the literature and meta-analysis. *Clinical Oral Implants Research, 27*(9), 1106–1122.
207. Fretwurst, T., et al. (2015). Dentoalveolar reconstruction: Modern approaches. *Current Opinion in Otolaryngology & Head and Neck Surgery, 23*(4), 316–322.
208. Nkenke, E., & Neukam, F. W. (2014). Autogenous bone harvesting and grafting in advanced jaw resorption: Morbidity, resorption and implant survival. *European Journal of Oral Implantology, 7*(Suppl 2), S203–S217.
209. Al-Nawas, B., & Schiegnitz, E. (2014). Augmentation procedures using bone substitute materials or autogenous bone—a systematic review and meta-analysis. *European Journal of Oral Implantology, 7*(Suppl 2), S219–S234.
210. Milinkovic, I., & Cordaro, L. (2014). Are there specific indications for the different alveolar bone augmentation procedures for implant placement? A systematic review. *International Journal of Oral and Maxillofacial Surgery, 43*(5), 606–625.
211. Reichert, J. C., et al. (2009). The challenge of establishing preclinical models for segmental bone defect research. *Biomaterials, 30*(12), 2149–2163.
212. Gugala, Z., R.W. Lindsey, and S. Gogolewski. New approaches in the treatment of critical-size segmental defects in long bones. In *Macromolecular symposia*. 2007. Wiley Online Library.
213. Li, Y., et al. (2015). Bone defect animal models for testing efficacy of bone substitute biomaterials. *The Journal of Orthopaedic Translation, 3*(3), 95–104.

214. Schmitz, J. P., & Hollinger, J. O. (1986). The critical size defect as an experimental model for craniomandibulofacial nonunions. *Clinical Orthopaedics and Related Research*, Apr(205), 299–308.
215. Bosch, C., Melsen, B., & Vargervik, K. (1998). Importance of the critical-size bone defect in testing bone-regenerating materials. *The Journal of Craniofacial Surgery, 9*(4), 310–316.
216. Ernst, M., et al. (2012). Evidence of bone remodeling in the rabbit jaw. Poster session presented at the AADR/CADR annual meeting & exhibition.
217. Gjerde, C., et al. (2017). Autologous porcine bone marrow mesenchymal cells for reconstruction of a resorbed alveolar bone: A preclinical model in mini-pigs. *International Journal of Stem cell Research & Therapy, 3*, 050.
218. Khojasteh, A., et al. (2013). The effect of PCL-TCP scaffold loaded with mesenchymal stem cells on vertical bone augmentation in dog mandible: A preliminary report. *Journal of Biomedical Materials Research Part B: Applied Biomaterials, 101*(5), 848–854.
219. Lopez, M. J. (2014). Bench to bedside: It's all about the model. *Stem Cell Research & Therapy, 5*(1), 11.
220. Khojasteh, A., et al. (2017). Bone engineering in dog mandible: Coculturing mesenchymal stem cells with endothelial progenitor cells in a composite scaffold containing vascular endothelial growth factor. *Journal of Biomedical Materials Research Part B: Applied Biomaterials, 105*(7), 1767–1777.
221. Tricker, N. (2002). Cortical bone turnover and mineral apposition in dentate bone mandible. In Bridging the gap between dental and orthopedic implants. Proceedings of the 3rd annual Indiana conference, 12–16 May 1998. School of Dentistry, Indiana University.
222. Khojasteh, A., et al. (2018). Antibody-mediated osseous regeneration for bone tissue engineering in canine segmental defects. *BioMed Research International, 2018, 1-10.*
223. Huja, S. S., et al. (2006). Remodeling dynamics in the alveolar process in skeletally mature dogs. *The Anatomical Record, 288*(12), 1243–1249.
224. Mardas, N., et al. (2014). Experimental model for bone regeneration in oral and cranio-maxillo-facial surgery. *Journal of Investigative Surgery, 27*(1), 32–49.
225. Willie, B. M., et al. (2004). Determining relevance of a weight-bearing ovine model for bone ingrowth assessment. *Journal of Biomedical Materials Research Part A, 69*(3), 567–576.
226. Koh, K. S., et al. (2018). Bone regeneration using silk hydroxyapatite hybrid composite in a rat alveolar defect model. *International Journal of Medical Sciences, 15*(1), 59.
227. Chierici, G., Harvold, E., & Dawson, W. (1970). Morphologic adaptations secondary to the production of experimental cleft palate in primates. *The Cleft Palate Journal, 7*, 59–67.
228. Dalia, E.-B., et al. (1993). New technique for creating permanent experimental alveolar clefts in a rabbit model. *The Cleft Palate-Craniofacial Journal, 30*(6), 542–547.
229. Jonsson, G., & Stenström, S. (1978). Maxillary growth after palatal surgery: An experimental study on dogs. *Scandinavian Journal of Plastic and Reconstructive Surgery, 12*(2), 131–137.
230. Quarto, N., et al. (2010). Origin matters: Differences in embryonic tissue origin and Wnt signaling determine the osteogenic potential and healing capacity of frontal and parietal calvarial bones. *Journal of Bone and Mineral Research, 25*(7), 1680–1694.
231. Ichikawa, Y., et al. (2015). Differences in the developmental origins of the periosteum may influence bone healing. *Journal of Periodontal Research, 50*(4), 468–478.
232. Liebschner, M. A. (2004). Biomechanical considerations of animal models used in tissue engineering of bone. *Biomaterials, 25*(9), 1697–1714.
233. Bagi, C. M., Berryman, E., & Moalli, M. R. (2011). Comparative bone anatomy of commonly used laboratory animals: Implications for drug discovery. *Comparative Medicine, 61*(1), 76–85.
234. Wang, S., et al. (2015). Comprehensive evaluation of cryopreserved bone-derived osteoblasts for the repair of segmental mandibular defects in canines. *Clinical Implant Dentistry and Related Research, 17*(4), 798–810.
235. Schliephake, H., et al. (2001). Use of cultivated osteoprogenitor cells to increase bone formation in segmental mandibular defects: An experimental pilot study in sheep. *International Journal of Oral and Maxillofacial Surgery, 30*(6), 531–537.

236. Chanchareonsook, N., et al. (2014). Segmental mandibular bone reconstruction with a carbonate-substituted hydroxyapatite-coated modular endoprosthetic poly (ε-caprolactone) scaffold in Macaca fascicularis. *Journal of Biomedical Materials Research Part B: Applied Biomaterials, 102*(5), 962–976.
237. Zhao, J., et al. (2009). Apatite-coated silk fibroin scaffolds to healing mandibular border defects in canines. *Bone, 45*(3), 517–527.
238. Wei, J., et al. (2011). Growth of Schwann cells in silk fibroin scaffolds with different pore sizes. *Journal of Clinical Rehabilitative Tissue Engineering Research, 15*(25), 4607–4610.
239. Xia, L., et al. (2011). Maxillary sinus floor elevation using BMP-2 and Nell-1 gene-modified bone marrow stromal cells and TCP in rabbits. *Calcified Tissue International, 89*(1), 53–64.
240. Sun, X.-J., et al. (2010). Maxillary sinus floor elevation using a tissue engineered bone complex with BMP-2 gene modified bMSCs and a novel porous ceramic scaffold in rabbits. *Archives of Oral Biology, 55*(3), 195–202.
241. Scarano, A., et al. (2017). Bone regeneration induced by bone porcine block with bone marrow stromal stem cells in a minipig model of mandibular "Critical Size" defect. *Stem Cells International, 2017, 1-9.*
242. Saka, B., et al. (2002). Experimental and comparative study of the blood supply to the mandibular cortex in Göttingen minipigs and in man. *Journal of Cranio-Maxillofacial Surgery, 30*(4), 219–225.
243. Ruehe, B., et al. (2009). Miniature pigs as an animal model for implant research: Bone regeneration in critical-size defects. *Oral Surgery, Oral Medicine, Oral Pathology, Oral Radiology, and Endodontics, 108*(5), 699–706.
244. Kamal, M., et al. (2017). Bone regeneration using composite non-demineralized xenogenic dentin with beta-tricalcium phosphate in experimental alveolar cleft repair in a rabbit model. *Journal of Translational Medicine, 15*(1), 263.
245. Ad De, R., et al. (2011). β-TCP versus autologous bone for repair of alveolar clefts in a goat model. *The Cleft Palate-Craniofacial Journal, 48*(6), 654–662.
246. Chung, V. H.-Y., et al. (2012). Engineered autologous bone marrow mesenchymal stem cells: Alternative to cleft alveolar bone graft surgery. *The Journal of Craniofacial Surgery, 23*(5), 1558–1563.
247. Caballero, M., et al. (2015). Juvenile swine surgical alveolar cleft model to test novel autologous stem cell therapies. *Tissue Engineering Part C: Methods, 21*(9), 898–908.
248. Xu, Y., Sun, J., & Chen, Z. (2015). Establishment of a rat model for alveolar cleft with bone wax. *Journal of Oral and Maxillofacial Surgery, 73*(4), 733. e1–733. e10.
249. Sawada, Y., et al. (2009). A trial of alveolar cleft bone regeneration by controlled release of bone morphogenetic protein: An experimental study in rabbits. *Oral Surgery, Oral Medicine, Oral Pathology, Oral Radiology, and Endodontics, 108*(6), 812–820.
250. Papadopoulos, M. A., et al. (2006). Three-dimensional cephalometric evaluation of maxillary growth following in utero repair of cleft lip and alveolar-like defects in the mid-gestational sheep model. *Fetal Diagnosis and Therapy, 21*(1), 105–114.
251. Koo, S.-H., et al. (2001). The transforming growth factor-β3 knock-out mouse: An animal model for cleft palate. *Plastic and Reconstructive Surgery, 108*(4), 938–947.
252. Wolf, Z. T., et al. (2014). A LINE-1 insertion in DLX6 is responsible for cleft palate and mandibular abnormalities in a canine model of Pierre Robin sequence. *PLoS Genetics, 10*(4), e1004257.
253. Caballero, M., et al. (2017). Tissue engineering strategies to improve osteogenesis in the juvenile swine alveolar cleft model. *Tissue Engineering Part C: Methods, 23*(12), 889–899.
254. De Ruiter, A., et al. (2015). Micro-structured beta-tricalcium phosphate for repair of the alveolar cleft in cleft lip and palate patients: A pilot study. *The Cleft Palate-Craniofacial Journal, 52*(3), 336–340.
255. Van Der Donk, S., et al. (2001). Similarity of bone ingrowth in rats and goats: A bone chamber study. *Comparative Medicine, 51*(4), 336–340.
256. Muschler, G. F., et al. (2010). The design and use of animal models for translational research in bone tissue engineering and regenerative medicine. *Tissue Engineering Part B: Reviews, 16*(1), 123–145.

257. Diewert, V. M., & Lozanoff, S. (2002). Animal models of facial clefting: Experimental, congenital, and transgenic. In *Understanding craniofacial anomalies* (pp. 251–272). Hoboken: Wiley.
258. Wilson, J. B., et al. (1993). Transgenic mouse model of X-linked cleft palate. *Cell Growth & Differentiation: The Molecular Biology Journal of the American Association for Cancer Research, 4*, 67.
259. Maddox, B. K., et al. (1998). Craniofacial and otic capsule abnormalities in a transgenic mouse strain with a Col2a1 mutation. *Journal of Craniofacial Genetics and Developmental Biology, 18*(4), 195–201.
260. Yon, J., et al. (2015). Pre-clinical evaluation of the osteogenic potential of bone morphogenetic protein-2 loaded onto a particulate porcine bone biomaterial. *Journal of Clinical Periodontology, 42*(1), 81–88.
261. Schlegel, K. A., et al. (2003). Histologic findings in sinus augmentation with autogenous bone chips versus a bovine bone substitute. *The International Journal of Oral & Maxillofacial Implants, 18*(1), 53–58.
262. Terheyden, H., et al. (1999). Sinus floor augmentation with simultaneous placement of dental implants using a combination of deproteinized bone xenografts and recombinant human osteogenic protein-l. A histometric study in miniature pigs. *Clinical Oral Implants Research, 10*(6), 510–521.
263. Philipp, A., et al. (2014). Comparison of SLA® or SLActive® implants placed in the maxillary sinus with or without synthetic bone graft materials–an animal study in sheep. *Clinical Oral Implants Research, 25*(10), 1142–1148.
264. Susin, C., et al. (2017). Sinus augmentation using a mini-pig model: Effect of ceramic and allogeneic bone biomaterials. *Journal of Clinical Periodontology*.
265. Asai, S., Shimizu, Y., & Ooya, K. (2002). Maxillary sinus augmentation model in rabbits: Effect of occluded nasal ostium on new bone formation. *Clinical Oral Implants Research, 13*(4), 405–409.
266. Lambert, F., et al. (2011). Influence of space-filling materials in subantral bone augmentation: Blood clot vs. autogenous bone chips vs. bovine hydroxyapatite. *Clinical Oral Implants Research, 22*(5), 538–545.
267. Xu, H., et al. (2004). Grafting of deproteinized bone particles inhibits bone resorption after maxillary sinus floor elevation. *Clinical Oral Implants Research, 15*(1), 126–133.
268. Scharf, K. E., et al. (1995). Pressure measurements in the normal and occluded rabbit maxillary sinus. *The Laryngoscope, 105*(6), 570–574.
269. Xia, L., et al. (2011). Maxillary sinus floor elevation using a tissue-engineered bone with rhBMP-2-loaded porous calcium phosphate cement scaffold and bone marrow stromal cells in rabbits. *Cells, Tissues, Organs, 194*(6), 481–493.
270. Grageda, E., et al. (2005). Bone formation in the maxillary sinus by using platelet-rich plasma: An experimental study in sheep. *The Journal of Oral Implantology, 31*(1), 2–17.
271. Walsh, W. R., et al. (2008). β-TCP bone graft substitutes in a bilateral rabbit tibial defect model. *Biomaterials, 29*(3), 266–271.
272. Calvo-Guirado, J., et al. (2012). Retracted: Histomorphometric and mineral degradation study of Ossceram®: A novel biphasic B-tricalcium phosphate, in critical size defects in rabbits. *Clinical Oral Implants Research, 23*(6), 667–675.
273. Komaki, H., et al. (2006). Repair of segmental bone defects in rabbit tibiae using a complex of β-tricalcium phosphate, type I collagen, and fibroblast growth factor-2. *Biomaterials, 27*(29), 5118–5126.
274. Gauthier, O., et al. (2005). In vivo bone regeneration with injectable calcium phosphate biomaterial: A three-dimensional micro-computed tomographic, biomechanical and SEM study. *Biomaterials, 26*(27), 5444–5453.
275. Wang, X. L., et al. (2013). Exogenous phytoestrogenic molecule icaritin incorporated into a porous scaffold for enhancing bone defect repair. *Journal of Orthopaedic Research, 31*(1), 164–172.

276. Liu, Y., et al. (2014). An animal experimental study of porous magnesium scaffold degradation and osteogenesis. *Brazilian Journal of Medical and Biological Research, 47*(8), 715–720.
277. Chen, S.-h., et al. (2014). Comparative study of poly (lactic-co-glycolic acid)/tricalcium phosphate scaffolds incorporated or coated with osteogenic growth factors for enhancement of bone regeneration. *The Journal of Orthopaedic Translation, 2*(2), 91–104.
278. Kokubo, S., et al. (2003). Bone regeneration by recombinant human bone morphogenetic protein-2 and a novel biodegradable carrier in a rabbit ulnar defect model. *Biomaterials, 24*(9), 1643–1651.
279. Kim, H.-W., et al. (2008). Bone formation on the apatite-coated zirconia porous scaffolds within a rabbit calvarial defect. *Journal of Biomaterials Applications, 22*(6), 485–504.
280. Lee, E.-H., et al. (2010). A combination graft of low-molecular-weight silk fibroin with Choukroun platelet-rich fibrin for rabbit calvarial defect. *Oral Surgery, Oral Medicine, Oral Pathology, Oral Radiology, and Endodontics, 109*(5), e33–e38.
281. Jiang, X., et al. (2006). The use of tissue-engineered bone with human bone morphogenetic protein-4-modified bone-marrow stromal cells in repairing mandibular defects in rabbits. *International Journal of Oral and Maxillofacial Surgery, 35*(12), 1133–1139.
282. Wei, J., et al. (2015). Enhanced osteogenic behavior of ADSCs produced by deproteinized antler cancellous bone and evidence for involvement of ERK signaling pathway. *Tissue Engineering Part A, 21*(11-12), 1810–1821.
283. Su, F., et al. (2015). Enhancement of periodontal tissue regeneration by transplantation of osteoprotegerin-engineered periodontal ligament stem cells. *Stem Cell Research & Therapy, 6*(1), 22.
284. Saad, K. A.-E., et al. (2015). Evaluation of the role of autogenous bone-marrow–derived mesenchymal stem cell transplantation for the repair of mandibular bone defects in rabbits. *Journal of Cranio-Maxillo-Facial Surgery, 43*(7), 1151–1160.
285. Park, J.-B., et al. (2013). Establishment of the chronic bone defect model in experimental model mandible and evaluation of the efficacy of the mesenchymal stem cells in enhancing bone regeneration. *Journal of Tissue Engineering and Regenerative Medicine, 10*(1), 18–24.
286. Zhang, C., et al. (2001). Replacement of segmental bone defects using porous bioceramic cylinders: A biomechanical and X-ray diffraction study. *Journal of Biomedical Materials Research Part A, 54*(3), 407–411.
287. Bruder, S. P., et al. (1998). The effect of implants loaded with autologous mesenchymal stem cells on the healing of canine segmental bone defects. *The Journal of Bone & Joint Surgery, 80*(7), 985–996.
288. Sarsilmaz, F., et al. (2007). A polyethylene-high proportion hydroxyapatite implant and its investigation in vivo. *Acta of Bioengineering and Biomechanics, 9*(2), 9.
289. Grundel, R., et al. (1991). Autogeneic bone marrow and porous biphasic calcium phosphate ceramic for segmental bone defects in the canine ulna. *Clinical Orthopaedics and Related Research*, May(266), 244–258.
290. Kim, J. M., et al. (2015). Bone regeneration of hydroxyapatite/alumina bilayered scaffold with 3 mm passage-like medullary canal in canine tibia model. *BioMed Research International, 2015, 1-6.*
291. Yoon, D., et al. (2015). Effect of serum-derived albumin scaffold and canine adipose tissue-derived mesenchymal stem cells on osteogenesis in canine segmental bone defect model. *Journal of Veterinary Science, 16*(4), 397–404.
292. Tuominen, T., et al. (2000). Native bovine bone morphogenetic protein improves the potential of biocoral to heal segmental canine ulnar defects. *International Orthopaedics, 24*(5), 289–294.
293. Cai, L., et al. (2011). Vascular and micro-environmental influences on MSC-coral hydroxyapatite construct-based bone tissue engineering. *Biomaterials, 32*(33), 8497–8505.
294. De Kok, I. J., et al. (2003). Investigation of allogeneic mesenchyrnal stem cell-based alveolar bone formation: Preliminary findings. *Clinical Oral Implants Research, 14*(4), 481–489.

295. Yamada, Y., et al. (2004). Autogenous injectable bone for regeneration with mesenchymal stem cells and platelet-rich plasma: Tissue-engineered bone regeneration. *Tissue Engineering, 10*(5-6), 955–964.
296. Jafarian, M., et al. (2008). Marrow-derived mesenchymal stem cells-directed bone regeneration in the dog mandible: A comparison between biphasic calcium phosphate and natural bone mineral. *Oral Surgery, Oral Medicine, Oral Pathology, Oral Radiology, and Endodontics, 105*(5), e14–e24.
297. Khojasteh, A., et al. (2013). Effects of different growth factors and carriers on bone regeneration: A systematic review. *Oral Surgery, Oral Medicine, Oral Pathology, Oral Radiology, 116*(6), e405–e423.
298. Behnia, A., et al. (2014). Transplantation of stem cells from human exfoliated deciduous teeth for bone regeneration in the dog mandibular defect. *World Journal of Stem Cells, 6*(4), 505.
299. Zhang, D., et al. (2011). Orthodontic tooth movement in alveolar cleft repaired with a tissue engineering bone: An experimental study in dogs. *Tissue Engineering Part A, 17*(9-10), 1313–1325.
300. Kondo, N., et al. (2005). Bone formation and resorption of highly purified β-tricalcium phosphate in the rat femoral condyle. *Biomaterials, 26*(28), 5600–5608.
301. Tielinen, L., et al. (2001). Inability of transforming growth factor-β1, combined with a bioabsorbable polymer paste, to promote healing of bone defects in the rat distal femur. *Archives of Orthopaedic and Trauma Surgery, 121*(4), 191–196.
302. Inzana, J. A., et al. (2014). 3D printing of composite calcium phosphate and collagen scaffolds for bone regeneration. *Biomaterials, 35*(13), 4026–4034.
303. Ohgushi, H., Goldberg, V. M., & Caplan, A. I. (1989). Repair of bone defects with marrow cells and porous ceramic: Experiments in rats. *Acta Orthopaedica Scandinavica, 60*(3), 334–339.
304. Kirker-Head, C., et al. (2007). BMP-silk composite matrices heal critically sized femoral defects. *Bone, 41*(2), 247–255.
305. Ye, J.-H., et al. (2011). Critical-size calvarial bone defects healing in a mouse model with silk scaffolds and SATB2-modified iPSCs. *Biomaterials, 32*(22), 5065–5076.
306. Yoon, E., et al. (2007). In vivo osteogenic potential of human adipose-derived stem cells/poly lactide-co-glycolic acid constructs for bone regeneration in a rat critical-sized calvarial defect model. *Tissue Engineering, 13*(3), 619–627.
307. Arosarena, O. A., & Collins, W. L. (2003). Defect repair in the rat mandible with bone morphogenic protein 5 and prostaglandin E1. *Archives of Otolaryngology – Head & Neck Surgery, 129*(10), 1125–1130.
308. Jiang, X., et al. (2009). Mandibular repair in rats with premineralized silk scaffolds and BMP-2-modified bMSCs. *Biomaterials, 30*(27), 4522–4532.
309. Mohammadi, R., & Amini, K. (2015). Guided bone regeneration of mandibles using chitosan scaffold seeded with characterized uncultured omental adipose–Derived stromal vascular fraction: An animal study. *The International Journal of Oral & Maxillofacial Implants, 30*(1), 216–222.
310. Riegger, C., et al. (2012). Quantitative assessment of bone defect healing by multidetector CT in a pig model. *Skeletal Radiology, 41*(5), 531–537.
311. Chang, S. C.-N., et al. (2009). Large-scale bicortical skull bone regeneration using ex vivo replication-defective adenoviral-mediated bone morphogenetic protein—2 gene—transferred bone marrow stromal cells and composite biomaterials. *Operative Neurosurgery, 65*(suppl_6), ons75–ons83.
312. Wehrhan, F., et al. (2012). PEG matrix enables cell-mediated local BMP-2 gene delivery and increased bone formation in a porcine critical size defect model of craniofacial bone regeneration. *Clinical Oral Implants Research, 23*(7), 805–813.
313. Buser, D., et al. (1998). Evaluation of filling materials in membrane-protected bone defects. A comparative histomorphometric study in the mandible of miniature pigs. *Clinical Oral Implants Research, 9*(3), 137–150.

314. Fuerst, G., et al. (2004). Effects of fibrin sealant protein concentrate with and without platelet-released growth factors on bony healing of cortical mandibular defects. *Clinical Oral Implants Research, 15*(3), 301–307.
315. Gröger, A., et al. (2003). Tissue engineering of bone for mandibular augmentation in immunocompetent minipigs: Preliminary study. *Scandinavian Journal of Plastic and Reconstructive Surgery and Hand Surgery, 37*(3), 129–133.
316. Zheng, Y., et al. (2009). Stem cells from deciduous tooth repair mandibular defect in swine. *Journal of Dental Research, 88*(3), 249–254.
317. Pieri, F., et al. (2009). Effect of mesenchymal stem cells and platelet-rich plasma on the healing of standardized bone defects in the alveolar ridge: A comparative histomorphometric study in minipigs. *Journal of Oral and Maxillofacial Surgery, 67*(2), 265–272.
318. Kuo, T.-f., et al. (2015). An in vivo swine study for xeno-grafts of calcium sulfate-based bone grafts with human dental pulp stem cells (hDPSCs). *Materials Science and Engineering: C, 50*, 19–23.
319. Chang, S. C.-N., et al. (2003). Ex vivo gene therapy in autologous critical-size craniofacial bone regeneration. *Plastic and Reconstructive Surgery, 112*(7), 1841–1850.
320. Bensaid, W., et al. (2005). De novo reconstruction of functional bone by tissue engineering in the metatarsal sheep model. *Tissue Engineering, 11*(5-6), 814–824.
321. Viateau, V., et al. (2007). Long-bone critical-size defects treated with tissue-engineered grafts: A study on sheep. *Journal of Orthopaedic Research, 25*(6), 741–749.
322. Berner, A., et al. (2017). Scaffold–cell bone engineering in a validated preclinical animal model: Precursors vs differentiated cell source. *Journal of Tissue Engineering and Regenerative Medicine, 11*(7), 2081–2089.
323. Reichert, J. C., et al. (2011). Custom-made composite scaffolds for segmental defect repair in long bones. *International Orthopaedics, 35*(8), 1229–1236.
324. Schneiders, W., et al. (2009). In vivo effects of modification of hydroxyapatite/collagen composites with and without chondroitin sulphate on bone remodeling in the sheep tibia. *Journal of Orthopaedic Research, 27*(1), 15–21.
325. Marcacci, M., et al. (1999). Reconstruction of extensive long-bone defects in sheep using porous hydroxyapatite sponges. *Calcified Tissue International, 64*(1), 83–90.
326. Kirker-Head, C. A., et al. (1995). Long-term healing of bone using recombinant human bone morphogenetic protein 2. *Clinical Orthopaedics and Related Research*, Sep(318), 222–230.
327. Nandi, S. K., et al. (2009). The repair of segmental bone defects with porous bioglass: An experimental study in goat. *Research in Veterinary Science, 86*(1), 162–173.
328. Decambron, A., et al. (2017). Low-dose BMP-2 and MSC dual delivery onto coral scaffold for critical-size bone defect regeneration in sheep. *Journal of Orthopaedic Research, 35*(12), 2637–2645.
329. Nair, M. B., et al. (2009). Treatment of goat femur segmental defects with silica-coated hydroxyapatite—one-year follow-up. *Tissue Engineering Part A, 16*(2), 385–391.
330. Zhu, L., et al. (2006). Tissue-engineered bone repair of goat-femur defects with osteogenically induced bone marrow stromal cells. *Tissue Engineering, 12*(3), 423–433.
331. Liu, G., et al. (2008). Repair of goat tibial defects with bone marrow stromal cells and β-tricalcium phosphate. *Journal of Materials Science: Materials in Medicine, 19*(6), 2367–2376.
332. Fan, H., et al. (2014). Efficacy of prevascularization for segmental bone defect repair using β-tricalcium phosphate scaffold in rhesus monkey. *Biomaterials, 35*(26), 7407–7415.
333. Masaoka, T., et al. (2016). Bone defect regeneration by a combination of a β-tricalcium phosphate scaffold and bone marrow stromal cells in a non-human primate model. *The Open Biomedical Engineering Journal, 10*, 2.
334. Huang, J., et al. (2015). Rapid maxillary expansion in alveolar cleft repaired with a tissue-engineered bone in a canine model. *Journal of the Mechanical Behavior of Biomedical Materials, 48*, 86–99.
335. Ren, Y., Maltha, J. C., & Kuijpers-Jagtman, A. M. (2004). The rat as a model for orthodontic tooth movement—a critical review and a proposed solution. *The European Journal of Orthodontics, 26*(5), 483–490.

336. Persson, M. (1995). The role of sutures in normal and abnormal craniofacial growth. *Acta Odontologica Scandinavica, 53*(3), 152–161.
337. Krishnan, V., & Davidovitch, Z. (2006). Cellular, molecular, and tissue-level reactions to orthodontic force. *American Journal of Orthodontics and Dentofacial Orthopedics, 129*(4), 469.e1–469.e32.
338. Meikle, M. C. (2006). The tissue, cellular, and molecular regulation of orthodontic tooth movement: 100 years after Carl Sandstedt. *The European Journal of Orthodontics, 28*(3), 221–240.
339. Braga, S. M., et al. (2011). Effect of diabetes on orthodontic tooth movement in a mouse model. *European Journal of Oral Sciences, 119*(1), 7–14.
340. Kouskoura, T., Katsaros, C., & von Gunten, S. (2017). The potential use of pharmacological agents to modulate orthodontic tooth movement (OTM). *Frontiers in Physiology, 8*, 67.
341. Abtahi, M., et al. (2014). Effect of corticosteroids on orthodontic tooth movement in a rabbit model. *Journal of Clinical Pediatric Dentistry, 38*(3), 285–289.
342. Al-Hamdany, A. K., Al-Khatib, A. R., & Al-Sadi, H. I. (2017). Influence of olive oil on alveolar bone response during orthodontic retention period: Rabbit model study. *Acta Odontologica Scandinavica, 75*(6), 413–422.
343. Choi, J., et al. (2010). Effects of clodronate on early alveolar bone remodeling and root resorption related to orthodontic forces: A histomorphometric analysis. *American Journal of Orthodontics and Dentofacial Orthopedics, 138*(5), 548.e1–548.e8.
344. Güleç, A., et al. (2017). Effects of local platelet-rich plasma injection on the rate of orthodontic tooth movement in a rat model: A histomorphometric study. *American Journal of Orthodontics and Dentofacial Orthopedics, 151*(1), 92–104.
345. Jettar, V., et al. (2018). Effects of photobiomodulation on SOFAT, a T-cell-derived cytokine, may explain accelerated orthodontic tooth movement. *Photochemistry and Photobiology, 94(3). 604-610.*
346. Dogru, M., et al. (2014). Examination of extremely low frequency electromagnetic fields on orthodontic tooth movement in rats. *Biotechnology & Biotechnological Equipment, 28*(1), 118–122.
347. Gomes, M. F., et al. (2017). Effects of the GaAlAs diode laser (780 nm) on the periodontal tissues during orthodontic tooth movement in diabetes rats: Histomorphological and immunohistochemical analysis. *Lasers in Medical Science, 32*(7), 1479–1487.
348. Sun, J., et al. (2017). Histological evidence that metformin reverses the adverse effects of diabetes on orthodontic tooth movement in rats. *Journal of Molecular Histology, 48*(2), 73–81.
349. Dibart, S., Sebaoun, J. D., & Surmenian, J. (2009). Piezocision: A minimally invasive, periodontally accelerated orthodontic tooth movement procedure. *Compendium of Continuing Education in Dentistry (Jamesburg, NJ: 1995), 30*(6), 342–344, 346, 348–50.
350. Ibrahim, A., et al. (2017). Resolving differences between animal models for expedited orthodontic tooth movement. *Orthodontics & Craniofacial Research, 20*(S1), 72–76.
351. Iino, S., et al. (2007). Acceleration of orthodontic tooth movement by alveolar corticotomy in the dog. *American Journal of Orthodontics and Dentofacial Orthopedics, 131*(4), 448.e1–448.e8.
352. Khan, N. (2015). Corticotomy-assisted orthodontics (Doctoral dissertation).
353. Alikhani, M., et al. (2015). Saturation of the biological response to orthodontic forces and its effect on the rate of tooth movement. *Orthodontics & Craniofacial Research, 18*, 8–17.
354. Viecilli, R., et al. (2013). Effects of initial stresses and time on orthodontic external root resorption. *Journal of Dental Research, 92*(4), 346–351.
355. Dibart, S., et al. (2013). Tissue response during Piezocision-assisted tooth movement: A histological study in rats. *European Journal of Orthodontics, 36*(4), 457–464.
356. Medeiros, M. A. B., et al. (2014). Effects of laser vs ultrasound on bone healing after distraction osteogenesis: A histomorphometric analysis. *The Angle Orthodontist, 85*(4), 555–561.
357. Taylor, B. A., et al. (2017). Effect of strontium citrate on bone consolidation during mandibular distraction osteogenesis. *The Laryngoscope, 127*(7), E212-E218.

358. Terheyden, H., et al. (2003). Acceleration of callus maturation using rhOP-1 in mandibular distraction osteogenesis in a rat model. *International Journal of Oral and Maxillofacial Surgery, 32*(5), 528–533.
359. Küçük, D., et al. (2011). Comparison of local and systemic alendronate on distraction osteogenesis. *International Journal of Oral and Maxillofacial Surgery, 40*(12), 1395–1400.
360. Yang, Z.-h., et al. (2016). Targeting P38 pathway regulates bony formation via MSC recruitment during mandibular distraction osteogenesis in rats. *International Journal of Medical Sciences, 13*(10), 783.
361. Al Ruhaimi, K. (2001). Effect of calcium sulphate on the rate of osteogenesis in distracted bone. *International Journal of Oral and Maxillofacial Surgery, 30*(3), 228–233.
362. Cao, J., et al. (2012). Local injection of nerve growth factor via a hydrogel enhances bone formation during mandibular distraction osteogenesis. *Oral Surgery, Oral Medicine, Oral Pathology, Oral Radiology, 113*(1), 48–53.
363. El-Bialy, T., et al. (2008). Effects of ultrasound modes on mandibular osteodistraction. *Journal of Dental Research, 87*(10), 953–957.
364. Pampu, A. A., et al. (2008). Histomorphometric evaluation of the effects of zoledronic acid on mandibular distraction osteogenesis in rabbits. *Journal of Oral and Maxillofacial Surgery, 66*(5), 905–910.
365. Pampu, A. A., et al. (2009). The effects of osteoformin on mineralisation and quality of newly formed bone during mandibular distraction osteogenesis in rabbits. *Oral Surgery, Oral Medicine, Oral Pathology, Oral Radiology, and Endodontics, 108*(6), 833–837.
366. Polat, H. B., et al. (2009). Effect of oil-based calcium hydroxide (Osteoinductal) on distraction osteogenesis in rabbit mandible. *Oral Surgery, Oral Medicine, Oral Pathology, Oral Radiology, and Endodontics, 107*(6), e30–e36.
367. Cho, B. C., et al. (2005). The effect of chitosan bead encapsulating calcium sulfate as an injectable bone substitute on consolidation in the mandibular distraction osteogenesis of a dog model. *Journal of Oral and Maxillofacial Surgery, 63*(12), 1753–1764.
368. Terbish, M., et al. (2015). Accelerated bone formation in distracted alveolar bone after injection of recombinant human bone morphogenetic protein-2. *Journal of Periodontology, 86*(9), 1078–1086.
369. Aykan, A., et al. (2013). Biomechanical analysis of the effect of mesenchymal stem cells on mandibular distraction osteogenesis. *The Journal of Craniofacial Surgery, 24*(2), e169–e175.
370. Sun, Z., et al. (2013). Scaffold-based delivery of autologous mesenchymal stem cells for mandibular distraction osteogenesis: Preliminary studies in a porcine model. *PLoS ONE, 8*(9), e74672.
371. Zhu, S., et al. (2006). Reconstruction of mandibular condyle by transport distraction osteogenesis: Experimental study in rhesus monkey. *Journal of Oral and Maxillofacial Surgery, 64*(10), 1487–1492.
372. Kılıç, E., et al. (2008). Effects of simvastatin on mandibular distraction osteogenesis. *Journal of Oral and Maxillofacial Surgery, 66*(11), 2233–2238.
373. Yang, Y., et al. (2017). Stem cell therapy for enhancement of bone consolidation in distraction osteogenesis: A contemporary review of experimental studies. *Bone & Joint Research, 6*(6), 385–390.
374. Gokce, S., et al. (2015). The effect of human amniotic fluid on mandibular distraction osteogenesis. *International Journal of Oral and Maxillofacial Surgery, 44*(3), 404–411.
375. Tee, B., & Sun, Z. (2015). Mandibular distraction osteogenesis assisted by cell-based tissue engineering: A systematic review. *Orthodontics & Craniofacial Research, 18*(S1), 39–49.
376. Andersen, K., et al. (2014). Effect of mandibular distraction osteogenesis on the temporomandibular joint: A systematic review of animal experimental studies. *Oral Surgery, Oral Medicine, Oral Pathology, Oral Radiology, 117*(4), 407–415.
377. Karp, N. S., et al. (1990). Bone lengthening in the craniofacial skeleton. *Annals of Plastic Surgery, 24*(3), 231–237.

378. Norris, S. A., et al. (2001). Calcium metabolism and bone mass in female rabbits during skeletal maturation: Effects of dietary calcium intake. *Bone, 29*(1), 62–69.
379. Utreja, A., et al. (2018). Maxillary expansion in an animal model with light, continuous force. *The Angle Orthodontist*, 88(3), 306-313.
380. Zhao, S., et al. (2015). Effects of strontium ranelate on bone formation in the mid-palatal suture after rapid maxillary expansion. *Drug Design, Development and Therapy, 9*, 2725.
381. Kobayashi, E., et al. (1999). Force-induced rapid changes in cell fate at midpalatal suture cartilage of growing rats. *Journal of Dental Research, 78*(9), 1495–1504.
382. Takahashi, I., et al. (1996). Effects of expansive force on the differentiation of midpalatal suture cartilage in rats. *Bone, 18*(4), 341–348.
383. Motamedian, S. R., et al. (2015). Smart scaffolds in bone tissue engineering: A systematic review of literature. *World Journal of Stem Cells, 7*(3), 657.
384. Uysal, T., et al. (2009). Effect of ED-71, a new active vitamin D analog, on bone formation in an orthopedically expanded suture in rats. A histomorphometric study. *European Journal of Dentistry, 3*(3), 165.
385. Uysal, T., et al. (2011). Effect of vitamin C on bone formation in the expanded inter-premaxillary suture. Early bone changes. *Journal of Orofacial Orthopedics/Fortschritte der Kieferorthopädie, 72*(4), 290.
386. Kara, M. I., et al. (2012). Thymoquinone accelerates new bone formation in the rapid maxillary expansion procedure. *Archives of Oral Biology, 57*(4), 357–363.
387. Lee, K., et al. (2001). Effects of bisphosphonate on the remodeling of rat sagittal suture after rapid expansion. *The Angle Orthodontist, 71*(4), 265–273.
388. Guiran, Z., et al. (2017). A new way to accelerate the distraction of the transpalatal suture in growing dogs using recombinant human bone morphogenetic protein-2. *The Cleft Palate-Craniofacial Journal, 54*(2), 193–201.
389. Lai, R.-F., Zhou, Z.-Y., & Chen, T. (2013). Accelerating bone generation and bone mineralization in the interparietal sutures of rats using an rhBMP-2/ACS composite after rapid expansion. *Experimental Animals, 62*(3), 189–196.
390. Saito, S., & Shimizu, N. (1997). Stimulatory effects of low-power laser irradiation on bone regeneration in midpalatal suture during expansion in the rat. *American Journal of Orthodontics and Dentofacial Orthopedics, 111*(5), 525–532.
391. Che, X., et al. (2016). Intramuscular injection of bone marrow mononuclear cells contributes to bone repair following midpalatal expansion in rats. *Molecular Medicine Reports, 13*(1), 681–688.
392. Le, M. H. T., et al. (2018). Adjunctive buccal and palatal corticotomy for adult maxillary expansion in an animal model. *The Korean Journal of Orthodontics, 48*(2), 98–106.
393. Kim, T., et al. (2002). Constriction of the maxillary dental arch by mucoperiosteal denudation of the palate. *The Cleft Palate-Craniofacial Journal, 39*(4), 425–431.
394. Irgin, C., et al. (2016). Does stinging nettle (Urtica dioica) have an effect on bone formation in the expanded inter-premaxillary suture? *Archives of Oral Biology, 69*, 13–18.
395. Kara, M. I., et al. (2012). Effects of Ginkgo biloba on experimental rapid maxillary expansion model: A histomorphometric study. *Oral Surgery, Oral Medicine, Oral Pathology, Oral Radiology, 114*(6), 712–718.
396. Murray, J. M. G., & Cleall, J. F. (1971). Early tissue response to rapid maxillary expansion in the midpalatal suture of the rhesus monkey. *Journal of Dental Research, 50*(6), 1654–1660.
397. Haugen, S., et al. (2017). Adiponectin prevents orthodontic tooth movement in rats. *Archives of Oral Biology, 83*, 304–311.
398. Liao, L.-S., et al. (2009). Animal experimental study on repairing alveolar clefts by using rectilinear distraction osteogenesis. *Journal of Plastic, Reconstructive & Aesthetic Surgery, 62*(12), 1573–1579.
399. Tong, F., et al. (2017). Effects of a magnetic palatal expansion appliance with reactivation system: An animal experiment. *American Journal of Orthodontics and Dentofacial Orthopedics, 151*(1), 132–142.

400. Brown, A. J., et al. (1993). Guidelines for animal surgery in research. *American Journal of Veterinary Research, 54*(9), 1544–1559.
401. Olfert, E., Cross, B., & McWilliam, A. (1993). *Guide to the care and use of experimental animals* (Vol. 1, p. 2011). Ottawa: Canadian Council on Animal Care.
402. Flecknell, P. A. (1987). *Laboratory animal anaesthesia. An introduction for research workers and technicians*. Amsterdam: Academic Press.
403. Anderson, L. C. (2007). Institutional and IACUC responsibilities for animal care and use education and training programs. *ILAR Journal, 48*(2), 90–95.
404. Akins, C. K., Panicker, S. E., & Cunningham, C. L. (2005). *Laboratory animals in research and teaching: Ethics, care, and methods*. Washington, D.C.: American Psychological Association.
405. Festing, S., & Wilkinson, R. (2007). The ethics of animal research: Talking point on the use of animals in scientific research. *EMBO Reports, 8*(6), 526–530.
406. Russell, W. M. S., Burch, R. L., & Hume, C. W. (1959). *The principles of humane experimental technique*. London: Methuen.
407. Foëx, B. A. (2007). The ethics of animal experimentation. *Emergency Medicine Journal, 24*(11), 750.
408. Kolar, R. (2006). Animal experimentation. *Science and Engineering Ethics, 12*(1), 111–122.
409. Sechzer, J. A. (1981). Historical issues concerning animal experimentation in the United States. *Social Science & Medicine. Part F, 15*(1), 13–17.
410. Thompson, P. B. (2008). Animal biotechnology: How not to presume. *The American Journal of Bioethics, 8*(6), 49–50.
411. Benam, K. H., et al. (2015). Engineered in vitro disease models. *Annual Review of Pathology: Mechanisms of Disease, 10*, 195–262.
412. Liu, Z., Han, X., & Qin, L. (2016). Recent progress of microfluidics in translational applications. *Advanced Healthcare Materials, 5*(8), 871–888.
413. Pagella, P., et al. (2015). Investigation of orofacial stem cell niches and their innervation through microfluidic devices. *European Cells & Materials, 29*, 213–223.
414. van de Stolpe, A., & den Toonder, J. (2013). Workshop meeting report Organs-on-Chips: Human disease models. *Lab on a Chip, 13*(18), 3449–3470.
415. Bersini, S., et al. (2014). A microfluidic 3D in vitro model for specificity of breast cancer metastasis to bone. *Biomaterials, 35*(8), 2454–2461.
416. Huh, D., et al. (2012). A human disease model of drug toxicity–induced pulmonary edema in a lung-on-a-chip microdevice. *Science Translational Medicine, 4*(159), 159ra147–159ra147.
417. Huh, D., et al. (2010). Reconstituting organ-level lung functions on a chip. *Science, 328*(5986), 1662–1668.
418. Jansson, K., et al. (2012). Endogenous concentrations of ouabain act as a cofactor to stimulate fluid secretion and cyst growth of in vitro ADPKD models via cAMP and EGFR-Src-MEK pathways. *American Journal of Physiology - Renal Physiology, 303*(7), F982–F990.
419. McCain, M. L., et al. (2013). Recapitulating maladaptive, multiscale remodeling of failing myocardium on a chip. *Proceedings of the National Academy of Sciences, 110*(24), 9770–9775.
420. Torisawa, Y.-s., et al. (2014). Bone marrow–on–a–chip replicates hematopoietic niche physiology in vitro. *Nature Methods, 11*(6), 663.
421. Westein, E., et al. (2013). Atherosclerotic geometries exacerbate pathological thrombus formation poststenosis in a von Willebrand factor-dependent manner. *Proceedings of the National Academy of Sciences, 110*(4), 1357–1362.
422. Shumi, W., et al. (2010). Environmental factors that affect Streptococcus mutans biofilm formation in a microfluidic device mimicking teeth. *BioChip Journal, 4*(4), 257–263.
423. Shumi, W., et al. (2013). Shear stress tolerance of Streptococcus mutans aggregates determined by microfluidic funnel device (μFFD). *Journal of Microbiological Methods, 93*(2), 85–89.

424. Nance, W. C., et al. (2013). A high-throughput microfluidic dental plaque biofilm system to visualize and quantify the effect of antimicrobials. *Journal of Antimicrobial Chemotherapy, 68*(11), 2550–2560.
425. Lam, R. H., et al. (2016). High-throughput dental biofilm growth analysis for multiparametric microenvironmental biochemical conditions using microfluidics. *Lab on a Chip, 16*(9), 1652–1662.
426. Kim, D., & Park, S.-H. (2016). A microfluidics-based pulpal arteriole blood flow phantom for validation of Doppler ultrasound devices in pulpal blood flow velocity measurement. *Journal of Endodontics, 42*(11), 1660–1666.
427. Pagella, P., et al. (2014). Microfluidics co-culture systems for studying tooth innervation. *Frontiers in Physiology, 5*, 326.
428. Kang, K.-J., et al. (2016). Indirect co-culture of stem cells from human exfoliated deciduous teeth and oral cells in a microfluidic platform. *Journal of Tissue Engineering and Regenerative Medicine, 13*(4), 428–436.

# Chapter 19
# Whole Tooth Engineering

**Leila Mohammadi Amirabad, Payam Zarrintaj, Amanda Lindemuth, and Lobat Tayebi**

## 1 Introduction

Total tooth loss due to traumatic injury, poor dental hygiene, periodontal or congenital diseases affects over 276 million people worldwide [1]. Today, removable dentures and artificial dental implants have been commonly utilized to restore occlusal function as tooth replacement therapy. Nevertheless, there are some challenges in using the artificial implants, including high risk of bone loss and fracture encircling artificial implants and high susceptibility to infection and inflammation, therefore leading to implant failure [2, 3]. Accordingly, finding alternative procedures to manufacture biologically replaced teeth is an essential demand to rehabilitate physiologically functional teeth.

Theoretically, the whole tooth would be generated by implanting the autologous stem/progenitor cell-seeded scaffolds at the site of tooth loss, where it can grow, erupt, and develop like a natural tooth. Actually, this approach would take place just in the presence of the appropriate cell source(s), scaffolds, and the cascade expression of special genes that are involved in tooth development in the presence of several growth factors. Mimicking such conditions is feasible by understanding the structure and steps of embryonic tooth development.

Interactions between dental epithelium—derived from ectoderm—and neural crest-derived mesenchymal stem cells (NC-MSCs) initiate tooth development. Briefly, at the sites of the future tooth, cascade expressions of homeobox genes—

L. Mohammadi Amirabad · A. Lindemuth · L. Tayebi (✉)
Marquette University School of Dentistry, Milwaukee, WI, USA
e-mail: lobat.tayebi@marquette.edu

P. Zarrintaj
Color and Polymer Research Center (CPRC), Amirkabir University of Technology, Tehran, Iran

Polymer Engineering Department, Faculty of Engineering, Urmia University, Urmia, Iran



L. Tayebi (ed.), *Applications of Biomedical Engineering in Dentistry*,
https://doi.org/10.1007/978-3-030-21583-5_19

such as Barx1, Lhx8, Msc1, and Msc2—and secretion of BMPs and FGFs induce the thickening of the dental lamina and therefore initiate tooth development. After that, the dental epithelium cells in the placode, a specific dental laminar domain, proliferate and invaginate into the region wherein NC-MSCs reside and form the tooth bud. The epithelial cells proliferate and extend further into the NC-MSC-including tissue and condense the mesenchyme more to form a cap structure. In the next stage, called "bell stage," primary, secondary, or tertiary enamel knots form—based on the number of cusps of the eventual tooth—before developing into the crown of the tooth. Then, by expression of a second cascade of genes in the epithelial cells of enamel knots (including BMPs, FGFs, Wnts, and Shh), epithelial cells differentiate into ameloblasts, producing enamel, and mesenchymal cells differentiate into the progenitor of odontoblasts, producing dentine and dental follicle. Dental follicle cells produce the periodontal ligament, cementum, and alveolar bone, and thereafter tooth eruption begins by elongation of the tooth root (Fig. 19.1).

Up until now, efforts have been made in rehabilitating lost teeth using whole tooth bioengineering and different methods of tissue engineering and organ regeneration. Recently, several techniques have been applied to engineer fully functional whole tooth from embryonic germ cells in different small and large animals, including mice, rats, pigs, and dogs [4, 5]. These studies demonstrate the feasibility of producing whole tooth at the site of tooth loss as a promising approach for tooth replacement therapy.

In this chapter, we will start by focusing on different cell sources and cell signaling through which the cells produce different parts of the tooth during development procedure. Then, current methods in whole tooth replacement will be discussed and followed by an explanation of the functionality of a whole bioengineered tooth and future prospects for whole tooth engineering.

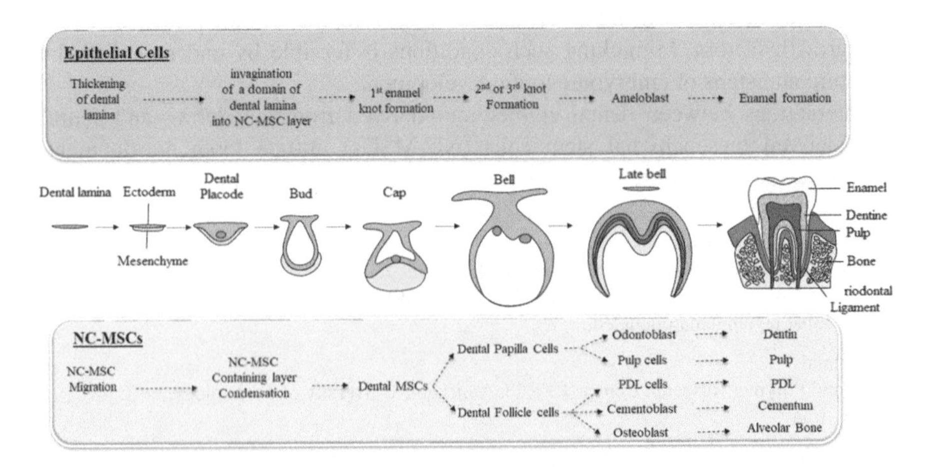


Fig. 19.1 Different stages in tooth development

## 2 Cell Sources for Whole Tooth Engineering

Tissue engineering using stem cells is a promising approach to restore lost or damaged craniofacial tissues. In whole tooth tissue engineering, different varieties of cells are used and investigated to detect the best source of cells that can be isolated, generated, and utilized for clinical applications. The findings achieved from these investigations can help us to understand how these cells can be utilized for whole tooth engineering. Recent studies, which used some scaffold-free methods for whole tooth bioengineering, manifested the importance of cell sources in the application of tooth regenerative studies [6, 7]. Two major types of stem cell sources are used in whole tooth engineering: pluripotent cells and adult stem cells. Pluripotent cells have the ability to differentiate into the cells of all three germ layers—including endoderm, mesoderm, and ectoderm. These cells, in the presence of appropriate stimuli, can differentiate into more than 200 adult cell types [8]. Adult stem cells are the other cell source, which are commonly used in engineering of different craniofacial tissues such as teeth. These cells are naturally responsible for normal tissue repair and healing after injuries [9]. Here, we will focus on the different cell types in each embryonic and adult stem cell categories and investigate their differentiation potential into different dental cells.

### *2.1 Embryonic Stem Cells*

Embryonic stem cells (ESs) are pluripotent stem cells that can give rise to cells of the different germ layers. However, using these cells in craniofacial tissue engineering for clinical purposes is limited due to ethical issues and immune rejection reaction.

Recently, with the appearance of a new generation of pluripotent stem cells, called induced pluripotent stem cells (iPSCs), it is possible to use pluripotent stem cells in tooth regeneration research. These cells can be generated from different patient-specific progenitor/differentiated cells including fibroblasts, gingival cells, SHED, SCAP, DSCPs, and periodontal ligament cells, therefore resolving the immune responses and rejection reactions [10–13]. Moreover, several studies have shown that iPSCs successfully differentiate into different cells of tooth tissue, such as ameloblast-like and odontoblast-like cells [14, 15].

### *2.2 Adult Stem Cells*

As described above, pluripotent stem cells, including ESs and iPSCs, are appropriate candidates to generate a successfully bioengineered tooth. However, using human ESs for tooth regeneration is impossible due to ethical issues and potential allogeneic immune rejection. Moreover, the procedure of producing of iPSCs is difficult, and the usual procedure to generate iPSCs using genetic manipulation and different kinds of viruses makes it harmful to use in clinical application. Therefore, autologous, multipotent adult stem cells are the putative source of the cells for craniofacial tissue engineering.

MSCs are standard stem cells that can be isolated from various tissues such as bone marrow, umbilical cord, and adipose and dental tissues [16, 17]. Postnatal dental pulp stem cells (DPSCs), the first and the most common source of dental MSCs in tooth tissue engineering, can be isolated easily from dental pulp [18]. Studies show that DPSCs can differentiate into odontoblasts and osteoblasts and thereby form pulp, dentin, and cementum tissues, respectively [20–23]. DPSCs also can differentiate into other cell lineages, such as neurons, chondrocytes, vascular tissues, osteocytes, and adipocytes [22–24].

The periodontal ligament was found to be another source of dental MSC population, called periodontal ligament stem cells (PDLSCs). The studies show that PDLSCs can differentiate into adipocytes, collagen-forming cells, cementoblast-like cells, and cementum-PDL-like structures in vitro, which contribute to periodontal tissue repair. Moreover, a study showed that co-culture of PDLSCs with DPSCs induces formation of rootlike and dentin-like structures [19].

Another promising source of stem cells is the pulp of primary human teeth (autologous baby teeth). The isolated stem cells, called human exfoliated deciduous teeth (SHEDs), can provide a sufficient number of the cells for dental tissue engineering applications. These highly proliferative cells can differentiate into neural cells, endothelium, chondrocytes, osteocytes, adipocytes, odontoblasts, and pulp-like and dentin-like tissues [20–22].

Dental follicle precursor cells (DFPCs) are the other type of mesenchymal stem cells that surround the developing tooth bud, which will differentiate into odontoblasts [23], cementoblasts (producing the cementum), and periodontal ligament-like tissues [24]. It has been shown that the DFPCs are remarkable undifferentiated lineage cells in the periodontium prior to, or even during, tooth eruption [24].

Stem cells from the apical papilla (SCAPs) are the other adult MSCs that are isolated from pulp tissue of developing baby teeth. They can differentiate into odontoblasts and osteoblasts, and form dentin-like structures [22]. Despite the fact that their proliferation rate is higher than DPSCs, their dentinogenic differentiation capacity is similar to DPSCs and BMSCs. Upon osteogenic differentiation, SHEDs show a higher alkaline phosphatase activity and osteocalcin expression compared with DPSC [18]. However, the studies show that their adipogenic differentiation capacity is less than BMSCs [25]. The SCAP growth factor receptor gene profiles—including FGFR1, TGFbRI, STRO-1, bone sialophosphoprotein, and osteocalcin—are similar to the gene profiles in DPSCs. Moreover, it has been shown that upon stimuli, SCAPs express a wide variety of neurogenic markers, such as nestin and neurofilament M [25].

Despite the potential of the aforementioned dental stem cells to create dental differentiated cells and structures, determining the best dental MSC for whole tooth engineering has been challenging. It is due to the difference in proliferation and clonogenicity, as well as the differentiation ability of the different types of MSCs. During distinct differentiation pathways, some specific surface markers are expressed on each dental stem cell type due to microenvironments of each cell lineage origin [26]. Even in the same population of the MSCs, the subpopulation of the cells shows heterogeneity in their differentiation potentials [27]. Moreover, to achieve an appropriate approach in whole tooth engineering, it is necessary to determine the factors that control the MSC differentiation fate during tooth development [26]. The mutual interaction between factors secreted from various types of dental epithelial cells (such as dental epithelial cell rests of Malassez (ERM), keratinocytes isolated from human foreskin and gingival epithelial cells, and factors secreted from dental MSCs) causes formation of odontoblasts, ameloblasts, cementoblasts, cementum, and enamel [28–30]. Combination of these epithelial cell sources with MSC sources could lead to a promising approach for effective whole tooth tissue engineering.

# 3 Cell Signaling

The signaling pathways are the part of a complex system of communication that organizes cell fate, activities, and interactions through cascade expressions of the genes. The signaling mechanisms in tooth development seem to be conservative among different species [31]. Investigation of tooth development in several models—such as zebra fish, snakes, lizards, ferrets, rats, mice, and humans—helps to detect the genes and signaling pathways involved in tooth development. These findings could suggest a promising approach to achieve successful whole tooth engineering [31, 32].

All signaling pathways take place in interactions between dental epithelium derived from ectoderm and NC-MSCs. The conserved signaling pathways in tooth development are Hedgehog (Hh), Wnt, fibroblast growth factor (FGF), transforming growth factor ® (Tgf ®), bone morphogenic protein (BMP), and ectodysplasin (Eda) (Fig. 19.2). There are three signaling centers in tooth development, including placodes, primary enamel knots, and secondary (or tertiary) enamel knots. Their formation is regulated by epithelial-mesenchymal interactions, and they all largely express the same array of multiple growth factors.

Transcription factor p63 is expressed throughout the surface ectoderm, which regulates placode formation. The function of this transcription factor was discovered when its function deletion caused the lack of teeth placodes and other ectodermal appendage development [33]. P53 plays a pivotal role in Eda, Notch, BMP, and FGF signaling pathways [33]. The studies show that impairing signaling pathways at the placode stage stops tooth development before epithelial budding [34].

Ectodysplasin (Eda), a tumor necrosis factor, affects the function of placodes and enamel knots through its receptor [35]. Human syndrome hypohidrotic ectodermal dysplasia (HED) is caused by mutations in the genes involving in Eda signaling. In this syndrome, multiple teeth are missing, and there are several defects in other

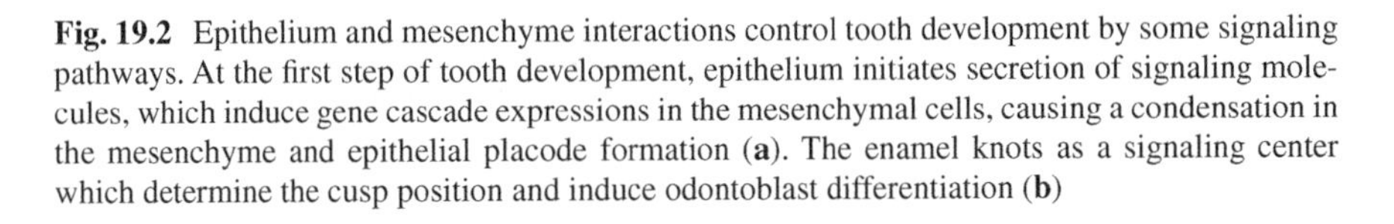


**Fig. 19.2** Epithelium and mesenchyme interactions control tooth development by some signaling pathways. At the first step of tooth development, epithelium initiates secretion of signaling molecules, which induce gene cascade expressions in the mesenchymal cells, causing a condensation in the mesenchyme and epithelial placode formation (**a**). The enamel knots as a signaling center which determine the cusp position and induce odontoblast differentiation (**b**)

ectodermal organs [35]. Impairing Eda function causes loss of third molars or incisal teeth, and the molar cusp pattern becomes abnormal [36], whereas overexpressing Eda in epithelium causes an extra tooth in front of the molars [37]. Eda signaling changes the gene expressions of the proteins involved in important signaling pathways in ectodermal organ development, including Dkk4, Fgf20, Shh, ctgf, and Follistatin [35].

Between the bud and cap stages, the primary enamel knot forms in the dental epithelium. The primary enamel knot manages crown formation and directs secondary enamel knot position, thereby determining the cusp tip position in the molar crown [38]. Wnt/b-catenin signaling in dental epithelium regulates Lef1 for *FGF4* expression in the enamel knots and induces new enamel knots and placodes [39]. The enamel knots induce cell proliferation in adjacent epithelium by secreting growth factors of FGF3, FGF4, FGF9, and FGF20. Because of expression lacking of P21 and FGF receptor in the epithelial cells of enamel knots, the epithelial cells remain nonproliferative. The FGF growth factors also induce NC-MSCs to express and secrete FGF3 and Runx2. Then, FGF3 and Runx2 attach to their receptors on the epithelial cells, thereby affecting the morphogenesis of tooth [40].

Shh, another factor secreted from the enamel knot, induces mesenchyme to produce factors that regulate morphogenesis of epithelium [41]. The signaling pathways conducted by *Shh, Bmp*, and *Tgf*® induce the proliferation activity of the stem cells and ameloblast differentiation, thereby producing the enamel.

Moreover, the studies show that TGF-® proteins, including BMPs, induce odontoblastic differentiation in the canonical TGF-® pathway, modulate smads, and thereby provoke dentin formation [42].

# 4 Approaches for Whole Tooth Organ

The procedure of whole tooth development is a highly complicated process, where transcription and growth factors express spatiotemporally and control cusp position and number, root formation, tooth length, crown size, and tooth development. To generate a functional whole bioengineered tooth with appropriate size and morphology, the proper interaction between different aforementioned factors is necessary. Recently, several approaches for whole bioengineered teeth have been suggested, including organ germ method, cell sheets, and dental tissue engineering using scaffolds.

## *4.1 Organ Germ Method*

A promising approach to bioengineer a whole tooth is mimicking organogenesis by inducing mutual epithelial-mesenchymal interconnection similar to what occurs in organ development. Here, we describe different approaches to bioengineer whole teeth using the organ germ method.

### 4.1.1 Embryonic Tooth Germ-Derived Epithelial and Mesenchymal Stem Cells

Embryonic tooth germ cells of the mouse are an appropriate candidate to develop a whole bioengineered tooth because they can make functional teeth by epithelial-mesenchymal interconnection [43]. Moreover, the organogenesis in this animal model takes place in a relatively short time frame, making it possible to achieve an accurate protocol. As described before, the primary enamel knot, acting as a second signaling center involved in the morphogenesis of the tooth crown, forms in the enamel organ, thus making it an important stage to producing functional reconstitutes of germ cells. In a study, dental mesenchyme and enamel organ were dissociated from the mouse's first lower molars at early cap stage (E14). Then, the dissociated cells from enamel organ were cultured and reassociated to either intact dental mesenchyme or dissociated mesenchymal cells in vitro. Although in teeth developed in both types of experiments, the tooth developed faster in intact dental mesenchyme than the dissociated mesenchymal cells due to cell history memorization in the intact mesenchymal tissue. However, progression duration in the initial steps of epithelial histogenesis is equal in both experiments, which shows that history reassociations in early stage are not memorized by mesenchymal tissue [44].

To bioengineer a whole tooth using embryonic tooth germ cells, reconstitution of tooth germ-like structures will be initiated by co-culturing the epithelial and mesenchymal stem cells in vitro for 5–7 days. In this stage, differentiation of odontoblasts, cusp morphogenesis, and crown formation will be started, and epithelial histogenesis will be completed [45, 46]. The construct will be then implanted under skin or the sub-renal capsule of adult mice, where vascular tissues, enamel and dentin, and toothlike structure will be formed [7, 47]. A study shows that this bioengineered toothlike structure with full function is produced in the case of an edentulous jaw using organ replacement therapy (Fig. 19.3) [6]. These methods can suggest a promising approach to achieve functional bioengineered whole teeth in the edentulous jaw.

There are no studies that show that human embryonic dental cells will produce bioengineered teeth, which tooth germ cells of mice produce. However, a study on the embryonic human dental epithelium (obtained from cap stage) and human embryonic lip mesenchyme shows that human embryonic dental tissues indeed possess similar tooth-inductive capability [49].

Recently, the main problems in the tooth organ method are discovering the appropriate cells and recapitulating the molecular processes of tooth development. Therefore, finding the molecular markers is necessary for detection of this molecular process. Even though the embryonic tooth cells seem to be good candidates for tooth bioengineering, their use in clinical application is challenging because of limitations, such as immunological rejection reactions and ethical concerns. Adult stem cells would be the alternative cell source for this purpose.

### 4.1.2 Non-embryonic Tooth Germ-Derived Epithelial and Mesenchymal Stem Cells

As described previously, tooth formation is induced by interconnections between epithelial and mesenchymal cells during the development process of a tooth [4]. Recently, different sources of cells, including non-embryonic cells, have been used based on this strategy. These cells can produce a plentiful amount of the cell population and are easy to access and isolate.

Bone marrow mesenchymal stem cells (BM-MSCs), showing similar properties of DPSCs, would be a good candidate as an alternative cell source. These cells can be isolated and harvested in an abundant amount at all ages and differentiate into a variety of cell types, including ameloblast-like cells [45]. A study shows that interconnection between BM-MSCs and oral epithelial cells from a mouse embryo (E10) induced bioengineered-like teeth after implantation in kidney capsules [50].

iPSCs are the other alternative cell source for tooth bioengineering because of their pluripotent characteristics similar to human embryonic stem cells. However, iPSCs do not have some limitations of human embryonic stem cells, such as ethical or immune rejection reaction problems [13]. Neural crest-like cells derived from

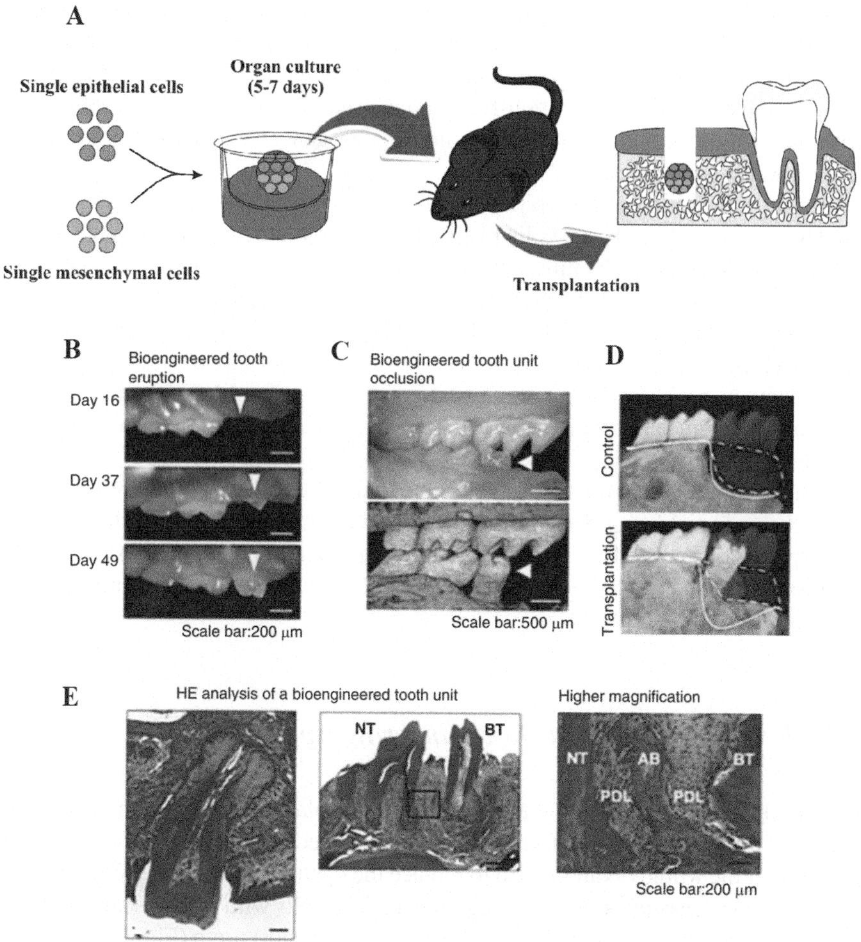


**Fig. 19.3** Producing a bioengineered tooth in a mouse jaw. (**a**) Schematic image of bioengineering a tooth in the jaw using reassociation of tooth germ. (**b**) Oral image of transplanted bioengineered tooth before and after eruption and after occlusion (top, center, and bottom, respectively). (**c**) The transplanted bioengineered tooth occluded with the opposing upper tooth after 40 days. (**d**) Micro CT images of normal (gray, double dotted line) and no transplantation (top image) and transplanted bioengineered tooth in an extensive bone defect at day 0 (red, straight line) and after 45 days (green, dotted line). Here, each line determines the superior edges of the recipient alveolar bone. (**e**) H&E analysis of bioengineered tooth after occlusion, which shows that engrafted bioengineered construct has the correct tooth structure. Abbreviations: NT natural tooth, BT bioengineered tooth, PDL periodontal ligament, AB alveolar bone. (Panels B, C, D, and E are reused from Ref. [48] with permission)

iPSCs in combination with incisor dental epithelium can undergo odontogenic differentiation [51]. A study shows co-culturing iPSCs with incisor mesenchymal cells causes toothlike structure formation with newly formed bone-like cells [52]. It has been demonstrated that integration-free human urine-derived iPSCs in combination with molar mesenchyme (form E14.5 mouse) can generate intact toothlike structures in a sub-renal culture [53].

Recently, in another study, epithelial cells obtained from adult human gingiva are used as a source of epithelial cells to engineer a whole bioengineered tooth. These cells, in combination with embryonic tooth mesenchymal cells of a mouse, produce a bioengineered tooth with different parts of a tooth, such as enamel with ameloblast-like cells, dentine, and the ERM of human origin after transplantation in kidney capsules [53].

It seems human keratinocytes can be a good source of epithelial cells, which in combination with embryonic mouse mesenchyme can differentiate into enamel-secreting ameloblasts [54].

Human umbilical cord mesenchymal stem cells (hUCMSCs) are another potential cell source to bioengineer the whole tooth with characteristics similar to those of pulp tissue stem cells. These cells can differentiate into odontoblast-like cells expressing dentine-related proteins, such as dentine sialoprotein and dentine matrix protein-1 [55].

## 4.2 *Scaffolds for Tooth Bioengineering Approach*

Organ substitution brings to light the whole tissue replacement of an impaired organ using in vitro cell-cultured 3D structures. It is supposed that future technologies will reconstruct the whole organ in vitro to replace the dysfunctional tissue. Whole tooth regeneration necessitates the accompaniment of the cells with proper scaffolding to regenerate the whole tooth to functional recovery of the lost tooth (Fig. 19.4). In this

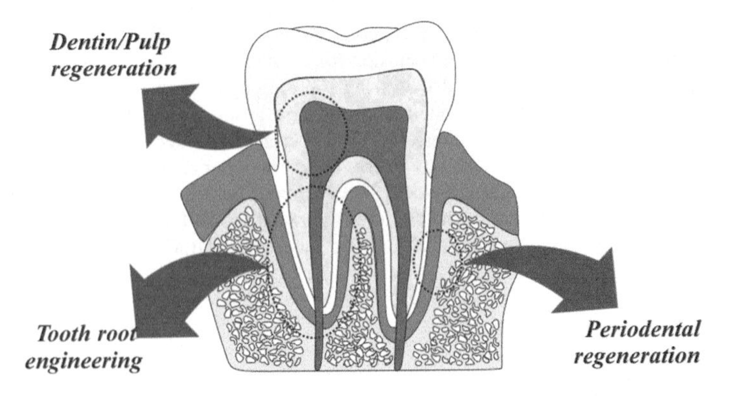


**Fig. 19.4** Whole tooth engineering

method, natural and synthetic polymers have been utilized to reconstruct the whole tissue, which clinical experiments have reported. In this section, whole tissue regeneration using scaffold will be discussed.

### 4.2.1 Synthetic Polymeric Scaffolds

Biomaterials play an important role in tissue engineering, in which incorporation of cells exhibits a synergistic effect on damaged tissue regeneration. Appropriate material selection has a strong impact on dental regeneration. For instance, scaffold modulus affects cellular adhesion, growth, proliferation, differentiation, and fate. Young et al. seeded cells on the PLGA scaffolds, which are appropriate for controlling the shape and size of the tooth, and successfully regenerated a tooth from dissociated tooth tissues, involving enamel and dentin [56]. However, scaffold residue in the tissue hindered the whole tooth regeneration. Precise arrangement of cells—such as ameloblasts, odontoblasts, and cementoblasts similar to native teeth—resulted in proper connection of enamel, dentin, and cementum, which leads to full regeneration of teeth [57]. In whole tooth engineering, root regeneration is the most important aspect. After root regeneration, the crown can regenerate on the constructed root. Bopp et al. loaded Cyclosporine A (CsA) in PLGA nanoparticles and embedded these cells into PCL electrospun scaffolds in which the local and sustained release of the nanoparticles was achieved.

It was reported that the in vivo implantation of such scaffolds did not alter tooth regeneration, and that 88% of the regenerated teeth were innervated [58]. Chen et al. electrospun the PLGA and gelatin to achieve aligned nanofibers and treated the nanofibers using dentin matrix and native dental pulp extracellular matrix for periodontal and dental pulp regeneration. Such scaffolding can simulate the ECM properties, which facilitates the odontogenic differentiation of dental stem cells after seeding with stem cells transplanted within the porcine jaws. It is observed that in dentin, an odontoblast-like layer forms between the predentin matrix and dental pulp-like tissues, along with blood vessel formation; moreover, in the periodontium, cellular cementum and periodontal ligament (PDL)-like tissues are formed [59]. Rasperini et al. bioprinted the PCL for periodontal repair. Adjustable degradation rate and high porosity results in tissue ingrowth and vascularization [60]. Zhang et al. synthesized chitosan–/collagen-containing growth factor for periodontal reconstruction. This scaffold induced the cellular proliferation and upregulation of collagen expression, and surrounding tissues grew within the scaffold, as well [61].

### 4.2.2 Decellularized Scaffold as Natural Scaffolds

Even though synthetic scaffolds can be constructed with desired properties, it is hard to perfectly recapitulate the ECM in dental tissues. In this regard, decellularized scaffolding can be utilized to enhance such simulation. Moreover, decellularized scaffolding reduces the inflammation, immune rejection, and foreign body rejection. Such scaffolds can maintain the structure, mechanical feature, shape, and molecular gradient to enhance cellular activities. Various methods such as physical, chemical, and enzymatic methods have been utilized for decellularization, in which the cell membranes were disrupted and rinsed away to achieve the decellularized scaffold. It is theorized that decellularized scaffolds can enhance tooth regeneration.

Zhang et al. utilized decellularized scaffolds for whole tissue regeneration. In their study, a porcine decellularized tooth bud is utilized to regenerate the whole tooth. A decellularized scaffold is seeded with porcine dental epithelial cells, human dental pulp cells, and human umbilical vein endothelial cells. The constructed scaffold exhibits a high degree of cellular activity, which was beneficial for whole tooth regeneration [62].

It is supposed that endodontic regeneration is an alternative procedure to treat the root canal of immature teeth. Song et al. decellularized human dental pulp and recellularized it with the stem cells of the apical papilla to regenerate the tooth. The decellularized scaffold supports the proliferation and differentiation of the stem cells of the apical papilla [63]. Traphagen et al. decellularized porcine molar tooth buds, maintaining the ECM proteins such as collagen, laminin, and fibronectin. A reseeded decellularized tooth contains higher content of collagen than decellularized tooth tissue. It was concluded that the natural decellularized scaffolds are proper for tooth regeneration to mimic the native tissue [64].

Hu et al. decellularized the swine dental pulp from the mandibular anterior teeth of swine and seeded with human dental pulp stem cells for pulp regeneration. It is observed that the bioscaffold maintained the natural shape and ECM components, which enhanced cellular activities, such as growth and proliferation [65]. Precisely controlling the bioengineered tooth shape and size, forming the functional tooth root, and removing abnormal mineralized tissue formation are the challenging issues in whole tissue engineering. Based on the reported studies, decellularized scaffolds can provide a niche-like environment with minimal immunological response.

## 4.3 *Cell Sheets for Tooth Regeneration*

Sheet engineering has been developed as a new effective approach to produce tissues in vitro. In sheet engineering, cell sheets are detached from culture plates using scrapers, thermos-responsive polymer coatings, magnetic force, ionic-induced dissolution, electrochemical polarization, electrochemically induced pH decrease, and UV illumination [66]. Using these techniques, the extracellular matrix formed by the cells perseveres. Herein, following implantation, the cells in the sheets can attach to the recipient tissues without any additional materials, which increases the survival rate of implanted tissues [67]. In the case of bioengineering a whole tooth, the cell sheet technology can be applied to investigate and establish an epithelial-mesenchymal interconnection. Moreover, studies show that it is possible to generate a functional bioengineered tooth using this technique in combination with scaffold-based tissue engineering.

In studies, it has been shown that human dental follicle cell sheets combined with dentin matrix scaffolds and autologous fibroblast multilayer cell sheets regenerate bio-root structures [68, 69]. 3D SCAP sheet-derived pellets also regenerate roots when they were implanted in the back of immunodeficient mice. Here, SCAP sheets induce generation of odontoblast-like cells and mineralized dentine-like tissue [70]. In another study, Vc-induced periodontal ligament stem cell sheets cover dental pulp stem cell-seeded root-shaped hydroxy-apatite scaffolds, which are then implanted into jaw bone implant sockets. After 6 months, by installing a crown on the bio-root, the whole functional tooth is generated [71].

# 5 Investigation the Functionality the Whole Bioengineered Teeth

The ultimate goal of tooth engineering is to achieve a fully functional bioengineered tooth. Recently, several studies report producing whole bioengineered teeth using cell aggregation methods [69], cell sheet engineering, and biocompatible scaffolds [71]. For successful whole tooth replacement therapy, the bioengineered teeth must be able to integrate with the bone and periodontal ligament tissues in the edentulous jaw area. Moreover, the bioengineered teeth should have sufficient strength against mechanical load during mastication and respond well to noxious stimulations in the maxillofacial region.

## 5.1 *Successful Transplantation*

The main concern about whole tooth bioengineering using the organ germ method is whether the implanted construct can erupt and occlude with the neighbor and opposing teeth in the oral environment. During tooth development, cell signaling and genetic and molecular mechanisms regulate tooth eruption and occlusion in the region of jaw bone from where the teeth will be erupted [72, 73]. Thus far, several studies indicate that transplanted in vitro germ constructs can erupt in an edentulous region of the oral cavity [6, 43, 50]. It seems that the bioengineered teeth, generated using the organ germ method, could erupt through bone/gingival remodeling induced by the genetic/molecular mechanisms similar to the process of natural tooth eruption. Moreover, the studies show that the bioengineered teeth generated by organ germ method occluded with the neighbor and opposing teeth after transplantation [6].

## 5.2 Integration with Periodontal Ligament Tissues

The tooth germ is surrounded by dental follicular cells during tooth development. These follicular cells will differentiate into osteoblasts, cementoblasts, and fibroblasts, and therefore produce alveolar bone, cementum, and the periodontal ligament [74]. One of the main concerns in bioengineering tooth therapy is whether transplanting an engineered tooth or construct will successfully fix and create periodontal ligament tissue around the implant in the edentulous area. Regarding transplantation of bioengineered immature tooth using the organ germ method, because the whole process of developing tooth will be established in the transplanted germ construct in the edental region, it is obviously the periodontal ligament that will be generated during tooth development in the appropriate area. But this is a bit different for transplantation of bioengineered mature tooth. The bioengineered mature tooth has a higher priority compared with bioengineered immature tooth, as the mature one would exhibit an in vivo immediate functional operation [75]. In a study, it has been shown that when a bioengineered mature tooth unit is transplanted into a murine jawbone, the bioengineered tooth (with its periodontal ligament tissues) was successfully engrafted and integrated into the jaw after 40 days [7]. Therefore, both the bioengineered mature and immature teeth would successfully restore the masticatory function related to integration of the periodontal ligament after transplantation.

## 5.3 Responses to Mechanical Load of Bioengineered Teeth

Biological response to mechanical stresses in the bioengineered whole tooth is another important factor that should be investigated. Oral function necessitates the harmonized cooperation of the maxillofacial region and teeth using the periodontal ligament. The physiological properties of the tooth—such as absorption of occlusal loadings, preserving the alveolar bone height, and orthodontic movement of the tooth—affect the periodontal properties. It has been theorized that preserving the periodontal tissue of the tooth root is crucial for ankylosis prevention. The PDL connection plays an important role in tooth function, as its absence in synthetic implants results in major drawbacks in tooth functionality. In this regards, biological therapies attract more attention than artificial options in tooth restoration [76, 77].

Since the periodontal ligament is an important component for implant restoration, the neural responses also need to be considered. The tissue-implant interface is an important region, which in proper conditions results in osseointegration. The fibro-osseous interface can be developed by micromovement of the implant. Bone not only provides strength, but also provides regulation of calcium homeostasis. It is hypothesized that the mechanical load on bone causes a chain of events that results in a biological response. In this regard, properly designing the implant provides an appropriate mechanical transfer to the bone and results in activity of bone cells [78]. Direction, degree, duration, and rate of loading to the tooth determine the biomechanical response. Mechano-transduction includes (1) mechanocoupling, which transduces the mechanical loading to the biosignal to be detectable for sensor cells; (2) biochemical coupling, which converts the mechanical signals to the biochemical signals to illuminate the cell response; (3) transfer the sensor cell biosignals to effector cells; and (4) final response of effector cell.

Osteocytes sense the mechanical forces and assist the translation of the mechanical forces to the biochemical signals. These cells are located in the lacunae of the bony matrix and are more resistant to mechanical forces than osteoblasts [79, 80]. Recent studies on bioengineered teeth show that functional tooth movement and bone regeneration have been attained [6, 7]. These results determine that bioengineered teeth could appropriately accommodate the mechanical forces, similar to natural teeth. This is because of PDL formation and integration in bioengineered teeth—in contrast to dental implants, where the lack of PDL tissue causes their lack of response to mechanical loads and subsequent failure of the whole implant.

## 5.4 Perceptive Potential for Noxious Stimuli in Bioengineered Teeth

Sympathetic, parasympathetic, and sensory nerves innervate the teeth, like other peripheral organs. Afferent nerves regulate the physiological function of tooth and noxious stimulation comprehension [81]. Moreover, it seems that the nervous system plays an important role in tooth development. In a study, it was determined that tooth regeneration with a lesioned nerve did not occur [82]. This proves that there is a close correlation between tooth formation and peripheral innervation. It is supposed that nerves produce signaling molecules that affect the interaction between mesenchyme and dental epithelium. During tooth development, trigeminal ganglion sensory endings near dental MCSs release Shh, which acts as a key signaling molecule in tooth growth [83].

Hence, it seems that after transplantation of a bioengineered or autologous tooth, the neuronal regeneration is necessary for successful whole tooth bioengineering therapy [84]. Here, neuronal regeneration causes nerve fibers to enter into the bioengineered tooth, which innervate the pulp cavity, odontoblastic layer, and periodontal ligament with blood vessel reconstruction [6, 7]. Lack of innervation in the periodontal tissues and the pulp cavity after transplantation of conventional dental implants causes them to not comprehend peripheral stimuli, such as injuries, excessive loading, and orthodontic movement [85].

Innervation of the bioengineered teeth from the alveolar nerve after transplantation is one of the main challenges in producing a functional tooth implant. Studies show that if bioengineered immature constructs, including mesenchymal-epithelial cells, implant in the correct position in the jaw, the regeneration of nerves will be conducted [6, 7, 86]. To investigate innervation of embryonic dental epithelium and neural crest-derived MSCs, the reassociations of the cells obtained from embryonic day 14 mouse molars were implanted underneath the skin along with dorsal root ganglia. The results show that the innervation of the dental mesenchyme was not observed. Then, cell reassociation implantation along with trigeminal ganglia caused extension of axon growth to surround the forming teeth. However, the axons are detected in the dental mesenchyme in just 2.5% of samples, showing a specific defect in entering trigeminal ganglia into the dental mesenchyme. It has been shown that inhibition of T cells using immunosuppressive reagents such as cyclosporin A improves axonal regeneration. Cyclosporin A also has a direct effect on axonal regeneration by enhancing growth associated protein-43 expression [87]. The coimplantation of cell reassociations and trigeminal ganglia in cyclosporin A-treated ICR and immunocompromised nude mice shows the innervation of the dental mesenchyme in both strains similarly. These results demonstrate that immunosuppression can impair the innervation process in the dental mesenchyme [88].

Despite previous studies showing that the bioengineered whole tooth would potentially restore neuronal responses, more research needs to be done in order to reach practically this achievement with high performance.

## 6 Summary

Although clinical prosthetics, such as dental implants, have been used for tooth replacement, there are many disadvantages in their use. Currently, whole tooth engineering can provide a promising alternative approach. The research attempts in the bioengineering field of teeth should focus on the molecular processes during the tooth development, finding a promising autologous cell source, appropriate bioactive materials, and other barriers that limit the development of clinically functional bioengineered whole teeth. Despite the high complexity of the tooth organ component, the accomplishments of previous studies show that whole tooth engineering for humans is possible and a solution is on the horizon.

## References

1. Kassebaum, N., et al. (2017). Global, regional, and national prevalence, incidence, and disability-adjusted life years for oral conditions for 195 countries, 1990–2015: A systematic analysis for the global burden of diseases, injuries, and risk factors. *Journal of Dental Research, 96*(4), 380–387.
2. Greenstein, G., Cavallaro, J., Romanos, G., & Tarnow, D. (2008). Clinical recommendations for avoiding and managing surgical complications associated with implant dentistry: A review. *Journal of Periodontology, 79*(8), 1317–1329.
3. Jung, R. E., Pjetursson, B. E., Glauser, R., Zembic, A., Zwahlen, M., & Lang, N. P. (2008). A systematic review of the 5-year survival and complication rates of implant-supported single crowns. *Clinical Oral Implants Research, 19*(2), 119–130.

4. Lai, W.-F., Lee, J.-M., & Jung, H.-S. (2014). Molecular and engineering approaches to regenerate and repair teeth in mammals. *Cellular and Molecular Life Sciences, 71*(9), 1691–1701.
5. Zhang, Y. D., Zhi, C., Song, Y. Q., Chao, L., & Chen, Y. P. (2005). Making a tooth: Growth factors, transcription factors, and stem cells. *Cell Research, 15*(5), 301.
6. Ikeda, E., et al. (2009). Fully functional bioengineered tooth replacement as an organ replacement therapy. *Proceedings of the National Academy of Sciences, 106*(32), 13475–13480.
7. Oshima, M., et al. (2011). Functional tooth regeneration using a bioengineered tooth unit as a mature organ replacement regenerative therapy. *PLoS One, 6*(7), e21531.
8. Gao, Z., et al. (2016). Bio-root and implant-based restoration as a tooth replacement alternative. *Journal of Dental Research, 95*(6), 642–649.
9. Young, C. S., et al. (2005). Tissue-engineered hybrid tooth and bone. *Tissue Engineering, 11*(9–10), 1599–1610.
10. Egusa, H., et al. (2010). Gingival fibroblasts as a promising source of induced pluripotent stem cells. *PLoS One, 5*(9), e12743.
11. Wada, N., Wang, B., Lin, N. H., Laslett, A. L., Gronthos, S., & Bartold, P. M. (2011). Induced pluripotent stem cell lines derived from human gingival fibroblasts and periodontal ligament fibroblasts. *Journal of Periodontal Research, 46*(4), 438–447.
12. Yan, X., Qin, H., Qu, C., Tuan, R. S., Shi, S., & Huang, G. T.-J. (2010). iPS cells reprogrammed from human mesenchymal-like stem/progenitor cells of dental tissue origin. *Stem Cells and Development, 19*(4), 469–480.
13. Amirabad, L. M., et al. (2017). Enhanced cardiac differentiation of human cardiovascular disease patient-specific induced pluripotent stem cells by applying unidirectional electrical pulses using aligned electroactive nanofibrous scaffolds. *ACS Applied Materials & Interfaces, 9*(8), 6849–6864.
14. Liu, L., Liu, Y. F., Zhang, J., Duan, Y. Z., & Jin, Y. (2016). Ameloblasts serum-free conditioned medium: Bone morphogenic protein 4-induced odontogenic differentiation of mouse induced pluripotent stem cells. *Journal of Tissue Engineering and Regenerative Medicine, 10*(6), 466–474.
15. Ozeki, N., et al. (2013). Mouse-induced pluripotent stem cells differentiate into odontoblast-like cells with induction of altered adhesive and migratory phenotype of integrin. *PLoS One, 8*(11), e80026.
16. Zamanlui, S., Amirabad, L. M., Soleimani, M., & Faghihi, S. (2018). Influence of hydrodynamic pressure on chondrogenic differentiation of human bone marrow mesenchymal stem cells cultured in perfusion system. *Biologicals, 56*, 1–8.
17. Amari, A., et al. (2015). In vitro generation of IL-35-expressing human Wharton's jelly-derived mesenchymal stem cells using lentiviral vector. *Iranian Journal of Allergy, Asthma, and Immunology, 14*(4), 416–426.
18. Gronthos, S., Mankani, M., Brahim, J., Robey, P. G., & Shi, S. (2000). Postnatal human dental pulp stem cells (DPSCs) in vitro and in vivo. *Proceedings of the National Academy of Sciences, 97*(25), 13625–13630.
19. Seo, B.-M., et al. (2004). Investigation of multipotent postnatal stem cells from human periodontal ligament. *The Lancet, 364*(9429), 149–155.
20. Miura, M., et al. (2003). SHED: Stem cells from human exfoliated deciduous teeth. *Proceedings of the National Academy of Sciences, 100*(10), 5807–5812.
21. Cordeiro, M. M., et al. (2008). Dental pulp tissue engineering with stem cells from exfoliated deciduous teeth. *Journal of Endodontics, 34*(8), 962–969.
22. Ge, J., et al. (2013). Distal C terminus of CaV1. 2 channels plays a crucial role in the neural differentiation of dental pulp stem cells. *PLoS One, 8*(11), e81332.
23. Guo, W., et al. (2009). The use of dentin matrix scaffold and dental follicle cells for dentin regeneration. *Biomaterials, 30*(35), 6708–6723.
24. Morsczeck, C., et al. (2005). Isolation of precursor cells (PCs) from human dental follicle of wisdom teeth. *Matrix Biology, 24*(2), 155–165.

25. Sonoyama, W., et al. (2008). Characterization of the apical papilla and its residing stem cells from human immature permanent teeth: A pilot study. *Journal of Endodontics, 34*(2), 166–171.
26. Saito, M. T., Silvério, K. G., Casati, M. Z., Sallum, E. A., & Nociti, F. H., Jr. (2015). Tooth-derived stem cells: Update and perspectives. *World Journal of Stem Cells, 7*(2), 399.
27. Okamoto, T., et al. (2002). Clonal heterogeneity in differentiation potential of immortalized human mesenchymal stem cells. *Biochemical and Biophysical Research Communications, 295*(2), 354–361.
28. Shinmura, Y., Tsuchiya, S., Hata, K., & Honda, M. J. (2008). Quiescent epithelial cell rests of Malassez can differentiate into ameloblast-like cells. *Journal of Cellular Physiology, 217*(3), 728–738.
29. Honda, M., Shinohara, Y., Hata, K., & Ueda, M. (2007). Subcultured odontogenic epithelial cells in combination with dental mesenchymal cells produce enamel–dentin-like complex structures. *Cell Transplantation, 16*(8), 833–847.
30. Liu, Y., et al. (2013). Skin epithelial cells as possible substitutes for ameloblasts during tooth regeneration. *Journal of Tissue Engineering and Regenerative Medicine, 7*(12), 934–943.
31. Jussila, M., Juuri, E., & Thesleff, I. (2013). Tooth morphogenesis and renewal. In *Stem cells in craniofacial development and regeneration* (pp. 109–134). Hoboken: Wiley-Blackwell.
32. Wu, P., et al. (2013). Specialized stem cell niche enables repetitive renewal of alligator teeth. *Proceedings of the National Academy of Sciences, 110*(22), E2009–E2018.
33. Laurikkala, J., Mikkola, M. L., James, M., Tummers, M., Mills, A. A., & Thesleff, I. (2006). p63 regulates multiple signalling pathways required for ectodermal organogenesis and differentiation. *Development, 133*(8), 1553–1563.
34. Bei, M. (2009). Molecular genetics of tooth development. *Current Opinion in Genetics & Development, 19*(5), 504–510.
35. Mikkola, M. L. (2009). Molecular aspects of hypohidrotic ectodermal dysplasia. *American Journal of Medical Genetics Part A, 149*(9), 2031–2036.
36. Pispa, J., et al. (1999). Cusp patterning defect in Tabby mouse teeth and its partial rescue by FGF. *Developmental Biology, 216*(2), 521–534.
37. Mustonen, T., et al. (2003). Stimulation of ectodermal organ development by Ectodysplasin-A1. *Developmental Biology, 259*(1), 123–136.
38. Jernvall, J., Keränen, S. V., & Thesleff, I. (2000). Evolutionary modification of development in mammalian teeth: Quantifying gene expression patterns and topography. *Proceedings of the National Academy of Sciences, 97*(26), 14444–14448.
39. Kratochwil, K., Galceran, J., Tontsch, S., Roth, W., & Grosschedl, R. (2002). FGF4, a direct target of LEF1 and Wnt signaling, can rescue the arrest of tooth organogenesis in Lef1−/− mice. *Genes & Development, 16*(24), 3173–3185.
40. Klein, O. D., et al. (2006). Sprouty genes control diastema tooth development via bidirectional antagonism of epithelial-mesenchymal FGF signaling. *Developmental Cell, 11*(2), 181–190.
41. Gritli-Linde, A., Bei, M., Maas, R., Zhang, X. M., Linde, A., & McMahon, A. P. (2002). Shh signaling within the dental epithelium is necessary for cell proliferation, growth and polarization. *Development, 129*(23), 5323–5337.
42. Nakashima, M., & Reddi, A. H. (2003). The application of bone morphogenetic proteins to dental tissue engineering. *Nature Biotechnology, 21*(9), 1025.
43. Nakao, K., et al. (2007). The development of a bioengineered organ germ method. *Nature Methods, 4*(3), 227.
44. Hu, B., Nadiri, A., Bopp-Kuchler, S., Perrin-Schmitt, F., Wang, S., & Lesot, H. (2005). Dental epithelial histo-morphogenesis in the mouse: Positional information versus cell history. *Archives of Oral Biology, 50*(2), 131–136.
45. Hu, B., Nadiri, A., Kuchler-Bopp, S., Perrin-Schmitt, F., Peters, H., & Lesot, H. (2006). Tissue engineering of tooth crown, root, and periodontium. *Tissue Engineering, 12*(8), 2069–2075.
46. Ikeda, E., & Tsuji, T. (2008). Growing bioengineered teeth from single cells: Potential for dental regenerative medicine. *Expert Opinion on Biological Therapy, 8*(6), 735–744.

47. Lechguer, A. N., et al. (2011). Cell differentiation and matrix organization in engineered teeth. *Journal of Dental Research, 90*(5), 583–589.
48. Oshima, M., & Tsuji, T. (2015). Whole tooth regeneration as a future dental treatment. In *Engineering Mineralized and Load Bearing Tissues* (pp. 255–269). Cham: Springer.
49. Hu, X., et al. (2014). Conserved odontogenic potential in embryonic dental tissues. *Journal of Dental Research, 93*(5), 490–495.
50. Ohazama, A., Modino, S., Miletich, I., & Sharpe, P. (2004). Stem-cell-based tissue engineering of murine teeth. *Journal of Dental Research, 83*(7), 518–522.
51. Otsu, K., et al. (2011). Differentiation of induced pluripotent stem cells into dental mesenchymal cells. *Stem Cells and Development, 21*(7), 1156–1164.
52. Wen, Y., et al. (2012). Application of induced pluripotent stem cells in generation of a tissue-engineered tooth-like structure. *Tissue Engineering Part A, 18*(15–16), 1677–1685.
53. Cai, J., et al. (2013). Generation of tooth-like structures from integration-free human urine induced pluripotent stem cells. *Cell Regeneration, 2*(1), 6.
54. Wang, B., et al. (2010). Induction of human keratinocytes into enamel-secreting ameloblasts. *Developmental Biology, 344*(2), 795–799.
55. Chen, Y., et al. (2015). Human umbilical cord mesenchymal stem cells: A new therapeutic option for tooth regeneration. *Stem Cells International, 2015*, 1.
56. Young, C., Terada, S., Vacanti, J., Honda, M., Bartlett, J., & Yelick, P. (2002). Tissue engineering of complex tooth structures on biodegradable polymer scaffolds. *Journal of Dental Research, 81*(10), 695–700.
57. Angelova Volponi, A., Kawasaki, M., & Sharpe, P. (2013). Adult human gingival epithelial cells as a source for whole-tooth bioengineering. *Journal of Dental Research, 92*(4), 329–334.
58. Kuchler-Bopp, S., et al. (2017). Promoting bioengineered tooth innervation using nanostructured and hybrid scaffolds. *Acta Biomaterialia, 50*, 493–501.
59. Chen, G., et al. (2015). Combination of aligned PLGA/Gelatin electrospun sheets, native dental pulp extracellular matrix and treated dentin matrix as substrates for tooth root regeneration. *Biomaterials, 52*, 56–70.
60. Rasperini, G., et al. (2015). 3D-printed bioresorbable scaffold for periodontal repair. *Journal of Dental Research, 94*(9_suppl), 153S–157S.
61. Zhang, Y., et al. (2006). Novel chitosan/collagen scaffold containing transforming growth factor-β1 DNA for periodontal tissue engineering. *Biochemical and Biophysical Research Communications, 344*(1), 362–369.
62. Zhang, W., Vazquez, B., Oreadi, D., & Yelick, P. (2017). Decellularized tooth bud scaffolds for tooth regeneration. *Journal of Dental Research, 96*(5), 516–523.
63. Song, J., Takimoto, K., Jeon, M., Vadakekalam, J., Ruparel, N., & Diogenes, A. (2017). Decellularized human dental pulp as a scaffold for regenerative endodontics. *Journal of Dental Research, 96*(6), 640–646.
64. Traphagen, S. B., et al. (2012). Characterization of natural, decellularized and reseeded porcine tooth bud matrices. *Biomaterials, 33*(21), 5287–5296.
65. Hu, L., et al. (2017). Decellularized swine dental pulp as a bioscaffold for pulp regeneration. *BioMed Research International, 2017*, 9342714.
66. Owaki, T., Shimizu, T., Yamato, M., & Okano, T. (2014). Cell sheet engineering for regenerative medicine: Current challenges and strategies. *Biotechnology Journal, 9*(7), 904–914.
67. Okano, T. (2014). Current progress of cell sheet tissue engineering and future perspective. *Tissue Engineering Part A, 20*(9–10), 1353–1354.
68. Yang, B., et al. (2012). Tooth root regeneration using dental follicle cell sheets in combination with a dentin matrix-based scaffold. *Biomaterials, 33*(8), 2449–2461.
69. Zhou, Y., Li, Y., Mao, L., & Peng, H. (2012). Periodontal healing by periodontal ligament cell sheets in a teeth replantation model. *Archives of Oral Biology, 57*(2), 169–176.
70. Na, S., et al. (2016). Regeneration of dental pulp/dentine complex with a three-dimensional and scaffold-free stem-cell sheet-derived pellet. *Journal of Tissue Engineering and Regenerative Medicine, 10*(3), 261–270.

71. Wei, F., et al. (2013). Functional tooth restoration by allogeneic mesenchymal stem cell-based bio-root regeneration in swine. *Stem Cells and Development, 22*(12), 1752–1762.
72. Wise, G., & King, G. (2008). Mechanisms of tooth eruption and orthodontic tooth movement. *Journal of Dental Research, 87*(5), 414–434.
73. Wise, G., Frazier-Bowers, S., & D'souza, R. (2002). Cellular, molecular, and genetic determinants of tooth eruption. *Critical Reviews in Oral Biology & Medicine, 13*(4), 323–335.
74. Hou, L.-T., et al. (1999). Characterization of dental follicle cells in developing mouse molar. *Archives of Oral Biology, 44*(9), 759–770.
75. Gridelli, B., & Remuzzi, G. (2000). Strategies for making more organs available for transplantation. *New England Journal of Medicine, 343*(6), 404–410.
76. Bas, O., De-Juan-Pardo, E. M., Catelas, I., & Hutmacher, D. W. (2018). The quest for mechanically and biologically functional soft biomaterials via soft network composites. *Advanced Drug Delivery Reviews, 132*, 214–234.
77. Nanci, A. (2017). *Ten Cate's oral histology: Development, structure, and function*. Elsevier Health Sciences, St. Louis, Missouri.
78. Jamal, H. (2016). Tooth organ bioengineering: Cell sources and innovative approaches. *Dentistry Journal, 4*(2), 18.
79. Saxena, S. (2015). Tissue response to mechanical load in dental implants. *International Journal of Oral & Maxillofacial Pathology, 6*(3), 02–06.
80. Xiu, P., et al. (2016). Tailored surface treatment of 3D printed porous Ti6Al4V by micro-arc oxidation for enhanced osseointegration via optimized bone in-growth patterns and interlocked bone/implant interface. *ACS Applied Materials & Interfaces, 8*(28), 17964–17975.
81. Luukko, K., Kvinnsland, I. H., & Kettunen, P. (2005). Tissue interactions in the regulation of axon pathfinding during tooth morphogenesis. *Developmental Dynamics, 234*(3), 482–488.
82. Tuisku, F., & Hildebrand, C. (1994). Evidence for a neural influence on tooth germ generation in a polyphyodont species. *Developmental Biology, 165*(1), 1–9.
83. Zhao, H., et al. (2014). Secretion of shh by a neurovascular bundle niche supports mesenchymal stem cell homeostasis in the adult mouse incisor. *Cell Stem Cell, 14*(2), 160–173.
84. Kjaer, M., Beyer, N., & Secher, N. (1999). Exercise and organ transplantation. *Scandinavian Journal of Medicine & Science in Sports, 9*(1), 1–14.
85. Burns, D. R., Beck, D. A., & Nelson, S. K. (2003). A review of selected dental literature on contemporary provisional fixed prosthodontic treatment: report of the Committee on Research in Fixed Prosthodontics of the Academy of Fixed Prosthodontics. *The Journal of Prosthetic Dentistry, 90*(5), 474–497.
86. Luukko, K., et al. (2008). Secondary induction and the development of tooth nerve supply. *Annals of Anatomy-Anatomischer Anzeiger, 190*(2), 178–187.
87. Ibarra, A., et al. (2007). Cyclosporin-A enhances non-functional axonal growing after complete spinal cord transection. *Brain Research, 1149*, 200–209.
88. Kökten, T., Bécavin, T., Keller, L., Weickert, J.-L., Kuchler-Bopp, S., & Lesot, H. (2014). Immunomodulation stimulates the innervation of engineered tooth organ. *PLoS One, 9*(1), e86011.

# Index





L. Tayebi (ed.), *Applications of Biomedical Engineering in Dentistry*,
https://doi.org/10.1007/978-3-030-21583-5

## L



## M

**P**

**Q**

Printed in the United States
By Bookmasters